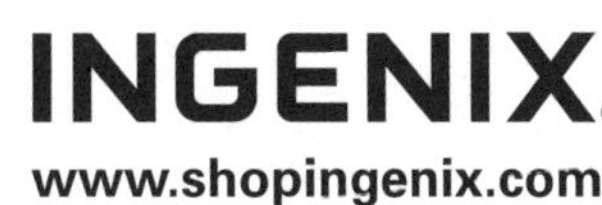

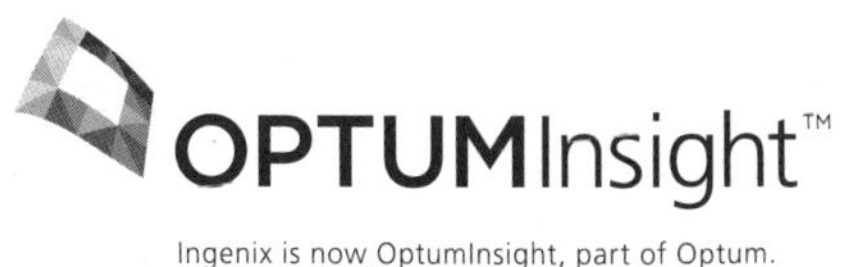

October 2011

Dear OptumInsight Customer:

This is your FY 2012 draft for the *ICD-10-PCS: The Complete Official Draft Code Set*.

The Centers for Medicare and Medicaid Services (CMS) is the agency charged with maintaining and updating the International Classification of Diseases 10th Revision Procedure Classification System (ICD-10-PCS). This FY 2012 draft represents the most current changes to the ICD-10-PCS as released by CMS.

Remember, the codes in ICD-10-PCS are not currently valid for any documentation or reporting of health care services. It is anticipated that CMS will make several updates and revisions to the draft prior to implementation of ICD-10-PCS; however, the basic structure will remain the same.

The Department of Health and Human Services (HHS) published the final rule regarding the adoption of both ICD-10-CM and ICD-10-PCS in the January 16, 2009, *Federal Register* (45 CFR part 162 [CMS—0013—F]). The compliance date for implementation of ICD-10-CM and ICD-10-PCS as a replacement for ICD-9-CM is October 1, 2013.

ICD-10-PCS will replace ICD-9-CM Volume 3, including the official coding guidelines, for the following procedures or other actions taken for diseases, injuries, and impairments on **hospital inpatients reported by hospitals**: prevention, diagnosis, treatment, and management.

We appreciate your choosing OptumInsight to meet your ICD-10-PCS conversion preparation and coding training needs. If you have any questions or comments concerning your draft *ICD-10-PCS: The Complete Official Draft Code Set*, please do not hesitate to call our customer service department. The toll-free number is 1-800-464-3649, option 1.

2525 Lake Park Blvd. • Salt Lake City, UT 84120 • 800.464.3649 • Fax 801.982.4033

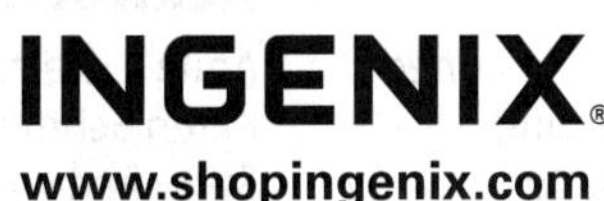

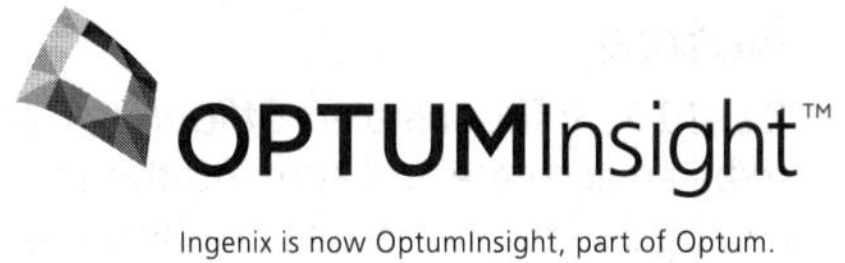

ICD-10-PCS
The Complete Official Draft Code Set

2012

Notice

ICD-10-PCS: The Complete Official Draft Code Set is designed to be an accurate and authoritative source regarding coding and every reasonable effort has been made to ensure accuracy and completeness of the content. However, OptumInsight makes no guarantee, warranty, or representation that this publication is accurate, complete, or without errors. It is understood that OptumInsight is not rendering any legal or other professional services or advice in this publication and that OptumInsight bears no liability for any results or consequences that may arise from the use of this book. Please address all correspondence to:

OptumInsight
2525 Lake Park Blvd
Salt Lake City, UT 84120

Our Commitment to Accuracy

OptumInsight is committed to producing accurate and reliable materials. To report corrections, please visit www.shopingenix.com/accuracy or email accuracy@ingenix.com. You can also reach customer service by calling 1.800.464.3649, option 1.

Copyright

ISBN 978-1-60151-607-7

Acknowledgments

Anita C. Hart, RHIA, CCS, CCS-P, *Product Manager*
Karen Schmidt, BSN, *Technical Director*
Stacy Perry, *Manager, Desktop Publishing*
Tracy Betzler, *Desktop Publishing Specialist*
Hope M. Dunn, *Desktop Publishing Specialist*
Kate Holden, *Editor*

Anita C. Hart, RHIA, CCS, CCS-P

Ms. Hart's experience includes 15 years conducting and publishing research in clinical medicine and human genetics for Yale University, Massachusetts General Hospital, and Massachusetts Institute of Technology. Her research conclusions have been published in several peer-reviewed journals. In addition, Ms. Hart has supervised medical records management, health information management, coding and reimbursement, and workers' compensation issues as the office manager for a physical therapy rehabilitation clinic. Ms. Hart is an expert in physician and facility coding, reimbursement systems, and compliance issues. She is also the author of the several OptumInsight publications and has served as subject matter advisor on numerous other publications for hospital and physician practices. Ms. Hart is the ICD-9-CM and ICD-10-CM/PCS subject matter expert for the OptumInsight, has served as the product manager for that product line for 15 years, and has presented at numerous national conferences. Ms. Hart is a member of the American Academy of Professional Coders (AAPC) and a fully credentialed active member of the American Health Information Management Association (AHIMA). Ms Hart is a current AHIMA Approved ICD-10-CM/PCS Trainer and leads the training initiatives within OptumInsight's Coding Solutions business unit.

Beth Ford, RHIT, CCS

Ms. Ford has more than 25 years of experience in physician and facility ICD-9-CM and CPT/HCPCS coding and compliance. She has extensive experience in a variety of health care settings, including acute and post-acute facilities, occupational health, and ambulatory care. Ms. Ford has provided coding education and consulting services to hospitals and physician practices, and has developed curriculum for medical terminology and ICD-9-CM and CPT coding education for a large health care system and multi-specialty physician groups. Formerly, she served as a coding specialist, coding manager, coding trainer/educator, coding consultant, and a health information management director. Her areas of specialization include coding, auditing, and training for DRG, inpatient, outpatient, and physician coding. She is credentialed by the American Health Information Management Association (AHIMA) as a Registered Health Information Technologist (RHIT) and a Certified Coding Specialist (CCS). She is an active member of AHIMA and is an AHIMA-approved ICD-10-CM/PCS trainer.

Contents

Preface

This draft of the International Classification of Diseases, 1Øth Revision, Procedure Classification System (ICD-1Ø-PCS) has been developed as a replacement for volume 3 of the International Classification of Diseases, Ninth Revision (ICD-9-CM). The development of ICD-1Ø-PCS was funded by the U.S. Centers for Medicare and Medicaid Services under contract nos. 9Ø-138, 91-223ØØ 5ØØ-95-ØØØ5 and HHSM-55Ø-2ØØ4-ØØØ11C to 3M Health Information Systems. ICD-1Ø-PCS has a multi-axial, seven-character, alphanumeric code structure that provides a unique code for all substantially different procedures and allows new procedures to be easily incorporated as new codes. The initial draft was formally tested and evaluated by an independent contractor; the final version was released in 1998, with annual updates since the final release.

What's New for 2012

The Centers for Medicare and Medicaid Services is the agency charged with maintaining and updating the ICD-10-PCS. The most current revisions were released by CMS in parallel with new ICD-9-CM codes valid October 1, 2011. A summary of the changes may be found on the CMS website at: http://www.cms.hhs.gov/ICD10/Downloads/pcs_whats_new_2012.pdf

The CMS website that contains all information and files related to both ICD-10-PCS and ICD-10-CM is: http://www.cms.gov/ICD10/11b15_2012_ICD10PCS.asp#TopOfPage

Due to the unique structure of ICD-10-PCS, a change in a character value may affect many individual codes and several Code Tables.

Change Summary Table

2011 Total	New Codes	Revised Titles	Deleted Codes	2012 Total
72,081	1,182	381	1,345	71,918

ICD-10-PCS Code 2011 Total, By Section

Medical and Surgical	61,896
Obstetrics	300
Placement	861
Administration	1,384
Measurement and Monitoring	339
Extracorporeal Assistance and Performance	41
Extracorporeal Therapies	42
Osteopathic	100
Other Procedures	60
Chiropractic	90
Imaging	2,934
Nuclear Medicine	463
Radiation Oncology	1,939
Rehabilitation and Diagnostic Audiology	1,380
Mental Health	30
Substance Abuse Treatment	59
Total	**71,918**

ICD-10-PCS Code Changes

The code revisions for FY 2012:

- Codes added in parallel with new ICD-9-CM codes valid October 1, 2011
- Codes deleted in parallel with ICD-9-CM changes or to enhance internal consistency in ICD-10-PCS
- Individual codes added, revised, or deleted
  - In response to public input, including:
    - In the Medical and Surgical section, add new qualifier Vertical in the Medical and Surgical section for the stomach body part to specify vertical sleeve gastrectomy
    - In the Medical and Surgical section, add new qualifier Left Atrial Appendage for the left atrium body part to specify procedures performed on the left atrial appendage
    - In the Introduction section, add new qualifier Anti-Infective Envelope to specify placing an antimicrobial envelope around device (e.g., pacemaker generator) inserted in the subcutaneous tissue
  - Based on internal review for clarity and ease of use, including:
    - Revise device values as needed to adhere to new device value maintenance standard
    - Add Respiratory, Breast, and Prostate body part values for **laser interstitial thermal therapy (LITT)** to be consistent with body parts specified in ICD-9-CM includes notes and index entries

ICD-10-PCS Device Classification Maintenance Standards Developed and Applied to FY 2012 update

Two new maintenance standards were developed based on industry feedback and internal review, to preserve the usability and maintainability of PCS

1. Device information is contained only in the device character.
2. ICD-10-PCS contains a PCS Device Aggregation Table that crosswalks the *specific* device character values that have been created for specific root operations and specific body part character values to the *general* device character value that would be used for root operations that represent a broad range of procedures and general body part character values, such as Removal and Revision.

First Maintenance Standard—Explanation and Example

Device information should not be split between the device and the qualifier characters. The qualifier should be reserved for essential detail about specific procedures that cannot be captured using any of the other existing values. If the seventh-character qualifier is used to further specify a sixth-character device value, then subsequent requests for additional specificity cannot be accommodated without adding information to the device value that is unrelated to the device. This makes the system imprecise as a classification and more difficult for both coders and secondary users of the data.

The public request presented at the March 2011 Coordination and Maintenance Committee meeting to add procedural detail to the hip, knee, and ankle replacement codes is an example of what can happen when device detail from a previous request has already "used up" the qualifier. All the CMS options presented at the C&M meeting attempted to accommodate the new request by adding the words "Cemented" and "Uncemented" to the device values because the qualifier values were already used to describe the device bearing surfaces, as shown on the next page.

Replacement of Hip Joint (ØSR)

Body Part	Approach	Device	Qualifier
9 Hip Joint, Right **B** Hip Joint, Left	**Ø** Open	**G** Synthetic Substitute, **Uncemented** **H** Synthetic Substitute, **Cemented** **J** Synthetic Substitute	**5** Metal on Polyethylene **6** Metal on Metal **7** Ceramic on Ceramic **8** Ceramic on Polyethylene **Z** No Qualifier

After internal review, a revised proposal was developed that would place all of the device detail in the device character and add the requested detail regarding the method used to affix the prosthetic joint in the qualifier as shown below.

Replacement of Hip Joint Table (ØBR), Revised for FY 2012

Body Part	Approach	Device	Qualifier
9 Hip Joint, Right **B** Hip Joint, Left	**Ø** Open	**1** Synthetic Substitute, Metal **2** Synthetic Substitute, Metal on Polyethylene **3** Synthetic Substitute, Ceramic **4** Synthetic Substitute, Ceramic on Polyethylene **J** Synthetic Substitute	**9** **Cemented** **A** **Uncemented** **Z** No Qualifier

Existing qualifier values containing device information were similarly revised in the classification to adhere to the new standard.

Second Maintenance Standard—Explanation and Example

ICD-10-PCS should contain information that correlates a specific device value used in the original root operation where the device was placed (Bypass, Dilation, Insertion, Occlusion, Replacement, and so on) with its more general device value used in other root operations. In root operations such as Removal and Revision, the device values are often the aggregate, general device of an entire family of specific device values.

This additional reference table directs coders and secondary data users from more specific device values used in the original root operations to root operations in the system where the selection of device values is less specific. Each specific device is assigned to its aggregate general device in the Device Aggregation Table, as shown in the example below.

Example of Device Values in Device Aggregation Table

Specific Device	for Operation	in Body System	General Device
Synthetic Substitute, Ceramic on Ceramic	Replacement	Lower Joints	J Synthetic Substitute
Synthetic Substitute, Ceramic on Polyethylene	Replacement	Lower Joints	J Synthetic Substitute
Synthetic Substitute, Metal	Replacement	Lower Joints	J Synthetic Substitute
Synthetic Substitute, Metal on Polyethylene	Replacement	Lower Joints	J Synthetic Substitute
Synthetic Substitute, Polyethylene	Replacement	Lower Joints	J Synthetic Substitute

New ICD-10-PCS Draft Device Key Added to ICD-10-PCS Core Content

- Contains more than 300 new entries in the PCS index and in standalone ICD-10-PCS reference tables
- Has two table listings, one arranged by device name (brand name or common name) and one by PCS device value, for ease of use as a printed document

New/Updated Files

New—ICD-10-PCS Tables/Index/Definitions in XML

- Provides ICD-10-PCS core content in unambiguous machine-readable format, in response to public comment
- Includes accompanying schema, one for each type of content (tabular, index, reference)

New—ICD-10-PCS Tabular Order Descriptions

- Defines an unambiguous order for all ICD-10-CM/PCS codes
- Is in text file format
- Provides a unique five-digit "order number" for each ICD-10-PCS table and code
- Includes accompanying documentation

Updated—ICD-10-PCS Tables/Index/Definitions

- In downloadable PDF format
- Includes the FY 2012 version of ICD-10-PCS
- **New:** Has two table listings for PCS Body Part Key, in response to public comment, for ease of use as a printed document: one list is arranged by anatomic site and the other by PCS body part value
- Contains new links added for ease of online navigation, in response to public comment

Updated—ICD-10-PCS Long Descriptions

- In text file format
- Includes the FY 2012 version of ICD-10-PCS
    - Accompanying readme file in PDF format

Updated—ICD-10-PCS Table Descriptions

- In machine-readable text file for developers
- Includes the FY 2012 version of ICD-10-PCS
  - Accompanying readme file in PDF format

Updated—ICD-10-PCS Short Descriptions

- In machine readable text file for developers
- Includes the FY 2012 version of ICD-10-PCS with 60-character maximum length descriptions
  - Accompanying readme file in PDF format

Updated —ICD-10-PCS 2011 Final Addenda

- Lists new code titles for FY 2012 in ICD-10-PCS standard tables (PDF format)
  - Accompanying list of revised 2011 code titles for comparison
- Lists invalid (deleted) 2011 code titles in ICD-10-PCS standard tables (PDF format)
  - Accompanying list of original 2011 code titles revised, for comparison with 2012 list
- Comprehensive file of new, revised and invalid code titles in machine readable text format for developers
  - Accompanying readme file in PDF format

Updated—ICD-10-PCS Reference Manual

- In downloadable PDF format
- Includes FY 2012 version of ICD-10-PCS
- Contains new coding practice examples that were added or revised in response to public input
- Includes streamlined appendix A:
  - PCS root operation and approach definitions only
    - In response to public input
    - Users referred to PCS core content references for complete definitions
- **New** appendix C: Discusses the distinguishing features of device, substance, and equipment as classified in ICD-10-PCS
  - Provides further guidance for correct identification and coding

Updated—ICD-10-PCS Official Coding Guidelines

- In downloadable PDF format
- Contains revisions in parallel with code changes in FY 2012 ICD-10-PCS
- Contains revisions in response to public comment and internal review

Updated—ICD-10-PCS Slide Presentation

- Contains reference slides available in PDF format

ICD-10-PCS and ICD-9-CM General Equivalence Mappings

- **Note**: The 2012 update of the ICD-10 general equivalence mappings were posted October 1, 2011, after changes based on public comment and internal review are complete for the FY 2012 versions of ICD-10-PCS and ICD-9-CM volume 3.

ICD-10 Reimbursement Mappings

- **Note**: The 2012 update of the ICD-10 reimbursement mappings will be posted after December 1, 2011, when the 2012 update of ICD-10-CM is scheduled to be posted.

Introduction

Volume 3 of the International Classification of Diseases Ninth Revision Clinical Modification (ICD-9-CM) has been used in the United States for reporting inpatient procedures since 1979. The structure of volume 3 of ICD-9-CM has not allowed new procedures associated with rapidly changing technology to be effectively incorporated as new codes. As a result, in 1992 the U.S. Centers for Medicare and Medicaid Services funded a project to design a replacement for volume 3 of ICD-9-CM. In 1995 CMS awarded 3M Health Information Systems a three-year contract to complete development of the replacement system. The new system is the ICD-10 Procedure Coding System (ICD-10-PCS).

History of ICD-10-PCS

The World Health Organization has maintained the International Classification of Diseases (ICD) for recording cause of death since 1893. It has updated the ICD periodically to reflect new discoveries in epidemiology and changes in medical understanding of disease.

The International Classification of Diseases Tenth Revision (ICD-10), published in 1992, is the latest revision of the ICD. The WHO authorized the National Center for Health Statistics (NCHS) to develop a clinical modification of ICD-10 for use in the United States. This version, called ICD-10-CM, is intended to replace the previous U.S. clinical modification, ICD-9-CM, that has been in use since 1979. ICD-9-CM contains a procedure classification; ICD-10-CM does not.

CMS, the agency responsible for maintaining the inpatient procedure code set in the United States, contracted with 3M Health Information Systems in 1993 to design and then develop a procedure classification system to replace volume 3 of ICD-9-CM.

The result, ICD-10-PCS, was initially completed in 1998. The code set has been updated annually since that time to ensure that ICD-10-PCS includes classifications for new procedures, devices, and technologies.

The development of ICD-10-PCS had as its goal the incorporation of the following major attributes:

- **Completeness:** There should be a unique code for all substantially different procedures. In volume 3 of ICD-9-CM, procedures on different body parts, with different approaches, or of different types are sometimes assigned to the same code.
- **Unique definitions:** Because ICD-10-PCS codes are constructed of individual values rather than lists of fixed codes and text descriptions, the unique, stable definition of a code in the system is retained. New values may be added to the system to represent a specific new approach or device or qualifier, but whole codes by design cannot be given new meanings and reused.
- **Expandability:** As new procedures are developed, the structure of ICD-10-PCS should allow them to be easily incorporated as unique codes.
- **Multi-axial codes:** ICD-10-PCS codes should consist of independent characters, with each individual component retaining its meaning across broad ranges of codes to the extent possible.
- **Standardized terminology:** ICD-10-PCS should include definitions of the terminology used. While the meaning of specific words varies in common usage, ICD-10-PCS should not include multiple meanings for the same term, and each term must be assigned a specific meaning. There are no eponyms or common procedure terms in ICD-10-PCS.
- **Structural integrity:** ICD-10-PCS can be easily expanded without disrupting the structure of the system. ICD-10-PCS allows unique new codes to be added to the system because values for the seven characters that make up a code can be combined as needed. The system can evolve as medical technology and clinical practice evolve, without disrupting the ICD-10-PCS structure.

In the development of ICD-10-PCS, several additional general characteristics were added:

- **Diagnostic information is not included in procedure description:** When procedures are performed for specific diseases or disorders, the disease or disorder is not contained in the procedure code. The diagnosis codes, not the procedure codes, specify the disease or disorder.
- **Explicit not otherwise specified (NOS) options are restricted:** Explicit "not otherwise specified," (NOS) options are restricted in ICD-10-PCS. A minimal level of specificity is required for each component of the procedure.
- **Limited use of not elsewhere classified (NEC) option:** Because all significant components of a procedure are specified in ICD-10-PCS, there is generally no need for a "not elsewhere classified" (NEC) code option. However, limited NEC options are incorporated into ICD-10-PCS where necessary. For example, new devices are frequently developed, and therefore it is necessary to provide an "other device" option for use until the new device can be explicitly added to the coding system.
- **Level of specificity:** All procedures currently performed can be specified in ICD-10-PCS. The frequency with which a procedure is performed was not a consideration in the development of the system. A unique code is available for variations of a procedure that can be performed.

ICD-10-PCS code structure results in qualities that optimize the performance of the system in electronic applications, and maximize the usefulness of the coded healthcare data. These qualities include:

- **Optimal search capability:** ICD-10-PCS is designed for maximum versatility in the ability to aggregate coded data. Values belonging to the same character as defined in a section or sections can be easily compared, since they occupy the same position in a code. This provides a high degree of flexibility and functionality for data mining.
- **Consistent characters and values:** Stability of characters and values across vast ranges of codes provides the maximum degree of functionality and flexibility for the collection and analysis of data. Because the character definition is consistent, and only the individual values assigned to that character differ as needed, meaningful comparisons of data over time can be conducted across a virtually infinite range of procedures.
- **Code readability:** ICD-10-PCS resembles a language in the sense that it is made up of semi-independent values combined by following the rules of the system, much the way a sentence is formed by combining words and following the rules of grammar and syntax. As with words in their context, the meaning of any

single value is a combination of its position in the code and any preceding values on which it may be dependent.

ICD-1Ø-PCS Code Structure

ICD-1Ø-PCS has a seven-character alphanumeric code structure. Each character contains up to 34 possible values. Each value represents a specific option for the general character definition. The 1Ø digits Ø–9 and the 24 letters A–H, J–N, and P–Z may be used in each character. The letters O and I are not used so as to avoid confusion with the digits Ø and 1. An ICD-1Ø-PCS code is the result of a process rather than as a single fixed set of digits or alphabetic characters. The process consists of combining semi-independent values from among a selection of values, according to the rules governing the construction of codes.

	Section	Body System	Root Operation	Body Part	Approach	Device	Qualifier
Characters:	1	2	3	4	5	6	7

A code is derived by choosing a specific value for each of the seven characters. Based on details about the procedure performed, values for each character specifying the section, body system, root operation, body part, approach, device, and qualifier are assigned. Because the definition of each character is also a function of its physical position in the code, the same letter or number placed in a different position in the code has different meaning.

The seven characters that make up a complete code have specific meanings that vary for each of the 16 sections of the manual. (The resource section of this manual lists character meanings for each section along with body-part definitions.)

Procedures are then divided into sections that identify the general type of procedure (e.g., Medical and Surgical, Obstetrics, Imaging). The first character of the procedure code always specifies the section. The second through seventh characters have the same meaning within each section, but may mean different things in other sections. In all sections, the third character specifies the general type of procedure performed (e.g., Resection, Transfusion, Fluoroscopy), while the other characters give additional information such as the body part and approach.

In ICD-1Ø-PCS, the term *procedure* refers to the complete specification of the seven characters.

Number of Codes in ICD-1Ø-PCS

At the time of this publication, there are 71,918 codes in the 2Ø11 ICD-1Ø-PCS. This is a substantial increase over the number of ICD-9-CM procedure codes. However, many codes have been eliminated from ICD-1Ø-PCS from the Medical and Surgical section as part of a planned streamlining and refinement initiated in 2ØØ6. This code reduction has also included the deletion of certain body system values specified as "other" in order to facilitate more selective body part and system values. For FY 2Ø12, 1,182 new codes were added to the system, combined with the deletion of 1,345 codes, resulting in a total of 71,918 ICD-1Ø-PCS codes.

The table structure of ICD-1Ø-PCS permits the specification of a large number of codes on a single page.

ICD-1Ø-PCS Manual

Index

Codes may be found in the index based on the general type of procedure (e.g., resection, transfusion, fluoroscopy), or a more commonly used term (e.g., appendectomy). For example, the code for percutaneous intraluminal dilation of the coronary arteries with an intraluminal device can be found in the Index under *Dilation*, or a synonym of *Dilation* (e.g., angioplasty). The Index then specifies the first three or four values of the code or directs the user to see another term.

Example:

Dilation
  Artery
    Coronary
      One Site Ø27Ø

Based on the first three values of the code provided in the Index, the corresponding table can be located. In the example above, the first three values indicate table Ø27 is to be referenced for code completion.

The tables and characters are arranged first by number and then by letter for each character (tables for ØØ-, Ø1-, Ø2-, etc., are followed by those for ØB-, ØC-, ØD-, etc., followed by ØB1, ØB2, etc., followed by ØBB, ØBC, ØBD, etc.).

Note: The Tables section must be used to construct a complete and valid code by specifying the last three or four values.

Tables

The Tables section is organized differently from ICD-9-CM. Each page in the section is composed of rows that specify the valid combinations of code values. In most sections of the system, the upper portion of each table contains a description of the first three characters of the procedure code. In the Medical and Surgical section, for example, the first three characters contain the name of the section, the body system, and the root operation performed.

For instance, the values *Ø27* specify the section *Medical and Surgical* (Ø), the body system *Heart and Great Vessels* (2) and the root operation *Dilation* (7). As shown in table Ø27, the root operation (*Dilation*) is accompanied by its definition.

The lower portion of the table specifies all the valid combinations of characters 4 through 7. The four columns in the table specify the last four characters. In the Medical and Surgical section they are labeled body part, approach, device and qualifier, respectively. Each row in the table specifies the valid combination of values for characters 4 through 7.

Ø Medical and Surgical
2 Heart and Great Vessels
7 Dilation Expanding an orifice or the lumen of a tubular body part

Body Part Character 4	Approach Character 5	Device Character 6	Qualifier Character 7
Ø Coronary Artery, One Site **1** Coronary Artery, Two Sites **2** Coronary Artery, Three Sites **3** Coronary Artery, Four or More Sites	**Ø** Open **3** Percutaneous **4** Percutaneous Endoscopic	**4** Intraluminal Device, Drug-eluting **D** Intraluminal Device **T** Intraluminal Device, Radioactive **Z** No Device	**6** Bifurcation **Z** No Qualifier
F Aortic Valve **G** Mitral Valve **H** Pulmonary Valve **J** Tricuspid Valve **K** Ventricle, Right **P** Pulmonary Trunk **Q** Pulmonary Artery, Right **S** Pulmonary Vein, Right **T** Pulmonary Vein, Left **V** Superior Vena Cava **W** Thoracic Aorta	**Ø** Open **3** Percutaneous **4** Percutaneous Endoscopic	**4** Intraluminal Device, Drug-eluting **D** Intraluminal Device **Z** No Device	**Z** No Qualifier
R Pulmonary Artery, Left	**Ø** Open **3** Percutaneous **4** Percutaneous Endoscopic	**4** Intraluminal Device, Drug-eluting **D** Intraluminal Device **Z** No Device	**T** Ductus Arteriosus **Z** No Qualifier

The rows of this table can be used to construct 213 unique procedure codes. For example, code Ø27Ø3DZ specifies the procedure for dilation of one coronary artery using an intraluminal device via percutaneous approach (i.e., percutaneous transluminal coronary angioplasty with stent).

Following are the 24 valid combinations of characters 5 through 7 for the Medical and Surgical procedure dilation of the heart and great vessels coronary artery, one site (Ø27Ø):

Ø27ØØ46	Dilation of Coronary Artery, One Site, Bifurcation, with Drug-eluting Intraluminal Device, Open Approach
Ø27ØØ4Z	Dilation of Coronary Artery, One Site with Drug-eluting Intraluminal Device, Open Approach
Ø27ØØD6	Dilation of Coronary Artery, One Site, Bifurcation, with Intraluminal Device, Open Approach
Ø27ØØDZ	Dilation of Coronary Artery, One Site with Intraluminal Device, Open Approach
Ø27ØØT6	Dilation of Coronary Artery, One Site, Bifurcation, with Radioactive Intraluminal Device, Open Approach
Ø27ØØTZ	Dilation of Coronary Artery, One Site with Radioactive Intraluminal Device, Open Approach
Ø27ØØZ6	Dilation of Coronary Artery, One Site, Bifurcation, Open Approach
Ø27ØØZZ	Dilation of Coronary Artery, One Site, Open Approach
Ø27Ø346	Dilation of Coronary Artery, One Site, Bifurcation, with Drug-eluting Intraluminal Device, Percutaneous Approach
Ø27Ø34Z	Dilation of Coronary Artery, One Site with Drug-eluting Intraluminal Device, Percutaneous Approach
Ø27Ø3D6	Dilation of Coronary Artery, One Site, Bifurcation, with Intraluminal Device, Percutaneous Approach
Ø27Ø3DZ	Dilation of Coronary Artery, One Site with Intraluminal Device, Percutaneous Approach
Ø27Ø3T6	Dilation of Coronary Artery, One Site, Bifurcation, with Radioactive Intraluminal Device, Percutaneous Approach
Ø27Ø3TZ	Dilation of Coronary Artery, One Site with Radioactive Intraluminal Device, Percutaneous Approach
Ø27Ø3Z6	Dilation of Coronary Artery, One Site, Bifurcation, Percutaneous Approach
Ø27Ø3ZZ	Dilation of Coronary Artery, One Site, Percutaneous Approach
Ø27Ø446	Dilation of Coronary Artery, One Site, Bifurcation, with Drug-eluting Intraluminal Device, Percutaneous Endoscopic Approach
Ø27Ø44Z	Dilation of Coronary Artery, One Site with Drug-eluting Intraluminal Device, Percutaneous Endoscopic Approach
Ø27Ø4D6	Dilation of Coronary Artery, One Site, Bifurcation, with Intraluminal Device, Percutaneous Endoscopic Approach
Ø27Ø4DZ	Dilation of Coronary Artery, One Site with Intraluminal Device, Percutaneous Endoscopic Approach
Ø27Ø4T6	Dilation of Coronary Artery, One Site, Bifurcation, with Radioactive Intraluminal Device, Percutaneous Endoscopic Approach
Ø27Ø4TZ	Dilation of Coronary Artery, One Site with Radioactive Intraluminal Device, Percutaneous Endoscopic Approach
Ø27Ø4Z6	Dilation of Coronary Artery, One Site, Bifurcation, Percutaneous Endoscopic Approach
Ø27Ø4ZZ	Dilation of Coronary Artery, One Site, Percutaneous Endoscopic Approach

Each table contains only those combinations of values that make up a valid procedure code. In some instances, the tables are split, indicating that there is a restriction in the combination of character choices. In table Ø27 above, character 7, qualifier 6 Bifurcation can be used only with coronary artery body part characters Ø–3. Character 7, qualifier T Ductus Arteriosus can be used only with body part character R Pulmonary Artery, Left.

The lower portion of table ØØ1, shown below, is split into two sections; values of characters must be selected from within the same section (row) of the table.

Ø Medical and Surgical
Ø Central Nervous System
1 Bypass Altering the route of passage of the contents of a tubular body part

Body Part Character 4	Approach Character 5	Device Character 6	Qualifier Character 7
6 Cerebral Ventricle	**Ø** Open **3** Percutaneous	**7** Autologous Tissue Substitute **J** Synthetic Substitute **K** Nonautologous Tissue Substitute	**Ø** Nasopharynx **1** Mastoid Sinus **2** Atrium **3** Blood Vessel **4** Pleural Cavity **5** Intestine **6** Peritoneal Cavity **7** Urinary Tract **8** Bone Marrow **B** Cerebral Cisterns
U Spinal Canal	**Ø** Open **3** Percutaneous	**7** Autologous Tissue Substitute **J** Synthetic Substitute **K** Nonautologous Tissue Substitute	**4** Pleural Cavity **6** Peritoneal Cavity **7** Urinary Tract **9** Fallopian Tube

Body part value *6* may be in combination with device values *7, J,* or *K.* Body part (character 4) value *U* may be used only in combination with qualifier (character 7) values of 4, 6, 7, and 9. In other words, code ØØ1UØ73 is invalid since the qualifier character appears above the line separating the two sections of the table.

Note: In this manual, there are instances in which some tables due to length must be continued on the next page. Each section must be used separately and value selection must be made within the same section (row) of the table.

Character Meanings

In each section each character has a specific meaning. Within a section all character meanings remain constant. The resource section of this manual lists character meanings for each section.

Sections

Procedures are divided into sections that identify the general type of procedure (e.g., Medical and Surgical, Obstetrics, Imaging). The first character of the procedure code always specifies the section.

The sections are listed below:

- Ø Medical and Surgical
- 1 Obstetrics
- 2 Placement
- 3 Administration
- 4 Measurement and Monitoring
- 5 Extracorporeal Assistance and Performance
- 6 Extracorporeal Therapies
- 7 Osteopathic
- 8 Other Procedures
- 9 Chiropractic
- B Imaging
- C Nuclear Medicine
- D Radiation Oncology
- F Physical Rehabilitation and Diagnostic Audiology
- G Mental Health
- H Substance Abuse Treatment

Medical and Surgical Section (Ø)

Character Meaning

The seven characters for Medical and Surgical procedures have the following meaning:

Character	Meaning
1	Section
2	Body System
3	Root Operation
4	Body Part
5	Approach
6	Device
7	Qualifier

The Medical and Surgical section constitutes the vast majority of procedures reported in an inpatient setting. Medical and Surgical procedure codes all have a first-character value of *Ø*. The second character indicates the general body system (e.g., Mouth and Throat, Gastrointestinal). The third character indicates the root operation, or specific objective, of the procedure (e.g., Excision). The fourth character indicates the specific body part on which the procedure was performed (e.g., Tonsils, Duodenum). The fifth character indicates the approach used to reach the procedure site (e.g., Open). The sixth character indicates whether a device was left in place during in the procedure (e.g., Synthetic Substitute). The seventh character is qualifier, which has a specific meaning for each root operation. For example, the qualifier can be used to identify the destination site of a *Bypass*. The first through fifth characters are always assigned a specific value, but the device (sixth character) and the qualifier (seventh character) are not applicable to all procedures. The value *Z* is used for the sixth and seventh characters to indicate that a specific device or qualifier does not apply to the procedure.

Section (Character 1)

Medical and Surgical procedure codes all have a first-character value of *Ø*.

Body Systems (Character 2)

Body systems for Medical and Surgical section codes are specified in the second character.

Body Systems

- Ø Central Nervous System
- 1 Peripheral Nervous System
- 2 Heart and Great Vessels
- 3 Upper Arteries
- 4 Lower Arteries
- 5 Upper Veins
- 6 Lower Veins
- 7 Lymphatic and Hemic Systems
- 8 Eye
- 9 Ear, Nose, Sinus
- B Respiratory System
- C Mouth and Throat
- D Gastrointestinal System
- F Hepatobiliary System and Pancreas
- G Endocrine System
- H Skin and Breast
- J Subcutaneous Tissue and Fascia
- K Muscles
- L Tendons
- M Bursae and Ligaments
- N Head and Facial Bones
- P Upper Bones
- Q Lower Bones
- R Upper Joints
- S Lower Joints
- T Urinary System
- U Female Reproductive System
- V Male Reproductive System
- W Anatomical Regions, General
- X Anatomical Regions, Upper Extremities
- Y Anatomical Regions, Lower Extremities

Root Operations (Character 3)

The root operation is specified in the third character. In the Medical and Surgical section there are 31 different root operations. The root operation identifies the objective of the procedure. Each root operation has a precise definition.

- *Alteration:* Modifying the natural anatomic structure of a body part without affecting the function of the body part
- *Bypass:* Altering the route of passage of the contents of a tubular body part
- *Change:* Taking out or off a device from a body part and putting back an identical or similar device in or on the same body part without cutting or puncturing the skin or a mucous membrane
- *Control:* Stopping, or attempting to stop, postprocedural bleeding
- *Creation:* Making a new genital structure that does not take over the function of a body part
- *Destruction:* Physical eradication of all or a portion of a body part by the direct use of energy, force, or a destructive agent
- *Detachment:* Cutting off all or a portion of the upper or lower extremities
- *Dilation:* Expanding an orifice or the lumen of a tubular body part
- *Division:* Cutting into a body part without draining fluids and/or gases from the body part in order to separate or transect a body part
- *Drainage:* Taking or letting out fluids and/or gases from a body part
- *Excision:* Cutting out or off, without replacement, a portion of a body part
- *Extirpation:* Taking or cutting out solid matter from a body part
- *Extraction:* Pulling or stripping out or off all or a portion of a body part by the use of force
- *Fragmentation:* Breaking solid matter in a body part into pieces
- *Fusion:* Joining together portions of an articular body part rendering the articular body part immobile
- *Insertion:* Putting in a nonbiological appliance that monitors, assists, performs, or prevents a physiological function but does not physically take the place of a body part
- *Inspection:* Visually and/or manually exploring a body part
- *Map:* Locating the route of passage of electrical impulses and/or locating functional areas in a body part
- *Occlusion:* Completely closing an orifice or lumen of a tubular body part
- *Reattachment:* Putting back in or on all or a portion of a separated body part to its normal location or other suitable location
- *Release:* Freeing a body part from an abnormal physical constraint by cutting or by use of force
- *Removal:* Taking out or off a device from a body part
- *Repair:* Restoring, to the extent possible, a body part to its normal anatomic structure and function
- *Replacement:* Putting in or on biological or synthetic material that physically takes the place and/or function of all or a portion of a body part
- *Reposition:* Moving to its normal location or other suitable location all or a portion of a body part
- *Resection:* Cutting out or off, without replacement, all of a body part
- *Restriction:* Partially closing an orifice or lumen of a tubular body part
- *Revision:* Correcting, to the extent possible, a portion of a malfunctioning device or the position of a displaced device
- *Supplement:* Putting in or on biological or synthetic material that physically reinforces and/or augments the function of a portion of a body part
- *Transfer:* Moving, without taking out, all or a portion of a body part to another location to take over the function of all or a portion of a body part
- *Transplantation:* Putting in or on all or a portion of a living body part taken from another individual or animal to physically take the place and/or function of all or a portion of a similar body part

The above definitions of root operation illustrate the precision of code values defined in the system. There is a clear distinction between each root operation.

A root operation specifies the objective of the procedure. The term *anastomosis* is not a root operation, because it is a means of joining and is always an integral part of another procedure (e.g., Bypass, Resection) with a specific objective. Similarly, *incision* is not a root operation, since it is always part of the objective of another procedure (e.g., Division, Drainage). The root operation *Repair* in the Medical and Surgical section functions as a "not elsewhere classified" option. *Repair* is used when the procedure performed is not one of the other specific root operations.

Appendix A provides additional explanation and representative examples of the Medical and Surgical root operations. Appendix B groups all root operations in the Medical and Surgical section into subcategories and provides an example of each root operation.

Body Part (Character 4)

The body part is specified in the fourth character. The body part indicates the specific part of the body system on which the procedure was performed (e.g., Duodenum). Tubular body parts are defined in ICD-10-PCS as those hollow body parts that provide a route of passage for solids, liquids, or gases. They include the cardiovascular system and body parts such as those contained in the gastrointestinal tract, genitourinary tract, biliary tract, and respiratory tract.

Approach (Character 5)

The technique used to reach the site of the procedure is specified in the fifth character. There are seven different approaches:

- *Open*: Cutting through the skin or mucous membrane and any other body layers necessary to expose the site of the procedure
- *Percutaneous:* Entry, by puncture or minor incision, of instrumentation through the skin or mucous membrane and any other body layers necessary to reach the site of the procedure
- *Percutaneous Endoscopic:* Entry, by puncture or minor incision, of instrumentation through the skin or mucous membrane and any other body layers necessary to reach and visualize the site of the procedure
- *Via Natural or Artificial Opening*: Entry of instrumentation through a natural or artificial external opening to reach the site of the procedure
- *Via Natural or Artificial Opening Endoscopic:* Entry of instrumentation through a natural or artificial external opening to reach and visualize the site of the procedure
- *Via Natural or Artificial Opening with Percutaneous Endoscopic Assistance:* Entry of instrumentation through a natural or artificial external opening and entry, by puncture or minor incision, of instrumentation through the skin or mucous membrane and any other body layers necessary to aid in the performance of the procedure
- *External:* Procedures performed directly on the skin or mucous membrane and procedures performed indirectly by the application of external force through the skin or mucous membrane

The approach comprises three components: the access location, method, and type of instrumentation.

Access location: For procedures performed on an internal body part, the access location specifies the external site through which the site of the procedure is reached. There are two general types of access locations: skin or mucous membranes, and external orifices. Every approach value except external includes one of these two access locations. The skin or mucous membrane can be cut or punctured to reach the procedure site. All open and percutaneous approach values use this access location. The site of a procedure can also be reached through an external opening. External openings can be natural (e.g., mouth) or artificial (e.g., colostomy stoma).

Method: For procedures performed on an internal body part, the method specifies how the external access location is entered. An open method specifies cutting through the skin or mucous membrane and any other intervening body layers necessary to expose the site of the procedure. An instrumentation method specifies the entry of instrumentation through the access location to the internal procedure site. Instrumentation can be introduced by puncture or minor incision, or through an external opening. The puncture or minor incision does not constitute an open approach because it does not expose the site of the procedure. An approach can define multiple methods. For example, *Via Natural or Artificial Opening with Percutaneous Endoscopic Assistance* includes both the initial entry of instrumentation to reach the site of the procedure, and the placement of additional percutaneous instrumentation into the body part to visualize and assist in the performance of the procedure.

Type of instrumentation: For procedures performed on an internal body part, instrumentation means that specialized equipment is used to perform the procedure. Instrumentation is used in all internal approaches other than the basic open approach. Instrumentation may or may not include the capacity to visualize the procedure site. For example, the instrumentation used to perform a sigmoidoscopy permits the internal site of the procedure to be visualized, while the instrumentation used to perform a needle biopsy of the liver does not. The term "endoscopic" as used in approach values refers to instrumentation that permits a site to be visualized.

Procedures performed directly on the skin or mucous membrane are identified by the external approach (e.g., skin excision). Procedures performed indirectly by the application of external force are also identified by the external approach (e.g., closed reduction of fracture).

Appendix E compares the components (access location, method, and type of instrumentation) of each approach and provides an example of each approach.

Device (Character 6)

The device is specified in the sixth character and is used only to specify devices that remain after the procedure is completed. There are four general types of devices:

- Grafts and Prostheses
- Implants
- Simple or Mechanical Appliances
- Electronic Appliances

While all devices can be removed, some cannot be removed without putting in another nonbiological appliance or body-part substitute.

When a specific device value is used to identify the device for a root operation, such as *Insertion* and that same device value is not an option for a more broad range root operation such as *Removal*, select the general device value. For example, in the body system Heart and Great Vessels, the specific device character for Cardiac Lead, Pacemaker in root operation *Insertion* is J. For the root operation *Removal*, the general device character M Cardiac Lead would be selected for the pacemaker lead.

ICD-10-PCS contains a PCS Device Aggregation Table (see appendix D) that crosswalks the *specific* device character values that have been created for specific root operations and specific body part character values to the *general* device character value that would be used for root operations that represent a broad range of procedures and general body part character values, such as Removal and Revision.

Instruments used to visualize the procedure site are specified in the approach, not the device, value.

If the objective of the procedure is to put in the device, then the root operation is *Insertion*. If the device is put in to meet an objective other than *Insertion*, then the root operation defining the underlying objective of the procedure is used, with the device specified in the device character. For example, if a procedure to replace the hip joint is performed, the root operation *Replacement* is coded, and the prosthetic device is specified in the device character. Materials that are incidental to a procedure such as clips, ligatures, and sutures are not specified in the device character. Because new devices can be developed, the value *Other Device* is provided as a temporary option for use until a specific device value is added to the system.

Qualifier (Character 7)

The qualifier is specified in the seventh character. The qualifier contains unique values for individual procedures. For example, the qualifier can be used to identify the destination site in a *Bypass*.

Medical and Surgical Section Principles

In developing the Medical and Surgical procedure codes, several specific principles were followed.

Composite Terms Are Not Root Operations

Composite terms such as colonoscopy, sigmoidectomy, or appendectomy do not describe root operations, but they do specify multiple components of a specific root operation. In ICD-10-PCS, the components of a procedure are defined separately by the characters making up the complete code. And the only component of a procedure specified in the root operation is the objective of the procedure. With each complete code the underlying objective of the procedure is specified by the root operation (third character), the precise part is specified by the body part (fourth character), and the method used to reach and visualize the procedure site is specified by the approach (fifth character). While colonoscopy, sigmoidectomy, and appendectomy are included in the Index, they do not constitute root operations in the Tables section. The objective of colonoscopy is the visualization of the colon and the root operation (character 3) is *Inspection*. Character 4 specifies the body part, which in this case is part of the colon. These composite terms, like colonoscopy or appendectomy, are included as cross-reference only. The index provides the correct root operation reference. Examples of other types of composite terms not representative of root operations are *partial* sigmoidectomy, *total* hysterectomy, and *partial* hip replacement. Always refer to the correct root operation in the Index and Tables section.

Root Operation Based on Objective of Procedure

The root operation is based on the objective of the procedure, such as *Resection* of transverse colon or *Dilation* of an artery. The assignment of the root operation is based on the procedure actually performed, which may or may not have been the intended procedure. If the intended procedure is modified or discontinued (e.g., excision instead of resection is performed), the root operation is determined by the procedure actually performed. If the desired result is not attained after completing the procedure (i.e., the artery does not remain expanded after the dilation procedure), the root operation is still determined by the procedure actually performed.

Examples:

- Dilating the urethra is coded as *Dilation* since the objective of the procedure is to dilate the urethra. If dilation of the urethra includes putting in an intraluminal stent, the root operation remains *Dilation* and not *Insertion* of the intraluminal device because the underlying objective of the procedure is dilation of the urethra. The stent is identified by the intraluminal device value in the sixth character of the dilation procedure code.
- If the objective is solely to put a radioactive element in the urethra, then the procedure is coded to the root operation *Insertion*, with the radioactive element identified in the sixth character of the code.
- If the objective of the procedure is to correct a malfunctioning or displaced device, then the procedure is coded to the root operation *Revision*. In the root operation *Revision*, the original device being revised is identified in the device character. *Revision* is typically performed on mechanical appliances (e.g., pacemaker) or materials used in replacement procedures (e.g., synthetic substitute). Typical revision procedures include adjustment of pacemaker position and correction of malfunctioning knee prosthesis.

Combination Procedures Are Coded Separately

If multiple procedures as defined by distinct objectives are performed during an operative episode, then multiple codes are used. For example, obtaining the vein graft used for coronary bypass surgery is coded as a separate procedure from the bypass itself.

Redo of Procedures

The complete or partial redo of the original procedure is coded to the root operation that identifies the procedure performed rather than *Revision*.

Example:

A complete redo of a hip replacement procedure that requires putting in a new prosthesis is coded to the root operation *Replacement* rather than *Revision*.

The correction of complications arising from the original procedure, other than device complications, is coded to the procedure performed. Correction of a malfunctioning or displaced device would be coded to the root operation *Revision*.

Example:

A procedure to control hemorrhage arising from the original procedure is coded to *Control* rather than *Revision*.

Examples of Procedures Coded in the Medical Surgical Section

The following are examples of procedures from the Medical and Surgical section, coded in ICD-10-PCS.

- Suture of skin laceration, left lower arm: 0HQEXZZ

  Medical and Surgical section (0), body system *Skin and Breast* (H), root operation *Repair* (Q), body part *Skin, Left Lower Arm* (E), *External* Approach (X) *No device* (Z), and *No qualifier* (Z).

- Laparoscopic appendectomy: 0DTJ4ZZ

  Medical and surgical section (0), body system *Gastrointestinal* (D), root operation *Resection* (T), body part *Appendix* (J), *Percutaneous Endoscopic* approach (4), No Device (Z), and No qualifier (Z).

- Sigmoidoscopy with biopsy: ØDBN8ZX

  Medical and Surgical section (Ø), body system *Gastrointestinal* (D), root operation *Excision* (B), body part *Sigmoid Colon* (N), *Via Natural or Artificial Opening Endoscopic* approach (8), *No Device* (Z), and with qualifier *Diagnostic* (X).

- Tracheostomy with tracheostomy tube: ØB11ØF4

  Medical and Surgical section (Ø), body system *Respiratory* (B), root operation *Bypass* (1), body part *Trachea* (1), *Open* approach (Ø), with *Tracheostomy Device* (F), and qualifier *Cutaneous* (4).

Obstetrics Section

Character Meanings

The seven characters in the Obstetrics section have the same meaning as in the Medical and Surgical section.

Character	Meaning
1	Section
2	Body System
3	Root Operation
4	Body Part
5	Approach
6	Device
7	Qualifier

The Obstetrics section includes procedures performed on the products of conception only. Procedures on the pregnant female are coded in the Medical and Surgical section (e.g., episiotomy). The term "products of conception" refers to all physical components of a pregnancy, including the fetus, amnion, umbilical cord, and placenta. There is no differentiation of the products of conception based on gestational age. Thus, the specification of the products of conception as a zygote, embryo or fetus, or the trimester of the pregnancy is not part of the procedure code but can be found in the diagnosis code.

Section (Character 1)

Obstetrics procedure codes have a first-character value of *1*.

Body System (Character 2)

The second-character value for body system is *Pregnancy*.

Root Operation (Character 3)

The root operations *Change, Drainage, Extraction, Insertion, Inspection, Removal, Repair, Reposition, Resection,* and *Transplantation* are used in the obstetrics section and have the same meaning as in the Medical and Surgical section.

The Obstetrics section also includes two additional root operations, *Abortion* and *Delivery*, defined below:

- *Abortion*: Artificially terminating a pregnancy
- *Delivery*: Assisting the passage of the products of conception from the genital canal

A cesarean section is not a separate root operation because the underlying objective is *Extraction* (i.e., pulling out all or a portion of a body part).

Body Part (Character 4)

The body-part values in the obstetrics section are:

- *Products of conception*
- *Products of conception, retained*
- *Products of conception, ectopic*

Approach (Character 5)

The fifth character specifies approaches and is defined as are those in the Medical and Surgical section. In the case of an abortion procedure that uses a laminaria or an abortifacient, the approach is *Via Natural or Artificial Opening*.

Device (Character 6)

The sixth character is used for devices such as fetal monitoring electrodes.

Qualifier (Character 7)

Qualifier values are specific to the root operation and are used to specify the type of extraction (e.g., low forceps, high forceps, etc.), the type of cesarean section (e.g., classical, low cervical, etc.), or the type of fluid taken out during a drainage procedure (e.g., amniotic fluid, fetal blood, etc.).

Placement Section

Character Meanings

The seven characters in the Placement section have the following meaning:

Character	Meaning
1	Section
2	Anatomical Region
3	Root Operation
4	Body Region/Orifice
5	Approach
6	Device
7	Qualifier

Placement section codes represent procedures for putting a device in or on a body region for the purpose of protection, immobilization, stretching, compression, or packing.

Section (Character 1)

Placement procedure codes have a first-character value of *2*.

Body System (Character 2)

The second character contains two values specifying either *Anatomical Regions* or *Anatomical Orifices*.

Root Operation (Character 3)

The root operations in the Placement section include only those procedures that are performed without making an incision or a puncture. The root operations *Change* and *Removal* are in the Placement section and have the same meaning as in the Medical and Surgical section.

The Placement section also includes five additional root operations, defined as follows:

- *Compression*: Putting pressure on a body region
- *Dressing*: Putting material on a body region for protection
- *Immobilization*: Limiting or preventing motion of an external body region
- *Packing*: Putting material in a body region or orifice
- *Traction*: Exerting a pulling force on a body region in a distal direction

Body Region (Character 4)
The fourth-character values are either body regions (e.g., *Upper Leg*) or natural orifices (e.g., *Ear*).

Approach (Character 5)
Since all placement procedures are performed directly on the skin or mucous membrane, or performed indirectly by applying external force through the skin or mucous membrane, the approach value is always *External*.

Device (Character 6)
The device character is always specified (except in the case of manual traction) and indicates the device placed during the procedure (e.g., cast, splint, bandage, etc.). Except for casts for fractures and dislocations, devices in the Placement section are off the shelf and do not require any extensive design, fabrication, or fitting. Placement of devices that require extensive design, fabrication, or fitting are coded in the Rehabilitation section.

Qualifier (Character 7)
The qualifier character is not specified in the Placement section; the qualifier value is always *No Qualifier*.

Administration Section

Character Meanings
The seven characters in the Administration section have the following meaning:

Character	Meaning
1	Section
2	Physiological System and Anatomical Region
3	Root Operation
4	Body System/Region
5	Approach
6	Substance
7	Qualifier

Administration section codes represent procedures for putting in or on a therapeutic, prophylactic, protective, diagnostic, nutritional, or physiological substance. The section includes transfusions, infusions, and injections, along with other similar services such as irrigation and tattooing.

Section (Character 1)
Administration procedure codes have a first-character value of *3*.

Body System (Character 2)
The body-system character contains only three values: *Indwelling Device, Physiological Systems and Anatomical Regions,* or *Circulatory System*. The *Circulatory System* is used for transfusion procedures.

Root Operation (Character 3)
There are three root operations in the Administration section.

- *Introduction*: Putting in or on a therapeutic, diagnostic, nutritional, physiological, or prophylactic substance except blood or blood products
- *Irrigation*: Putting in or on a cleansing substance
- *Transfusion*: Putting in blood or blood products

Body/System Region (Character 4)
The fourth character specifies the body system/region. The fourth character identifies the site where the substance is administered, not the site where the substance administered takes effect. Sites include *Skin and Mucous Membrane, Subcutaneous Tissue* and *Muscle*. These differentiate intradermal, subcutaneous, and intramuscular injections, respectively. Other sites include *Eye, Respiratory Tract, Peritoneal Cavity,* and *Epidural Space*.

The body systems/regions for arteries and veins are *Peripheral Artery, Central Artery, Peripheral Vein,* and *Central Vein*. The *Peripheral Artery* or *Vein* is typically used when a substance is introduced locally into an artery or vein. For example, chemotherapy is the introduction of an antineoplastic substance into a peripheral artery or vein by a percutaneous approach. In general, the substance introduced into a peripheral artery or vein has a systemic effect.

The *Central Artery* or *Vein* is typically used when the site where the substance is introduced is distant from the point of entry into the artery or vein. For example, the introduction of a substance directly at the site of a clot within an artery or vein using a catheter is coded as an introduction of a thrombolytic substance into a central artery or vein by a percutaneous approach. In general, the substance introduced into a central artery or vein has a local effect.

Approach (Character 5)
The fifth character specifies approaches as defined in the Medical and Surgical section. The approach for intradermal, subcutaneous, and intramuscular introductions (i.e., injections) is *Percutaneous*. If a catheter is placed to introduce a substance into an internal site within the circulatory system, then the approach is also *Percutaneous*. For example, if a catheter is used to introduce contrast directly into the heart for angiography, then the procedure would be coded as a percutaneous introduction of contrast into the heart.

Substance (Character 6)
The sixth character specifies the substance being introduced. Broad categories of substances are defined, such as anesthetic, contrast, dialysate, and blood products such as platelets.

Qualifier (Character 7)
The seventh character is a qualifier and is used to indicate whether the substance is *Autologous* or *Nonautologous*, or to further specify the substance.

Measurement and Monitoring Section

Character Meanings

The seven characters in the Measurement and Monitoring section have the following meaning:

Character	Meaning
1	Section
2	Physiological System
3	Root Operation
4	Body System
5	Approach
6	Function/Device
7	Qualifier

Measurement and Monitoring section codes represent procedures for determining the level of a physiological or physical function.

Section (Character 1)

Measurement and Monitoring procedure codes have a first-character value of *4*.

Body System (Character 2)

The second-character values for body system are A, *Physiological Systems* or *B, Physiological Devices*.

Root Operation (Character 3)

There are two root operations in the Measurement and Monitoring section, as defined below:

- *Measurement*: Determining the level of a physiological or physical function at a point in time
- *Monitoring*: Determining the level of a physiological or physical function repetitively over a period of time

Body System (Character 4)

The fourth character specifies the specific body system measured or monitored.

Approach (Character 5)

The fifth character specifies approaches as defined in the Medical and Surgical section.

Function/Device (Character 6)

The sixth character specifies the physiological or physical function being measured or monitored. Examples of physiological or physical functions are *Conductivity, Metabolism, Pulse, Temperature,* and *Volume*. If a device used to perform the measurement or monitoring is inserted and left in, then insertion of the device is coded as a separate Medical and Surgical procedure.

Qualifier (Character 7)

The seventh-character qualifier contains specific values as needed to further specify the body part (e.g., central, portal, pulmonary) or a variation of the procedure performed (e.g., ambulatory, stress). Examples of typical procedures coded in this section are EKG, EEG, and cardiac catheterization. An EKG is the measurement of cardiac electrical activity, while an EEG is the measurement of electrical activity of the central nervous system. A cardiac catheterization performed to measure the pressure in the heart is coded as the measurement of cardiac pressure by percutaneous approach.

Extracorporeal Assistance and Performance Section

Character Meanings

The seven characters in the Extracorporeal Assistance and Performance section have the following meaning:

Character	Meaning
1	Section
2	Physiological System
3	Root Operation
4	Body System
5	Duration
6	Function
7	Qualifier

In Extracorporeal Assistance and Performance procedures, equipment outside the body is used to assist or perform a physiological function. The section includes procedures performed in a critical care setting, such as mechanical ventilation and cardioversion; it also includes other services such as hyperbaric oxygen treatment and hemodialysis.

Section (Character 1)

Extracorporeal Assistance and Performance procedure codes have a first-character value of *5*.

Body System (Character 2)

The second-character value for body system is A, *Physiological Systems*.

Root Operation (Character 3)

There are three root operations in the Extracorporeal Assistance and Performance section, as defined below.

- *Assistance*: Taking over a portion of a physiological function by extracorporeal means
- *Performance*: Completely taking over a physiological function by extracorporeal means
- *Restoration*: Returning, or attempting to return, a physiological function to its natural state by extracorporeal means

The root operation *Restoration* contains a single procedure code that identifies extracorporeal cardioversion.

Body System (Character 4)

The fourth character specifies the body system (e.g., cardiac, respiratory) to which extracorporeal assistance or performance is applied.

Duration (Character 5)

The fifth character specifies the duration of the procedure—*Single, Intermittent*, or *Continuous*. For respiratory ventilation assistance or performance, the duration is specified in hours— *< 24 Consecutive Hours, 24–96 Consecutive Hours*, or *> 96 Consecutive Hours*. Value 6, *Multiple* identifies serial procedure treatment.

Function (Character 6)

The sixth character specifies the physiological function assisted or performed (e.g., oxygenation, ventilation) during the procedure.

Qualifier (Character 7)

The seventh-character qualifier specifies the type of equipment used, if any.

Extracorporeal Therapies Section

Character Meanings

The seven characters in the Extracorporeal Therapies section have the following meaning:

Character	Meaning
1	Section
2	Physiological Systems
3	Root Operation
4	Body System
5	Duration
6	Qualifier
7	Qualifier

In extracorporeal therapy, equipment outside the body is used for a therapeutic purpose that does not involve the assistance or performance of a physiological function.

Section (Character 1)

Extracorporeal Therapy procedure codes have a first-character value of 6.

Body System (Character 2)

The second-character value for body system is *Physiological Systems*.

Root Operation (Character 3)

There are 10 root operations in the Extracorporeal Therapy section, as defined below.

- *Atmospheric Control*: Extracorporeal control of atmospheric pressure and composition
- *Decompression*: Extracorporeal elimination of undissolved gas from body fluids

  Coding note: The root operation *Decompression* involves only one type of procedure: treatment for decompression sickness (the bends) in a hyperbaric chamber.
- *Electromagnetic Therapy*: Extracorporeal treatment by electromagnetic rays
- *Hyperthermia*: Extracorporeal raising of body temperature

  Coding note: The term hyperthermia is used to describe both a temperature imbalance treatment and also as an adjunct radiation treatment for cancer. When treating the temperature imbalance, it is coded to this section; for the cancer treatment, it is coded in section *D Radiation Oncology.*
- *Hypothermia*: Extracorporeal lowering of body temperature
- *Pheresis*: Extracorporeal separation of blood products

  Coding note: Pheresis may be used for two main purposes: to treat diseases when too much of a blood component is produced (e.g., leukemia) and to remove a blood product such as platelets from a donor, for transfusion into another patient.
- *Phototherapy*: Extracorporeal treatment by light rays

  Coding note: Phototherapy involves using a machine that exposes the blood to light rays outside the body, recirculates it, and then returns it to the body.
- *Shock Wave Therapy*: Extracorporeal treatment by shock waves
- *Ultrasound Therapy*: Extracorporeal treatment by ultrasound
- *Ultraviolet Light Therapy*: Extracorporeal treatment by ultraviolet light

Body System (Character 4)

The fourth character specifies the body system on which the extracorporeal therapy is performed (e.g., skin, circulatory).

Duration (Character 5)

The fifth character specifies the duration of the procedure (e.g., single or intermittent).

Qualifier (Character 6)

The sixth character is not specified for Extracorporeal Therapies and always has the value *No Qualifier.*

Qualifier (Character 7)

The seventh-character qualifier is used in the root operation *Pheresis* to specify the blood component on which pheresis is performed and in the root operation *Ultrasound Therapy* to specify site of treatment.

Osteopathic Section

Character Meanings

The seven characters in the Osteopathic section have the following meaning:

Character	Meaning
1	Section
2	Anatomical Region
3	Root Operation
4	Body Region
5	Approach
6	Method
7	Qualifier

Section (Character 1)

Osteopathic procedure codes have a first-character value of *7*.

Body System (Character 2)

The body-system character contains the value *Anatomical Regions*.

Root Operation (Character 3)

There is only one root operation in the Osteopathic section.

- *Treatment*: Manual treatment to eliminate or alleviate somatic dysfunction and related disorders

Body Region (Character 4)

The fourth character specifies the body region on which the osteopathic treatment is performed.

Approach (Character 5)

The approach for osteopathic treatment is always *External.*

Method (Character 6)

The sixth character specifies the method by which the treatment is accomplished.

Qualifier (Character 7)

The seventh character is not specified in the Osteopathic section and always has the value *None*.

Other Procedures Section

Character Meanings

The seven characters in the Other Procedures section have the following meaning:

Character	Meaning
1	Section
2	Body System
3	Root Operation
4	Body Region
5	Approach
6	Method
7	Qualifier

The Other Procedures section includes acupuncture, suture removal, and in vitro fertilization.

Section (Character 1)

Other Procedure section codes have a first-character value of *8*.

Body System (Character 2)

The second-character values for body systems are *Physiological Systems and Anatomical Regions* and *Indwelling Device*.

Root Operation (Character 3)

The Other Procedures section has only one root operation, defined as follows:

- *Other Procedures*: Methodologies that attempt to remediate or cure a disorder or disease.

Body Region (Character 4)

The fourth character contains specified body-region values, and also the body-region value *None* for Extracorporeal Procedures.

Approach (Character 5)

The fifth character specifies approaches as defined in the Medical and Surgical section.

Method (Character 6)

The sixth character specifies the method (e.g., *Acupuncture, Therapeutic Massage*).

Qualifier (Character 7)

The seventh character is a qualifier and contains specific values as needed.

Chiropractic Section

Character Meanings

The seven characters in the Chiropractic section have the following meaning:

Character	Meaning
1	Section
2	Anatomical Regions
3	Root Operation
4	Body Region
5	Approach
6	Method
7	Qualifier

Section (Character 1)

Chiropractic section procedure codes have a first-character value of *9*.

Body System (Character 2)

The second-character value for body system is *Anatomical Regions*.

Root Operation (Character 3)

There is only one root operation in the *Chiropractic* section.

- *Manipulation:* Manual procedure that involves a directed thrust to move a joint past the physiological range of motion, without exceeding the anatomical limit.

Body Region (Character 4)

The fourth character specifies the body region on which the chiropractic manipulation is performed.

Approach (Character 5)

The approach for chiropractic manipulation is always *External*.

Method (Character 6)

The sixth character is the method by which the manipulation is accomplished.

Qualifier (Character 7)

The seventh character is not specified in the Chiropractic section and always has the value *None*.

Imaging Section

Character Meanings

The seven characters in Imaging procedures have the following meaning:

Character	Meaning
1	Section
2	Body System
3	Root Type
4	Body Part
5	Contrast
6	Qualifier
7	Qualifier

Imaging procedures include plain radiography, fluoroscopy, CT, MRI, and ultrasound. Nuclear medicine procedures, including PET, uptakes, and scans, are in the nuclear medicine section. Therapeutic radiation procedure codes are in a separate radiation oncology section.

Section (Character 1)

Imaging procedure codes have a first-character value of *B*.

Body System (Character 2)

In the Imaging section, the second character defines the body system, such as *Heart* or *Gastrointestinal System*.

Root Type (Character 3)

The third character defines the type of imaging procedure (e.g., MRI, ultrasound). The following list includes all types in the *Imaging* section with a definition of each type:

- *Computerized Tomography (CT Scan)* : Computer-reformatted digital display of multiplanar images developed from the capture of multiple exposures of external ionizing radiation
- *Fluoroscopy*: Single plane or bi-plane real-time display of an image developed from the capture of external ionizing radiation on fluorescent screen. The image may also be stored by either digital or analog means
- *Magnetic Resonance Imaging (MRI)* : Computer reformatted digital display of multiplanar images developed from the capture of radiofrequency signals emitted by nuclei in a body site excited within a magnetic field
- *Plain Radiography*: Planar display of an image developed from the capture of external ionizing radiation on photographic or photoconductive plate
- *Ultrasonography*: Real-time display of images of anatomy or flow information developed from the capture of reflected and attenuated high-frequency sound waves

Body Part(Character 4)

The fourth character defines the body part with different values for each body system (character 2) value.

Contrast (Character 5)

The fifth character specifies whether the contrast material used in the imaging procedure is *High* or *Low Osmolar*, when applicable.

Qualifier (Character 6)

The sixth-character qualifier provides further detail regarding the nature of the substance or technologies used, such as *Unenhanced and Enhanced (contrast), Laser, or Intravascular Optical Coherence*.

Qualifier (Character 7)

The seventh character is a qualifier that may be used to specify certain procedural circumstances, the method by which the procedure was performed, or technologies utilized, such as *Intraoperative, Intravascular, or Transesophageal*.

Nuclear Medicine Section

Character Meanings

The seven characters in the Nuclear Medicine section have the following meaning:

Character	Meaning
1	Section
2	Body System
3	Root Type
4	Body Part
5	Radionuclide
6	Qualifier
7	Qualifier

Nuclear Medicine is the introduction of radioactive material into the body to create an image, to diagnose and treat pathologic conditions, or to assess metabolic functions. The Nuclear Medicine section does not include the introduction of encapsulated radioactive material for the treatment of cancer. These procedures are included in the Radiation Oncology section.

Section (Character 1)

Nuclear Medicine procedure codes have a first-character value of *C*.

Body System (Character 2)

The second character specifies the body system on which the nuclear medicine procedure is performed.

Root Type (Character 3)

The third character indicates the type of nuclear medicine procedure (e.g., planar imaging or nonimaging uptake). The following list includes the types of nuclear medicine procedures with a definition of each type.

- *Nonimaging Uptake:* Introduction of radioactive materials into the body for measurements of organ function, from the detection of radioactive emissions
- *Nonimaging Probe:* Introduction of radioactive materials into the body for the study of distribution and fate of certain substances by the detection of radioactive emissions; or alternatively, measurement of absorption of radioactive emissions from an external source
- *Nonimaging Assay:* Introduction of radioactive materials into the body for the study of body fluids and blood elements, by the detection of radioactive emissions
- *Planar Imaging*: Introduction of radioactive materials into the body for single-plane display of images developed from the capture of radioactive emissions
- *Positron Emission Tomography (PET):* Introduction of radioactive materials into the body for three-dimensional display of images developed from the simultaneous capture, 180 degrees apart, of radioactive emissions
- *Systemic Therapy:* Introduction of unsealed radioactive materials into the body for treatment
- *Tomographic (Tomo) Imaging*: Introduction of radioactive materials into the body for three dimensional display of images developed from the capture of radioactive emissions

Body Part (Character 4)

The fourth character indicates the body part or body region studied. *Regional* (e.g., lower extremity veins) and *Combination* (e.g., liver and spleen) body parts are commonly used in this section.

Radionuclide (Character 5)

The fifth character specifies the radionuclide, the radiation source. The option *Other Radionuclide* is provided in the nuclear medicine section for newly approved radionuclides until they can be added to the coding system. If more than one radiopharmaceutical is given to perform the procedure, then more than one code is used.

Qualifier (Character 6 and 7)

The sixth and seventh characters are qualifiers but are not specified in the *Nuclear Medicine* section; the value is always *None.*

Radiation Oncology Section

Character Meanings

The seven characters in the Radiation Oncology section have the following meaning:

Character	Meaning
1	Section
2	Body System
3	Root Type
4	Treatment Site
5	Modality Qualifier
6	Isotope
7	Qualifier

Section (Character 1)

Radiation oncology procedure codes have a first-character value of *D.*

Body System (Character 2)

The second character specifies the body system (e.g., central nervous system, musculoskeletal) irradiated.

Root Type (Character 3)

The third character specifies the general modality used (e.g., beam radiation).

Treatment Site (Character 4)

The fourth character specifies the body part that is the focus of the radiation therapy.

Modality Qualifier (Character 5)

The fifth character further specifies the radiation modality used (e.g., photons, electrons).

Isotope (Character 6)

The sixth character specifies the isotopes introduced into the body, if applicable.

Qualifier (Character 7)

The seventh character may specify whether the procedure was performed intraoperatively.

Physical Rehabilitation and Diagnostic Audiology Section

Character Meanings

The seven characters in the Physical Rehabilitation and Diagnostic Audiology section have the following meaning:

Character	Meaning
1	Section
2	Section Qualifier
3	Root Type
4	Body System & Region
5	Type Qualifier
6	Equipment
7	Qualifier

Physical rehabilitation procedures include physical therapy, occupational therapy, and speech-language pathology. Osteopathic procedures and chiropractic procedures are in separate sections.

Section (Character 1)

Physical Rehabilitation and Diagnostic Audiology procedure codes have a first-character value of *F.*

Section Qualifier (Character 2)

The section qualifier *Rehabilitation* or *Diagnostic Audiology* is specified in the second character.

Root Type (Character 3)

The third character specifies the root type. There are 14 different root type values, which can be classified into four basic types of rehabilitation and diagnostic audiology procedures, defined as follows:

- *Assessment*: Includes a determination of the patient's diagnosis when appropriate, need for treatment, planning for treatment, periodic assessment, and documentation related to these activities
- *Caregiver Training*: Educating caregiver with the skills and knowledge used to interact with and assist the patient
- *Fitting(s)*: Design, fabrication, modification, selection, and/or application of splint, orthosis, prosthesis, hearing aids, and/or other rehabilitation device
- *Treatment*: Use of specific activities or methods to develop, improve, and/or restore the performance of necessary functions, compensate for dysfunction and/or minimize debilitation

The type of treatment includes training as well as activities that restore function.

Body System & Region (Character 4)

The fourth character specifies the body region and/or system on which the procedure is performed.

Type Qualifier (Character 5)

The fifth character is a type qualifier that further specifies the procedure performed. Examples include therapy to improve the range of motion and training for bathing techniques. Refer to appendix D for definitions of these types of procedures.

Equipment (Character 6)

The sixth character specifies the equipment used. Specific equipment is not defined in the equipment value. Instead, broad categories of equipment are specified (e.g., aerobic endurance and conditioning, assistive/adaptive/supportive, etc.)

Qualifier (Character 7)

The seventh character is not specified in the Physical Rehabilitation and Diagnostic Audiology section and always has the value *None*.

Mental Health Section

Character Meanings

The seven characters in the Mental Health section have the following meaning:

Character	Meaning
1	Section
2	Body System
3	Root Type
4	Type Qualifier
5	Qualifier
6	Qualifier
7	Qualifier

Section (Character 1)

Mental health procedure codes have a first-character value of *G*.

Body System (Character 2)

The second character is used to identify the body system elsewhere in ICD-10-PCS. In this section it always has the value *None*.

Root Type (Character 3)

The third character specifies the procedure type, such as crisis intervention or counseling. There are 12 types of mental health procedures, some of which are defined below.

Psychological Tests:

- Developmental: Age-normed developmental status of cognitive, social, and adaptive behavior skills
- Intellectual and Psychoeducational: Intellectual abilities, academic achievement, and learning capabilities (including behavior and emotional factors affecting learning)
- Neurobehavioral and Cognitive Status: Includes neurobehavioral status exam, interview(s), and observation for the clinical assessment of thinking, reasoning, and judgment, acquired knowledge, attention, memory, visual spatial abilities, language functions, and planning
- Neuropsychological: Thinking, reasoning and judgment, acquired knowledge, attention, memory, visual spatial abilities, language functions, planning
- Personality and Behavioral: Mood, emotion, behavior, social functioning, psychopathological conditions, personality traits, and characteristics

Crisis intervention: Includes defusing, debriefing, counseling, psychotherapy, and/or coordination of care with other providers or agencies

Individual Psychotherapy:

- Behavior: Primarily to modify behavior. Includes modeling and role playing, positive reinforcement of target behaviors, response cost, and training of self-management skills
- Cognitive/behavioral: Combining cognitive and behavioral treatment strategies to improve functioning. Maladaptive responses are examined to determine how cognitions relate to behavior patterns in response to an event. Uses learning principles and information-processing models
- Cognitive: Primarily to correct cognitive distortions and errors
- Interactive: Uses primarily physical aids and other forms of nonoral interaction with a patient who is physically, psychologically, or developmentally unable to use ordinary language for communication (e.g., the use of toys in symbolic play)
- Interpersonal: Helps an individual make changes in interpersonal behaviors to reduce psychological dysfunction. Includes exploratory techniques, encouragement of affective expression, clarification of patient statements, analysis of communication patterns, use of therapy relationship, and behavior change techniques.
- Psychoanalysis: Methods of obtaining a detailed account of past and present mental and emotional experiences to determine the source and eliminate or diminish the undesirable effects of unconscious conflicts by making the individual aware of their existence, origin, and inappropriate expression in emotions and behavior.
- Psychodynamic: Exploration of past and present emotional experiences to understand motives and drives using insight-oriented techniques (e.g., empathetic listening, clarifying self-defeating behavior patterns, and exploring adaptive alternatives) to reduce the undesirable effects of internal conflicts on emotions and behavior
- Psychophysiological: Monitoring and alternation of physiological processes to help the individual associate physiological reactions combined with cognitive and behavioral strategies to gain improved control of these processes to help the individual cope more effectively
- Supportive: Formation of therapeutic relationship primarily for providing emotional support to prevent further deterioration in functioning during periods of particular stress. Often used in conjunction with other therapeutic approaches

Counseling:

- Vocational: Exploration of vocational interest, aptitudes, and required adaptive behavior skills to develop and carry out a plan for achieving a successful vocational placement, enhancing work-related adjustment, and/or pursuing viable options in training education or preparation

Family Psychotherapy:

- Remediation of emotional or behavioral problems presented by one or more family members when psychotherapy with more than one family member is indicated

Electroconvulsive Therapy: Includes appropriate sedation and other preparation of the individual

Biofeedback: Includes electroencephalogram (EEG), blood pressure, skin temperature or peripheral blood flow, electrocardiogram (ECG), electrooculogram, electromyogram (EMG), respirometry or capnometry, galvanic skin response (GSR) or electrodermal response (EDR), perineometry to monitor and regulate bowel or bladder activity, and electrogastrogram to monitor and regulate gastric motility

Other Mental Health procedures include *Hypnosis, Narcosynthesis, Group Psychotherapy, Light Therapy* and *Medication Management*. There are no ICD-10-PCS definitions of these procedures at this time.

Type Qualifier (Character 4)

The fourth character is a type qualifier (e.g., to indicate that counseling was educational or vocational).

Qualifier (Character 5, 6 and 7)

The fifth, sixth, and seventh characters are not specified and always have the value *None*.

Substance Abuse Treatment Section

Character Meanings

The seven characters in the Substance Abuse Treatment section have the following meaning:

Character	Meaning
1	Section
2	Body System
3	Root Type
4	Type Qualifier
5	Qualifier
6	Qualifier
7	Qualifier

Section (Character 1)

Substance Abuse Treatment codes have a first-character value of *H*.

Body System (Character 2)

The second character is used to identify the body system elsewhere in ICD-10-PCS. In this section, it always has the value *None*.

Root Type (Character 3)

The third character specifies the procedure. There are seven root type values classified in this section, as listed below:

- *Detoxification Services:* Not a treatment modality but helps the patient stabilize physically and psychologically until the body becomes free of drugs and the effects of alcohol
- *Individual Counseling:* Comprising several techniques, which apply various strategies to address drug addiction
- *Group Counseling:* Provides structured group counseling sessions and healing power through the connection with others
- *Family Counseling:* Provides support and education for family members of addicted individuals. Family member participation seen as critical to substance abuse treatment
- Other root type values in this section include *Individual Psychotherapy, Medication Management,* and *Pharmacotherapy*; there are no ICD-10-PCS definitions of these procedures at this time.

Type Qualifier (Character 4)

The fourth character further specifies the procedure type. Type Qualifier values vary dependent upon the Root Type procedure (Character 3). Root type 2, *Detoxification Services* contains only the value Z, *None* and Root type 6, *Family Counseling* contains only the value 3, *Other Family Counseling* , whereas the remainder Root Type procedures include nine to twelve total possible values.

Qualifier (Character 5, 6 and 7)

The fifth through seventh characters are designated as qualifiers but are never specified, so they always have the value *None*.

Comparison of ICD-10-PCS and ICD-9-CM

In 1993, the National Committee on Vital and Health Statistics (NCVHS) issued a report specifying recommendations for a new procedure classification system. NCVHS identified the essential characteristics that a procedure classification system should possess. Those characteristics include hierarchical structure, expandability, comprehensive, nonoverlapping, ease of use, setting and provider neutrality, multi-axial structure, and limited to classification of procedures.

ICD-10-PCS meets virtually all NCVHS characteristics, while ICD-9-CM fails to meet many NCVHS characteristics. In addition to the NCVHS characteristics, there are several other attributes of a procedure coding system that should be taken into consideration when comparing systems.

Completeness and Accuracy of Codes

The procedures coded in ICD-10-PCS provided a much more complete and accurate description of the procedure performed. The specification of the procedures performed not only affects payment, but is integral to internal management systems, external performance comparisons, and the assessment of quality of care. The detail and completeness of ICD-10-PCS is essential in today's health care environment.

General Equivalence Mappings

Due to the complexities of ICD-10-PCS and the drastic structural differences between the two coding systems, a direct code crosswalk is not possible. However, a general "mapping" of similar code choices has been developed. This network of relationships between the two code sets may be referred to as general equivalence mappings (GEMs). The purpose of these mappings, from ICD-9-CM to ICD-10-PCS, and vice versa, is to attempt to find corresponding procedure codes in lieu of a direct translation. For example:

- The ICD-9-CM to ICD-10-PCS GEM may help with analyzing or comparing data coded using the ICD-9-CM system to facilitate "forward mapping" to ICD-10-PCS.
- The ICD-10-PCS to ICD-9-CM GEM may help in comparing coded data using the ICD-10-PCS system to facilitate "backward mapping" to ICD-9-CM.

The 2012 update of the ICD-10 general equivalence mappings are posted for reference on the CMS website at the URL below: https://www.cms.gov/ICD10/11b15_2012_ICD10PCS.asp#TopOfPage.

Communications with Physicians

ICD-9-CM procedure codes often poorly describe the precise procedure performed. Physicians or others reviewing or analyzing data coded in ICD-9-CM may have difficulty developing clinical pathways, evaluating the coding for possible fraud and abuse, or conducting research. The ICD-10-PCS codes provide more clinically relevant procedure descriptions that can be more readily understood and used by physicians.

Independent evaluation of ICD-1Ø-PCS demonstrated that there is a learning curve associated with ICD-1Ø-PCS. Because of the additional specificity in ICD-1Ø-PCS, it probably takes longer to attain a minimum level of coding proficiency for ICD-1Ø-PCS than for ICD-9-CM. However, it should take less time to become *highly* proficient with ICD-1Ø-PCS than with ICD-9-CM. ICD-9-CM lacks clear definitions, and many substantially different procedures are coded with the same code. Therefore, identifying the correct code requires extensive knowledge of the American Hospital Association's *Coding Clinic for ICD-9-CM* and other coding guidelines. Becoming completely familiar with all the conventions associated with ICD-9-CM requires extensive and continued effort. As a result, becoming highly proficient in ICD-9-CM can take a long time.

Conclusion

ICD-1Ø-PCS has been developed as a replacement for volume 3 of ICD-9-CM. The system has evolved during its development based on extensive input from many segments of the health care industry. The multi-axial structure of the system, combined with its detailed definition of terminology, permits a precise specification of procedures for use in health services research, epidemiology, statistical analysis, and administrative areas. ICD-1Ø-PCS will also allow health information coders to assign accurate procedure codes with minimal effort.

Sources

All material contained in this manual is derived from the ICD-1Ø-PCS Coding System and Training Manual and related files revised and distributed by the Centers for Medicare and Medicaid Services, FY 2Ø12.

ICD-1Ø-PCS Draft Coding Guidelines

Conventions

A1. ICD-1Ø-PCS codes are composed of seven characters. Each character is an axis of classification that specifies information about the procedure performed. Within a defined code range, a character specifies the same type of information in that axis of classification.

Example: The fifth axis of classification specifies the approach in sections Ø through 4 and 7 through 9 of the system.

A2. One of 34 possible values can be assigned to each axis of classification in the seven-character code: they are the numbers Ø through 9 and the alphabet (except I and O because they are easily confused with the numbers 1 and Ø). The number of unique values used in an axis of classification differs as needed.

Example: Where the fifth axis of classification specifies the approach, seven different approach values are currently used to specify the approach.

A3. The valid values for an axis of classification can be added to as needed.

Example: If a significantly distinct type of device is used in a new procedure, a new device value can be added to the system.

A4. As with words in their context, the meaning of any single value is a combination of its axis of classification and any preceding values on which it may be dependent.

Example: The meaning of a body part value in the Medical and Surgical section is always dependent on the body system value. The body part value Ø in the Central Nervous body system specifies Brain and the body part value Ø in the Peripheral Nervous body system specifies Cervical Plexus.

A5. As the system is expanded to become increasingly detailed, over time more values will depend on preceding values for their meaning.

Example: In the Lower Joints body system, the device value 3 in the root operation Insertion specifies Infusion Device and the device value 3 in the root operation Fusion specifies Interbody Fusion Device.

[**Editor's Note:** Due to changes in the 2Ø12 draft code set, the above example is no longer valid. A current example of this guideline is found in the Heart and Great Vessels body system; the device character J in root operation Insertion specifies Cardiac Lead, Pacemaker, in root operation Removal device character J specifies Synthetic Substitute.]

A6. The purpose of the alphabetic index is to locate the appropriate table that contains all information necessary to construct a procedure code. The PCS Tables should always be consulted to find the most appropriate valid code.

A7. It is not required to consult the index first before proceeding to the tables to complete the code. A valid code may be chosen directly from the tables.

A8. All seven characters must be specified to be a valid code. If the documentation is incomplete for coding purposes, the physician should be queried for the necessary information.

A9. Within a PCS table, valid codes include all combinations of choices in characters 4 through 7 contained in the same row of the table. In the example below, ØJHT3VZ is a valid code, and ØJHW3VZ is *not* a valid code.

A10. "And," when used in a code description, means "and/or."

Example: Lower Arm and Wrist Muscle means lower arm and/or wrist muscle.

A11. Many of the terms used to construct PCS codes are defined within the system. It is the coder's responsibility to determine what the documentation in the medical record equates to in the PCS definitions. The physician is not expected to use the terms used in PCS code descriptions, nor is the coder required to query the physician when the correlation between the documentation and the defined PCS terms is clear.

Example: When the physician documents "partial resection" the coder can independently correlate "partial resection" to the root operation Excision without querying the physician for clarification.

Sample ICD-1Ø-PCS Table

Ø Medical and Surgical
J Subcutaneous Tissue and Fascia
H Insertion Putting in a nonbiological appliance that monitors, assists, performs, or prevents a physiological function but does not physically take the place of a body part

Body Part Character 4	Approach Character 5	Device Character 6	Qualifier Character 7
S Subcutaneous Tissue and Fascia, Head and Neck **V** Subcutaneous Tissue and Fascia, Upper Extremity **W** Subcutaneous Tissue and Fascia, Lower Extremity	**Ø** Open **3** Percutaneous	**1** Radioactive Element **3** Infusion Device	**Z** No Qualifier
T Subcutaneous Tissue and Fascia, Trunk	**Ø** Open **3** Percutaneous	**1** Radioactive Element **3** Infusion Device **V** Infusion Pump	**Z** No Qualifier

Medical and Surgical Section Guidelines (section Ø)

B2. Body System

General guidelines

B2.1a. The procedure codes in the general anatomical regions body systems should only be used when the procedure is performed on an anatomical region rather than a specific body part (e.g., root operations Control and Detachment, drainage of a body cavity) or on the rare occasion when no information is available to support assignment of a code to a specific body part.

Example: Control of postoperative hemorrhage is coded to the root operation Control found in the general anatomical regions body systems.

B2.1b. Body systems designated as upper or lower contain body parts located above or below the diaphragm respectively.

Example: Vein body parts above the diaphragm are found in the Upper Veins body system; vein body parts below the diaphragm are found in the Lower Veins body system.

The procedure codes in the general anatomical regions body systems should only be used when the procedure is performed on an anatomical region rather than a specific body part (e.g., root operations Control and Detachment, drainage of a body cavity) or on the rare occasion when no information is available to support assignment of a code to a specific body part.

Example: Control of postoperative hemorrhage is coded to the root operation Control found in the general anatomical regions body systems.

B2.1b. Body systems designated as upper or lower contain body parts located above or below the diaphragm respectively.

Example: Vein body parts above the diaphragm are found in the Upper Veins body system; vein body parts below the diaphragm are found in the Lower Veins body system.

B3. Root Operation

General guidelines

B3.1a. In order to determine the appropriate root operation, the full definition of the root operation as contained in the PCS Tables must be applied.

B3.1b. Components of a procedure specified in the root operation definition and explanation are not coded separately. Procedural steps necessary to reach the operative site and close the operative site are also not coded separately.

Example: Resection of a joint as part of a joint replacement procedure is included in the root operation definition of Replacement and is not coded separately. Laparotomy performed to reach the site of an open liver biopsy is not coded separately.

Multiple procedures

B3.2. During the same operative episode, multiple procedures are coded if:

a. The same root operation is performed on different body parts as defined by distinct values of the body part character.

   Example: Diagnostic excision of liver and pancreas are coded separately.

b. The same root operation is repeated at different body sites that are included in the same body part value.

   Example: Excision of the sartorius muscle and excision of the gracilis muscle are both included in the upper leg muscle body part value, and multiple procedures are coded.

c. Multiple root operations with distinct objectives are performed on the same body part.

   Example: Destruction of sigmoid lesion and bypass of sigmoid colon are coded separately.

d. The intended root operation is attempted using one approach, but is converted to a different approach.

   Example: Laparoscopic cholecystectomy converted to an open cholecystectomy is coded as percutaneous endoscopic Inspection and open Resection.

Discontinued procedures

B3.3. If the intended procedure is discontinued, code the procedure to the root operation performed. If a procedure is discontinued before any other root operation is performed, code the root operation Inspection of the body part or anatomical region inspected.

Example: A planned aortic valve replacement procedure is discontinued after the initial thoracotomy and before any incision is made in the heart muscle, when the patient becomes hemodynamically unstable. This procedure is coded as an open Inspection of the mediastinum.

Biopsy followed by more definitive treatment

B3.4. If a diagnostic Excision, Extraction, or Drainage procedure (biopsy) is followed by a more definitive procedure, such as Destruction, Excision or Resection at the same procedure site, both the biopsy and the more definitive treatment are coded.

Example: Biopsy of breast followed by partial mastectomy at the same procedure site, both the biopsy and the partial mastectomy procedure are coded.

Overlapping body layers

B3.5. If the root operations Excision, Repair or Inspection are performed on overlapping layers of the musculoskeletal system, the body part specifying the deepest layer is coded. *Example*: Excisional debridement that includes skin and subcutaneous tissue and muscle is coded to the muscle body part.

Bypass procedures

B3.6a. Bypass procedures are coded by identifying the body part bypassed "from" and the body part bypassed "to." The fourth character body part specifies the body part bypassed from, and the qualifier specifies the body part bypassed to.

Example: Bypass from stomach to jejunum, stomach is the body part and jejunum is the qualifier.

B3.6b. Coronary arteries are classified by number of distinct sites treated, rather than number of coronary arteries or anatomic name of a coronary artery (e.g., left anterior descending). Coronary artery bypass procedures are coded differently than other bypass procedures as described in the previous guideline. Rather than identifying the body part bypassed from, the body part identifies the number of coronary artery sites bypassed to, and the qualifier specifies the vessel bypassed from.

Example: Aortocoronary artery bypass of one site on the left anterior descending coronary artery and one site on the obtuse marginal coronary artery is classified in the body part axis of classification as two coronary artery sites and the qualifier specifies the aorta as the body part bypassed from.

B3.6c. If multiple coronary artery sites are bypassed, a separate procedure is coded for each coronary artery site that uses a different device and/or qualifier.

Example: Aortocoronary artery bypass and internal mammary coronary artery bypass are coded separately.

Control vs. more definitive root operations

B3.7. The root operation Control is defined as, "Stopping, or attempting to stop, postprocedural bleeding." If an attempt to stop postprocedural bleeding is initially unsuccessful, and to stop the bleeding requires performing any of the definitive root operations Bypass, Detachment, Excision, Extraction, Reposition, Replacement, or Resection, then that root operation is coded instead of Control.

Example: Resection of spleen to stop postprocedural bleeding is coded to Resection instead of Control.

Excision vs. Resection

B3.8. PCS contains specific body parts for anatomical subdivisions of a body part, such as lobes of the lungs or liver and regions of the intestine. Resection of the specific body part is coded whenever all of the body part is cut out or off, rather than coding Excision of a less specific body part.

Example: Left upper lung lobectomy is coded to Resection of Upper Lung Lobe, Left rather than Excision of Lung, Left.

Excision for graft

B3.9. If an autograft is obtained from a different body part in order to complete the objective of the procedure, a separate procedure is coded.

Example: Coronary bypass with excision of saphenous vein graft, excision of saphenous vein is coded separately.

Fusion procedures of the spine

B3.10a. The body part coded for a spinal vertebral joint(s) rendered immobile by a spinal fusion procedure is classified by the level of the spine (e.g. thoracic). There are distinct body part values for a single vertebral joint and for multiple vertebral joints at each spinal level.

Example: Body part values specify Lumbar Vertebral Joint, Lumbar Vertebral Joints, 2 or More and Lumbosacral Vertebral Joint.

B3.10b. If multiple vertebral joints are fused, a separate procedure is coded for each vertebral joint that uses a different device and/or qualifier.

Example: Fusion of lumbar vertebral joint, posterior approach, anterior column and fusion of lumbar vertebral joint, posterior approach, posterior column are coded separately.

B3.10c. Combinations of devices and materials are often used on a vertebral joint to render the joint immobile. When combinations of devices are used on the same vertebral joint, the device value coded for the procedure is as follows:

- If an interbody fusion device is used to render the joint immobile (alone or containing other material like bone graft), the procedure is coded with the device value Interbody Fusion Device
- If bone graft is the *only* device used to render the joint immobile, the procedure is coded with the device value Nonautologous Tissue Substitute or Autologous Tissue Substitute
- If a mixture of autologous and nonautologous bone graft (with or without biological or synthetic extenders or binders) is used to render the joint immobile, code the procedure with the device value Autologous Tissue Substitute

Examples: Fusion of a vertebral joint using a cage style interbody fusion device containing morsellized bone graft is coded to the device Interbody Fusion Device.

Fusion of a vertebral joint using a bone dowel interbody fusion device made of cadaver bone and packed with a mixture of local morsellized bone and demineralized bone matrix is coded to the device Interbody Fusion Device.

Fusion of a vertebral joint using both autologous bone graft and bone bank bone graft is coded to the device Autologous Tissue Substitute.

Inspection procedures

B3.11a. Inspection of a body part(s) performed in order to achieve the objective of a procedure is not coded separately.

Example: Fiberoptic bronchoscopy performed for irrigation of bronchus, only the irrigation procedure is coded.

B3.11b. If multiple tubular body parts are inspected, the most distal body part inspected is coded. If multiple non-tubular body parts in a region are inspected, the body part that specifies the entire area inspected is coded.

Examples: Cystoureteroscopy with inspection of bladder and ureters is coded to the ureter body part value.

Exploratory laparotomy with general inspection of abdominal contents is coded to the peritoneal cavity body part value.

B3.11c. When both an Inspection procedure and another procedure are performed on the same body part during the same episode, if the Inspection procedure is performed using a different approach than the other procedure, the Inspection procedure is coded separately.

Example: Endoscopic Inspection of the duodenum is coded separately when open Excision of the duodenum is performed during the same procedural episode.

Occlusion vs. Restriction for vessel embolization procedures

B3.12. If the objective of an embolization procedure is to completely close a vessel, the root operation Occlusion is coded. If the objective of an embolization procedure is to narrow the lumen of a vessel, the root operation Restriction is coded.

Examples: Tumor embolization is coded to the root operation Occlusion, because the objective of the procedure is to cut off the blood supply to the vessel.

Embolization of a cerebral aneurysm is coded to the root operation Restriction, because the objective of the procedure is not to close off the vessel entirely, but to narrow the lumen of the vessel at the site of the aneurysm where it is abnormally wide.

Release procedures

B3.13. In the root operation Release, the body part value coded is the body part being freed and not the tissue being manipulated or cut to free the body part.

Example: Lysis of intestinal adhesions is coded to the specific intestine body part value.

Release vs. Division

B3.14. If the sole objective of the procedure is freeing a body part without cutting the body part, the root operation is Release. If the sole objective of the procedure is separating or transecting a body part, the root operation is Division.

Examples: Freeing a nerve root from surrounding scar tissue to relieve pain is coded to the root operation Release. Severing a nerve root to relieve pain is coded to the root operation Division.

Reposition for fracture treatment

B3.15. Reduction of a displaced fracture is coded to the root operation Reposition and the application of a cast or splint in conjunction with the Reposition procedure is not coded separately. Treatment of a nondisplaced fracture is coded to the procedure performed.

Examples: Putting a pin in a nondisplaced fracture is coded to the root operation Insertion.

Casting of a nondisplaced fracture is coded to the root operation Immobilization in the Placement section.

Transplantation vs. Administration

B3.16. Putting in a mature and functioning living body part taken from another individual or animal is coded to the root operation Transplantation. Putting in autologous or nonautologous cells is coded to the Administration section.

Example: Putting in autologous or nonautologous bone marrow, pancreatic islet cells or stem cells is coded to the Administration section.

B4. Body Part

General guidelines

B4.1a. If a procedure is performed on a portion of a body part that does not have a separate body part value, code the body part value corresponding to the whole body part.

Example: A procedure performed on the alveolar process of the mandible is coded to the mandible body part.

B4.1b. If the prefix "peri" is combined with a body part to identify the site of the procedure, the procedure is coded to the body part named.

Example: A procedure site identified as perirenal is coded to the kidney body part.

Branches of body parts

B4.2. Where a specific branch of a body part does not have its own body part value in PCS, the body part is coded to the closest proximal branch that has a specific body part value.

Example: A procedure performed on the mandibular branch of the trigeminal nerve is coded to the trigeminal nerve body part value

Bilateral body part values

B4.3. Bilateral body part values are available for a limited number of body parts. If the identical procedure is performed on contralateral body parts, and a bilateral body part value exists for that body part, a single procedure is coded using the bilateral body part value. If no bilateral body part value exists, each procedure is coded separately using the appropriate body part value.

Example: The identical procedure performed on both fallopian tubes is coded once using the body part value Fallopian Tube, Bilateral. The identical procedure performed on both knee joints is coded twice using the body part values Knee Joint, Right and Knee Joint, Left.

Coronary arteries

B4.4. The coronary arteries are classified as a single body part that is further specified by number of sites treated and not by name or number of arteries. Separate body part values are used to specify the number of sites treated when the same procedure is performed on multiple sites in the coronary arteries.

Examples: Angioplasty of two distinct sites in the left anterior descending coronary artery with placement of two stents is coded as Dilation of Coronary Arteries, Two Sites, with Intraluminal Device.

Angioplasty of two distinct sites in the left anterior descending coronary artery, one with stent placed and one without, is coded separately as Dilation of Coronary Artery, One Site with Intraluminal Device, and Dilation of Coronary Artery, One Site with no device.

Tendons, ligaments, bursae and fascia near a joint

B4.5. Procedures performed on tendons, ligaments, bursae and fascia supporting a joint are coded to the body part in the respective body system that is the focus of the procedure. Procedures performed on joint structures themselves are coded to the body part in the joint body systems.

Example: Repair of the anterior cruciate ligament of the knee is coded to the knee bursae and ligament body part in the bursae and ligaments body system. Knee arthroscopy with shaving of articular cartilage is coded to the knee joint body part in the Lower Joints body system.

Skin, subcutaneous tissue and fascia overlying a joint

B4.6. If a procedure is performed on the skin, subcutaneous tissue or fascia overlying a joint, the procedure is coded to the following body part:

- Shoulder is coded to Upper Arm
- Elbow is coded to Lower Arm
- Wrist is coded to Lower Arm
- Hip is coded to Upper Leg
- Knee is coded to Lower Leg
- Ankle is coded to Foot

Fingers and toes

B4.7. If a body system does not contain a separate body part value for fingers, procedures performed on the fingers are coded to the body part value for the hand. If a body system does not contain a separate body part value for toes, procedures performed on the toes are coded to the body part value for the foot.

Example: Excision of finger muscle is coded to one of the hand muscle body part values in the Muscles body system.

B6. Device

General guidelines

B6.1a. A device is coded only if a device remains after the procedure is completed. If no device remains, the device value No Device is coded.

B6.1b. Materials such as sutures, ligatures, radiological markers and temporary post-operative wound drains are considered integral to the performance of a procedure and are not coded as devices.

B6.1c. Procedures performed on a device only and not on a body part are specified in the root operations Change, Irrigation, Removal and Revision, and are coded to the procedure performed.

Example: Irrigation of percutaneous nephrostomy tube is coded to the root operation Irrigation of indwelling device in the Administration section.

Drainage device

B6.2. A separate procedure to put in a drainage device is coded to the root operation Drainage with the device value Drainage Device.

Obstetric Section Guidelines (section 1)

C. Obstetrics Section

Products of conception

C1. Procedures performed on the products of conception are coded to the Obstetrics section. Procedures performed on the pregnant female other than the products of conception are coded to the appropriate root operation in the Medical and Surgical section.

Example: Amniocentesis is coded to the products of conception body part in the Obstetrics section. Repair of obstetric urethral laceration is coded to the urethra body part in the Medical and Surgical section.

Procedures following delivery or abortion [end ital]

C2. Procedures performed following a delivery or abortion for curettage of the endometrium or evacuation of retained products of conception are all coded in the Obstetrics section, to the root operation Extraction and the body part Products of Conception, Retained. Diagnostic or therapeutic dilation and curettage performed during times other than the postpartum or post-abortion period are all coded in the Medical and Surgical section, to the root operation Extraction and the body part Endometrium.

Coding Exercises

Using the ICD-10-PCS tables construct the code that accurately represents the procedure performed. Answers to these coding exercises may be found in appendix G.

Medical Surgical Section

Procedure	Code
Excision of malignant melanoma from skin of right ear	
Laparoscopy with excision of endometrial implant from left ovary	
Percutaneous needle core biopsy of right kidney	
EGD with gastric biopsy	
Open endarterectomy of left common carotid artery	
Excision of basal cell carcinoma of lower lip	
Open excision of tail of pancreas	
Percutaneous biopsy of right gastrocnemius muscle	
Sigmoidoscopy with sigmoid polypectomy	
Open excision of lesion from right Achilles tendon	
Open resection of cecum	
Total excision of pituitary gland, open	
Explantation of left failed kidney, open	
Open left axillary total lymphadenectomy	
Laparoscopic-assisted total vaginal hysterectomy	
Right total mastectomy, open	
Open resection of papillary muscle	
Radical retropubic prostatectomy, open	
Laparoscopic cholecystectomy	
Endoscopic bilateral total maxillary sinusectomy	
Amputation at right elbow level	
Right below-knee amputation, proximal tibia/fibula	
Fifth ray carpometacarpal joint amputation, left hand	
Right leg and hip amputation through ischium	
DIP joint amputation of right thumb	
Right wrist joint amputation	
Trans-metatarsal amputation of foot at left big toe	
Mid-shaft amputation, right humerus	
Left fourth toe amputation, mid-proximal phalanx	
Right above-knee amputation, distal femur	
Cryotherapy of wart on left hand	
Percutaneous radiofrequency ablation of right vocal cord lesion	

Medical Surgical Section (Continued)

Procedure	Code
Left heart catheterization with laser destruction of arrhythmogenic focus, A-V node	
Cautery of nosebleed	
Transurethral endoscopic laser ablation of prostate	
Cautery of oozing varicose vein, left calf	
Laparoscopy with destruction of endometriosis, bilateral ovaries	
Laser coagulation of right retinal vessel hemorrhage, percutaneous	
Thoracoscopic talc instillation pleurodesis, left side	
Percutaneous talc injection pleurodesis, left side	
Sclerotherapy of brachial plexus lesion, alcohol injection	
Forceps total mouth extraction, upper and lower teeth	
Removal of left thumbnail	
Extraction of right intraocular lens without replacement, percutaneous	
Laparoscopy with needle aspiration of ova for in vitro fertilization	
Nonexcisional debridement of skin ulcer, right foot	
Open stripping of abdominal fascia, right side	
Hysteroscopy with D&C, diagnostic	
Liposuction for medical purposes, left upper arm	
Removal of tattered right ear drum fragments with tweezers	
Microincisional phlebectomy of spider veins, right lower leg	
Routine Foley catheter placement	
Incision and drainage of external perianal abscess	
Percutaneous drainage of ascites	
Laparoscopy with left ovarian cystotomy and drainage	
Laparotomy with hepatotomy and drain placement for liver abscess, right lobe	
Right knee arthrotomy with drain placement	
Thoracentesis of left pleural effusion	
Phlebotomy of left median cubital vein for polycythemia vera	
Percutaneous chest tube placement for right pneumothorax	
Endoscopic drainage of left ethmoid sinus	
Thoracentesis of left pleural effusion	
Arterial blood gas sample from right brachial artery line	

Medical Surgical Section (Continued)

Procedure	Code
Percutaneous chest tube placement for right pneumothorax	
Endoscopic drainage of left ethmoid sinus	
Removal of foreign body, right cornea	
Percutaneous mechanical thrombectomy, left brachial artery	
Esophagogastroscopy with removal of bezoar from stomach	
Foreign body removal, skin of left thumb	
Transurethral cystoscopy with removal of bladder stone	
Forceps removal of foreign body in right nostril	
Laparoscopy with excision of old suture from mesentery	
Incision and removal of right lacrimal duct stone	
Nonincisional removal of intraluminal foreign body from vagina	
Open excision of retained sliver, subcutaneous tissue of left foot	
Extracorporeal shock-wave lithotripsy (ESWL), bilateral ureters	
Endoscopic retrograde cholangiopancreatography (ERCP) with lithotripsy of common bile duct stone	
Thoracotomy with crushing of pericardial calcifications	
Transurethral cystoscopy with fragmentation of bladder calculus	
Hysteroscopy with intraluminal lithotripsy of left fallopian tube calcification	
Division of right foot tendon, percutaneous	
Left heart catheterization with division of bundle of HIS	
Open osteotomy of capitate, left hand	
EGD with esophagotomy of esophagogastric junction	
Sacral rhizotomy for pain control, percutaneous	
Laparotomy with exploration and adhesiolysis of right ureter	
Incision of scar contracture, right elbow	
Frenulotomy for treatment of tongue-tie syndrome	
Right shoulder arthroscopy with coracoacromial ligament release	
Mitral valvulotomy for release of fused leaflets, open approach	
Percutaneous left Achilles tendon release	
Laparoscopy with lysis of peritoneal adhesions	
Manual rupture of right shoulder joint adhesions under general anesthesia	
Open posterior tarsal tunnel release	
Laparoscopy with freeing of left ovary and fallopian tube	
Liver transplant with donor matched liver	

Medical Surgical Section (Continued)

Procedure	Code
Orthotopic heart transplant using porcine heart	
Right lung transplant, open, using organ donor match	
Left kidney/pancreas organ bank transplant	
Replantation of avulsed scalp	
Reattachment of severed right ear	
Reattachment of traumatic left gastrocnemius avulsion, open	
Closed replantation of three avulsed teeth, lower jaw	
Reattachment of severed left hand	
Right hand open palmaris longus tendon transfer	
Endoscopic radial to median nerve transfer	
Fasciocutaneous flap closure of left thigh, open	
Transfer left index finger to left thumb position, open	
Percutaneous fascia transfer to fill defect, anterior neck	
Trigeminal to facial nerve transfer, percutaneous endoscopic	
Endoscopic left leg flexor hallucis longus tendon transfer	
Right scalp advancement flap to right temple	
Bilateral TRAM pedicle flap reconstruction status post mastectomy, muscle only, open	
Skin transfer flap closure of complex open wound, left lower back	
Open fracture reduction, right tibia	
Laparoscopy with gastropexy for malrotation	
Left knee arthroscopy with reposition of anterior cruciate ligament	
Open transposition of ulnar nerve	
Closed reduction with percutaneous internal fixation of right femoral neck fracture	
Trans-vaginal intraluminal cervical cerclage	
Cervical cerclage using Shirodkar technique	
Thoracotomy with banding of left pulmonary artery using extraluminal device	
Restriction of thoracic duct with intraluminal stent, percutaneous	
Craniotomy with clipping of cerebral aneurysm	
Nonincisional, transnasal placement of restrictive stent in right lacrimal duct	
Percutaneous ligation of esophageal vein	
Percutaneous embolization of left internal carotid-cavernous fistula	
Laparoscopy with bilateral occlusion of fallopian tubes using Hulka extraluminal clips	
Open suture ligation of failed A-V graft, left brachial artery	
Percutaneous embolization of vascular supply, intracranial meningioma	

Medical Surgical Section (Continued)

Procedure	Code
ERCP with balloon dilation of common bile duct	
PTCA of two coronary arteries, LAD with stent placement, RCA with no stent	
Cystoscopy with intraluminal dilation of bladder neck stricture	
Open dilation of old anastomosis, left femoral artery	
Dilation of upper esophageal stricture, direct visualization, with Bougie sound	
PTA of right brachial artery stenosis	
Transnasal dilation and stent placement in right lacrimal duct	
Hysteroscopy with balloon dilation of bilateral fallopian tubes	
Tracheoscopy with intraluminal dilation of tracheal stenosis	
Cystoscopy with dilation of left ureteral stricture, with stent placement	
Open gastric bypass with Roux-en-Y limb to jejunum	
Right temporal artery to intracranial artery bypass using Gore-Tex graft, open	
Tracheostomy formation with tracheostomy tube placement, percutaneous	
PICVA (percutaneous in situ coronary venous arterialization) of single coronary artery	
Open left femoral-popliteal artery bypass using cadaver vein graft	
Shunting of intrathecal cerebrospinal fluid to peritoneal cavity using synthetic shunt	
Colostomy formation, open, transverse colon to abdominal wall	
Open urinary diversion, left ureter, using ileal conduit to skin	
CABG of LAD using left internal mammary artery, open off-bypass	
Open pleuroperitoneal shunt, right pleural cavity, using synthetic device	
End-of-life replacement of spinal neurostimulator generator, multiple array, in lower abdomen	
Percutaneous insertion of spinal neurostimulator lead, lumbar spinal cord	
Percutaneous placement of pacemaker lead in left atrium	
Open placement of dual chamber pacemaker generator in chest wall	
Percutaneous placement of venous central line in right internal jugular	
Open insertion of multiple channel cochlear implant, left ear	
Percutaneous placement of Swan-Ganz catheter in superior vena cava	
Bronchoscopy with insertion of brachytherapy seeds, right main bronchus	

Medical Surgical Section (Continued)

Procedure	Code
Placement of intrathecal infusion pump for pain management, percutaneous	
Open insertion of interspinous process device into lumbar vertebral joint	
Open placement of bone growth stimulator, left femoral shaft	
Cystoscopy with placement of brachytherapy seeds in prostate gland	
Full-thickness skin graft to right lower arm, autograft (do not code graft harvest for this exercise)	
Excision of necrosed left femoral head with bone bank bone graft to fill the defect, open	
Penetrating keratoplasty of right cornea with donor matched cornea, percutaneous approach	
Bilateral mastectomy with concomitant saline breast implants, open	
Excision of abdominal aorta with Gore-Tex graft replacement, open	
Total right knee arthroplasty with insertion of total knee prosthesis	
Bilateral mastectomy with free TRAM flap reconstruction	
Tenonectomy with graft to right ankle using cadaver graft, open	
Mitral valve replacement using porcine valve, open	
Percutaneous phacoemulsification of right eye cataract with prosthetic lens insertion	
Aortic valve annuloplasty using ring, open	
Laparoscopic repair of left inguinal hernia with marlex plug	
Autograft nerve graft to right median nerve, percutaneous endoscopic (do not code graft harvest for this exercise)	
Exchange of liner in femoral component of previous left hip replacement, open approach	
Anterior colporrhaphy with polypropylene mesh reinforcement, open approach	
Implantation of CorCap cardiac support device, open approach	
Abdominal wall herniorrhaphy, open, using synthetic mesh	
Tendon graft to strengthen injured left shoulder using autograft, open (do not code graft harvest for this exercise)	
Onlay lamellar keratoplasty of left cornea using autograft, external approach	
Resurfacing procedure on right femoral head, open approach	
Exchange of drainage tube from right hip joint	
Tracheostomy tube exchange	
Change chest tube for left pneumothorax	
Exchange of cerebral ventriculostomy drainage tube	
Foley urinary catheter exchange	

Medical Surgical Section (Continued)

Procedure	Code
Open removal of lumbar sympathetic neurostimulator lead	
Nonincisional removal of Swan-Ganz catheter from right pulmonary artery	
Laparotomy with removal of pancreatic drain	
Extubation, endotracheal tube	
Nonincisional PEG tube removal	
Transvaginal removal of extraluminal cervical cerclage	
Incision with removal of K-wire fixation, right first metatarsal	
Cystoscopy with retrieval of left ureteral stent	
Removal of nasogastric drainage tube for decompression	
Removal of external fixator, left radial fracture	
Reposition of Swan-Ganz catheter insertion to superior vena cava	
Open revision of right hip replacement, with readjustment of prosthesis	
Adjustment of position, pacemaker lead in left ventricle, percutaneous	
External repositioning of Foley catheter to bladder	
Revision of VAD reservoir placement in chest wall, causing patient discomfort, open	
Thoracotomy with exploration of right pleural cavity	
Diagnostic laryngoscopy	
Exploratory arthrotomy of left knee	
Colposcopy with diagnostic hysteroscopy	
Digital rectal exam	
Diagnostic arthroscopy of right shoulder	
Endoscopy of bilateral maxillary sinus	
Laparotomy with palpation of liver	
Transurethral diagnostic cystoscopy	
Colonoscopy, abandoned at sigmoid colon	
Percutaneous mapping of basal ganglia	
Heart catheterization with cardiac mapping	
Intraoperative whole brain mapping via craniotomy	
Mapping of left cerebral hemisphere, percutaneous endoscopic	
Intraoperative cardiac mapping during open heart surgery	
Hysteroscopy with cautery of post-hysterectomy oozing and evacuation of clot	
Open exploration and ligation of post-op arterial bleeder, left forearm	
Control of postoperative retroperitoneal bleeding via laparotomy	
Reopening of thoracotomy site with drainage and control of post-op hemopericardium	

Medical Surgical Section (Continued)

Procedure	Code
Arthroscopy with drainage of hemarthrosis at previous operative site, right knee	
Radiocarpal fusion of left hand with internal fixation, open	
Posterior spinal fusion at L1–L3 level with BAK cage interbody fusion device, open	
Intercarpal fusion of right hand with bone bank bone graft, open	
Sacrococcygeal fusion with bone graft from same operative site, open	
Interphalangeal fusion of left great toe, percutaneous pin fixation	
Suture repair of left radial nerve laceration	
Laparotomy with suture repair of blunt force duodenal laceration	
Cosmetic face lift, open, no other information available	
Bilateral breast augmentation with silicone implants, open	
Cosmetic rhinoplasty with septal reduction and tip elevation using local tissue graft, open	
Abdominoplasty (tummy tuck), open	
Liposuction of bilateral thighs	
Creation of penis in female patient using tissue bank donor graft	
Creation of vagina in male patient using synthetic material	

Obstetrics

Procedure	Code
Abortion by dilation and evacuation following laminaria insertion	
Manually assisted spontaneous abortion	
Abortion by abortifacient insertion	
Bimanual pregnancy examination	
Extraperitoneal C-section, low transverse incision	
Fetal spinal tap, percutaneous	
Fetal kidney transplant, laparoscopic	
Open in utero repair of congenital diaphragmatic hernia	
Laparoscopy with total excision of tubal pregnancy	
Transvaginal removal of fetal monitoring electrode	

Placement

Procedure	Code
Placement of packing material, right ear	
Mechanical traction of entire left leg	
Removal of splint, right shoulder	
Placement of neck brace	
Change of vaginal packing	
Packing of wound, chest wall	
Sterile dressing placement to left groin region	
Removal of packing material from pharynx	
Placement of intermittent pneumatic compression device, covering entire right arm	
Exchange of pressure dressing to left thigh	

Administration

Procedure	Code
Peritoneal dialysis via indwelling catheter	
Transvaginal artificial insemination	
Infusion of total parenteral nutrition via central venous catheter	
Esophagogastroscopy with Botox injection into esophageal sphincter	
Percutaneous irrigation of knee joint	
Epidural injection of mixed steroid and local anesthetic for pain control	
Chemical pleurodesis using injection of tetracycline	
Transfusion of antihemophilic factor, (nonautologous) via arterial central line	
Transabdominal in vitro fertilization, implantation of donor ovum	
Autologous bone marrow transplant via central venous line	

Measurement and Monitoring

Procedure	Code
Cardiac stress test, single measurement	
EGD with biliary flow measurement	
Temperature monitoring, rectal	
Peripheral venous pulse, external, single measurement	
Holter monitoring	
Respiratory rate, external, single measurement	

Measurement and Monitoring

Procedure	Code
Fetal heart rate monitoring, transvaginal	
Visual mobility test, single measurement	
Pulmonary artery wedge pressure monitoring from Swan-Ganz catheter	
Olfactory acuity test, single measurement	

Extracorporeal Assistance and Performance

Procedure	Code
Mechanical ventilation, 16 hours	
Liver dialysis, single encounter	
Cardiac countershock with successful conversion to sinus rhythm	
IPPB (intermittent positive pressure breathing) for mobilization of secretions, 22 hours	
Measurement and monitoring of intracranial pressure, percutaneous approach	
Renal dialysis, series of encounters	
IABP (intra-aortic balloon pump) continuous	
Intra-operative cardiac pacing, continuous	
ECMO (extracorporeal membrane oxygenation), continuous	
Controlled mechanical ventilation (CMV), 45 hours	
Pulsatile compression boot with intermittent inflation	

Extracorporeal Therapies

Procedure	Code
Donor thrombocytapheresis, single encounter	
Bili-lite UV phototherapy, series treatment	
Whole body hypothermia, single treatment	
Circulatory phototherapy, single encounter	
Shock wave therapy of plantar fascia, single treatment	
Antigen-free air conditioning, series treatment	
TMS (transcranial magnetic stimulation), series treatment	
Therapeutic ultrasound of peripheral vessels, single treatment	
Plasmapheresis, series treatment	
Extracorporeal electromagnetic stimulation (EMS) for urinary incontinence, single treatment	

Osteopathic

Procedures	Code
Isotonic muscle energy treatment of right leg	
Low velocity-high amplitude osteopathic treatment of head	
Lymphatic pump osteopathic treatment of left axilla	
Indirect osteopathic treatment of sacrum	
Articulatory osteopathic treatment of cervical region	

Other Procedures

Procedure	Code
Near infrared spectroscopy of leg vessels	
CT computer assisted sinus surgery	
Suture removal, abdominal wall	
Isolation after infectious disease exposure	
Robotic assisted open prostatectomy	

Chiropractic

Procedure	Code
Chiropractic treatment of lumbar region using long lever specific contact	
Chiropractic manipulation of abdominal region, indirect visceral	
Chiropractic extra-articular treatment of hip region	
Chiropractic treatment of sacrum using long and short lever specific contact	
Mechanically-assisted chiropractic manipulation of head	

Imaging

Procedure	Code
Noncontrast CT of abdomen and pelvis	
Ultrasound guidance for catheter placement, left subclavian artery	
Chest x-ray, AP/PA and lateral views	
Endoluminal ultrasound of gallbladder and bile ducts	
MRI of thyroid gland, contrast unspecified	
Esophageal videofluoroscopy study with oral barium contrast	

Imaging

Procedure	Code
Portable x-ray study of right radius/ulna shaft, standard series	
Routine fetal ultrasound, second trimester twin gestation	
CT scan of bilateral lungs, high osmolar contrast with densitometry	
Fluoroscopic guidance for percutaneous transluminal angioplasty (PTA) of left common femoral artery, low osmolar contrast	

Nuclear Medicine

Procedure	Code
Tomo scan of right and left heart, unspecified radiopharmaceutical, qualitative gated rest	
Technetium pentetate assay of kidneys, ureters, and bladder	
Uniplanar scan of spine using technetium oxidronate, with first-pass study	
Thallous chloride tomographic scan of bilateral breasts	
PET scan of myocardium using rubidium	
Gallium citrate scan of head and neck, single plane imaging	
Xenon gas nonimaging probe of brain	
Upper GI scan, radiopharmaceutical unspecified, for gastric emptying	
Carbon 11 PET scan of brain with quantification	
Iodinated albumin nuclear medicine assay, blood plasma volume study	

Radiation Oncology

Procedure	Code
Plaque radiation of left eye, single port	
8 MeV photon beam radiation to brain	
IORT of colon, 3 ports	
HDR brachytherapy of prostate using palladium-103	
Electron radiation treatment of right breast, with custom device	
Hyperthermia oncology treatment of pelvic region	
Contact radiation of tongue	
Heavy particle radiation treatment of pancreas, four risk sites	
LDR brachytherapy to spinal cord using iodine	
Whole body phosphorus-32 administration with risk to hematopoetic system	

Physical Rehabilitation and Diagnostic Audiology

Procedure	Code
Bekesy assessment using audiometer	
Individual fitting of left eye prosthesis	
Physical therapy for range of motion and mobility, patient right hip, no special equipment	
Bedside swallow assessment using assessment kit	
Caregiver training in airway clearance techniques	
Application of short arm cast in rehabilitation setting	
Verbal assessment of patient's pain level	
Caregiver training in communication skills using manual communication board	
Group musculoskeletal balance training exercises, whole body, no special equipment	
Individual therapy for auditory processing using tape recorder	

Mental Health

Procedure	Code
Cognitive-behavioral psychotherapy, individual	
Narcosynthesis	
Light therapy	
ECT (electroconvulsive therapy), unilateral, multiple seizure	
Crisis intervention	

Mental Health

Procedure	Code
Neuropsychological testing	
Hypnosis	
Developmental testing	
Vocational counseling	
Family psychotherapy	

Substance Abuse Treatment

Procedure	Code
Naltrexone treatment for drug dependency	
Substance abuse treatment family counseling	
Medication monitoring of patient on methadone maintenance	
Individual interpersonal psychotherapy for drug abuse	
Patient in for alcohol detoxification treatment	
Group motivational counseling	
Individual 12-step psychotherapy for substance abuse	
Post-test infectious disease counseling for IV drug abuser	
Psychodynamic psychotherapy for drug-dependent patient	
Group cognitive-behavioral counseling for substance abuse	

A

B

C

D

E

Index

Extirpation — Extirpation

F

G

H

I

J

K

L

N

O

Q

R

S

T

U

V

W

X

Tables

Central Nervous System ØØ1–ØØX

Ø Medical and Surgical
Ø Central Nervous System
1 Bypass Altering the route of passage of the contents of a tubular body part

Body Part Character 4	Approach Character 5	Device Character 6	Qualifier Character 7
6 Cerebral Ventricle	**Ø** Open **3** **Percutaneous**	**7** Autologous Tissue Substitute **J** Synthetic Substitute **K** Nonautologous Tissue Substitute	**Ø** Nasopharynx **1** Mastoid Sinus **2** Atrium **3** Blood Vessel **4** Pleural Cavity **5** Intestine **6** Peritoneal Cavity **7** Urinary Tract **8** Bone Marrow **B** Cerebral Cisterns
U Spinal Canal	**Ø** Open **3** **Percutaneous**	**7** Autologous Tissue Substitute **J** Synthetic Substitute **K** Nonautologous Tissue Substitute	**4** Pleural Cavity **6** Peritoneal Cavity **7** Urinary Tract **9** Fallopian Tube

Ø Medical and Surgical
Ø Central Nervous System
2 Change Taking out or off a device from a body part and putting back an identical or similar device in or on the same body part without cutting or puncturing the skin or a mucous membrane

Body Part Character 4	Approach Character 5	Device Character 6	Qualifier Character 7
Ø Brain **E** Cranial Nerve **U** Spinal Canal	**X** External	**Ø** Drainage Device **Y** Other Device	**Z** No Qualifier

Ø Medical and Surgical
Ø Central Nervous System
5 Destruction Physical eradication of all or a portion of a body part by the direct use of energy, force, or a destructive agent

Body Part Character 4	Approach Character 5	Device Character 6	Qualifier Character 7
Ø Brain **1** Cerebral Meninges **2** Dura Mater **6** Cerebral Ventricle **7** Cerebral Hemisphere **8** Basal Ganglia **9** Thalamus **A** Hypothalamus **B** Pons **C** Cerebellum **D** Medulla Oblongata **F** Olfactory Nerve **G** Optic Nerve **H** Oculomotor Nerve **J** Trochlear Nerve **K** Trigeminal Nerve **L** Abducens Nerve **M** Facial Nerve **N** Acoustic Nerve **P** Glossopharyngeal Nerve **Q** Vagus Nerve **R** Accessory Nerve **S** Hypoglossal Nerve **T** Spinal Meninges **W** Cervical Spinal Cord **X** Thoracic Spinal Cord **Y** Lumbar Spinal Cord	**Ø** Open **3** Percutaneous **4** Percutaneous Endoscopic	**Z** No Device	**Z** No Qualifier

Ø Medical and Surgical
Ø Central Nervous System
8 Division Cutting into a body part without draining fluids and/or gases from the body part in order to separate or transect a body part

Body Part Character 4	Approach Character 5	Device Character 6	Qualifier Character 7
Ø Brain **7** Cerebral Hemisphere **8** Basal Ganglia **F** Olfactory Nerve **G** Optic Nerve **H** Oculomotor Nerve **J** Trochlear Nerve **K** Trigeminal Nerve **L** Abducens Nerve **M** Facial Nerve **N** Acoustic Nerve **P** Glossopharyngeal Nerve **Q** Vagus Nerve **R** Accessory Nerve **S** Hypoglossal Nerve **W** Cervical Spinal Cord **X** Thoracic Spinal Cord **Y** Lumbar Spinal Cord	**Ø** Open **3** Percutaneous **4** Percutaneous Endoscopic	**Z** No Device	**Z** No Qualifier

Ø Medical and Surgical
Ø Central Nervous System
9 Drainage Taking or letting out fluids and/or gases from a body part

Body Part Character 4	Approach Character 5	Device Character 6	Qualifier Character 7
Ø Brain **1** Cerebral Meninges **2** Dura Mater **3** Epidural Space **4** Subdural Space **5** Subarachnoid Space **6** Cerebral Ventricle **7** Cerebral Hemisphere **8** Basal Ganglia **9** Thalamus **A** Hypothalamus **B** Pons **C** Cerebellum **D** Medulla Oblongata **F** Olfactory Nerve **G** Optic Nerve **H** Oculomotor Nerve **J** Trochlear Nerve **K** Trigeminal Nerve **L** Abducens Nerve **M** Facial Nerve **N** Acoustic Nerve **P** Glossopharyngeal Nerve **Q** Vagus Nerve **R** Accessory Nerve **S** Hypoglossal Nerve **T** Spinal Meninges **U** Spinal Canal **W** Cervical Spinal Cord **X** Thoracic Spinal Cord **Y** Lumbar Spinal Cord	**Ø** Open **3** Percutaneous **4** Percutaneous Endoscopic	**Ø** Drainage Device	**Z** No Qualifier

ØØ9 Continued on next page

0 Medical and Surgical
0 Central Nervous System
9 Drainage Taking or letting out fluids and/or gases from a body part

009 Continued

Body Part Character 4	Approach Character 5	Device Character 6	Qualifier Character 7
0 Brain 1 Cerebral Meninges 2 Dura Mater 3 Epidural Space 4 Subdural Space 5 Subarachnoid Space 6 Cerebral Ventricle 7 Cerebral Hemisphere 8 Basal Ganglia 9 Thalamus A Hypothalamus B Pons C Cerebellum D Medulla Oblongata F Olfactory Nerve G Optic Nerve H Oculomotor Nerve J Trochlear Nerve K Trigeminal Nerve L Abducens Nerve M Facial Nerve N Acoustic Nerve P Glossopharyngeal Nerve Q Vagus Nerve R Accessory Nerve S Hypoglossal Nerve T Spinal Meninges U Spinal Canal W Cervical Spinal Cord X Thoracic Spinal Cord Y Lumbar Spinal Cord	0 Open 3 Percutaneous 4 Percutaneous Endoscopic	Z No Device	X Diagnostic Z No Qualifier

0 Medical and Surgical
0 Central Nervous System
B Excision Cutting out or off, without replacement, a portion of a body part

Body Part Character 4	Approach Character 5	Device Character 6	Qualifier Character 7
0 Brain 1 Cerebral Meninges 2 Dura Mater 6 Cerebral Ventricle 7 Cerebral Hemisphere 8 Basal Ganglia 9 Thalamus A Hypothalamus B Pons C Cerebellum D Medulla Oblongata F Olfactory Nerve G Optic Nerve H Oculomotor Nerve J Trochlear Nerve K Trigeminal Nerve L Abducens Nerve M Facial Nerve N Acoustic Nerve P Glossopharyngeal Nerve Q Vagus Nerve R Accessory Nerve S Hypoglossal Nerve T Spinal Meninges W Cervical Spinal Cord X Thoracic Spinal Cord Y Lumbar Spinal Cord	0 Open 3 Percutaneous 4 Percutaneous Endoscopic	Z No Device	X Diagnostic Z No Qualifier

Ø Medical and Surgical
Ø Central Nervous System
C Extirpation Taking or cutting out solid matter from a body part

Body Part Character 4	Approach Character 5	Device Character 6	Qualifier Character 7
Ø Brain	**Ø** Open	**Z** No Device	**Z** No Qualifier
1 Cerebral Meninges	**3** Percutaneous		
2 Dura Mater	**4** Percutaneous Endoscopic		
3 Epidural Space			
4 Subdural Space			
5 Subarachnoid Space			
6 Cerebral Ventricle			
7 Cerebral Hemisphere			
8 Basal Ganglia			
9 Thalamus			
A Hypothalamus			
B Pons			
C Cerebellum			
D Medulla Oblongata			
F Olfactory Nerve			
G Optic Nerve			
H Oculomotor Nerve			
J Trochlear Nerve			
K Trigeminal Nerve			
L Abducens Nerve			
M Facial Nerve			
N Acoustic Nerve			
P Glossopharyngeal Nerve			
Q Vagus Nerve			
R Accessory Nerve			
S Hypoglossal Nerve			
T Spinal Meninges			
W Cervical Spinal Cord			
X Thoracic Spinal Cord			
Y Lumbar Spinal Cord			

Ø Medical and Surgical
Ø Central Nervous System
D Extraction Pulling or stripping out or off all or a portion of a body part by the use of force

Body Part Character 4	Approach Character 5	Device Character 6	Qualifier Character 7
1 Cerebral Meninges	**Ø** Open	**Z** No Device	**Z** No Qualifier
2 Dura Mater	**3** Percutaneous		
F Olfactory Nerve	**4** Percutaneous Endoscopic		
G Optic Nerve			
H Oculomotor Nerve			
J Trochlear Nerve			
K Trigeminal Nerve			
L Abducens Nerve			
M Facial Nerve			
N Acoustic Nerve			
P Glossopharyngeal Nerve			
Q Vagus Nerve			
R Accessory Nerve			
S Hypoglossal Nerve			
T Spinal Meninges			

Ø Medical and Surgical
Ø Central Nervous System
F Fragmentation Breaking solid matter in a body part into pieces

Body Part Character 4	Approach Character 5	Device Character 6	Qualifier Character 7
3 Epidural Space	**Ø** Open	**Z** No Device	**Z** No Qualifier
4 Subdural Space	**3** Percutaneous		
5 Subarachnoid Space	**4** Percutaneous Endoscopic		
6 Cerebral Ventricle	**X** External		
U Spinal Canal			

0 Medical and Surgical
0 Central Nervous System
H Insertion Putting in a nonbiological appliance that monitors, assists, performs, or prevents a physiological function but does not physically take the place of a body part

Body Part Character 4	Approach Character 5	Device Character 6	Qualifier Character 7
0 Brain **6** Cerebral Ventricle **E** Cranial Nerve **U** Spinal Canal **V** Spinal Cord	**0** Open **3** Percutaneous **4** Percutaneous Endoscopic	**2** Monitoring Device **3** Infusion Device **M** Neurostimulator Lead	**Z** No Qualifier

0 Medical and Surgical
0 Central Nervous System
J Inspection Visually and/or manually exploring a body part

Body Part Character 4	Approach Character 5	Device Character 6	Qualifier Character 7
0 Brain **E** Cranial Nerve **U** Spinal Canal **V** Spinal Cord	**0** Open **3** Percutaneous **4** Percutaneous Endoscopic	**Z** No Device	**Z** No Qualifier

0 Medical and Surgical
0 Central Nervous System
K Map Locating the route of passage of electrical impulses and/or locating functional areas in a body part

Body Part Character 4	Approach Character 5	Device Character 6	Qualifier Character 7
0 Brain **7** Cerebral Hemisphere **8** Basal Ganglia **9** Thalamus **A** Hypothalamus **B** Pons **C** Cerebellum **D** Medulla Oblongata	**0** Open **3** Percutaneous **4** Percutaneous Endoscopic	**Z** No Device	**Z** No Qualifier

0 Medical and Surgical
0 Central Nervous System
N Release Freeing a body part from an abnormal physical constraint

Body Part Character 4	Approach Character 5	Device Character 6	Qualifier Character 7
0 Brain **1** Cerebral Meninges **2** Dura Mater **6** Cerebral Ventricle **7** Cerebral Hemisphere **8** Basal Ganglia **9** Thalamus **A** Hypothalamus **B** Pons **C** Cerebellum **D** Medulla Oblongata **F** Olfactory Nerve **G** Optic Nerve **H** Oculomotor Nerve **J** Trochlear Nerve **K** Trigeminal Nerve **L** Abducens Nerve **M** Facial Nerve **N** Acoustic Nerve **P** Glossopharyngeal Nerve **Q** Vagus Nerve **R** Accessory Nerve **S** Hypoglossal Nerve **T** Spinal Meninges **W** Cervical Spinal Cord **X** Thoracic Spinal Cord **Y** Lumbar Spinal Cord	**0** Open **3** Percutaneous **4** Percutaneous Endoscopic	**Z** No Device	**Z** No Qualifier

Ø Medical and Surgical
Ø Central Nervous System
P Removal Taking out or off a device from a body part

Body Part Character 4	Approach Character 5	Device Character 6	Qualifier Character 7
Ø Brain **6** Cerebral Ventricle **E** Cranial Nerve **U** Spinal Canal **V** Spinal Cord	**X** External	**Ø** Drainage Device **2** Monitoring Device **3** Infusion Device **M** Neurostimulator Lead	**Z** No Qualifier
Ø Brain **V** Spinal Cord	**Ø** Open **3** Percutaneous **4** Percutaneous Endoscopic	**Ø** Drainage Device **2** Monitoring Device **3** Infusion Device **7** Autologous Tissue Substitute **J** Synthetic Substitute **K** Nonautologous Tissue Substitute **M** Neurostimulator Lead	**Z** No Qualifier
6 Cerebral Ventricle **U** Spinal Canal	**Ø** Open **3** Percutaneous **4** Percutaneous Endoscopic	**Ø** Drainage Device **2** Monitoring Device **3** Infusion Device **J** Synthetic Substitute **M** Neurostimulator Lead	**Z** No Qualifier
E Cranial Nerve	**Ø** Open **3** Percutaneous **4** Percutaneous Endoscopic	**Ø** Drainage Device **2** Monitoring Device **3** Infusion Device **7** Autologous Tissue Substitute **M** Neurostimulator Lead	**Z** No Qualifier

Ø Medical and Surgical
Ø Central Nervous System
Q Repair Restoring, to the extent possible, a body part to its normal anatomic structure and function

Body Part Character 4	Approach Character 5	Device Character 6	Qualifier Character 7
Ø Brain **1** Cerebral Meninges **2** Dura Mater **6** Cerebral Ventricle **7** Cerebral Hemisphere **8** Basal Ganglia **9** Thalamus **A** Hypothalamus **B** Pons **C** Cerebellum **D** Medulla Oblongata **F** Olfactory Nerve **G** Optic Nerve **H** Oculomotor Nerve **J** Trochlear Nerve **K** Trigeminal Nerve **L** Abducens Nerve **M** Facial Nerve **N** Acoustic Nerve **P** Glossopharyngeal Nerve **Q** Vagus Nerve **R** Accessory Nerve **S** Hypoglossal Nerve **T** Spinal Meninges **W** Cervical Spinal Cord **X** Thoracic Spinal Cord **Y** Lumbar Spinal Cord	**Ø** Open **3** Percutaneous **4** Percutaneous Endoscopic	**Z** No Device	**Z** No Qualifier

0 Medical and Surgical
0 Central Nervous System
S Reposition Moving to its normal location or other suitable location all or a portion of a body part

Body Part Character 4	Approach Character 5	Device Character 6	Qualifier Character 7
F Olfactory Nerve G Optic Nerve H Oculomotor Nerve J Trochlear Nerve K Trigeminal Nerve L Abducens Nerve M Facial Nerve N Acoustic Nerve P Glossopharyngeal Nerve Q Vagus Nerve R Accessory Nerve S Hypoglossal Nerve W Cervical Spinal Cord X Thoracic Spinal Cord Y Lumbar Spinal Cord	0 Open 3 Percutaneous 4 Percutaneous Endoscopic	Z No Device	Z No Qualifier

0 Medical and Surgical
0 Central Nervous System
T Resection Cutting out or off, without replacement, all of a body part

Body Part Character 4	Approach Character 5	Device Character 6	Qualifier Character 7
7 Cerebral Hemisphere	0 Open 3 Percutaneous 4 Percutaneous Endoscopic	Z No Device	Z No Qualifier

0 Medical and Surgical
0 Central Nervous System
U Supplement Putting in or on biological or synthetic material that physically reinforces and/or augments the function of a portion of a body part

Body Part Character 4	Approach Character 5	Device Character 6	Qualifier Character 7
1 Cerebral Meninges 2 Dura Mater T Spinal Meninges	0 Open 3 Percutaneous 4 Percutaneous Endoscopic	7 Autologous Tissue Substitute J Synthetic Substitute K Nonautologous Tissue Substitute	Z No Qualifier
F Olfactory Nerve G Optic Nerve H Oculomotor Nerve J Trochlear Nerve K Trigeminal Nerve L Abducens Nerve M Facial Nerve N Acoustic Nerve P Glossopharyngeal Nerve Q Vagus Nerve R Accessory Nerve S Hypoglossal Nerve	0 Open 3 Percutaneous 4 Percutaneous Endoscopic	7 Autologous Tissue Substitute	Z No Qualifier

0 Medical and Surgical
0 Central Nervous System
W Revision Correcting, to the extent possible, a portion of a malfunctioning device or the position of a displaced device

Body Part Character 4	Approach Character 5	Device Character 6	Qualifier Character 7
0 Brain V Spinal Cord	0 Open 3 Percutaneous 4 Percutaneous Endoscopic X External	0 Drainage Device 2 Monitoring Device 3 Infusion Device 7 Autologous Tissue Substitute J Synthetic Substitute K Nonautologous Tissue Substitute M Neurostimulator Lead	Z No Qualifier
6 Cerebral Ventricle U Spinal Canal	0 Open 3 Percutaneous 4 Percutaneous Endoscopic X External	0 Drainage Device 2 Monitoring Device 3 Infusion Device J Synthetic Substitute M Neurostimulator Lead	Z No Qualifier
E Cranial Nerve	0 Open 3 Percutaneous 4 Percutaneous Endoscopic X External	0 Drainage Device 2 Monitoring Device 3 Infusion Device 7 Autologous Tissue Substitute M Neurostimulator Lead	Z No Qualifier

Ø Medical and Surgical
Ø Central Nervous System
X Transfer Moving, without taking out, all or a portion of a body part to another location to take over the function of all or a portion of a body part

Body Part Character 4	Approach Character 5	Device Character 6	Qualifier Character 7
F Olfactory Nerve **G** Optic Nerve **H** Oculomotor Nerve **J** Trochlear Nerve **K** Trigeminal Nerve **L** Abducens Nerve **M** Facial Nerve **N** Acoustic Nerve **P** Glossopharyngeal Nerve **Q** Vagus Nerve **R** Accessory Nerve **S** Hypoglossal Nerve	**Ø** Open **4** Percutaneous Endoscopic	**Z** No Device	**F** Olfactory Nerve **G** Optic Nerve **H** Oculomotor Nerve **J** Trochlear Nerve **K** Trigeminal Nerve **L** Abducens Nerve **M** Facial Nerve **N** Acoustic Nerve **P** Glossopharyngeal Nerve **Q** Vagus Nerve **R** Accessory Nerve **S** Hypoglossal Nerve

Peripheral Nervous System 012–01X

0 Medical and Surgical
1 Peripheral Nervous System
2 Change Taking out or off a device from a body part and putting back an identical or similar device in or on the same body part without cutting or puncturing the skin or a mucous membrane

Body Part Character 4	Approach Character 5	Device Character 6	Qualifier Character 7
Y Peripheral Nerve	**X** External	**0** Drainage Device **Y** Other Device	**Z** No Qualifier

0 Medical and Surgical
1 Peripheral Nervous System
5 Destruction Physical eradication of all or a portion of a body part by the direct use of energy, force, or a destructive agent

Body Part Character 4	Approach Character 5	Device Character 6	Qualifier Character 7
0 Cervical Plexus **1** Cervical Nerve **2** Phrenic Nerve **3** Brachial Plexus **4** Ulnar Nerve **5** Median Nerve **6** Radial Nerve **8** Thoracic Nerve **9** Lumbar Plexus **A** Lumbosacral Plexus **B** Lumbar Nerve **C** Pudendal Nerve **D** Femoral Nerve **F** Sciatic Nerve **G** Tibial Nerve **H** Peroneal Nerve **K** Head and Neck Sympathetic Nerve **L** Thoracic Sympathetic Nerve **M** Abdominal Sympathetic Nerve **N** Lumbar Sympathetic Nerve **P** Sacral Sympathetic Nerve **Q** Sacral Plexus **R** Sacral Nerve	**0** Open **3** Percutaneous **4** Percutaneous Endoscopic	**Z** No Device	**Z** No Qualifier

0 Medical and Surgical
1 Peripheral Nervous System
8 Division Cutting into a body part without draining fluids and/or gases from the body part in order to separate or transect a body part

Body Part Character 4	Approach Character 5	Device Character 6	Qualifier Character 7
0 Cervical Plexus **1** Cervical Nerve **2** Phrenic Nerve **3** Brachial Plexus **4** Ulnar Nerve **5** Median Nerve **6** Radial Nerve **8** Thoracic Nerve **9** Lumbar Plexus **A** Lumbosacral Plexus **B** Lumbar Nerve **C** Pudendal Nerve **D** Femoral Nerve **F** Sciatic Nerve **G** Tibial Nerve **H** Peroneal Nerve **K** Head and Neck Sympathetic Nerve **L** Thoracic Sympathetic Nerve **M** Abdominal Sympathetic Nerve **N** Lumbar Sympathetic Nerve **P** Sacral Sympathetic Nerve **Q** Sacral Plexus **R** Sacral Nerve	**0** Open **3** Percutaneous **4** Percutaneous Endoscopic	**Z** No Device	**Z** No Qualifier

Ø Medical and Surgical
1 Peripheral Nervous System
9 Drainage Taking or letting out fluids and/or gases from a body part

Body Part Character 4	Approach Character 5	Device Character 6	Qualifier Character 7
Ø Cervical Plexus **1** Cervical Nerve **2** Phrenic Nerve **3** Brachial Plexus **4** Ulnar Nerve **5** Median Nerve **6** Radial Nerve **8** Thoracic Nerve **9** Lumbar Plexus **A** Lumbosacral Plexus **B** Lumbar Nerve **C** Pudendal Nerve **D** Femoral Nerve **F** Sciatic Nerve **G** Tibial Nerve **H** Peroneal Nerve **K** Head and Neck Sympathetic Nerve **L** Thoracic Sympathetic Nerve **M** Abdominal Sympathetic Nerve **N** Lumbar Sympathetic Nerve **P** Sacral Sympathetic Nerve **Q** Sacral Plexus **R** Sacral Nerve	**Ø** Open **3** Percutaneous **4** Percutaneous Endoscopic	**Ø** Drainage Device	**Z** No Qualifier
Ø Cervical Plexus **1** Cervical Nerve **2** Phrenic Nerve **3** Brachial Plexus **4** Ulnar Nerve **5** Median Nerve **6** Radial Nerve **8** Thoracic Nerve **9** Lumbar Plexus **A** Lumbosacral Plexus **B** Lumbar Nerve **C** Pudendal Nerve **D** Femoral Nerve **F** Sciatic Nerve **G** Tibial Nerve **H** Peroneal Nerve **K** Head and Neck Sympathetic Nerve **L** Thoracic Sympathetic Nerve **M** Abdominal Sympathetic Nerve **N** Lumbar Sympathetic Nerve **P** Sacral Sympathetic Nerve **Q** Sacral Plexus **R** Sacral Nerve	**Ø** Open **3** Percutaneous **4** Percutaneous Endoscopic	**Z** No Device	**X** Diagnostic **Z** No Qualifier

0 Medical and Surgical
1 Peripheral Nervous System
B Excision Cutting out or off, without replacement, a portion of a body part

Body Part Character 4	Approach Character 5	Device Character 6	Qualifier Character 7
0 Cervical Plexus **1** Cervical Nerve **2** Phrenic Nerve **3** Brachial Plexus **4** Ulnar Nerve **5** Median Nerve **6** Radial Nerve **8** Thoracic Nerve **9** Lumbar Plexus **A** Lumbosacral Plexus **B** Lumbar Nerve **C** Pudendal Nerve **D** Femoral Nerve **F** Sciatic Nerve **G** Tibial Nerve **H** Peroneal Nerve **K** Head and Neck Sympathetic Nerve **L** Thoracic Sympathetic Nerve **M** Abdominal Sympathetic Nerve **N** Lumbar Sympathetic Nerve **P** Sacral Sympathetic Nerve **Q** Sacral Plexus **R** Sacral Nerve	**0** Open **3** Percutaneous **4** Percutaneous Endoscopic	**Z** No Device	**X** Diagnostic **Z** No Qualifier

0 Medical and Surgical
1 Peripheral Nervous System
C Extirpation Taking or cutting out solid matter from a body part

Body Part Character 4	Approach Character 5	Device Character 6	Qualifier Character 7
0 Cervical Plexus **1** Cervical Nerve **2** Phrenic Nerve **3** Brachial Plexus **4** Ulnar Nerve **5** Median Nerve **6** Radial Nerve **8** Thoracic Nerve **9** Lumbar Plexus **A** Lumbosacral Plexus **B** Lumbar Nerve **C** Pudendal Nerve **D** Femoral Nerve **F** Sciatic Nerve **G** Tibial Nerve **H** Peroneal Nerve **K** Head and Neck Sympathetic Nerve **L** Thoracic Sympathetic Nerve **M** Abdominal Sympathetic Nerve **N** Lumbar Sympathetic Nerve **P** Sacral Sympathetic Nerve **Q** Sacral Plexus **R** Sacral Nerve	**0** Open **3** Percutaneous **4** Percutaneous Endoscopic	**Z** No Device	**Z** No Qualifier

0 Medical and Surgical
1 Peripheral Nervous System
D Extraction Pulling or stripping out or off all or a portion of a body part by the use of force

Body Part Character 4	Approach Character 5	Device Character 6	Qualifier Character 7
0 Cervical Plexus **1** Cervical Nerve **2** Phrenic Nerve **3** Brachial Plexus **4** Ulnar Nerve **5** Median Nerve **6** Radial Nerve **8** Thoracic Nerve **9** Lumbar Plexus **A** Lumbosacral Plexus **B** Lumbar Nerve **C** Pudendal Nerve **D** Femoral Nerve **F** Sciatic Nerve **G** Tibial Nerve **H** Peroneal Nerve **K** Head and Neck Sympathetic Nerve **L** Thoracic Sympathetic Nerve **M** Abdominal Sympathetic Nerve **N** Lumbar Sympathetic Nerve **P** Sacral Sympathetic Nerve **Q** Sacral Plexus **R** Sacral Nerve	**0** Open **3** Percutaneous **4** Percutaneous Endoscopic	**Z** No Device	**Z** No Qualifier

0 Medical and Surgical
1 Peripheral Nervous System
H Insertion Putting in a nonbiological appliance that monitors, assists, performs, or prevents a physiological function but does not physically take the place of a body part

Body Part Character 4	Approach Character 5	Device Character 6	Qualifier Character 7
Y Peripheral Nerve	**0** Open **3** Percutaneous **4** Percutaneous Endoscopic	**2** Monitoring Device **M** Neurostimulator Lead	**Z** No Qualifier

0 Medical and Surgical
1 Peripheral Nervous System
J Inspection Visually and/or manually exploring a body part

Body Part Character 4	Approach Character 5	Device Character 6	Qualifier Character 7
Y Peripheral Nerve	**0** Open **3** Percutaneous **4** Percutaneous Endoscopic	**Z** No Device	**Z** No Qualifier

0 Medical and Surgical
1 Peripheral Nervous System
N Release Freeing a body part from an abnormal physical constraint

Body Part Character 4	Approach Character 5	Device Character 6	Qualifier Character 7
0 Cervical Plexus **1** Cervical Nerve **2** Phrenic Nerve **3** Brachial Plexus **4** Ulnar Nerve **5** Median Nerve **6** Radial Nerve **8** Thoracic Nerve **9** Lumbar Plexus **A** Lumbosacral Plexus **B** Lumbar Nerve **C** Pudendal Nerve **D** Femoral Nerve **F** Sciatic Nerve **G** Tibial Nerve **H** Peroneal Nerve **K** Head and Neck Sympathetic Nerve **L** Thoracic Sympathetic Nerve **M** Abdominal Sympathetic Nerve **N** Lumbar Sympathetic Nerve **P** Sacral Sympathetic Nerve **Q** Sacral Plexus **R** Sacral Nerve	**0** Open **3** Percutaneous **4** Percutaneous Endoscopic	**Z** No Device	**Z** No Qualifier

0 Medical and Surgical
1 Peripheral Nervous System
P Removal Taking out or off a device from a body part

Body Part Character 4	Approach Character 5	Device Character 6	Qualifier Character 7
Y Peripheral Nerve	**0** Open **3** Percutaneous **4** Percutaneous Endoscopic	**0** Drainage Device **2** Monitoring Device **7** Autologous Tissue Substitute **M** Neurostimulator Lead	**Z** No Qualifier
Y Peripheral Nerve	**X** External	**0** Drainage Device **2** Monitoring Device **M** Neurostimulator Lead	**Z** No Qualifier

0 Medical and Surgical
1 Peripheral Nervous System
Q Repair Restoring, to the extent possible, a body part to its normal anatomic structure and function

Body Part Character 4	Approach Character 5	Device Character 6	Qualifier Character 7
0 Cervical Plexus **1** Cervical Nerve **2** Phrenic Nerve **3** Brachial Plexus **4** Ulnar Nerve **5** Median Nerve **6** Radial Nerve **8** Thoracic Nerve **9** Lumbar Plexus **A** Lumbosacral Plexus **B** Lumbar Nerve **C** Pudendal Nerve **D** Femoral Nerve **F** Sciatic Nerve **G** Tibial Nerve **H** Peroneal Nerve **K** Head and Neck Sympathetic Nerve **L** Thoracic Sympathetic Nerve **M** Abdominal Sympathetic Nerve **N** Lumbar Sympathetic Nerve **P** Sacral Sympathetic Nerve **Q** Sacral Plexus **R** Sacral Nerve	**0** Open **3** Percutaneous **4** Percutaneous Endoscopic	**Z** No Device	**Z** No Qualifier

Ø Medical and Surgical
1 Peripheral Nervous System
S Reposition Moving to its normal location or other suitable location all or a portion of a body part

Body Part Character 4	Approach Character 5	Device Character 6	Qualifier Character 7
Ø Cervical Plexus **1** Cervical Nerve **2** Phrenic Nerve **3** Brachial Plexus **4** Ulnar Nerve **5** Median Nerve **6** Radial Nerve **8** Thoracic Nerve **9** Lumbar Plexus **A** Lumbosacral Plexus **B** Lumbar Nerve **C** Pudendal Nerve **D** Femoral Nerve **F** Sciatic Nerve **G** Tibial Nerve **H** Peroneal Nerve **Q** Sacral Plexus **R** Sacral Nerve	**Ø** Open **3** Percutaneous **4** Percutaneous Endoscopic	**Z** No Device	**Z** No Qualifier

Ø Medical and Surgical
1 Peripheral Nervous System
U Supplement Putting in or on biological or synthetic material that physically reinforces and/or augments the function of a portion of a body part

Body Part Character 4	Approach Character 5	Device Character 6	Qualifier Character 7
1 Cervical Nerve **2** Phrenic Nerve **4** Ulnar Nerve **5** Median Nerve **6** Radial Nerve **8** Thoracic Nerve **B** Lumbar Nerve **C** Pudendal Nerve **D** Femoral Nerve **F** Sciatic Nerve **G** Tibial Nerve **H** Peroneal Nerve **R** Sacral Nerve	**Ø** Open **3** Percutaneous **4** Percutaneous Endoscopic	**7** Autologous Tissue Substitute	**Z** No Qualifier

Ø Medical and Surgical
1 Peripheral Nervous System
W Revision Correcting, to the extent possible, a portion of a malfunctioning device or the position of a displaced device

Body Part Character 4	Approach Character 5	Device Character 6	Qualifier Character 7
Y Peripheral Nerve	**Ø** Open **3** Percutaneous **4** Percutaneous Endoscopic **X** External	**Ø** Drainage Device **2** Monitoring Device **7** Autologous Tissue Substitute **M** Neurostimulator Lead	**Z** No Qualifier

Ø Medical and Surgical
1 Peripheral Nervous System
X Transfer Moving, without taking out, all or a portion of a body part to another location to take over the function of all or a portion of a body part

Body Part Character 4	Approach Character 5	Device Character 6	Qualifier Character 7
1 Cervical Nerve **2** Phrenic Nerve	**Ø** Open **4** Percutaneous Endoscopic	**Z** No Device	**1** Cervical Nerve **2** Phrenic Nerve
4 Ulnar Nerve **5** Median Nerve **6** Radial Nerve	**Ø** Open **4** Percutaneous Endoscopic	**Z** No Device	**4** Ulnar Nerve **5** Median Nerve **6** Radial Nerve
8 Thoracic Nerve	**Ø** Open **4** Percutaneous Endoscopic	**Z** No Device	**8** Thoracic Nerve
B Lumbar Nerve **C** Pudendal Nerve	**Ø** Open **4** Percutaneous Endoscopic	**Z** No Device	**B** Lumbar Nerve **C** Perineal Nerve
D Femoral Nerve **F** Sciatic Nerve **G** Tibial Nerve **H** Peroneal Nerve	**Ø** Open **4** Percutaneous Endoscopic	**Z** No Device	**D** Femoral Nerve **F** Sciatic Nerve **G** Tibial Nerve **H** Peroneal Nerve

Heart and Great Vessels 021–02Y

0 Medical and Surgical
2 Heart and Great Vessels
1 Bypass Altering the route of passage of the contents of a tubular body part

Body Part Character 4	Approach Character 5	Device Character 6	Qualifier Character 7
0 Coronary Artery, One Site **1** Coronary Artery, Two Sites **2** Coronary Artery, Three Sites **3** Coronary Artery, Four or More Sites	**0** Open **4** Percutaneous Endoscopic	**9** Autologous Venous Tissue **A** Autologous Arterial Tissue **J** Synthetic Substitute **K** Nonautologous Tissue Substitute	**3** Coronary Artery **8** Internal Mammary, Right **9** Internal Mammary, Left **C** Thoracic Artery **F** Abdominal Artery **W** Aorta
0 Coronary Artery, One Site **1** Coronary Artery, Two Sites **2** Coronary Artery, Three Sites **3** Coronary Artery, Four or More Sites	**0** Open **4** Percutaneous Endoscopic	**Z** No Device	**3** Coronary Artery **8** Internal Mammary, Right **9** Internal Mammary, Left **C** Thoracic Artery **F** Abdominal Artery
0 Coronary Artery, One Site **1** Coronary Artery, Two Sites **2** Coronary Artery, Three Sites **3** Coronary Artery, Four or More Sites	**3** Percutaneous **4** Percutaneous Endoscopic	**4** Drug-eluting Intraluminal Device **D** Intraluminal Device	**4** Coronary Vein
6 Atrium, Right	**0** Open **4** Percutaneous Endoscopic	**Z** No Device	**7** Atrium, Left **P** Pulmonary Trunk **Q** Pulmonary Artery, Right **R** Pulmonary Artery, Left
6 Atrium, Right **K** Ventricle, Right **L** Ventricle, Left	**0** Open **4** Percutaneous Endoscopic	**9** Autologous Venous Tissue **A** Autologous Arterial Tissue **J** Synthetic Substitute **K** Nonautologous Tissue Substitute	**P** Pulmonary Trunk **Q** Pulmonary Artery, Right **R** Pulmonary Artery, Left
7 Atrium, Left **V** Superior Vena Cava	**0** Open **4** Percutaneous Endoscopic	**9** Autologous Venous Tissue **A** Autologous Arterial Tissue **J** Synthetic Substitute **K** Nonautologous Tissue Substitute **Z** No Device	**P** Pulmonary Trunk **Q** Pulmonary Artery, Right **R** Pulmonary Artery, Left
K Ventricle, Right **L** Ventricle, Left	**0** Open **4** Percutaneous Endoscopic	**Z** No Device	**5** Coronary Circulation **8** Internal Mammary, Right **9** Internal Mammary, Left **C** Thoracic Artery **F** Abdominal Artery **P** Pulmonary Trunk **Q** Pulmonary Artery, Right **R** Pulmonary Artery, Left **W** Aorta
W Thoracic Aorta	**0** Open **4** Percutaneous Endoscopic	**9** Autologous Venous Tissue **A** Autologous Arterial Tissue **J** Synthetic Substitute **K** Nonautologous Tissue Substitute **Z** No Device	**B** Subclavian **D** Carotid **P** Pulmonary Trunk **Q** Pulmonary Artery, Right **R** Pulmonary Artery, Left

Ø Medical and Surgical
2 Heart and Great Vessels
5 Destruction Physical eradication of all or a portion of a body part by the direct use of energy, force, or a destructive agent

Body Part Character 4	Approach Character 5	Device Character 6	Qualifier Character 7
4 Coronary Vein **5** Atrial Septum **6** Atrium, Right **8** Conduction Mechanism **9** Chordae Tendineae **D** Papillary Muscle **F** Aortic Valve **G** Mitral Valve **H** Pulmonary Valve **J** Tricuspid Valve **K** Ventricle, Right **L** Ventricle, Left **M** Ventricular Septum **N** Pericardium **P** Pulmonary Trunk **Q** Pulmonary Artery, Right **R** Pulmonary Artery, Left **S** Pulmonary Vein, Right **T** Pulmonary Vein, Left **V** Superior Vena Cava **W** Thoracic Aorta	**Ø** Open **3** Percutaneous **4** Percutaneous Endoscopic	**Z** No Device	**Z** No Qualifier
7 Atrium, Left	**Ø** Open **3** Percutaneous **4** Percutaneous Endoscopic	**Z** No Device	**K Left Atrial Appendage** **Z** No Qualifier

Ø Medical and Surgical
2 Heart and Great Vessels
7 Dilation Expanding an orifice or the lumen of a tubular body part

Body Part Character 4	Approach Character 5	Device Character 6	Qualifier Character 7
Ø Coronary Artery, One Site **1** Coronary Artery, Two Sites **2** Coronary Artery, Three Sites **3** Coronary Artery, Four or More Sites	**Ø** Open **3** Percutaneous **4** Percutaneous Endoscopic	**4** Intraluminal Device, Drug-eluting **D** Intraluminal Device **T** Radioactive Intraluminal Device **Z** No Device	**6** Bifurcation **Z** No Qualifier
F Aortic Valve **G** Mitral Valve **H** Pulmonary Valve **J** Tricuspid Valve **K** Ventricle, Right **P** Pulmonary Trunk **Q** Pulmonary Artery, Right **S** Pulmonary Vein, Right **T** Pulmonary Vein, Left **V** Superior Vena Cava **W** Thoracic Aorta	**Ø** Open **3** Percutaneous **4** Percutaneous Endoscopic	**4** Intraluminal Device, Drug-eluting **D** Intraluminal Device **Z** No Device	**Z** No Qualifier
R Pulmonary Artery, Left	**Ø** Open **3** Percutaneous **4** Percutaneous Endoscopic	**4** Intraluminal Device, Drug-eluting **D** Intraluminal Device **Z** No Device	**T** Ductus Arteriosus **Z** No Qualifier

Ø Medical and Surgical
2 Heart and Great Vessels
8 Division Cutting into a body part without draining fluids and/or gases from the body part in order to separate or transect a body part

Body Part Character 4	Approach Character 5	Device Character 6	Qualifier Character 7
8 Conduction Mechanism **9** Chordae Tendineae **D** Papillary Muscle	**Ø** Open **3** Percutaneous **4** Percutaneous Endoscopic	**Z** No Device	**Z** No Qualifier

0 Medical and Surgical
2 Heart and Great Vessels
B Excision Cutting out or off, without replacement, a portion of a body part

Body Part Character 4	Approach Character 5	Device Character 6	Qualifier Character 7
4 Coronary Vein 5 Atrial Septum 6 Atrium, Right 8 Conduction Mechanism 9 Chordae Tendineae D Papillary Muscle F Aortic Valve G Mitral Valve H Pulmonary Valve J Tricuspid Valve K Ventricle, Right L Ventricle, Left M Ventricular Septum N Pericardium P Pulmonary Trunk Q Pulmonary Artery, Right R Pulmonary Artery, Left S Pulmonary Vein, Right T Pulmonary Vein, Left V Superior Vena Cava W Thoracic Aorta	0 Open 3 Percutaneous 4 Percutaneous Endoscopic	Z No Device	X Diagnostic Z No Qualifier
7 Atrium, Left	0 Open 3 Percutaneous 4 Percutaneous Endoscopic	Z No Device	**K Left Atrial Appendage** X Diagnostic Z No Qualifier

0 Medical and Surgical
2 Heart and Great Vessels
C Extirpation Taking or cutting out solid matter from a body part

Body Part Character 4	Approach Character 5	Device Character 6	Qualifier Character 7
0 Coronary Artery, One Site 1 Coronary Artery, Two Sites 2 Coronary Artery, Three Sites 3 Coronary Artery, Four or More Sites 4 Coronary Vein 5 Atrial Septum 6 Atrium, Right 7 Atrium, Left 8 Conduction Mechanism 9 Chordae Tendineae D Papillary Muscle F Aortic Valve G Mitral Valve H Pulmonary Valve J Tricuspid Valve K Ventricle, Right L Ventricle, Left M Ventricular Septum N Pericardium P Pulmonary Trunk Q Pulmonary Artery, Right R Pulmonary Artery, Left S Pulmonary Vein, Right T Pulmonary Vein, Left V Superior Vena Cava W Thoracic Aorta	0 Open 3 Percutaneous 4 Percutaneous Endoscopic	Z No Device	Z No Qualifier

0 Medical and Surgical
2 Heart and Great Vessels
F Fragmentation Breaking solid matter in a body part into pieces

Body Part Character 4	Approach Character 5	Device Character 6	Qualifier Character 7
N Pericardium	0 Open 3 Percutaneous 4 Percutaneous Endoscopic X External	Z No Device	Z No Qualifier

Ø Medical and Surgical
2 Heart and Great Vessels
H Insertion Putting in a nonbiological appliance that monitors, assists, performs, or prevents a physiological function but does not physically take the place of a body part

Body Part Character 4	Approach Character 5	Device Character 6	Qualifier Character 7
4 Coronary Vein **6** Atrium, Right **7** Atrium, Left **K** Ventricle, Right **L** Ventricle, Left	**Ø** Open **3** Percutaneous **4** Percutaneous Endoscopic	**Ø Monitoring Device, Pressure Sensor** **2** Monitoring Device **3** Infusion Device **D** Intraluminal Device **J Cardiac Lead, Pacemaker** **K Cardiac Lead, Defibrillator** **M** Cardiac Lead	**Z** No Qualifier
A Heart	**Ø** Open **3** Percutaneous **4** Percutaneous Endoscopic	**Q** Implantable Heart Assist System	**Z** No Qualifier
A Heart	**Ø** Open **3** Percutaneous **4** Percutaneous Endoscopic	**R** External Heart Assist System	**S** Biventricular **Z** No Qualifier
N Pericardium	**Ø** Open **3** Percutaneous **4** Percutaneous Endoscopic	**Ø Monitoring Device, Pressure Sensor** **2** Monitoring Device **J Cardiac Lead, Pacemaker** **K Cardiac Lead, Defibrillator** **M** Cardiac Lead	**Z** No Qualifier
P Pulmonary Trunk **Q** Pulmonary Artery, Right **R** Pulmonary Artery, Left **S** Pulmonary Vein, Right **T** Pulmonary Vein, Left **V** Superior Vena Cava **W** Thoracic Aorta	**Ø** Open **3** Percutaneous **4** Percutaneous Endoscopic	**Ø Monitoring Device, Pressure Sensor** **2** Monitoring Device **3** Infusion Device **D** Intraluminal Device	**Z** No Qualifier

Ø Medical and Surgical
2 Heart and Great Vessels
J Inspection Visually and/or manually exploring a body part

Body Part Character 4	Approach Character 5	Device Character 6	Qualifier Character 7
A Heart **Y** Great Vessel	**Ø** Open **3** Percutaneous **4** Percutaneous Endoscopic	**Z** No Device	**Z** No Qualifier

Ø Medical and Surgical
2 Heart and Great Vessels
K Map Locating the route of passage of electrical impulses and/or locating functional areas in a body part

Body Part Character 4	Approach Character 5	Device Character 6	Qualifier Character 7
8 Conduction Mechanism	**Ø** Open **3** Percutaneous **4** Percutaneous Endoscopic	**Z** No Device	**Z** No Qualifier

Ø Medical and Surgical
2 Heart and Great Vessels
L Occlusion Completely closing an orifice or the lumen of a tubular body part

Body Part Character 4	Approach Character 5	Device Character 6	Qualifier Character 7
7 Atrium, Left	**Ø Open** **3 Percutaneous** **4 Percutaneous Endoscopic**	**C Extraluminal Device** **D Intraluminal Device** **Z No Device**	**K Left Atrial Appendage**
R Pulmonary Artery, Left	**Ø** Open **3** Percutaneous **4** Percutaneous Endoscopic	**C** Extraluminal Device **D** Intraluminal Device **Z** No Device	**T** Ductus Arteriosus
S Pulmonary Vein, Right **T** Pulmonary Vein, Left **V** Superior Vena Cava	**Ø** Open **3** Percutaneous **4** Percutaneous Endoscopic	**C** Extraluminal Device **D** Intraluminal Device **Z** No Device	**Z** No Qualifier

0 Medical and Surgical
2 Heart and Great Vessels
N Release Freeing a body part from an abnormal physical constraint

Body Part Character 4	Approach Character 5	Device Character 6	Qualifier Character 7
4 Coronary Vein **5** Atrial Septum **6** Atrium, Right **7** Atrium, Left **8** Conduction Mechanism **9** Chordae Tendineae **D** Papillary Muscle **F** Aortic Valve **G** Mitral Valve **H** Pulmonary Valve **J** Tricuspid Valve **K** Ventricle, Right **L** Ventricle, Left **M** Ventricular Septum **N** Pericardium **P** Pulmonary Trunk **Q** Pulmonary Artery, Right **R** Pulmonary Artery, Left **S** Pulmonary Vein, Right **T** Pulmonary Vein, Left **V** Superior Vena Cava **W** Thoracic Aorta	**0** Open **3** Percutaneous **4** Percutaneous Endoscopic	**Z** No Device	**Z** No Qualifier

0 Medical and Surgical
2 Heart and Great Vessels
P Removal Taking out or off a device from a body part

Body Part Character 4	Approach Character 5	Device Character 6	Qualifier Character 7
A Heart	**0** Open **3** Percutaneous **4** Percutaneous Endoscopic	**2** Monitoring Device **3** Infusion Device **7** Autologous Tissue Substitute **8** Zooplastic Tissue **C** Extraluminal Device **D** Intraluminal Device **J** Synthetic Substitute **K** Nonautologous Tissue Substitute **M** Cardiac Lead **Q** Implantable Heart Assist System **R** External Heart Assist System	**Z** No Qualifier
A Heart	**X** External	**2** Monitoring Device **3** Infusion Device **D** Intraluminal Device **M** Cardiac Lead	**Z** No Qualifier
Y Great Vessel	**0** Open **3** Percutaneous **4** Percutaneous Endoscopic	**2** Monitoring Device **3** Infusion Device **7** Autologous Tissue Substitute **8** Zooplastic Tissue **C** Extraluminal Device **D** Intraluminal Device **J** Synthetic Substitute **K** Nonautologous Tissue Substitute	**Z** No Qualifier
Y Great Vessel	**X** External	**2** Monitoring Device **3** Infusion Device **D** Intraluminal Device	**Z** No Qualifier

Ø Medical and Surgical
2 Heart and Great Vessels
Q Repair Restoring, to the extent possible, a body part to its normal anatomic structure and function

Body Part Character 4	Approach Character 5	Device Character 6	Qualifier Character 7
Ø Coronary Artery, One Site **1** Coronary Artery, Two Sites **2** Coronary Artery, Three Sites **3** Coronary Artery, Four or More Sites **4** Coronary Vein **5** Atrial Septum **6** Atrium, Right **7** Atrium, Left **8** Conduction Mechanism **9** Chordae Tendineae **A** Heart **B** Heart, Right **C** Heart, Left **D** Papillary Muscle **F** Aortic Valve **G** Mitral Valve **H** Pulmonary Valve **J** Tricuspid Valve **K** Ventricle, Right **L** Ventricle, Left **M** Ventricular Septum **N** Pericardium **P** Pulmonary Trunk **Q** Pulmonary Artery, Right **R** Pulmonary Artery, Left **S** Pulmonary Vein, Right **T** Pulmonary Vein, Left **V** Superior Vena Cava **W** Thoracic Aorta	**Ø** Open **3** Percutaneous **4** Percutaneous Endoscopic	**Z** No Device	**Z** No Qualifier

Ø Medical and Surgical
2 Heart and Great Vessels
R Replacement Putting in or on biological or synthetic material that physically takes the place and/or function of all or a portion of a body part

Body Part Character 4	Approach Character 5	Device Character 6	Qualifier Character 7
5 Atrial Septum **6** Atrium, Right **7** Atrium, Left **9** Chordae Tendineae **D** Papillary Muscle **J** Tricuspid Valve **K** Ventricle, Right **L** Ventricle, Left **M** Ventricular Septum **N** Pericardium **P** Pulmonary Trunk **Q** Pulmonary Artery, Right **R** Pulmonary Artery, Left **S** Pulmonary Vein, Right **T** Pulmonary Vein, Left **V** Superior Vena Cava **W** Thoracic Aorta	**Ø** Open **4** Percutaneous Endoscopic	**7** Autologous Tissue Substitute **8** Zooplastic Tissue **J** Synthetic Substitute **K** Nonautologous Tissue Substitute	**Z** No Qualifier
F Aortic Valve **G** Mitral Valve **H** Pulmonary Valve	**Ø** Open **4** Percutaneous Endoscopic	**7** Autologous Tissue Substitute **8** Zooplastic Tissue **J** Synthetic Substitute **K** Nonautologous Tissue Substitute	**Z** No Qualifier
F Aortic Valve **G** Mitral Valve **H** Pulmonary Valve	**3** Percutaneous	**7** Autologous Tissue Substitute **8** Zooplastic Tissue **J** Synthetic Substitute **K** Nonautologous Tissue Substitute	**H** **Transapical** **Z** No Qualifier

0 Medical and Surgical
2 Heart and Great Vessels
S Reposition Moving to its normal location or other suitable location all or a portion of a body part

Body Part Character 4	Approach Character 5	Device Character 6	Qualifier Character 7
P Pulmonary Trunk **Q** Pulmonary Artery, Right **R** Pulmonary Artery, Left **S** Pulmonary Vein, Right **T** Pulmonary Vein, Left **V** Superior Vena Cava **W** Thoracic Aorta	**0** Open	**Z** No Device	**Z** No Qualifier

0 Medical and Surgical
2 Heart and Great Vessels
T Resection Cutting out or off, without replacement, all of a body part

Body Part Character 4	Approach Character 5	Device Character 6	Qualifier Character 7
5 Atrial Septum **8** Conduction Mechanism **9** Chordae Tendineae **D** Papillary Muscle **H** Pulmonary Valve **M** Ventricular Septum **N** Pericardium	**0** Open **3** Percutaneous **4** Percutaneous Endoscopic	**Z** No Device	**Z** No Qualifier

0 Medical and Surgical
2 Heart and Great Vessels
U Supplement Putting in or on biological or synthetic material that physically reinforces and/or augments the function of a portion of a body part

Body Part Character 4	Approach Character 5	Device Character 6	Qualifier Character 7
5 Atrial Septum **6** Atrium, Right **7** Atrium, Left **9** Chordae Tendineae **A** Heart **D** Papillary Muscle **F** Aortic Valve **G** Mitral Valve **H** Pulmonary Valve **J** Tricuspid Valve **K** Ventricle, Right **L** Ventricle, Left **M** Ventricular Septum **N** Pericardium **P** Pulmonary Trunk **Q** Pulmonary Artery, Right **R** Pulmonary Artery, Left **S** Pulmonary Vein, Right **T** Pulmonary Vein, Left **V** Superior Vena Cava **W** Thoracic Aorta	**0** Open **3** Percutaneous **4** Percutaneous Endoscopic	**7** Autologous Tissue Substitute **8** Zooplastic Tissue **J** Synthetic Substitute **K** Nonautologous Tissue Substitute	**Z** No Qualifier

Ø Medical and Surgical
2 Heart and Great Vessels
V Restriction Partially closing an orifice or the lumen of a tubular body part

Body Part Character 4	Approach Character 5	Device Character 6	Qualifier Character 7
A Heart	**Ø** Open **3** Percutaneous **4** Percutaneous Endoscopic	**C** Extraluminal Device **Z** No Device	**Z** No Qualifier
P Pulmonary Trunk **Q** Pulmonary Artery, Right **S** Pulmonary Vein, Right **T** Pulmonary Vein, Left **V** Superior Vena Cava	**Ø** Open **3** Percutaneous **4** Percutaneous Endoscopic	**C** Extraluminal Device **D** Intraluminal Device **Z** No Device	**Z** No Qualifier
R Pulmonary Artery, Left	**Ø** Open **3** Percutaneous **4** Percutaneous Endoscopic	**C** Extraluminal Device **D** Intraluminal Device **Z** No Device	**T** Ductus Arteriosus **Z** No Qualifier
W Thoracic Aorta	**Ø** Open **3** Percutaneous **4** Percutaneous Endoscopic	**C** Extraluminal Device **Z** No Device	**Z** No Qualifier
W Thoracic Aorta	**Ø** Open **3** Percutaneous **4** Percutaneous Endoscopic	**D** Intraluminal Device	**J** **Temporary** **Z** No Qualifier

Ø Medical and Surgical
2 Heart and Great Vessels
W Revision Correcting, to the extent possible, a portion of a malfunctioning device or the position of a displaced device

Body Part Character 4	Approach Character 5	Device Character 6	Qualifier Character 7
5 Atrial Septum **M** Ventricular Septum	**Ø** Open **4** Percutaneous Endoscopic	**J** Synthetic Substitute	**Z** No Qualifier
A Heart	**Ø** Open **3** Percutaneous **4** Percutaneous Endoscopic **X** External	**2** Monitoring Device **3** Infusion Device **7** Autologous Tissue Substitute **8** Zooplastic Tissue **C** Extraluminal Device **D** Intraluminal Device **J** Synthetic Substitute **K** Nonautologous Tissue Substitute **M** Cardiac Lead **Q** Implantable Heart Assist System **R** External Heart Assist System	**Z** No Qualifier
F Aortic Valve **G** Mitral Valve **H** Pulmonary Valve **J** Tricuspid Valve	**Ø** Open **4** Percutaneous Endoscopic	**7** Autologous Tissue Substitute **8** Zooplastic Tissue **J** Synthetic Substitute **K** Nonautologous Tissue Substitute	**Z** No Qualifier
Y Great Vessel	**Ø** Open **3** Percutaneous **4** Percutaneous Endoscopic **X** External	**2** Monitoring Device **3** Infusion Device **7** Autologous Tissue Substitute **8** Zooplastic Tissue **C** Extraluminal Device **D** Intraluminal Device **J** Synthetic Substitute **K** Nonautologous Tissue Substitute	**Z** No Qualifier

Ø Medical and Surgical
2 Heart and Great Vessels
Y Transplantation Putting in or on all or a portion of a living body part taken from another individual or animal to physically take the place and/or function of all or a portion of a similar body part

Body Part Character 4	Approach Character 5	Device Character 6	Qualifier Character 7
A Heart	**Ø** Open	**Z** No Device	**Ø** Allogeneic **1** Syngeneic **2** Zooplastic

Upper Arteries 031–03W

0 Medical and Surgical
3 Upper Arteries
1 Bypass Altering the route of passage of the contents of a tubular body part

Body Part Character 4	Approach Character 5	Device Character 6	Qualifier Character 7
2 Innominate Artery **5** Axillary Artery, Right **6** Axillary Artery, Left	**0** Open	**9** Autologous Venous Tissue **A** Autologous Arterial Tissue **J** Synthetic Substitute **K** Nonautologous Tissue Substitute **Z** No Device	**0** Upper Arm Artery, Right **1** Upper Arm Artery, Left **2** Upper Arm Artery, Bilateral **3** Lower Arm Artery, Right **4** Lower Arm Artery, Left **5** Lower Arm Artery, Bilateral **6** Upper Leg Artery, Right **7** Upper Leg Artery, Left **8** Upper Leg Artery, Bilateral **9** Lower Leg Artery, Right **B** Lower Leg Artery, Left **C** Lower Leg Artery, Bilateral **D** Upper Arm Vein **F** Lower Arm Vein **J** Extracranial Artery, Right **K** Extracranial Artery, Left
3 Subclavian Artery, Right **4** Subclavian Artery, Left	**0** Open	**9** Autologous Venous Tissue **A** Autologous Arterial Tissue **J** Synthetic Substitute **K** Nonautologous Tissue Substitute **Z** No Device	**0** Upper Arm Artery, Right **1** Upper Arm Artery, Left **2** Upper Arm Artery, Bilateral **3** Lower Arm Artery, Right **4** Lower Arm Artery, Left **5** Lower Arm Artery, Bilateral **6** Upper Leg Artery, Right **7** Upper Leg Artery, Left **8** Upper Leg Artery, Bilateral **9** Lower Leg Artery, Right **B** Lower Leg Artery, Left **C** Lower Leg Artery, Bilateral **D** Upper Arm Vein **F** Lower Arm Vein **J** Extracranial Artery, Right **K** Extracranial Artery, Left **M** Pulmonary Artery, Right **N** Pulmonary Artery, Left
7 Brachial Artery, Right	**0** Open	**9** Autologous Venous Tissue **A** Autologous Arterial Tissue **J** Synthetic Substitute **K** Nonautologous Tissue Substitute **Z** No Device	**0** Upper Arm Artery, Right **3** Lower Arm Artery, Right **D** Upper Arm Vein **F** Lower Arm Vein
8 Brachial Artery, Left	**0** Open	**9** Autologous Venous Tissue **A** Autologous Arterial Tissue **J** Synthetic Substitute **K** Nonautologous Tissue Substitute **Z** No Device	**1** Upper Arm Artery, Left **4** Lower Arm Artery, Left **D** Upper Arm Vein **F** Lower Arm Vein
9 Ulnar Artery, Right **B** Radial Artery, Right	**0** Open	**9** Autologous Venous Tissue **A** Autologous Arterial Tissue **J** Synthetic Substitute **K** Nonautologous Tissue Substitute **Z** No Device	**3** Lower Arm Artery, Right **F** Lower Arm Vein
A Ulnar Artery, Left **C** Radial Artery, Left	**0** Open	**9** Autologous Venous Tissue **A** Autologous Arterial Tissue **J** Synthetic Substitute **K** Nonautologous Tissue Substitute **Z** No Device	**4** Lower Arm Artery, Left **F** Lower Arm Vein
G Intracranial Artery **S** Temporal Artery, Right **T** Temporal Artery, Left	**0** Open	**9** Autologous Venous Tissue **A** Autologous Arterial Tissue **J** Synthetic Substitute **K** Nonautologous Tissue Substitute **Z** No Device	**G** Intracranial Artery
H Common Carotid Artery, Right	**0** Open	**9** Autologous Venous Tissue **A** Autologous Arterial Tissue **J** Synthetic Substitute **K** Nonautologous Tissue Substitute **Z** No Device	**G Intracranial Artery** **J** Extracranial Artery, Right

031 Continued on next page

Ø31 Continued

Ø Medical and Surgical
3 Upper Arteries
1 Bypass Altering the route of passage of the contents of a tubular body part

Body Part Character 4	Approach Character 5	Device Character 6	Qualifier Character 7
J Common Carotid Artery, Left	**Ø** Open	**9** Autologous Venous Tissue **A** Autologous Arterial Tissue **J** Synthetic Substitute **K** Nonautologous Tissue Substitute **Z** No Device	**G** **Intracranial Artery** **J** Extracranial Artery, Left
K Internal Carotid Artery, Right **M** External Carotid Artery, Right	**Ø** Open	**9** Autologous Venous Tissue **A** Autologous Arterial Tissue **J** Synthetic Substitute **K** Nonautologous Tissue Substitute **Z** No Device	**J** Extracranial Artery, Right
L Internal Carotid Artery, Left **N** External Carotid Artery, Left	**Ø** Open	**9** Autologous Venous Tissue **A** Autologous Arterial Tissue **J** Synthetic Substitute **K** Nonautologous Tissue Substitute **Z** No Device	**K** Extracranial Artery, Left

Ø Medical and Surgical
3 Upper Arteries
5 Destruction Physical eradication of all or a portion of a body part by the direct use of energy, force, or a destructive agent

Body Part Character 4	Approach Character 5	Device Character 6	Qualifier Character 7
Ø Internal Mammary Artery, Right **1** Internal Mammary Artery, Left **2** Innominate Artery **3** Subclavian Artery, Right **4** Subclavian Artery, Left **5** Axillary Artery, Right **6** Axillary Artery, Left **7** Brachial Artery, Right **8** Brachial Artery, Left **9** Ulnar Artery, Right **A** Ulnar Artery, Left **B** Radial Artery, Right **C** Radial Artery, Left **D** Hand Artery, Right **F** Hand Artery, Left **G** Intracranial Artery **H** Common Carotid Artery, Right **J** Common Carotid Artery, Left **K** Internal Carotid Artery, Right **L** Internal Carotid Artery, Left **M** External Carotid Artery, Right **N** External Carotid Artery, Left **P** Vertebral Artery, Right **Q** Vertebral Artery, Left **R** Face Artery **S** Temporal Artery, Right **T** Temporal Artery, Left **U** Thyroid Artery, Right **V** Thyroid Artery, Left **Y** Upper Artery	**Ø** Open **3** Percutaneous **4** Percutaneous Endoscopic	**Z** No Device	**Z** No Qualifier

0 Medical and Surgical
3 Upper Arteries
7 Dilation Expanding an orifice or the lumen of a tubular body part

Body Part Character 4	Approach Character 5	Device Character 6	Qualifier Character 7
0 Internal Mammary Artery, Right **1** Internal Mammary Artery, Left **2** Innominate Artery **3** Subclavian Artery, Right **4** Subclavian Artery, Left **5** Axillary Artery, Right **6** Axillary Artery, Left **7** Brachial Artery, Right **8** Brachial Artery, Left **9** Ulnar Artery, Right **A** Ulnar Artery, Left **B** Radial Artery, Right **C** Radial Artery, Left **D** Hand Artery, Right **F** Hand Artery, Left **G** Intracranial Artery **H** Common Carotid Artery, Right **J** Common Carotid Artery, Left **K** Internal Carotid Artery, Right **L** Internal Carotid Artery, Left **M** External Carotid Artery, Right **N** External Carotid Artery, Left **P** Vertebral Artery, Right **Q** Vertebral Artery, Left **R** Face Artery **S** Temporal Artery, Right **T** Temporal Artery, Left **U** Thyroid Artery, Right **V** Thyroid Artery, Left **Y** Upper Artery	**0** Open **3** Percutaneous **4** Percutaneous Endoscopic	**4** Drug-eluting Intraluminal Device **D** Intraluminal Device **Z** No Device	**Z** No Qualifier

0 Medical and Surgical
3 Upper Arteries
9 Drainage Taking or letting out fluids and/or gases from a body part

Body Part Character 4	Approach Character 5	Device Character 6	Qualifier Character 7
0 Internal Mammary Artery, Right **1** Internal Mammary Artery, Left **2** Innominate Artery **3** Subclavian Artery, Right **4** Subclavian Artery, Left **5** Axillary Artery, Right **6** Axillary Artery, Left **7** Brachial Artery, Right **8** Brachial Artery, Left **9** Ulnar Artery, Right **A** Ulnar Artery, Left **B** Radial Artery, Right **C** Radial Artery, Left **D** Hand Artery, Right **F** Hand Artery, Left **G** Intracranial Artery **H** Common Carotid Artery, Right **J** Common Carotid Artery, Left **K** Internal Carotid Artery, Right **L** Internal Carotid Artery, Left **M** External Carotid Artery, Right **N** External Carotid Artery, Left **P** Vertebral Artery, Right **Q** Vertebral Artery, Left **R** Face Artery **S** Temporal Artery, Right **T** Temporal Artery, Left **U** Thyroid Artery, Right **V** Thyroid Artery, Left **Y** Upper Artery	**0** Open **3** Percutaneous **4** Percutaneous Endoscopic	**0** Drainage Device	**Z** No Qualifier

039 Continued on next page

039 Continued

0 Medical and Surgical
3 Upper Arteries
9 Drainage Taking or letting out fluids and/or gases from a body part

Body Part Character 4	Approach Character 5	Device Character 6	Qualifier Character 7
0 Internal Mammary Artery, Right **1** Internal Mammary Artery, Left **2** Innominate Artery **3** Subclavian Artery, Right **4** Subclavian Artery, Left **5** Axillary Artery, Right **6** Axillary Artery, Left **7** Brachial Artery, Right **8** Brachial Artery, Left **9** Ulnar Artery, Right **A** Ulnar Artery, Left **B** Radial Artery, Right **C** Radial Artery, Left **D** Hand Artery, Right **F** Hand Artery, Left **G** Intracranial Artery **H** Common Carotid Artery, Right **J** Common Carotid Artery, Left **K** Internal Carotid Artery, Right **L** Internal Carotid Artery, Left **M** External Carotid Artery, Right **N** External Carotid Artery, Left **P** Vertebral Artery, Right **Q** Vertebral Artery, Left **R** Face Artery **S** Temporal Artery, Right **T** Temporal Artery, Left **U** Thyroid Artery, Right **V** Thyroid Artery, Left **Y** Upper Artery	**0** Open **3** Percutaneous **4** Percutaneous Endoscopic	**Z** No Device	**X** Diagnostic **Z** No Qualifier

0 Medical and Surgical
3 Upper Arteries
B Excision Cutting out or off, without replacement, a portion of a body part

Body Part Character 4	Approach Character 5	Device Character 6	Qualifier Character 7
0 Internal Mammary Artery, Right **1** Internal Mammary Artery, Left **2** Innominate Artery **3** Subclavian Artery, Right **4** Subclavian Artery, Left **5** Axillary Artery, Right **6** Axillary Artery, Left **7** Brachial Artery, Right **8** Brachial Artery, Left **9** Ulnar Artery, Right **A** Ulnar Artery, Left **B** Radial Artery, Right **C** Radial Artery, Left **D** Hand Artery, Right **F** Hand Artery, Left **G** Intracranial Artery **H** Common Carotid Artery, Right **J** Common Carotid Artery, Left **K** Internal Carotid Artery, Right **L** Internal Carotid Artery, Left **M** External Carotid Artery, Right **N** External Carotid Artery, Left **P** Vertebral Artery, Right **Q** Vertebral Artery, Left **R** Face Artery **S** Temporal Artery, Right **T** Temporal Artery, Left **U** Thyroid Artery, Right **V** Thyroid Artery, Left **Y** Upper Artery	**0** Open **3** Percutaneous **4** Percutaneous Endoscopic	**Z** No Device	**X** Diagnostic **Z** No Qualifier

0 Medical and Surgical
3 Upper Arteries
C Extirpation Taking or cutting out solid matter from a body part

Body Part Character 4	Approach Character 5	Device Character 6	Qualifier Character 7
0 Internal Mammary Artery, Right 1 Internal Mammary Artery, Left 2 Innominate Artery 3 Subclavian Artery, Right 4 Subclavian Artery, Left 5 Axillary Artery, Right 6 Axillary Artery, Left 7 Brachial Artery, Right 8 Brachial Artery, Left 9 Ulnar Artery, Right A Ulnar Artery, Left B Radial Artery, Right C Radial Artery, Left D Hand Artery, Right F Hand Artery, Left G Intracranial Artery H Common Carotid Artery, Right J Common Carotid Artery, Left K Internal Carotid Artery, Right L Internal Carotid Artery, Left M External Carotid Artery, Right N External Carotid Artery, Left P Vertebral Artery, Right Q Vertebral Artery, Left R Face Artery S Temporal Artery, Right T Temporal Artery, Left U Thyroid Artery, Right V Thyroid Artery, Left Y Upper Artery	0 Open 3 Percutaneous 4 Percutaneous Endoscopic	Z No Device	Z No Qualifier

0 Medical and Surgical
3 Upper Arteries
H Insertion Putting in a nonbiological appliance that monitors, assists, performs, or prevents a physiological function but does not physically take the place of a body part

Body Part Character 4	Approach Character 5	Device Character 6	Qualifier Character 7
0 Internal Mammary Artery, Right 1 Internal Mammary Artery, Left 2 Innominate Artery 3 Subclavian Artery, Right 4 Subclavian Artery, Left 5 Axillary Artery, Right 6 Axillary Artery, Left 7 Brachial Artery, Right 8 Brachial Artery, Left 9 Ulnar Artery, Right A Ulnar Artery, Left B Radial Artery, Right C Radial Artery, Left D Hand Artery, Right F Hand Artery, Left G Intracranial Artery H Common Carotid Artery, Right J Common Carotid Artery, Left M External Carotid Artery, Right N External Carotid Artery, Left P Vertebral Artery, Right Q Vertebral Artery, Left R Face Artery S Temporal Artery, Right T Temporal Artery, Left U Thyroid Artery, Right V Thyroid Artery, Left	0 Open 3 Percutaneous 4 Percutaneous Endoscopic	3 Infusion Device D Intraluminal Device	Z No Qualifier
K Internal Carotid Artery, Right L Internal Carotid Artery, Left	0 Open 3 Percutaneous 4 Percutaneous Endoscope	3 Infusion Device D Intraluminal Device M Stimulator Lead	Z No Qualifier
Y Upper Artery	0 Open 3 Percutaneous 4 Percutaneous Endoscopic	2 Monitoring Device 3 Infusion Device D Intraluminal Device	Z No Qualifier

Ø Medical and Surgical
3 Upper Arteries
J Inspection Visually and/or manually exploring a body part

Body Part Character 4	Approach Character 5	Device Character 6	Qualifier Character 7
Y Upper Artery	**Ø** Open **3** Percutaneous **4** Percutaneous Endoscopic **X** External	**Z** No Device	**Z** No Qualifier

Ø Medical and Surgical
3 Upper Arteries
L Occlusion Completely closing an orifice or the lumen of a tubular body part

Body Part Character 4	Approach Character 5	Device Character 6	Qualifier Character 7
Ø Internal Mammary Artery, Right **1** Internal Mammary Artery, Left **2** Innominate Artery **3** Subclavian Artery, Right **4** Subclavian Artery, Left **5** Axillary Artery, Right **6** Axillary Artery, Left **7** Brachial Artery, Right **8** Brachial Artery, Left **9** Ulnar Artery, Right **A** Ulnar Artery, Left **B** Radial Artery, Right **C** Radial Artery, Left **D** Hand Artery, Right **F** Hand Artery, Left **R** Face Artery **S** Temporal Artery, Right **T** Temporal Artery, Left **U** Thyroid Artery, Right **V** Thyroid Artery, Left **Y** Upper Artery	**Ø** Open **3** Percutaneous **4** Percutaneous Endoscopic	**C** Extraluminal Device **D** Intraluminal Device **Z** No Device	**Z** No Qualifier
G Intracranial Artery **H** Common Carotid Artery, Right **J** Common Carotid Artery, Left **K** Internal Carotid Artery, Right **L** Internal Carotid Artery, Left **M** External Carotid Artery, Right **N** External Carotid Artery, Left **P** Vertebral Artery, Right **Q** Vertebral Artery, Left	**Ø** Open **3** Percutaneous **4** Percutaneous Endoscopic	**B** Bioactive Intraluminal Device **C** Extraluminal Device **D** Intraluminal Device **Z** No Device	**Z** No Qualifier

0 Medical and Surgical
3 Upper Arteries
N Release Freeing a body part from an abnormal physical constraint

Body Part Character 4	Approach Character 5	Device Character 6	Qualifier Character 7
0 Internal Mammary Artery, Right **1** Internal Mammary Artery, Left **2** Innominate Artery **3** Subclavian Artery, Right **4** Subclavian Artery, Left **5** Axillary Artery, Right **6** Axillary Artery, Left **7** Brachial Artery, Right **8** Brachial Artery, Left **9** Ulnar Artery, Right **A** Ulnar Artery, Left **B** Radial Artery, Right **C** Radial Artery, Left **D** Hand Artery, Right **F** Hand Artery, Left **G** Intracranial Artery **H** Common Carotid Artery, Right **J** Common Carotid Artery, Left **K** Internal Carotid Artery, Right **L** Internal Carotid Artery, Left **M** External Carotid Artery, Right **N** External Carotid Artery, Left **P** Vertebral Artery, Right **Q** Vertebral Artery, Left **R** Face Artery **S** Temporal Artery, Right **T** Temporal Artery, Left **U** Thyroid Artery, Right **V** Thyroid Artery, Left **Y** Upper Artery	**0** Open **3** Percutaneous **4** Percutaneous Endoscopic	**Z** No Device	**Z** No Qualifier

0 Medical and Surgical
3 Upper Arteries
P Removal Taking out or off a device from a body part

Body Part Character 4	Approach Character 5	Device Character 6	Qualifier Character 7
Y Upper Artery	**0** Open **3** Percutaneous **4** Percutaneous Endoscopic	**0** Drainage Device **2** Monitoring Device **3** Infusion Device **7** Autologous Tissue Substitute **C** Extraluminal Device **D** Intraluminal Device **J** Synthetic Substitute **K** Nonautologous Tissue Substitute **M** Stimulator Lead	**Z** No Qualifier
Y Upper Artery	**X** External	**0** Drainage Device **2** Monitoring Device **3** Infusion Device **D** Intraluminal Device **M** Stimulator Lead	**Z** No Qualifier

Ø Medical and Surgical
3 Upper Arteries
Q Repair Restoring, to the extent possible, a body part to its normal anatomic structure and function

Body Part Character 4	Approach Character 5	Device Character 6	Qualifier Character 7
Ø Internal Mammary Artery, Right **1** Internal Mammary Artery, Left **2** Innominate Artery **3** Subclavian Artery, Right **4** Subclavian Artery, Left **5** Axillary Artery, Right **6** Axillary Artery, Left **7** Brachial Artery, Right **8** Brachial Artery, Left **9** Ulnar Artery, Right **A** Ulnar Artery, Left **B** Radial Artery, Right **C** Radial Artery, Left **D** Hand Artery, Right **F** Hand Artery, Left **G** Intracranial Artery **H** Common Carotid Artery, Right **J** Common Carotid Artery, Left **K** Internal Carotid Artery, Right **L** Internal Carotid Artery, Left **M** External Carotid Artery, Right **N** External Carotid Artery, Left **P** Vertebral Artery, Right **Q** Vertebral Artery, Left **R** Face Artery **S** Temporal Artery, Right **T** Temporal Artery, Left **U** Thyroid Artery, Right **V** Thyroid Artery, Left **Y** Upper Artery	**Ø** Open **3** Percutaneous **4** Percutaneous Endoscopic	**Z** No Device	**Z** No Qualifier

Ø Medical and Surgical
3 Upper Arteries
R Replacement Putting in or on biological or synthetic material that physically takes the place and/or function of all or a portion of a body part

Body Part Character 4	Approach Character 5	Device Character 6	Qualifier Character 7
Ø Internal Mammary Artery, Right **1** Internal Mammary Artery, Left **2** Innominate Artery **3** Subclavian Artery, Right **4** Subclavian Artery, Left **5** Axillary Artery, Right **6** Axillary Artery, Left **7** Brachial Artery, Right **8** Brachial Artery, Left **9** Ulnar Artery, Right **A** Ulnar Artery, Left **B** Radial Artery, Right **C** Radial Artery, Left **D** Hand Artery, Right **F** Hand Artery, Left **G** Intracranial Artery **H** Common Carotid Artery, Right **J** Common Carotid Artery, Left **K** Internal Carotid Artery, Right **L** Internal Carotid Artery, Left **M** External Carotid Artery, Right **N** External Carotid Artery, Left **P** Vertebral Artery, Right **Q** Vertebral Artery, Left **R** Face Artery **S** Temporal Artery, Right **T** Temporal Artery, Left **U** Thyroid Artery, Right **V** Thyroid Artery, Left **Y** Upper Artery	**Ø** Open **4** Percutaneous Endoscopic	**7** Autologous Tissue Substitute **J** Synthetic Substitute **K** Nonautologous Tissue Substitute	**Z** No Qualifier

0 Medical and Surgical
3 Upper Arteries
S Reposition Moving to its normal location or other suitable location all or a portion of a body part

Body Part Character 4	Approach Character 5	Device Character 6	Qualifier Character 7
0 Internal Mammary Artery, Right 1 Internal Mammary Artery, Left 2 Innominate Artery 3 Subclavian Artery, Right 4 Subclavian Artery, Left 5 Axillary Artery, Right 6 Axillary Artery, Left 7 Brachial Artery, Right 8 Brachial Artery, Left 9 Ulnar Artery, Right A Ulnar Artery, Left B Radial Artery, Right C Radial Artery, Left D Hand Artery, Right F Hand Artery, Left G Intracranial Artery H Common Carotid Artery, Right J Common Carotid Artery, Left K Internal Carotid Artery, Right L Internal Carotid Artery, Left M External Carotid Artery, Right N External Carotid Artery, Left P Vertebral Artery, Right Q Vertebral Artery, Left R Face Artery S Temporal Artery, Right T Temporal Artery, Left U Thyroid Artery, Right V Thyroid Artery, Left Y Upper Artery	0 Open 3 Percutaneous 4 Percutaneous Endoscopic	Z No Device	Z No Qualifier

0 Medical and Surgical
3 Upper Arteries
U Supplement Putting in or on biological or synthetic material that physically reinforces and/or augments the function of a portion of a body part

Body Part Character 4	Approach Character 5	Device Character 6	Qualifier Character 7
0 Internal Mammary Artery, Right 1 Internal Mammary Artery, Left 2 Innominate Artery 3 Subclavian Artery, Right 4 Subclavian Artery, Left 5 Axillary Artery, Right 6 Axillary Artery, Left 7 Brachial Artery, Right 8 Brachial Artery, Left 9 Ulnar Artery, Right A Ulnar Artery, Left B Radial Artery, Right C Radial Artery, Left D Hand Artery, Right F Hand Artery, Left G Intracranial Artery H Common Carotid Artery, Right J Common Carotid Artery, Left K Internal Carotid Artery, Right L Internal Carotid Artery, Left M External Carotid Artery, Right N External Carotid Artery, Left P Vertebral Artery, Right Q Vertebral Artery, Left R Face Artery S Temporal Artery, Right T Temporal Artery, Left U Thyroid Artery, Right V Thyroid Artery, Left Y Upper Artery	0 Open 3 Percutaneous 4 Percutaneous Endoscopic	7 Autologous Tissue Substitute J Synthetic Substitute K Nonautologous Tissue Substitute	Z No Qualifier

Ø Medical and Surgical
3 Upper Arteries
V Restriction Partially closing an orifice or the lumen of a tubular body part

Body Part Character 4	Approach Character 5	Device Character 6	Qualifier Character 7
Ø Internal Mammary Artery, Right **1** Internal Mammary Artery, Left **2** Innominate Artery **3** Subclavian Artery, Right **4** Subclavian Artery, Left **5** Axillary Artery, Right **6** Axillary Artery, Left **7** Brachial Artery, Right **8** Brachial Artery, Left **9** Ulnar Artery, Right **A** Ulnar Artery, Left **B** Radial Artery, Right **C** Radial Artery, Left **D** Hand Artery, Right **F** Hand Artery, Left **R** Face Artery **S** Temporal Artery, Right **T** Temporal Artery, Left **U** Thyroid Artery, Right **V** Thyroid Artery, Left **Y** Upper Artery	**Ø** Open **3** Percutaneous **4** Percutaneous Endoscopic	**C** Extraluminal Device **D** Intraluminal Device **Z** No Device	**Z** No Qualifier
G Intracranial Artery **H** Common Carotid Artery, Right **J** Common Carotid Artery, Left **K** Internal Carotid Artery, Right **L** Internal Carotid Artery, Left **M** External Carotid Artery, Right **N** External Carotid Artery, Left **P** Vertebral Artery, Right **Q** Vertebral Artery, Left	**Ø** Open **3** Percutaneous **4** Percutaneous Endoscopic	**B** Bioactive Intraluminal Device **C** Extraluminal Device **D** Intraluminal Device **Z** No Device	**Z** No Qualifier

Ø Medical and Surgical
3 Upper Arteries
W Revision Correcting, to the extent possible, a portion of a malfunctioning device or the position of a displaced device

Body Part Character 4	Approach Character 5	Device Character 6	Qualifier Character 7
Y Upper Artery	**Ø** Open **3** Percutaneous **4** Percutaneous Endoscopic **X** External	**Ø** Drainage Device **2** Monitoring Device **3** Infusion Device **7** Autologous Tissue Substitute **C** Extraluminal Device **D** Intraluminal Device **J** Synthetic Substitute **K** Nonautologous Tissue Substitute **M** Stimulator Lead	**Z** No Qualifier

Lower Arteries Ø41–Ø4W

Ø Medical and Surgical
4 Lower Arteries
1 Bypass Altering the route of passage of the contents of a tubular body part

Body Part Character 4	Approach Character 5	Device Character 6	Qualifier Character 7
Ø Abdominal Aorta **C** Common Iliac Artery, Right **D** Common Iliac Artery, Left	**Ø** Open **4** Percutaneous Endoscopic	**9** Autologous Venous Tissue **A** Autologous Arterial Tissue **J** Synthetic Substitute **K** Nonautologous Tissue Substitute **Z** No Device	**Ø** Abdominal Aorta **1** Celiac Artery **2** Mesenteric Artery **3** Renal Artery, Right **4** Renal Artery, Left **5** Renal Artery, Bilateral **6** Common Iliac Artery, Right **7** Common Iliac Artery, Left **8** Common Iliac Arteries, Bilateral **9** Internal Iliac Artery, Right **B** Internal Iliac Artery, Left **C** Internal Iliac Arteries, Bilateral **D** External Iliac Artery, Right **F** External Iliac Artery, Left **G** External Iliac Arteries, Bilateral **H** Femoral Artery, Right **J** Femoral Artery, Left **K** Femoral Arteries, Bilateral **Q** Lower Extremity Artery **R** Lower Artery
4 Splenic Artery	**Ø** Open **4** Percutaneous Endoscopic	**9** Autologous Venous Tissue **A** Autologous Arterial Tissue **J** Synthetic Substitute **K** Nonautologous Tissue Substitute **Z** No Device	**3** Renal Artery, Right **4** Renal Artery, Left **5** Renal Artery, Bilateral
E Internal Iliac Artery, Right **F** Internal Iliac Artery, Left **H** External Iliac Artery, Right **J** External Iliac Artery, Left	**Ø** Open **4** Percutaneous Endoscopic	**9** Autologous Venous Tissue **A** Autologous Arterial Tissue **J** Synthetic Substitute **K** Nonautologous Tissue Substitute **Z** No Device	**9** Internal Iliac Artery, Right **B** Internal Iliac Artery, Left **C** Internal Iliac Arteries, Bilateral **D** External Iliac Artery, Right **F** External Iliac Artery, Left **G** External Iliac Arteries, Bilateral **H** Femoral Artery, Right **J** Femoral Artery, Left **K** Femoral Arteries, Bilateral **P** Foot Artery **Q** Lower Extremity Artery
K Femoral Artery, Right **L** Femoral Artery, Left	**Ø** Open **4** Percutaneous Endoscopic	**9** Autologous Venous Tissue **A** Autologous Arterial Tissue **J** Synthetic Substitute **K** Nonautologous Tissue Substitute **Z** No Device	**H** Femoral Artery, Right **J** Femoral Artery, Left **K** Femoral Arteries, Bilateral **L** Popliteal Artery **M** Peroneal Artery **N** Posterior Tibial Artery **P** Foot Artery **Q** Lower Extremity Artery **S** Lower Extremity Vein
M Popliteal Artery, Right **N** Popliteal Artery, Left	**Ø** Open **4** Percutaneous Endoscopic	**9** Autologous Venous Tissue **A** Autologous Arterial Tissue **J** Synthetic Substitute **K** Nonautologous Tissue Substitute **Z** No Device	**L** Popliteal Artery **M** Peroneal Artery **P** Foot Artery **Q** Lower Extremity Artery **S** Lower Extremity Vein

Ø Medical and Surgical
4 Lower Arteries
5 Destruction Physical eradication of all or a portion of a body part by the direct use of energy, force, or a destructive agent

Body Part Character 4	Approach Character 5	Device Character 6	Qualifier Character 7
Ø Abdominal Aorta **1** Celiac Artery **2** Gastric Artery **3** Hepatic Artery **4** Splenic Artery **5** Superior Mesenteric Artery **6** Colic Artery, Right **7** Colic Artery, Left **8** Colic Artery, Middle **9** Renal Artery, Right **A** Renal Artery, Left **B** Inferior Mesenteric Artery **C** Common Iliac Artery, Right **D** Common Iliac Artery, Left **E** Internal Iliac Artery, Right **F** Internal Iliac Artery, Left **H** External Iliac Artery, Right **J** External Iliac Artery, Left **K** Femoral Artery, Right **L** Femoral Artery, Left **M** Popliteal Artery, Right **N** Popliteal Artery, Left **P** Anterior Tibial Artery, Right **Q** Anterior Tibial Artery, Left **R** Posterior Tibial Artery, Right **S** Posterior Tibial Artery, Left **T** Peroneal Artery, Right **U** Peroneal Artery, Left **V** Foot Artery, Right **W** Foot Artery, Left **Y** Lower Artery	**Ø** Open **3** Percutaneous **4** Percutaneous Endoscopic	**Z** No Device	**Z** No Qualifier

Ø Medical and Surgical
4 Lower Arteries
7 Dilation Expanding an orifice or the lumen of a tubular body part

Body Part Character 4	Approach Character 5	Device Character 6	Qualifier Character 7
Ø Abdominal Aorta **1** Celiac Artery **2** Gastric Artery **3** Hepatic Artery **4** Splenic Artery **5** Superior Mesenteric Artery **6** Colic Artery, Right **7** Colic Artery, Left **8** Colic Artery, Middle **9** Renal Artery, Right **A** Renal Artery, Left **B** Inferior Mesenteric Artery **C** Common Iliac Artery, Right **D** Common Iliac Artery, Left **E** Internal Iliac Artery, Right **F** Internal Iliac Artery, Left **H** External Iliac Artery, Right **J** External Iliac Artery, Left **K** Femoral Artery, Right **L** Femoral Artery, Left **M** Popliteal Artery, Right **N** Popliteal Artery, Left **P** Anterior Tibial Artery, Right **Q** Anterior Tibial Artery, Left **R** Posterior Tibial Artery, Right **S** Posterior Tibial Artery, Left **T** Peroneal Artery, Right **U** Peroneal Artery, Left **V** Foot Artery, Right **W** Foot Artery, Left **Y** Lower Artery	**Ø** Open **3** Percutaneous **4** Percutaneous Endoscopic	**4** Drug-eluting Intraluminal Device **D** Intraluminal Device **Z** No Device	**Z** No Qualifier

0 Medical and Surgical
4 Lower Arteries
9 Drainage Taking or letting out fluids and/or gases from a body part

Body Part Character 4	Approach Character 5	Device Character 6	Qualifier Character 7
0 Abdominal Aorta **1** Celiac Artery **2** Gastric Artery **3** Hepatic Artery **4** Splenic Artery **5** Superior Mesenteric Artery **6** Colic Artery, Right **7** Colic Artery, Left **8** Colic Artery, Middle **9** Renal Artery, Right **A** Renal Artery, Left **B** Inferior Mesenteric Artery **C** Common Iliac Artery, Right **D** Common Iliac Artery, Left **E** Internal Iliac Artery, Right **F** Internal Iliac Artery, Left **H** External Iliac Artery, Right **J** External Iliac Artery, Left **K** Femoral Artery, Right **L** Femoral Artery, Left **M** Popliteal Artery, Right **N** Popliteal Artery, Left **P** Anterior Tibial Artery, Right **Q** Anterior Tibial Artery, Left **R** Posterior Tibial Artery, Right **S** Posterior Tibial Artery, Left **T** Peroneal Artery, Right **U** Peroneal Artery, Left **V** Foot Artery, Right **W** Foot Artery, Left **Y** Lower Artery	**0** Open **3** Percutaneous **4** Percutaneous Endoscopic	**0** Drainage Device	**Z** No Qualifier
0 Abdominal Aorta **1** Celiac Artery **2** Gastric Artery **3** Hepatic Artery **4** Splenic Artery **5** Superior Mesenteric Artery **6** Colic Artery, Right **7** Colic Artery, Left **8** Colic Artery, Middle **9** Renal Artery, Right **A** Renal Artery, Left **B** Inferior Mesenteric Artery **C** Common Iliac Artery, Right **D** Common Iliac Artery, Left **E** Internal Iliac Artery, Right **F** Internal Iliac Artery, Left **H** External Iliac Artery, Right **J** External Iliac Artery, Left **K** Femoral Artery, Right **L** Femoral Artery, Left **M** Popliteal Artery, Right **N** Popliteal Artery, Left **P** Anterior Tibial Artery, Right **Q** Anterior Tibial Artery, Left **R** Posterior Tibial Artery, Right **S** Posterior Tibial Artery, Left **T** Peroneal Artery, Right **U** Peroneal Artery, Left **V** Foot Artery, Right **W** Foot Artery, Left **Y** Lower Artery	**0** Open **3** Percutaneous **4** Percutaneous Endoscopic	**Z** No Device	**X** Diagnostic **Z** No Qualifier

Ø Medical and Surgical
4 Lower Arteries
B Excision Cutting out or off, without replacement, a portion of a body part

Body Part Character 4	Approach Character 5	Device Character 6	Qualifier Character 7
Ø Abdominal Aorta **1** Celiac Artery **2** Gastric Artery **3** Hepatic Artery **4** Splenic Artery **5** Superior Mesenteric Artery **6** Colic Artery, Right **7** Colic Artery, Left **8** Colic Artery, Middle **9** Renal Artery, Right **A** Renal Artery, Left **B** Inferior Mesenteric Artery **C** Common Iliac Artery, Right **D** Common Iliac Artery, Left **E** Internal Iliac Artery, Right **F** Internal Iliac Artery, Left **H** External Iliac Artery, Right **J** External Iliac Artery, Left **K** Femoral Artery, Right **L** Femoral Artery, Left **M** Popliteal Artery, Right **N** Popliteal Artery, Left **P** Anterior Tibial Artery, Right **Q** Anterior Tibial Artery, Left **R** Posterior Tibial Artery, Right **S** Posterior Tibial Artery, Left **T** Peroneal Artery, Right **U** Peroneal Artery, Left **V** Foot Artery, Right **W** Foot Artery, Left **Y** Lower Artery	**Ø** Open **3** Percutaneous **4** Percutaneous Endoscopic	**Z** No Device	**X** Diagnostic **Z** No Qualifier

Ø Medical and Surgical
4 Lower Arteries
C Extirpation Taking or cutting out solid matter from a body part

Body Part Character 4	Approach Character 5	Device Character 6	Qualifier Character 7
Ø Abdominal Aorta **1** Celiac Artery **2** Gastric Artery **3** Hepatic Artery **4** Splenic Artery **5** Superior Mesenteric Artery **6** Colic Artery, Right **7** Colic Artery, Left **8** Colic Artery, Middle **9** Renal Artery, Right **A** Renal Artery, Left **B** Inferior Mesenteric Artery **C** Common Iliac Artery, Right **D** Common Iliac Artery, Left **E** Internal Iliac Artery, Right **F** Internal Iliac Artery, Left **H** External Iliac Artery, Right **J** External Iliac Artery, Left **K** Femoral Artery, Right **L** Femoral Artery, Left **M** Popliteal Artery, Right **N** Popliteal Artery, Left **P** Anterior Tibial Artery, Right **Q** Anterior Tibial Artery, Left **R** Posterior Tibial Artery, Right **S** Posterior Tibial Artery, Left **T** Peroneal Artery, Right **U** Peroneal Artery, Left **V** Foot Artery, Right **W** Foot Artery, Left **Y** Lower Artery	**Ø** Open **3** Percutaneous **4** Percutaneous Endoscopic	**Z** No Device	**Z** No Qualifier

0 Medical and Surgical
4 Lower Arteries
H Insertion Putting in a nonbiological appliance that monitors, assists, performs, or prevents a physiological function but does not physically take the place of a body part

Body Part Character 4	Approach Character 5	Device Character 6	Qualifier Character 7
0 Abdominal Aorta Y Lower Artery	0 Open 3 Percutaneous 4 Percutaneous Endoscopic	2 Monitoring Device 3 Infusion Device D Intraluminal Device	Z No Qualifier
1 Celiac Artery 2 Gastric Artery 3 Hepatic Artery 4 Splenic Artery 5 Superior Mesenteric Artery 6 Colic Artery, Right 7 Colic Artery, Left 8 Colic Artery, Middle 9 Renal Artery, Right A Renal Artery, Left B Inferior Mesenteric Artery C Common Iliac Artery, Right D Common Iliac Artery, Left E Internal Iliac Artery, Right F Internal Iliac Artery, Left H External Iliac Artery, Right J External Iliac Artery, Left K Femoral Artery, Right L Femoral Artery, Left M Popliteal Artery, Right N Popliteal Artery, Left P Anterior Tibial Artery, Right Q Anterior Tibial Artery, Left R Posterior Tibial Artery, Right S Posterior Tibial Artery, Left T Peroneal Artery, Right U Peroneal Artery, Left V Foot Artery, Right W Foot Artery, Left	0 Open 3 Percutaneous 4 Percutaneous Endoscopic	3 Infusion Device **D Intraluminal Device**	Z No Qualifier

0 Medical and Surgical
4 Lower Arteries
J Inspection Visually and/or manually exploring a body part

Body Part Character 4	Approach Character 5	Device Character 6	Qualifier Character 7
Y Lower Artery	0 Open 3 Percutaneous 4 Percutaneous Endoscopic X External	Z No Device	Z No Qualifier

Ø Medical and Surgical
4 Lower Arteries
L Occlusion Completely closing an orifice or the lumen of a tubular body part

Body Part Character 4	Approach Character 5	Device Character 6	Qualifier Character 7
Ø Abdominal Aorta **1** Celiac Artery **2** Gastric Artery **3** Hepatic Artery **4** Splenic Artery **5** Superior Mesenteric Artery **6** Colic Artery, Right **7** Colic Artery, Left **8** Colic Artery, Middle **9** Renal Artery, Right **A** Renal Artery, Left **B** Inferior Mesenteric Artery **C** Common Iliac Artery, Right **D** Common Iliac Artery, Left **H** External Iliac Artery, Right **J** External Iliac Artery, Left **K** Femoral Artery, Right **L** Femoral Artery, Left **M** Popliteal Artery, Right **N** Popliteal Artery, Left **P** Anterior Tibial Artery, Right **Q** Anterior Tibial Artery, Left **R** Posterior Tibial Artery, Right **S** Posterior Tibial Artery, Left **T** Peroneal Artery, Right **U** Peroneal Artery, Left **V** Foot Artery, Right **W** Foot Artery, Left **Y** Lower Artery	**Ø** Open **3** Percutaneous **4** Percutaneous Endoscopic	**C** Extraluminal Device **D** Intraluminal Device **Z** No Device	**Z** No Qualifier
E Internal Iliac Artery, Right	**Ø** Open **3** Percutaneous **4** Percutaneous Endoscopic	**C** Extraluminal Device **D** Intraluminal Device **Z** No Device	**T Uterine Artery, Right** **Z** No Qualifier
F Internal Iliac Artery, Left	**Ø** Open **3** Percutaneous **4** Percutaneous Endoscopic	**C** Extraluminal Device **D** Intraluminal Device **Z** No Device	**U Uterine Artery, Left** **Z** No Qualifier

Ø Medical and Surgical
4 Lower Arteries
N Release Freeing a body part from an abnormal physical constraint

Body Part Character 4	Approach Character 5	Device Character 6	Qualifier Character 7
Ø Abdominal Aorta **1** Celiac Artery **2** Gastric Artery **3** Hepatic Artery **4** Splenic Artery **5** Superior Mesenteric Artery **6** Colic Artery, Right **7** Colic Artery, Left **8** Colic Artery, Middle **9** Renal Artery, Right **A** Renal Artery, Left **B** Inferior Mesenteric Artery **C** Common Iliac Artery, Right **D** Common Iliac Artery, Left **E** Internal Iliac Artery, Right **F** Internal Iliac Artery, Left **H** External Iliac Artery, Right **J** External Iliac Artery, Left **K** Femoral Artery, Right **L** Femoral Artery, Left **M** Popliteal Artery, Right **N** Popliteal Artery, Left **P** Anterior Tibial Artery, Right **Q** Anterior Tibial Artery, Left **R** Posterior Tibial Artery, Right **S** Posterior Tibial Artery, Left **T** Peroneal Artery, Right **U** Peroneal Artery, Left **V** Foot Artery, Right **W** Foot Artery, Left **Y** Lower Artery	**Ø** Open **3** Percutaneous **4** Percutaneous Endoscopic	**Z** No Device	**Z** No Qualifier

0 Medical and Surgical
4 Lower Arteries
P Removal Taking out or off a device from a body part

Body Part Character 4	Approach Character 5	Device Character 6	Qualifier Character 7
Y Lower Artery	**0** Open **3** Percutaneous **4** Percutaneous Endoscopic	**0** Drainage Device **2** Monitoring Device **3** Infusion Device **7** Autologous Tissue Substitute **C** Extraluminal Device **D** Intraluminal Device **J** Synthetic Substitute **K** Nonautologous Tissue Substitute	**Z** No Qualifier
Y Lower Artery	**X** External	**0** Drainage Device **1** Radioactive Element **2** Monitoring Device **3** Infusion Device **D** Intraluminal Device	**Z** No Qualifier

0 Medical and Surgical
4 Lower Arteries
Q Repair Restoring, to the extent possible, a body part to its normal anatomic structure and function

Body Part Character 4	Approach Character 5	Device Character 6	Qualifier Character 7
0 Abdominal Aorta **1** Celiac Artery **2** Gastric Artery **3** Hepatic Artery **4** Splenic Artery **5** Superior Mesenteric Artery **6** Colic Artery, Right **7** Colic Artery, Left **8** Colic Artery, Middle **9** Renal Artery, Right **A** Renal Artery, Left **B** Inferior Mesenteric Artery **C** Common Iliac Artery, Right **D** Common Iliac Artery, Left **E** Internal Iliac Artery, Right **F** Internal Iliac Artery, Left **H** External Iliac Artery, Right **J** External Iliac Artery, Left **K** Femoral Artery, Right **L** Femoral Artery, Left **M** Popliteal Artery, Right **N** Popliteal Artery, Left **P** Anterior Tibial Artery, Right **Q** Anterior Tibial Artery, Left **R** Posterior Tibial Artery, Right **S** Posterior Tibial Artery, Left **T** Peroneal Artery, Right **U** Peroneal Artery, Left **V** Foot Artery, Right **W** Foot Artery, Left **Y** Lower Artery	**0** Open **3** Percutaneous **4** Percutaneous Endoscopic	**Z** No Device	**Z** No Qualifier

Ø Medical and Surgical
4 Lower Arteries
R Replacement Putting in or on biological or synthetic material that physically takes the place and/or function of all or a portion of a body part

Body Part Character 4	Approach Character 5	Device Character 6	Qualifier Character 7
Ø Abdominal Aorta **1** Celiac Artery **2** Gastric Artery **3** Hepatic Artery **4** Splenic Artery **5** Superior Mesenteric Artery **6** Colic Artery, Right **7** Colic Artery, Left **8** Colic Artery, Middle **9** Renal Artery, Right **A** Renal Artery, Left **B** Inferior Mesenteric Artery **C** Common Iliac Artery, Right **D** Common Iliac Artery, Left **E** Internal Iliac Artery, Right **F** Internal Iliac Artery, Left **H** External Iliac Artery, Right **J** External Iliac Artery, Left **K** Femoral Artery, Right **L** Femoral Artery, Left **M** Popliteal Artery, Right **N** Popliteal Artery, Left **P** Anterior Tibial Artery, Right **Q** Anterior Tibial Artery, Left **R** Posterior Tibial Artery, Right **S** Posterior Tibial Artery, Left **T** Peroneal Artery, Right **U** Peroneal Artery, Left **V** Foot Artery, Right **W** Foot Artery, Left **Y** Lower Artery	**Ø** Open **4** Percutaneous Endoscopic	**7** Autologous Tissue Substitute **J** Synthetic Substitute **K** Nonautologous Tissue Substitute	**Z** No Qualifier

Ø Medical and Surgical
4 Lower Arteries
S Reposition Moving to its normal location or other suitable location all or a portion of a body part

Body Part Character 4	Approach Character 5	Device Character 6	Qualifier Character 7
Ø Abdominal Aorta **1** Celiac Artery **2** Gastric Artery **3** Hepatic Artery **4** Splenic Artery **5** Superior Mesenteric Artery **6** Colic Artery, Right **7** Colic Artery, Left **8** Colic Artery, Middle **9** Renal Artery, Right **A** Renal Artery, Left **B** Inferior Mesenteric Artery **C** Common Iliac Artery, Right **D** Common Iliac Artery, Left **E** Internal Iliac Artery, Right **F** Internal Iliac Artery, Left **H** External Iliac Artery, Right **J** External Iliac Artery, Left **K** Femoral Artery, Right **L** Femoral Artery, Left **M** Popliteal Artery, Right **N** Popliteal Artery, Left **P** Anterior Tibial Artery, Right **Q** Anterior Tibial Artery, Left **R** Posterior Tibial Artery, Right **S** Posterior Tibial Artery, Left **T** Peroneal Artery, Right **U** Peroneal Artery, Left **V** Foot Artery, Right **W** Foot Artery, Left **Y** Lower Artery	**Ø** Open **3** Percutaneous **4** Percutaneous Endoscopic	**Z** No Device	**Z** No Qualifier

0 Medical and Surgical
4 Lower Arteries
U Supplement Putting in or on biological or synthetic material that physically reinforces and/or augments the function of a portion of a body part

Body Part Character 4	Approach Character 5	Device Character 6	Qualifier Character 7
0 Abdominal Aorta 1 Celiac Artery 2 Gastric Artery 3 Hepatic Artery 4 Splenic Artery 5 Superior Mesenteric Artery 6 Colic Artery, Right 7 Colic Artery, Left 8 Colic Artery, Middle 9 Renal Artery, Right A Renal Artery, Left B Inferior Mesenteric Artery C Common Iliac Artery, Right D Common Iliac Artery, Left E Internal Iliac Artery, Right F Internal Iliac Artery, Left H External Iliac Artery, Right J External Iliac Artery, Left K Femoral Artery, Right L Femoral Artery, Left M Popliteal Artery, Right N Popliteal Artery, Left P Anterior Tibial Artery, Right Q Anterior Tibial Artery, Left R Posterior Tibial Artery, Right S Posterior Tibial Artery, Left T Peroneal Artery, Right U Peroneal Artery, Left V Foot Artery, Right W Foot Artery, Left Y Lower Artery	0 Open 3 Percutaneous 4 Percutaneous Endoscopic	7 Autologous Tissue Substitute J Synthetic Substitute K Nonautologous Tissue Substitute	Z No Qualifier

0 Medical and Surgical
4 Lower Arteries
V Restriction Partially closing an orifice or the lumen of a tubular body part

Body Part Character 4	Approach Character 5	Device Character 6	Qualifier Character 7
0 Abdominal Aorta 1 Celiac Artery 2 Gastric Artery 3 Hepatic Artery 4 Splenic Artery 5 Superior Mesenteric Artery 6 Colic Artery, Right 7 Colic Artery, Left 8 Colic Artery, Middle 9 Renal Artery, Right A Renal Artery, Left B Inferior Mesenteric Artery C Common Iliac Artery, Right D Common Iliac Artery, Left E Internal Iliac Artery, Right F Internal Iliac Artery, Left H External Iliac Artery, Right J External Iliac Artery, Left K Femoral Artery, Right L Femoral Artery, Left M Popliteal Artery, Right N Popliteal Artery, Left P Anterior Tibial Artery, Right Q Anterior Tibial Artery, Left R Posterior Tibial Artery, Right S Posterior Tibial Artery, Left T Peroneal Artery, Right U Peroneal Artery, Left V Foot Artery, Right W Foot Artery, Left Y Lower Artery	0 Open 3 Percutaneous 4 Percutaneous Endoscopic	C Extraluminal Device D Intraluminal Device Z No Device	Z No Qualifier

Ø Medical and Surgical
4 Lower Arteries
W Revision Correcting, to the extent possible, a portion of a malfunctioning device or the position of a displaced device

Body Part Character 4	Approach Character 5	Device Character 6	Qualifier Character 7
Y Lower Artery	**Ø** Open **3** Percutaneous **4** Percutaneous Endoscopic **X** External	**Ø** Drainage Device **2** Monitoring Device **3** Infusion Device **7** Autologous Tissue Substitute **C** Extraluminal Device **D** Intraluminal Device **J** Synthetic Substitute **K** Nonautologous Tissue Substitute	**Z** No Qualifier

Upper Veins 051–05W

0 Medical and Surgical
5 Upper Veins
1 Bypass Altering the route of passage of the contents of a tubular body part

Body Part Character 4	Approach Character 5	Device Character 6	Qualifier Character 7
0 Azygos Vein 1 Hemiazygos Vein 3 Innominate Vein, Right 4 Innominate Vein, Left 5 Subclavian Vein, Right 6 Subclavian Vein, Left 7 Axillary Vein, Right 8 Axillary Vein, Left 9 Brachial Vein, Right A Brachial Vein, Left B Basilic Vein, Right C Basilic Vein, Left D Cephalic Vein, Right F Cephalic Vein, Left G Hand Vein, Right H Hand Vein, Left L Intracranial Vein M Internal Jugular Vein, Right N Internal Jugular Vein, Left P External Jugular Vein, Right Q External Jugular Vein, Left R Vertebral Vein, Right S Vertebral Vein, Left T Face Vein, Right V Face Vein, Left	0 Open 4 Percutaneous Endoscopic	7 Autologous Tissue Substitute 9 Autologous Venous Tissue A Autologous Arterial Tissue J Synthetic Substitute K Nonautologous Tissue Substitute Z No Device	Y Upper Vein

0 Medical and Surgical
5 Upper Veins
5 Destruction Physical eradication of all or a portion of a body part by the direct use of energy, force, or a destructive agent

Body Part Character 4	Approach Character 5	Device Character 6	Qualifier Character 7
0 Azygos Vein 1 Hemiazygos Vein 3 Innominate Vein, Right 4 Innominate Vein, Left 5 Subclavian Vein, Right 6 Subclavian Vein, Left 7 Axillary Vein, Right 8 Axillary Vein, Left 9 Brachial Vein, Right A Brachial Vein, Left B Basilic Vein, Right C Basilic Vein, Left D Cephalic Vein, Right F Cephalic Vein, Left G Hand Vein, Right H Hand Vein, Left L Intracranial Vein M Internal Jugular Vein, Right N Internal Jugular Vein, Left P External Jugular Vein, Right Q External Jugular Vein, Left R Vertebral Vein, Right S Vertebral Vein, Left T Face Vein, Right V Face Vein, Left Y Upper Vein	0 Open 3 Percutaneous 4 Percutaneous Endoscopic	Z No Device	Z No Qualifier

Ø Medical and Surgical
5 Upper Veins
7 Dilation Expanding an orifice or the lumen of a tubular body part

Body Part Character 4	Approach Character 5	Device Character 6	Qualifier Character 7
Ø Azygos Vein **1** Hemiazygos Vein **3** Innominate Vein, Right **4** Innominate Vein, Left **5** Subclavian Vein, Right **6** Subclavian Vein, Left **7** Axillary Vein, Right **8** Axillary Vein, Left **9** Brachial Vein, Right **A** Brachial Vein, Left **B** Basilic Vein, Right **C** Basilic Vein, Left **D** Cephalic Vein, Right **F** Cephalic Vein, Left **G** Hand Vein, Right **H** Hand Vein, Left **L** Intracranial Vein **M** Internal Jugular Vein, Right **N** Internal Jugular Vein, Left **P** External Jugular Vein, Right **Q** External Jugular Vein, Left **R** Vertebral Vein, Right **S** Vertebral Vein, Left **T** Face Vein, Right **V** Face Vein, Left **Y** Upper Vein	**Ø** Open **3** Percutaneous **4** Percutaneous Endoscopic	**D** Intraluminal Device **Z** No Device	**Z** No Qualifier

Ø Medical and Surgical
5 Upper Veins
9 Drainage Taking or letting out fluids and/or gases from a body part

Body Part Character 4	Approach Character 5	Device Character 6	Qualifier Character 7
Ø Azygos Vein **1** Hemiazygos Vein **3** Innominate Vein, Right **4** Innominate Vein, Left **5** Subclavian Vein, Right **6** Subclavian Vein, Left **7** Axillary Vein, Right **8** Axillary Vein, Left **9** Brachial Vein, Right **A** Brachial Vein, Left **B** Basilic Vein, Right **C** Basilic Vein, Left **D** Cephalic Vein, Right **F** Cephalic Vein, Left **G** Hand Vein, Right **H** Hand Vein, Left **L** Intracranial Vein **M** Internal Jugular Vein, Right **N** Internal Jugular Vein, Left **P** External Jugular Vein, Right **Q** External Jugular Vein, Left **R** Vertebral Vein, Right **S** Vertebral Vein, Left **T** Face Vein, Right **V** Face Vein, Left **Y** Upper Vein	**Ø** Open **3** Percutaneous **4** Percutaneous Endoscopic	**Ø** Drainage Device	**Z** No Qualifier

Ø59 Continued on next page

0 Medical and Surgical
5 Upper Veins
9 Drainage Taking or letting out fluids and/or gases from a body part

059 Continued

Body Part Character 4	Approach Character 5	Device Character 6	Qualifier Character 7
0 Azygos Vein **1** Hemiazygos Vein **3** Innominate Vein, Right **4** Innominate Vein, Left **5** Subclavian Vein, Right **6** Subclavian Vein, Left **7** Axillary Vein, Right **8** Axillary Vein, Left **9** Brachial Vein, Right **A** Brachial Vein, Left **B** Basilic Vein, Right **C** Basilic Vein, Left **D** Cephalic Vein, Right **F** Cephalic Vein, Left **G** Hand Vein, Right **H** Hand Vein, Left **L** Intracranial Vein **M** Internal Jugular Vein, Right **N** Internal Jugular Vein, Left **P** External Jugular Vein, Right **Q** External Jugular Vein, Left **R** Vertebral Vein, Right **S** Vertebral Vein, Left **T** Face Vein, Right **V** Face Vein, Left **Y** Upper Vein	**0** Open **3** Percutaneous **4** Percutaneous Endoscopic	**Z** No Device	**X** Diagnostic **Z** No Qualifier

0 Medical and Surgical
5 Upper Veins
B Excision Cutting out or off, without replacement, a portion of a body part

Body Part Character 4	Approach Character 5	Device Character 6	Qualifier Character 7
0 Azygos Vein **1** Hemiazygos Vein **3** Innominate Vein, Right **4** Innominate Vein, Left **5** Subclavian Vein, Right **6** Subclavian Vein, Left **7** Axillary Vein, Right **8** Axillary Vein, Left **9** Brachial Vein, Right **A** Brachial Vein, Left **B** Basilic Vein, Right **C** Basilic Vein, Left **D** Cephalic Vein, Right **F** Cephalic Vein, Left **G** Hand Vein, Right **H** Hand Vein, Left **L** Intracranial Vein **M** Internal Jugular Vein, Right **N** Internal Jugular Vein, Left **P** External Jugular Vein, Right **Q** External Jugular Vein, Left **R** Vertebral Vein, Right **S** Vertebral Vein, Left **T** Face Vein, Right **V** Face Vein, Left **Y** Upper Vein	**0** Open **3** Percutaneous **4** Percutaneous Endoscopic	**Z** No Device	**X** Diagnostic **Z** No Qualifier

Ø Medical and Surgical
5 Upper Veins
C Extirpation Taking or cutting out solid matter from a body part

Body Part Character 4	Approach Character 5	Device Character 6	Qualifier Character 7
Ø Azygos Vein **1** Hemiazygos Vein **3** Innominate Vein, Right **4** Innominate Vein, Left **5** Subclavian Vein, Right **6** Subclavian Vein, Left **7** Axillary Vein, Right **8** Axillary Vein, Left **9** Brachial Vein, Right **A** Brachial Vein, Left **B** Basilic Vein, Right **C** Basilic Vein, Left **D** Cephalic Vein, Right **F** Cephalic Vein, Left **G** Hand Vein, Right **H** Hand Vein, Left **L** Intracranial Vein **M** Internal Jugular Vein, Right **N** Internal Jugular Vein, Left **P** External Jugular Vein, Right **Q** External Jugular Vein, Left **R** Vertebral Vein, Right **S** Vertebral Vein, Left **T** Face Vein, Right **V** Face Vein, Left **Y** Upper Vein	**Ø** Open **3** Percutaneous **4** Percutaneous Endoscopic	**Z** No Device	**Z** No Qualifier

Ø Medical and Surgical
5 Upper Veins
D Extraction Pulling or stripping out or off all or a portion of a body part by the use of force

Body Part Character 4	Approach Character 5	Device Character 6	Qualifier Character 7
9 Brachial Vein, Right **A** Brachial Vein, Left **B** Basilic Vein, Right **C** Basilic Vein, Left **D** Cephalic Vein, Right **F** Cephalic Vein, Left **G** Hand Vein, Right **H** Hand Vein, Left **Y** Upper Vein	**Ø** Open **3** Percutaneous	**Z** No Device	**Z** No Qualifier

0 Medical and Surgical
5 Upper Veins
H Insertion Putting in a nonbiological appliance that monitors, assists, performs, or prevents a physiological function but does not physically take the place of a body part

Body Part Character 4	Approach Character 5	Device Character 6	Qualifier Character 7
0 Azygos Vein **1** Hemiazygos Vein **3** Innominate Vein, Right **4** Innominate Vein, Left **5** Subclavian Vein, Right **6** Subclavian Vein, Left **7** Axillary Vein, Right **8** Axillary Vein, Left **9** Brachial Vein, Right **A** Brachial Vein, Left **B** Basilic Vein, Right **C** Basilic Vein, Left **D** Cephalic Vein, Right **F** Cephalic Vein, Left **G** Hand Vein, Right **H** Hand Vein, Left **L** Intracranial Vein **M** Internal Jugular Vein, Right **N** Internal Jugular Vein, Left **P** External Jugular Vein, Right **Q** External Jugular Vein, Left **R** Vertebral Vein, Right **S** Vertebral Vein, Left **T** Face Vein, Right **V** Face Vein, Left	**0** Open **3** Percutaneous **4** Percutaneous Endoscopic	**3** Infusion Device **D** Intraluminal Device	**Z** No Qualifier
Y Upper Vein	**0** Open **3** Percutaneous **4** Percutaneous Endoscopic	**2** Monitoring Device **3** Infusion Device **D** Intraluminal Device	**Z** No Qualifier

0 Medical and Surgical
5 Upper Veins
J Inspection Visually and/or manually exploring a body part

Body Part Character 4	Approach Character 5	Device Character 6	Qualifier Character 7
Y Upper Vein	**0** Open **3** Percutaneous **4** Percutaneous Endoscopic **X** External	**Z** No Device	**Z** No Qualifier

0 Medical and Surgical
5 Upper Veins
L Occlusion Completely closing an orifice or the lumen of a tubular body part

Body Part Character 4	Approach Character 5	Device Character 6	Qualifier Character 7
0 Azygos Vein **1** Hemiazygos Vein **3** Innominate Vein, Right **4** Innominate Vein, Left **5** Subclavian Vein, Right **6** Subclavian Vein, Left **7** Axillary Vein, Right **8** Axillary Vein, Left **9** Brachial Vein, Right **A** Brachial Vein, Left **B** Basilic Vein, Right **C** Basilic Vein, Left **D** Cephalic Vein, Right **F** Cephalic Vein, Left **G** Hand Vein, Right **H** Hand Vein, Left **L** Intracranial Vein **M** Internal Jugular Vein, Right **N** Internal Jugular Vein, Left **P** External Jugular Vein, Right **Q** External Jugular Vein, Left **R** Vertebral Vein, Right **S** Vertebral Vein, Left **T** Face Vein, Right **V** Face Vein, Left **Y** Upper Vein	**0** Open **3** Percutaneous **4** Percutaneous Endoscopic	**C** Extraluminal Device **D** Intraluminal Device **Z** No Device	**Z** No Qualifier

Ø Medical and Surgical
5 Upper Veins
N Release Freeing a body part from an abnormal physical constraint

Body Part Character 4	Approach Character 5	Device Character 6	Qualifier Character 7
Ø Azygos Vein **1** Hemiazygos Vein **3** Innominate Vein, Right **4** Innominate Vein, Left **5** Subclavian Vein, Right **6** Subclavian Vein, Left **7** Axillary Vein, Right **8** Axillary Vein, Left **9** Brachial Vein, Right **A** Brachial Vein, Left **B** Basilic Vein, Right **C** Basilic Vein, Left **D** Cephalic Vein, Right **F** Cephalic Vein, Left **G** Hand Vein, Right **H** Hand Vein, Left **L** Intracranial Vein **M** Internal Jugular Vein, Right **N** Internal Jugular Vein, Left **P** External Jugular Vein, Right **Q** External Jugular Vein, Left **R** Vertebral Vein, Right **S** Vertebral Vein, Left **T** Face Vein, Right **V** Face Vein, Left **Y** Upper Vein	**Ø** Open **3** Percutaneous **4** Percutaneous Endoscopic	**Z** No Device	**Z** No Qualifier

Ø Medical and Surgical
5 Upper Veins
P Removal Taking out or off a device from a body part

Body Part Character 4	Approach Character 5	Device Character 6	Qualifier Character 7
Y Upper Vein	**Ø** Open **3** Percutaneous **4** Percutaneous Endoscopic	**Ø** Drainage Device **2** Monitoring Device **3** Infusion Device **7** Autologous Tissue Substitute **C** Extraluminal Device **D** Intraluminal Device **J** Synthetic Substitute **K** Nonautologous Tissue Substitute	**Z** No Qualifier
Y Upper Vein	**X** External	**Ø** Drainage Device **2** Monitoring Device **3** Infusion Device **D** Intraluminal Device	**Z** No Qualifier

0 Medical and Surgical
5 Upper Veins
Q Repair Restoring, to the extent possible, a body part to its normal anatomic structure and function

Body Part Character 4	Approach Character 5	Device Character 6	Qualifier Character 7
0 Azygos Vein 1 Hemiazygos Vein 3 Innominate Vein, Right 4 Innominate Vein, Left 5 Subclavian Vein, Right 6 Subclavian Vein, Left 7 Axillary Vein, Right 8 Axillary Vein, Left 9 Brachial Vein, Right A Brachial Vein, Left B Basilic Vein, Right C Basilic Vein, Left D Cephalic Vein, Right F Cephalic Vein, Left G Hand Vein, Right H Hand Vein, Left L Intracranial Vein M Internal Jugular Vein, Right N Internal Jugular Vein, Left P External Jugular Vein, Right Q External Jugular Vein, Left R Vertebral Vein, Right S Vertebral Vein, Left T Face Vein, Right V Face Vein, Left Y Upper Vein	0 Open 3 Percutaneous 4 Percutaneous Endoscopic	Z No Device	Z No Qualifier

0 Medical and Surgical
5 Upper Veins
R Replacement Putting in or on biological or synthetic material that physically takes the place and/or function of all or a portion of a body part

Body Part Character 4	Approach Character 5	Device Character 6	Qualifier Character 7
0 Azygos Vein 1 Hemiazygos Vein 3 Innominate Vein, Right 4 Innominate Vein, Left 5 Subclavian Vein, Right 6 Subclavian Vein, Left 7 Axillary Vein, Right 8 Axillary Vein, Left 9 Brachial Vein, Right A Brachial Vein, Left B Basilic Vein, Right C Basilic Vein, Left D Cephalic Vein, Right F Cephalic Vein, Left G Hand Vein, Right H Hand Vein, Left L Intracranial Vein M Internal Jugular Vein, Right N Internal Jugular Vein, Left P External Jugular Vein, Right Q External Jugular Vein, Left R Vertebral Vein, Right S Vertebral Vein, Left T Face Vein, Right V Face Vein, Left Y Upper Vein	0 Open 4 Percutaneous Endoscopic	7 Autologous Tissue Substitute J Synthetic Substitute K Nonautologous Tissue Substitute	Z No Qualifier

Ø Medical and Surgical
5 Upper Veins
S Reposition Moving to its normal location or other suitable location all or a portion of a body part

Body Part Character 4	Approach Character 5	Device Character 6	Qualifier Character 7
Ø Azygos Vein **1** Hemiazygos Vein **3** Innominate Vein, Right **4** Innominate Vein, Left **5** Subclavian Vein, Right **6** Subclavian Vein, Left **7** Axillary Vein, Right **8** Axillary Vein, Left **9** Brachial Vein, Right **A** Brachial Vein, Left **B** Basilic Vein, Right **C** Basilic Vein, Left **D** Cephalic Vein, Right **F** Cephalic Vein, Left **G** Hand Vein, Right **H** Hand Vein, Left **L** Intracranial Vein **M** Internal Jugular Vein, Right **N** Internal Jugular Vein, Left **P** External Jugular Vein, Right **Q** External Jugular Vein, Left **R** Vertebral Vein, Right **S** Vertebral Vein, Left **T** Face Vein, Right **V** Face Vein, Left **Y** Upper Vein	**Ø** Open **3** Percutaneous **4** Percutaneous Endoscopic	**Z** No Device	**Z** No Qualifier

Ø Medical and Surgical
5 Upper Veins
U Supplement Putting in or on biological or synthetic material that physically reinforces and/or augments the function of a portion of a body part

Body Part Character 4	Approach Character 5	Device Character 6	Qualifier Character 7
Ø Azygos Vein **1** Hemiazygos Vein **3** Innominate Vein, Right **4** Innominate Vein, Left **5** Subclavian Vein, Right **6** Subclavian Vein, Left **7** Axillary Vein, Right **8** Axillary Vein, Left **9** Brachial Vein, Right **A** Brachial Vein, Left **B** Basilic Vein, Right **C** Basilic Vein, Left **D** Cephalic Vein, Right **F** Cephalic Vein, Left **G** Hand Vein, Right **H** Hand Vein, Left **L** Intracranial Vein **M** Internal Jugular Vein, Right **N** Internal Jugular Vein, Left **P** External Jugular Vein, Right **Q** External Jugular Vein, Left **R** Vertebral Vein, Right **S** Vertebral Vein, Left **T** Face Vein, Right **V** Face Vein, Left **Y** Upper Vein	**Ø** Open **3** Percutaneous **4** Percutaneous Endoscopic	**7** Autologous Tissue Substitute **J** Synthetic Substitute **K** Nonautologous Tissue Substitute	**Z** No Qualifier

0 Medical and Surgical
5 Upper Veins
V Restriction Partially closing an orifice or the lumen of a tubular body part

Body Part Character 4	Approach Character 5	Device Character 6	Qualifier Character 7
0 Azygos Vein **1** Hemiazygos Vein **3** Innominate Vein, Right **4** Innominate Vein, Left **5** Subclavian Vein, Right **6** Subclavian Vein, Left **7** Axillary Vein, Right **8** Axillary Vein, Left **9** Brachial Vein, Right **A** Brachial Vein, Left **B** Basilic Vein, Right **C** Basilic Vein, Left **D** Cephalic Vein, Right **F** Cephalic Vein, Left **G** Hand Vein, Right **H** Hand Vein, Left **L** Intracranial Vein **M** Internal Jugular Vein, Right **N** Internal Jugular Vein, Left **P** External Jugular Vein, Right **Q** External Jugular Vein, Left **R** Vertebral Vein, Right **S** Vertebral Vein, Left **T** Face Vein, Right **V** Face Vein, Left **Y** Upper Vein	**0** Open **3** Percutaneous **4** Percutaneous Endoscopic	**C** Extraluminal Device **D** Intraluminal Device **Z** No Device	**Z** No Qualifier

0 Medical and Surgical
5 Upper Veins
W Revision Correcting, to the extent possible, a portion of a malfunctioning device or the position of a displaced device

Body Part Character 4	Approach Character 5	Device Character 6	Qualifier Character 7
Y Upper Vein	**0** Open **3** Percutaneous **4** Percutaneous Endoscopic **X** External	**0** Drainage Device **2** Monitoring Device **3** Infusion Device **7** Autologous Tissue Substitute **C** Extraluminal Device **D** Intraluminal Device **J** Synthetic Substitute **K** Nonautologous Tissue Substitute	**Z** No Qualifier

Lower Veins Ø61–Ø6W

Ø Medical and Surgical
6 Lower Veins
1 Bypass Altering the route of passage of the contents of a tubular body part

Body Part Character 4	Approach Character 5	Device Character 6	Qualifier Character 7
Ø Inferior Vena Cava	**Ø** Open **4** Percutaneous Endoscopic	**7** Autologous Tissue Substitute **9** Autologous Venous Tissue **A** Autologous Arterial Tissue **J** Synthetic Substitute **K** Nonautologous Tissue Substitute **Z** No Device	**5** Superior Mesenteric Vein **6** Inferior Mesenteric Vein **Y** Lower Vein
1 Splenic Vein **8** Portal Vein	**Ø** Open **4** Percutaneous Endoscopic	**7** Autologous Tissue Substitute **9** Autologous Venous Tissue **A** Autologous Arterial Tissue **J** Synthetic Substitute **K** Nonautologous Tissue Substitute **Z** No Device	**9** Renal Vein, Right **B** Renal Vein, Left **Y** Lower Vein
2 Gastric Vein **3** Esophageal Vein **4** Hepatic Vein **5** Superior Mesenteric Vein **6** Inferior Mesenteric Vein **7** Colic Vein **9** Renal Vein, Right **B** Renal Vein, Left **C** Common Iliac Vein, Right **D** Common Iliac Vein, Left **F** External Iliac Vein, Right **G** External Iliac Vein, Left **H** Hypogastric Vein, Right **J** Hypogastric Vein, Left **M** Femoral Vein, Right **N** Femoral Vein, Left **P** Greater Saphenous Vein, Right **Q** Greater Saphenous Vein, Left **R** Lesser Saphenous Vein, Right **S** Lesser Saphenous Vein, Left **T** Foot Vein, Right **V** Foot Vein, Left	**Ø** Open **4** Percutaneous Endoscopic	**7** Autologous Tissue Substitute **9** Autologous Venous Tissue **A** Autologous Arterial Tissue **J** Synthetic Substitute **K** Nonautologous Tissue Substitute **Z** No Device	**Y** Lower Vein
8 Portal Vein	**3** Percutaneous **4** Percutaneous Endoscopic	**D** Intraluminal Device	**Y** Lower Vein

0 Medical and Surgical
6 Lower Veins
5 Destruction Physical eradication of all or a portion of a body part by the direct use of energy, force, or a destructive agent

Body Part Character 4	Approach Character 5	Device Character 6	Qualifier Character 7
0 Inferior Vena Cava 1 Splenic Vein 2 Gastric Vein 3 Esophageal Vein 4 Hepatic Vein 5 Superior Mesenteric Vein 6 Inferior Mesenteric Vein 7 Colic Vein 8 Portal Vein 9 Renal Vein, Right B Renal Vein, Left C Common Iliac Vein, Right D Common Iliac Vein, Left F External Iliac Vein, Right G External Iliac Vein, Left H Hypogastric Vein, Right J Hypogastric Vein, Left M Femoral Vein, Right N Femoral Vein, Left P Greater Saphenous Vein, Right Q Greater Saphenous Vein, Left R Lesser Saphenous Vein, Right S Lesser Saphenous Vein, Left T Foot Vein, Right V Foot Vein, Left	0 Open 3 Percutaneous 4 Percutaneous Endoscopic	Z No Device	Z No Qualifier
Y Lower Vein	0 Open 3 Percutaneous 4 Percutaneous Endoscopic	Z No Device	C Hemorrhoidal Plexus Z No Qualifier

0 Medical and Surgical
6 Lower Veins
7 Dilation Expanding an orifice or the lumen of a tubular body part

Body Part Character 4	Approach Character 5	Device Character 6	Qualifier Character 7
0 Inferior Vena Cava 1 Splenic Vein 2 Gastric Vein 3 Esophageal Vein 4 Hepatic Vein 5 Superior Mesenteric Vein 6 Inferior Mesenteric Vein 7 Colic Vein 8 Portal Vein 9 Renal Vein, Right B Renal Vein, Left C Common Iliac Vein, Right D Common Iliac Vein, Left F External Iliac Vein, Right G External Iliac Vein, Left H Hypogastric Vein, Right J Hypogastric Vein, Left M Femoral Vein, Right N Femoral Vein, Left P Greater Saphenous Vein, Right Q Greater Saphenous Vein, Left R Lesser Saphenous Vein, Right S Lesser Saphenous Vein, Left T Foot Vein, Right V Foot Vein, Left Y Lower Vein	0 Open 3 Percutaneous 4 Percutaneous Endoscopic	D Intraluminal Device Z No Device	Z No Qualifier

Ø Medical and Surgical
6 Lower Veins
9 Drainage Taking or letting out fluids and/or gases from a body part

Body Part Character 4	Approach Character 5	Device Character 6	Qualifier Character 7
Ø Inferior Vena Cava **1** Splenic Vein **2** Gastric Vein **3** Esophageal Vein **4** Hepatic Vein **5** Superior Mesenteric Vein **6** Inferior Mesenteric Vein **7** Colic Vein **8** Portal Vein **9** Renal Vein, Right **B** Renal Vein, Left **C** Common Iliac Vein, Right **D** Common Iliac Vein, Left **F** External Iliac Vein, Right **G** External Iliac Vein, Left **H** Hypogastric Vein, Right **J** Hypogastric Vein, Left **M** Femoral Vein, Right **N** Femoral Vein, Left **P** Greater Saphenous Vein, Right **Q** Greater Saphenous Vein, Left **R** Lesser Saphenous Vein, Right **S** Lesser Saphenous Vein, Left **T** Foot Vein, Right **V** Foot Vein, Left **Y** Lower Vein	**Ø** Open **3** Percutaneous **4** Percutaneous Endoscopic	**Ø** Drainage Device	**Z** No Qualifier
Ø Inferior Vena Cava **1** Splenic Vein **2** Gastric Vein **3** Esophageal Vein **4** Hepatic Vein **5** Superior Mesenteric Vein **6** Inferior Mesenteric Vein **7** Colic Vein **8** Portal Vein **9** Renal Vein, Right **B** Renal Vein, Left **C** Common Iliac Vein, Right **D** Common Iliac Vein, Left **F** External Iliac Vein, Right **G** External Iliac Vein, Left **H** Hypogastric Vein, Right **J** Hypogastric Vein, Left **M** Femoral Vein, Right **N** Femoral Vein, Left **P** Greater Saphenous Vein, Right **Q** Greater Saphenous Vein, Left **R** Lesser Saphenous Vein, Right **S** Lesser Saphenous Vein, Left **T** Foot Vein, Right **V** Foot Vein, Left **Y** Lower Vein	**Ø** Open **3** Percutaneous **4** Percutaneous Endoscopic	**Z** No Device	**X** Diagnostic **Z** No Qualifier

Ø Medical and Surgical
6 Lower Veins
B Excision Cutting out or off, without replacement, a portion of a body part

Body Part Character 4	Approach Character 5	Device Character 6	Qualifier Character 7
Ø Inferior Vena Cava **1** Splenic Vein **2** Gastric Vein **3** Esophageal Vein **4** Hepatic Vein **5** Superior Mesenteric Vein **6** Inferior Mesenteric Vein **7** Colic Vein **8** Portal Vein **9** Renal Vein, Right **B** Renal Vein, Left **C** Common Iliac Vein, Right **D** Common Iliac Vein, Left **F** External Iliac Vein, Right **G** External Iliac Vein, Left **H** Hypogastric Vein, Right **J** Hypogastric Vein, Left **M** Femoral Vein, Right **N** Femoral Vein, Left **P** Greater Saphenous Vein, Right **Q** Greater Saphenous Vein, Left **R** Lesser Saphenous Vein, Right **S** Lesser Saphenous Vein, Left **T** Foot Vein, Right **V** Foot Vein, Left	**Ø** Open **3** Percutaneous **4** Percutaneous Endoscopic	**Z** No Device	**X** Diagnostic **Z** No Qualifier
Y Lower Vein	**Ø** Open **3** Percutaneous **4** Percutaneous Endoscopic	**Z** No Device	**C** Hemorrhoidal Plexus **X** Diagnostic **Z** No Qualifier

Ø Medical and Surgical
6 Lower Veins
C Extirpation Taking or cutting out solid matter from a body part

Body Part Character 4	Approach Character 5	Device Character 6	Qualifier Character 7
Ø Inferior Vena Cava **1** Splenic Vein **2** Gastric Vein **3** Esophageal Vein **4** Hepatic Vein **5** Superior Mesenteric Vein **6** Inferior Mesenteric Vein **7** Colic Vein **8** Portal Vein **9** Renal Vein, Right **B** Renal Vein, Left **C** Common Iliac Vein, Right **D** Common Iliac Vein, Left **F** External Iliac Vein, Right **G** External Iliac Vein, Left **H** Hypogastric Vein, Right **J** Hypogastric Vein, Left **M** Femoral Vein, Right **N** Femoral Vein, Left **P** Greater Saphenous Vein, Right **Q** Greater Saphenous Vein, Left **R** Lesser Saphenous Vein, Right **S** Lesser Saphenous Vein, Left **T** Foot Vein, Right **V** Foot Vein, Left **Y** Lower Vein	**Ø** Open **3** Percutaneous **4** Percutaneous Endoscopic	**Z** No Device	**Z** No Qualifier

Ø Medical and Surgical
6 Lower Veins
D Extraction Pulling or stripping out or off all or a portion of a body part by the use of force

Body Part Character 4	Approach Character 5	Device Character 6	Qualifier Character 7
M Femoral Vein, Right **N** Femoral Vein, Left **P** Greater Saphenous Vein, Right **Q** Greater Saphenous Vein, Left **R** Lesser Saphenous Vein, Right **S** Lesser Saphenous Vein, Left **T** Foot Vein, Right **V** Foot Vein, Left **Y** Lower Vein	**Ø** Open **3** Percutaneous **4** Percutaneous Endoscopic	**Z** No Device	**Z** No Qualifier

Ø Medical and Surgical
6 Lower Veins
H Insertion Putting in a nonbiological appliance that monitors, assists, performs, or prevents a physiological function but does not physically take the place of a body part

Body Part Character 4	Approach Character 5	Device Character 6	Qualifier Character 7
Ø Inferior Vena Cava	**Ø** Open **3** Percutaneous	**3** Infusion Device	**T** Via Umbilical Vein **Z** No Qualifier
Ø Inferior Vena Cava	**Ø** Open **3** Percutaneous	**D** Intraluminal Device	**Z** No Qualifier
Ø Inferior Vena Cava	**4** Percutaneous Endoscopic	**3** Infusion Device **D** Intraluminal Device	**Z** No Qualifier
1 Splenic Vein **2** Gastric Vein **3** Esophageal Vein **4** Hepatic Vein **5** Superior Mesenteric Vein **6** Inferior Mesenteric Vein **7** Colic Vein **8** Portal Vein **9** Renal Vein, Right **B** Renal Vein, Left **C** Common Iliac Vein, Right **D** Common Iliac Vein, Left **F** External Iliac Vein, Right **G** External Iliac Vein, Left **H** Hypogastric Vein, Right **J** Hypogastric Vein, Left **M** Femoral Vein, Right **N** Femoral Vein, Left **P** Greater Saphenous Vein, Right **Q** Greater Saphenous Vein, Left **R** Lesser Saphenous Vein, Right **S** Lesser Saphenous Vein, Left **T** Foot Vein, Right **V** Foot Vein, Left	**Ø** Open **3** Percutaneous **4** Percutaneous Endoscopic	**3** Infusion Device **D** Intraluminal Device	**Z** No Qualifier
Y Lower Vein	**Ø** Open **3** Percutaneous **4** Percutaneous Endoscopic	**2** Monitoring Device **3** Infusion Device **D** Intraluminal Device	**Z** No Qualifier

Ø Medical and Surgical
6 Lower Veins
J Inspection Visually and/or manually exploring a body part

Body Part Character 4	Approach Character 5	Device Character 6	Qualifier Character 7
Y Lower Vein	**Ø** Open **3** Percutaneous **4** Percutaneous Endoscopic **X** External	**Z** No Device	**Z** No Qualifier

0 Medical and Surgical
6 Lower Veins
L Occlusion Completely closing an orifice or the lumen of a tubular body part

Body Part Character 4	Approach Character 5	Device Character 6	Qualifier Character 7
0 Inferior Vena Cava 1 Splenic Vein 2 Gastric Vein 3 Esophageal Vein 4 Hepatic Vein 5 Superior Mesenteric Vein 6 Inferior Mesenteric Vein 7 Colic Vein 8 Portal Vein 9 Renal Vein, Right B Renal Vein, Left C Common Iliac Vein, Right D Common Iliac Vein, Left F External Iliac Vein, Right G External Iliac Vein, Left H Hypogastric Vein, Right J Hypogastric Vein, Left M Femoral Vein, Right N Femoral Vein, Left P Greater Saphenous Vein, Right Q Greater Saphenous Vein, Left R Lesser Saphenous Vein, Right S Lesser Saphenous Vein, Left T Foot Vein, Right V Foot Vein, Left	0 Open 3 Percutaneous 4 Percutaneous Endoscopic	C Extraluminal Device D Intraluminal Device Z No Device	Z No Qualifier
Y Lower Vein	0 Open 3 Percutaneous 4 Percutaneous Endoscopic	C Extraluminal Device D Intraluminal Device Z No Device	C Hemorrhoidal Plexus Z No Qualifier

0 Medical and Surgical
6 Lower Veins
N Release Freeing a body part from an abnormal physical constraint

Body Part Character 4	Approach Character 5	Device Character 6	Qualifier Character 7
0 Inferior Vena Cava 1 Splenic Vein 2 Gastric Vein 3 Esophageal Vein 4 Hepatic Vein 5 Superior Mesenteric Vein 6 Inferior Mesenteric Vein 7 Colic Vein 8 Portal Vein 9 Renal Vein, Right B Renal Vein, Left C Common Iliac Vein, Right D Common Iliac Vein, Left F External Iliac Vein, Right G External Iliac Vein, Left H Hypogastric Vein, Right J Hypogastric Vein, Left M Femoral Vein, Right N Femoral Vein, Left P Greater Saphenous Vein, Right Q Greater Saphenous Vein, Left R Lesser Saphenous Vein, Right S Lesser Saphenous Vein, Left T Foot Vein, Right V Foot Vein, Left Y Lower Vein	0 Open 3 Percutaneous 4 Percutaneous Endoscopic	Z No Device	Z No Qualifier

Ø Medical and Surgical
6 Lower Veins
P Removal Taking out or off a device from a body part

Body Part Character 4	Approach Character 5	Device Character 6	Qualifier Character 7
Y Lower Vein	**Ø** Open **3** Percutaneous **4** Percutaneous Endoscopic	**Ø** Drainage Device **2** Monitoring Device **3** Infusion Device **7** Autologous Tissue Substitute **C** Extraluminal Device **D** Intraluminal Device **J** Synthetic Substitute **K** Nonautologous Tissue Substitute	**Z** No Qualifier
Y Lower Vein	**X** External	**Ø** Drainage Device **2** Monitoring Device **3** Infusion Device **D** Intraluminal Device	**Z** No Qualifier

Ø Medical and Surgical
6 Lower Veins
Q Repair Restoring, to the extent possible, a body part to its normal anatomic structure and function

Body Part Character 4	Approach Character 5	Device Character 6	Qualifier Character 7
Ø Inferior Vena Cava **1** Splenic Vein **2** Gastric Vein **3** Esophageal Vein **4** Hepatic Vein **5** Superior Mesenteric Vein **6** Inferior Mesenteric Vein **7** Colic Vein **8** Portal Vein **9** Renal Vein, Right **B** Renal Vein, Left **C** Common Iliac Vein, Right **D** Common Iliac Vein, Left **F** External Iliac Vein, Right **G** External Iliac Vein, Left **H** Hypogastric Vein, Right **J** Hypogastric Vein, Left **M** Femoral Vein, Right **N** Femoral Vein, Left **P** Greater Saphenous Vein, Right **Q** Greater Saphenous Vein, Left **R** Lesser Saphenous Vein, Right **S** Lesser Saphenous Vein, Left **T** Foot Vein, Right **V** Foot Vein, Left **Y** Lower Vein	**Ø** Open **3** Percutaneous **4** Percutaneous Endoscopic	**Z** No Device	**Z** No Qualifier

0 Medical and Surgical
6 Lower Veins
R Replacement Putting in or on biological or synthetic material that physically takes the place and/or function of all or a portion of a body part

Body Part Character 4	Approach Character 5	Device Character 6	Qualifier Character 7
0 Inferior Vena Cava **1** Splenic Vein **2** Gastric Vein **3** Esophageal Vein **4** Hepatic Vein **5** Superior Mesenteric Vein **6** Inferior Mesenteric Vein **7** Colic Vein **8** Portal Vein **9** Renal Vein, Right **B** Renal Vein, Left **C** Common Iliac Vein, Right **D** Common Iliac Vein, Left **F** External Iliac Vein, Right **G** External Iliac Vein, Left **H** Hypogastric Vein, Right **J** Hypogastric Vein, Left **M** Femoral Vein, Right **N** Femoral Vein, Left **P** Greater Saphenous Vein, Right **Q** Greater Saphenous Vein, Left **R** Lesser Saphenous Vein, Right **S** Lesser Saphenous Vein, Left **T** Foot Vein, Right **V** Foot Vein, Left **Y** Lower Vein	**0** Open **4** Percutaneous Endoscopic	**7** Autologous Tissue Substitute **J** Synthetic Substitute **K** Nonautologous Tissue Substitute	**Z** No Qualifier

0 Medical and Surgical
6 Lower Veins
S Reposition Moving to its normal location or other suitable location all or a portion of a body part

Body Part Character 4	Approach Character 5	Device Character 6	Qualifier Character 7
0 Inferior Vena Cava **1** Splenic Vein **2** Gastric Vein **3** Esophageal Vein **4** Hepatic Vein **5** Superior Mesenteric Vein **6** Inferior Mesenteric Vein **7** Colic Vein **8** Portal Vein **9** Renal Vein, Right **B** Renal Vein, Left **C** Common Iliac Vein, Right **D** Common Iliac Vein, Left **F** External Iliac Vein, Right **G** External Iliac Vein, Left **H** Hypogastric Vein, Right **J** Hypogastric Vein, Left **M** Femoral Vein, Right **N** Femoral Vein, Left **P** Greater Saphenous Vein, Right **Q** Greater Saphenous Vein, Left **R** Lesser Saphenous Vein, Right **S** Lesser Saphenous Vein, Left **T** Foot Vein, Right **V** Foot Vein, Left **Y** Lower Vein	**0** Open **3** Percutaneous **4** Percutaneous Endoscopic	**Z** No Device	**Z** No Qualifier

Ø Medical and Surgical
6 Lower Veins
U Supplement Putting in or on biological or synthetic material that physically reinforces and/or augments the function of a portion of a body part

Body Part Character 4	Approach Character 5	Device Character 6	Qualifier Character 7
Ø Inferior Vena Cava **1** Splenic Vein **2** Gastric Vein **3** Esophageal Vein **4** Hepatic Vein **5** Superior Mesenteric Vein **6** Inferior Mesenteric Vein **7** Colic Vein **8** Portal Vein **9** Renal Vein, Right **B** Renal Vein, Left **C** Common Iliac Vein, Right **D** Common Iliac Vein, Left **F** External Iliac Vein, Right **G** External Iliac Vein, Left **H** Hypogastric Vein, Right **J** Hypogastric Vein, Left **M** Femoral Vein, Right **N** Femoral Vein, Left **P** Greater Saphenous Vein, Right **Q** Greater Saphenous Vein, Left **R** Lesser Saphenous Vein, Right **S** Lesser Saphenous Vein, Left **T** Foot Vein, Right **V** Foot Vein, Left **Y** Lower Vein	**Ø** Open **3** Percutaneous **4** Percutaneous Endoscopic	**7** Autologous Tissue Substitute **J** Synthetic Substitute **K** Nonautologous Tissue Substitute	**Z** No Qualifier

Ø Medical and Surgical
6 Lower Veins
V Restriction Partially closing an orifice or the lumen of a tubular body part

Body Part Character 4	Approach Character 5	Device Character 6	Qualifier Character 7
Ø Inferior Vena Cava **1** Splenic Vein **2** Gastric Vein **3** Esophageal Vein **4** Hepatic Vein **5** Superior Mesenteric Vein **6** Inferior Mesenteric Vein **7** Colic Vein **8** Portal Vein **9** Renal Vein, Right **B** Renal Vein, Left **C** Common Iliac Vein, Right **D** Common Iliac Vein, Left **F** External Iliac Vein, Right **G** External Iliac Vein, Left **H** Hypogastric Vein, Right **J** Hypogastric Vein, Left **M** Femoral Vein, Right **N** Femoral Vein, Left **P** Greater Saphenous Vein, Right **Q** Greater Saphenous Vein, Left **R** Lesser Saphenous Vein, Right **S** Lesser Saphenous Vein, Left **T** Foot Vein, Right **V** Foot Vein, Left **Y** Lower Vein	**Ø** Open **3** Percutaneous **4** Percutaneous Endoscopic	**C** Extraluminal Device **D** Intraluminal Device **Z** No Device	**Z** No Qualifier

0 Medical and Surgical
6 Lower Veins
W Revision Correcting, to the extent possible, a portion of a malfunctioning device or the position of a displaced device

Body Part Character 4	Approach Character 5	Device Character 6	Qualifier Character 7
Y Lower Vein	**0** Open **3** Percutaneous **4** Percutaneous Endoscopic **X** External	**0** Drainage Device **2** Monitoring Device **3** Infusion Device **7** Autologous Tissue Substitute **C** Extraluminal Device **D** Intraluminal Device **J** Synthetic Substitute **K** Nonautologous Tissue Substitute	**Z** No Qualifier

Lymphatic and Hemic Systems Ø72–Ø7Y

Ø Medical and Surgical
7 Lymphatic and Hemic Systems
2 Change Taking out or off a device from a body part and putting back an identical or similar device in or on the same body part without cutting or puncturing the skin or a mucous membrane

Body Part Character 4	Approach Character 5	Device Character 6	Qualifier Character 7
K Thoracic Duct **L** Cisterna Chyli **M** Thymus **N** Lymphatic **P** Spleen **T** Bone Marrow	**X** External	**Ø** Drainage Device **Y** Other Device	**Z** No Qualifier

Ø Medical and Surgical
7 Lymphatic and Hemic Systems
5 Destruction Physical eradication of all or a portion of a body part by the direct use of energy, force, or a destructive agent

Body Part Character 4	Approach Character 5	Device Character 6	Qualifier Character 7
Ø Lymphatic, Head **1** Lymphatic, Right Neck **2** Lymphatic, Left Neck **3** Lymphatic, Right Upper Extremity **4** Lymphatic, Left Upper Extremity **5** Lymphatic, Right Axillary **6** Lymphatic, Left Axillary **7** Lymphatic, Thorax **8** Lymphatic, Internal Mammary, Right **9** Lymphatic, Internal Mammary, Left **B** Lymphatic, Mesenteric **C** Lymphatic, Pelvis **D** Lymphatic, Aortic **F** Lymphatic, Right Lower Extremity **G** Lymphatic, Left Lower Extremity **H** Lymphatic, Right Inguinal **J** Lymphatic, Left Inguinal **K** Thoracic Duct **L** Cisterna Chyli **M** Thymus **P** Spleen	**Ø** Open **3** Percutaneous **4** Percutaneous Endoscopic	**Z** No Device	**Z** No Qualifier

Ø Medical and Surgical
7 Lymphatic and Hemic Systems
9 Drainage Taking or letting out fluids and/or gases from a body part

Body Part Character 4	Approach Character 5	Device Character 6	Qualifier Character 7
Ø Lymphatic, Head **1** Lymphatic, Right Neck **2** Lymphatic, Left Neck **3** Lymphatic, Right Upper Extremity **4** Lymphatic, Left Upper Extremity **5** Lymphatic, Right Axillary **6** Lymphatic, Left Axillary **7** Lymphatic, Thorax **8** Lymphatic, Internal Mammary, Right **9** Lymphatic, Internal Mammary, Left **B** Lymphatic, Mesenteric **C** Lymphatic, Pelvis **D** Lymphatic, Aortic **F** Lymphatic, Right Lower Extremity **G** Lymphatic, Left Lower Extremity **H** Lymphatic, Right Inguinal **J** Lymphatic, Left Inguinal **K** Thoracic Duct **L** Cisterna Chyli **M** Thymus **P** Spleen **T** Bone Marrow	**Ø** Open **3** Percutaneous **4** Percutaneous Endoscopic	**Ø** Drainage Device	**Z** No Qualifier

Ø79 Continued on next page

079 Continued

0 Medical and Surgical
7 Lymphatic and Hemic Systems
9 Drainage Taking or letting out fluids and/or gases from a body part

Body Part Character 4	Approach Character 5	Device Character 6	Qualifier Character 7
0 Lymphatic, Head 1 Lymphatic, Right Neck 2 Lymphatic, Left Neck 3 Lymphatic, Right Upper Extremity 4 Lymphatic, Left Upper Extremity 5 Lymphatic, Right Axillary 6 Lymphatic, Left Axillary 7 Lymphatic, Thorax 8 Lymphatic, Internal Mammary, Right 9 Lymphatic, Internal Mammary, Left B Lymphatic, Mesenteric C Lymphatic, Pelvis D Lymphatic, Aortic F Lymphatic, Right Lower Extremity G Lymphatic, Left Lower Extremity H Lymphatic, Right Inguinal J Lymphatic, Left Inguinal K Thoracic Duct L Cisterna Chyli M Thymus P Spleen T Bone Marrow	0 Open 3 Percutaneous 4 Percutaneous Endoscopic	Z No Device	X Diagnostic Z No Qualifier

0 Medical and Surgical
7 Lymphatic and Hemic Systems
B Excision Cutting out or off, without replacement, a portion of a body part

Body Part Character 4	Approach Character 5	Device Character 6	Qualifier Character 7
0 Lymphatic, Head 1 Lymphatic, Right Neck 2 Lymphatic, Left Neck 3 Lymphatic, Right Upper Extremity 4 Lymphatic, Left Upper Extremity 5 Lymphatic, Right Axillary 6 Lymphatic, Left Axillary 7 Lymphatic, Thorax 8 Lymphatic, Internal Mammary, Right 9 Lymphatic, Internal Mammary, Left B Lymphatic, Mesenteric C Lymphatic, Pelvis D Lymphatic, Aortic F Lymphatic, Right Lower Extremity G Lymphatic, Left Lower Extremity H Lymphatic, Right Inguinal J Lymphatic, Left Inguinal K Thoracic Duct L Cisterna Chyli M Thymus P Spleen	0 Open 3 Percutaneous 4 Percutaneous Endoscopic	Z No Device	X Diagnostic Z No Qualifier

0 Medical and Surgical
7 Lymphatic and Hemic Systems
C Extirpation Taking or cutting out solid matter from a body part

Body Part Character 4	Approach Character 5	Device Character 6	Qualifier Character 7
0 Lymphatic, Head **1** Lymphatic, Right Neck **2** Lymphatic, Left Neck **3** Lymphatic, Right Upper Extremity **4** Lymphatic, Left Upper Extremity **5** Lymphatic, Right Axillary **6** Lymphatic, Left Axillary **7** Lymphatic, Thorax **8** Lymphatic, Internal Mammary, Right **9** Lymphatic, Internal Mammary, Left **B** Lymphatic, Mesenteric **C** Lymphatic, Pelvis **D** Lymphatic, Aortic **F** Lymphatic, Right Lower Extremity **G** Lymphatic, Left Lower Extremity **H** Lymphatic, Right Inguinal **J** Lymphatic, Left Inguinal **K** Thoracic Duct **L** Cisterna Chyli **M** Thymus **P** Spleen	**0** Open **3** Percutaneous **4** Percutaneous Endoscopic	**Z** No Device	**Z** No Qualifier

0 Medical and Surgical
7 Lymphatic and Hemic Systems
D Extraction Pulling or stripping out or off all or a portion of a body part by the use of force

Body Part Character 4	Approach Character 5	Device Character 6	Qualifier Character 7
Q Bone Marrow, Sternum **R** Bone Marrow, Iliac **S** Bone Marrow, Vertebral	**0** Open **3** Percutaneous	**Z** No Device	**X** Diagnostic **Z** No Qualifier

0 Medical and Surgical
7 Lymphatic and Hemic Systems
H Insertion Putting in a nonbiological appliance that monitors, assists, performs, or prevents a physiological function but does not physically take the place of a body part

Body Part Character 4	Approach Character 5	Device Character 6	Qualifier Character 7
K Thoracic Duct **L** Cisterna Chyli **M** Thymus **N** Lymphatic **P** Spleen	**0** Open **3** Percutaneous **4** Percutaneous Endoscopic	**3** Infusion Device	**Z** No Qualifier

0 Medical and Surgical
7 Lymphatic and Hemic Systems
J Inspection Visually and/or manually exploring a body part

Body Part Character 4	Approach Character 5	Device Character 6	Qualifier Character 7
K Thoracic Duct **L** Cisterna Chyli **M** Thymus **T** Bone Marrow	**0** Open **3** Percutaneous **4** Percutaneous Endoscopic	**Z** No Device	**Z** No Qualifier
N Lymphatic **P** Spleen	**0** Open **3** Percutaneous **4** Percutaneous Endoscopic **X** External	**Z** No Device	**Z** No Qualifier

0 Medical and Surgical
7 Lymphatic and Hemic Systems
L Occlusion Completely closing an orifice or the lumen of a tubular body part

Body Part Character 4	Approach Character 5	Device Character 6	Qualifier Character 7
0 Lymphatic, Head 1 Lymphatic, Right Neck 2 Lymphatic, Left Neck 3 Lymphatic, Right Upper Extremity 4 Lymphatic, Left Upper Extremity 5 Lymphatic, Right Axillary 6 Lymphatic, Left Axillary 7 Lymphatic, Thorax 8 Lymphatic, Internal Mammary, Right 9 Lymphatic, Internal Mammary, Left B Lymphatic, Mesenteric C Lymphatic, Pelvis D Lymphatic, Aortic F Lymphatic, Right Lower Extremity G Lymphatic, Left Lower Extremity H Lymphatic, Right Inguinal J Lymphatic, Left Inguinal K Thoracic Duct L Cisterna Chyli	0 Open 3 Percutaneous 4 Percutaneous Endoscopic	C Extraluminal Device D Intraluminal Device Z No Device	Z No Qualifier

0 Medical and Surgical
7 Lymphatic and Hemic Systems
N Release Freeing a body part from an abnormal physical constraint

Body Part Character 4	Approach Character 5	Device Character 6	Qualifier Character 7
0 Lymphatic, Head 1 Lymphatic, Right Neck 2 Lymphatic, Left Neck 3 Lymphatic, Right Upper Extremity 4 Lymphatic, Left Upper Extremity 5 Lymphatic, Right Axillary 6 Lymphatic, Left Axillary 7 Lymphatic, Thorax 8 Lymphatic, Internal Mammary, Right 9 Lymphatic, Internal Mammary, Left B Lymphatic, Mesenteric C Lymphatic, Pelvis D Lymphatic, Aortic F Lymphatic, Right Lower Extremity G Lymphatic, Left Lower Extremity H Lymphatic, Right Inguinal J Lymphatic, Left Inguinal K Thoracic Duct L Cisterna Chyli M Thymus P Spleen	0 Open 3 Percutaneous 4 Percutaneous Endoscopic	Z No Device	Z No Qualifier

0 Medical and Surgical
7 Lymphatic and Hemic Systems
P Removal Taking out or off a device from a body part

Body Part Character 4	Approach Character 5	Device Character 6	Qualifier Character 7
K Thoracic Duct L Cisterna Chyli N Lymphatic	0 Open 3 Percutaneous 4 Percutaneous Endoscopic	0 Drainage Device 3 Infusion Device 7 Autologous Tissue Substitute C Extraluminal Device D Intraluminal Device J Synthetic Substitute K Nonautologous Tissue Substitute	Z No Qualifier
K Thoracic Duct L Cisterna Chyli N Lymphatic	X External	0 Drainage Device 3 Infusion Device D Intraluminal Device	Z No Qualifier
M Thymus P Spleen	0 Open 3 Percutaneous 4 Percutaneous Endoscopic X External	0 Drainage Device 3 Infusion Device	Z No Qualifier

07P Continued on next page

Ø7P Continued

Ø Medical and Surgical
7 Lymphatic and Hemic Systems
P Removal Taking out or off a device from a body part

Body Part Character 4	Approach Character 5	Device Character 6	Qualifier Character 7
T Bone Marrow	Ø Open 3 Percutaneous 4 Percutaneous Endoscopic X External	Ø Drainage Device	Z No Qualifier

Ø Medical and Surgical
7 Lymphatic and Hemic Systems
Q Repair Restoring, to the extent possible, a body part to its normal anatomic structure and function

Body Part Character 4	Approach Character 5	Device Character 6	Qualifier Character 7
Ø Lymphatic, Head 1 Lymphatic, Right Neck 2 Lymphatic, Left Neck 3 Lymphatic, Right Upper Extremity 4 Lymphatic, Left Upper Extremity 5 Lymphatic, Right Axillary 6 Lymphatic, Left Axillary 7 Lymphatic, Thorax 8 Lymphatic, Internal Mammary, Right 9 Lymphatic, Internal Mammary, Left B Lymphatic, Mesenteric C Lymphatic, Pelvis D Lymphatic, Aortic F Lymphatic, Right Lower Extremity G Lymphatic, Left Lower Extremity H Lymphatic, Right Inguinal J Lymphatic, Left Inguinal K Thoracic Duct L Cisterna Chyli M Thymus P Spleen	Ø Open 3 Percutaneous 4 Percutaneous Endoscopic	Z No Device	Z No Qualifier

Ø Medical and Surgical
7 Lymphatic and Hemic Systems
S Reposition Moving to its normal location or other suitable location all or a portion of a body part

Body Part Character 4	Approach Character 5	Device Character 6	Qualifier Character 7
M Thymus P Spleen	Ø Open	Z No Device	Z No Qualifier

Ø Medical and Surgical
7 Lymphatic and Hemic Systems
T Resection Cutting out or off, without replacement, all of a body part

Body Part Character 4	Approach Character 5	Device Character 6	Qualifier Character 7
Ø Lymphatic, Head 1 Lymphatic, Right Neck 2 Lymphatic, Left Neck 3 Lymphatic, Right Upper Extremity 4 Lymphatic, Left Upper Extremity 5 Lymphatic, Right Axillary 6 Lymphatic, Left Axillary 7 Lymphatic, Thorax 8 Lymphatic, Internal Mammary, Right 9 Lymphatic, Internal Mammary, Left B Lymphatic, Mesenteric C Lymphatic, Pelvis D Lymphatic, Aortic F Lymphatic, Right Lower Extremity G Lymphatic, Left Lower Extremity H Lymphatic, Right Inguinal J Lymphatic, Left Inguinal K Thoracic Duct L Cisterna Chyli M Thymus P Spleen	Ø Open 4 Percutaneous Endoscopic	Z No Device	Z No Qualifier

0 Medical and Surgical
7 Lymphatic and Hemic Systems
U Supplement Putting in or on biological or synthetic material that physically reinforces and/or augments the function of a portion of a body part

Body Part Character 4	Approach Character 5	Device Character 6	Qualifier Character 7
0 Lymphatic, Head **1** Lymphatic, Right Neck **2** Lymphatic, Left Neck **3** Lymphatic, Right Upper Extremity **4** Lymphatic, Left Upper Extremity **5** Lymphatic, Right Axillary **6** Lymphatic, Left Axillary **7** Lymphatic, Thorax **8** Lymphatic, Internal Mammary, Right **9** Lymphatic, Internal Mammary, Left **B** Lymphatic, Mesenteric **C** Lymphatic, Pelvis **D** Lymphatic, Aortic **F** Lymphatic, Right Lower Extremity **G** Lymphatic, Left Lower Extremity **H** Lymphatic, Right Inguinal **J** Lymphatic, Left Inguinal **K** Thoracic Duct **L** Cisterna Chyli	**0** Open **4** Percutaneous Endoscopic	**7** Autologous Tissue Substitute **J** Synthetic Substitute **K** Nonautologous Tissue Substitute	**Z** No Qualifier

0 Medical and Surgical
7 Lymphatic and Hemic Systems
V Restriction Partially closing an orifice or the lumen of a tubular body part

Body Part Character 4	Approach Character 5	Device Character 6	Qualifier Character 7
0 Lymphatic, Head **1** Lymphatic, Right Neck **2** Lymphatic, Left Neck **3** Lymphatic, Right Upper Extremity **4** Lymphatic, Left Upper Extremity **5** Lymphatic, Right Axillary **6** Lymphatic, Left Axillary **7** Lymphatic, Thorax **8** Lymphatic, Internal Mammary, Right **9** Lymphatic, Internal Mammary, Left **B** Lymphatic, Mesenteric **C** Lymphatic, Pelvis **D** Lymphatic, Aortic **F** Lymphatic, Right Lower Extremity **G** Lymphatic, Left Lower Extremity **H** Lymphatic, Right Inguinal **J** Lymphatic, Left Inguinal **K** Thoracic Duct **L** Cisterna Chyli	**0** Open **3** Percutaneous **4** Percutaneous Endoscopic	**C** Extraluminal Device **D** Intraluminal Device **Z** No Device	**Z** No Qualifier

0 Medical and Surgical
7 Lymphatic and Hemic Systems
W Revision Correcting, to the extent possible, a portion of a malfunctioning device or the position of a displaced device

Body Part Character 4	Approach Character 5	Device Character 6	Qualifier Character 7
K Thoracic Duct **L** Cisterna Chyli **N** Lymphatic	**0** Open **3** Percutaneous **4** Percutaneous Endoscopic **X** External	**0** Drainage Device **3** Infusion Device **7** Autologous Tissue Substitute **C** Extraluminal Device **D** Intraluminal Device **J** Synthetic Substitute **K** Nonautologous Tissue Substitute	**Z** No Qualifier
M Thymus **P** Spleen	**0** Open **3** Percutaneous **4** Percutaneous Endoscopic **X** External	**0** Drainage Device **3** Infusion Device	**Z** No Qualifier
T Bone Marrow	**0** Open **3** Percutaneous **4** Percutaneous Endoscopic **X** External	**0** Drainage Device	**Z** No Qualifier

Ø Medical and Surgical
7 Lymphatic and Hemic Systems
Y Transplantation Putting in or on all or a portion of a living body part taken from another individual or animal to physically take the place and/or function of all or a portion of a similar body part

Body Part Character 4	Approach Character 5	Device Character 6	Qualifier Character 7
M Thymus **P** Spleen	**Ø** Open	**Z** No Device	**Ø** Allogeneic **1** Syngeneic **2** Zooplastic

Eye 080–08X

0 Medical and Surgical
8 Eye
0 Alteration Modifying the anatomic structure of a body part without affecting the function of the body part

Body Part Character 4	Approach Character 5	Device Character 6	Qualifier Character 7
N Upper Eyelid, Right **P** Upper Eyelid, Left **Q** Lower Eyelid, Right **R** Lower Eyelid, Left	**0** Open **3** Percutaneous **X** External	**7** Autologous Tissue Substitute **J** Synthetic Substitute **K** Nonautologous Tissue Substitute **Z** No Device	**Z** No Qualifier

0 Medical and Surgical
8 Eye
1 Bypass Altering the route of passage of the contents of a tubular body part

Body Part Character 4	Approach Character 5	Device Character 6	Qualifier Character 7
2 Anterior Chamber, Right **3** Anterior Chamber, Left	**3** Percutaneous	**J** Synthetic Substitute **K** Nonautologous Tissue Substitute **Z** No Device	**4** Sclera
X Lacrimal Duct, Right **Y** Lacrimal Duct, Left	**0** Open **3** Percutaneous	**J** Synthetic Substitute **K** Nonautologous Tissue Substitute **Z** No Device	**3** Nasal Cavity

0 Medical and Surgical
8 Eye
2 Change Taking out or off a device from a body part and putting back an identical or similar device in or on the same body part without cutting or puncturing the skin or a mucous membrane

Body Part Character 4	Approach Character 5	Device Character 6	Qualifier Character 7
0 Eye, Right **1** Eye, Left	**X** External	**0** Drainage Device **Y** Other Device	**Z** No Qualifier

0 Medical and Surgical
8 Eye
5 Destruction Physical eradication of all or a portion of a body part by the direct use of energy, force, or a destructive agent

Body Part Character 4	Approach Character 5	Device Character 6	Qualifier Character 7
0 Eye, Right **1** Eye, Left **6** Sclera, Right **7** Sclera, Left **8** Cornea, Right **9** Cornea, Left **S** Conjunctiva, Right **T** Conjunctiva, Left	**X** External	**Z** No Device	**Z** No Qualifier
2 Anterior Chamber, Right **3** Anterior Chamber, Left **4** Vitreous, Right **5** Vitreous, Left **C** Iris, Right **D** Iris, Left **E** Retina, Right **F** Retina, Left **G** Retinal Vessel, Right **H** Retinal Vessel, Left **J** Lens, Right **K** Lens, Left	**3** Percutaneous	**Z** No Device	**Z** No Qualifier
A Choroid, Right **B** Choroid, Left **L** Extraocular Muscle, Right **M** Extraocular Muscle, Left **V** Lacrimal Gland, Right **W** Lacrimal Gland, Left	**0** Open **3** Percutaneous	**Z** No Device	**Z** No Qualifier
N Upper Eyelid, Right **P** Upper Eyelid, Left **Q** Lower Eyelid, Right **R** Lower Eyelid, Left	**0** Open **3** Percutaneous **X** External	**Z** No Device	**Z** No Qualifier

085 Continued on next page

Ø85 Continued

Ø Medical and Surgical
8 Eye
5 Destruction Physical eradication of all or a portion of a body part by the direct use of energy, force, or a destructive agent

Body Part Character 4	Approach Character 5	Device Character 6	Qualifier Character 7
X Lacrimal Duct, Right **Y** Lacrimal Duct, Left	**Ø** Open **3** Percutaneous **7** Via Natural or Artificial Opening **8** Via Natural or Artificial Opening Endoscopic	**Z** No Device	**Z** No Qualifier

Ø Medical and Surgical
8 Eye
7 Dilation Expanding an orifice or the lumen of a tubular body part

Body Part Character 4	Approach Character 5	Device Character 6	Qualifier Character 7
X Lacrimal Duct, Right **Y** Lacrimal Duct, Left	**Ø** Open **3** Percutaneous **7** Via Natural or Artificial Opening **8** Via Natural or Artificial Opening Endoscopic	**D** Intraluminal Device **Z** No Device	**Z** No Qualifier

Ø Medical and Surgical
8 Eye
9 Drainage Taking or letting out fluids and/or gases from a body part

Body Part Character 4	Approach Character 5	Device Character 6	Qualifier Character 7
Ø Eye, Right **1** Eye, Left **6** Sclera, Right **7** Sclera, Left **8** Cornea, Right **9** Cornea, Left **S** Conjunctiva, Right **T** Conjunctiva, Left	**X** External	**Ø** Drainage Device	**Z** No Qualifier
Ø Eye, Right **1** Eye, Left **6** Sclera, Right **7** Sclera, Left **8** Cornea, Right **9** Cornea, Left **S** Conjunctiva, Right **T** Conjunctiva, Left	**X** External	**Z** No Device	**X** Diagnostic **Z** No Qualifier
2 Anterior Chamber, Right **3** Anterior Chamber, Left **4** Vitreous, Right **5** Vitreous, Left **C** Iris, Right **D** Iris, Left **E** Retina, Right **F** Retina, Left **G** Retinal Vessel, Right **H** Retinal Vessel, Left **J** Lens, Right **K** Lens, Left	**3** Percutaneous	**Ø** Drainage Device	**Z** No Qualifier
2 Anterior Chamber, Right **3** Anterior Chamber, Left **4** Vitreous, Right **5** Vitreous, Left **C** Iris, Right **D** Iris, Left **E** Retina, Right **F** Retina, Left **G** Retinal Vessel, Right **H** Retinal Vessel, Left **J** Lens, Right **K** Lens, Left	**3** Percutaneous	**Z** No Device	**X** Diagnostic **Z** No Qualifier
A Choroid, Right **B** Choroid, Left **L** Extraocular Muscle, Right **M** Extraocular Muscle, Left **V** Lacrimal Gland, Right **W** Lacrimal Gland, Left	**Ø** Open **3** Percutaneous	**Ø** Drainage Device	**Z** No Qualifier

Ø89 Continued on next page

Ø Medical and Surgical
8 Eye
9 Drainage Taking or letting out fluids and/or gases from a body part

Ø89 Continued

Body Part Character 4	Approach Character 5	Device Character 6	Qualifier Character 7
A Choroid, Right B Choroid, Left L Extraocular Muscle, Right M Extraocular Muscle, Left V Lacrimal Gland, Right W Lacrimal Gland, Left	Ø Open 3 Percutaneous	Z No Device	X Diagnostic Z No Qualifier
N Upper Eyelid, Right P Upper Eyelid, Left Q Lower Eyelid, Right R Lower Eyelid, Left	Ø Open 3 Percutaneous X External	Ø Drainage Device	Z No Qualifier
N Upper Eyelid, Right P Upper Eyelid, Left Q Lower Eyelid, Right R Lower Eyelid, Left	Ø Open 3 Percutaneous X External	Z No Device	X Diagnostic Z No Qualifier
X Lacrimal Duct, Right Y Lacrimal Duct, Left	Ø Open 3 Percutaneous 7 Via Natural or Artificial Opening 8 Via Natural or Artificial Opening Endoscopic	Ø Drainage Device	Z No Qualifier
X Lacrimal Duct, Right Y Lacrimal Duct, Left	Ø Open 3 Percutaneous 7 Via Natural or Artificial Opening 8 Via Natural or Artificial Opening Endoscopic	Z No Device	X Diagnostic Z No Qualifier

Ø Medical and Surgical
8 Eye
B Excision Cutting out or off, without replacement, a portion of a body part

Body Part Character 4	Approach Character 5	Device Character 6	Qualifier Character 7
Ø Eye, Right 1 Eye, Left N Upper Eyelid, Right P Upper Eyelid, Left Q Lower Eyelid, Right R Lower Eyelid, Left	Ø Open 3 Percutaneous X External	Z No Device	X Diagnostic Z No Qualifier
4 Vitreous, Right 5 Vitreous, Left C Iris, Right D Iris, Left E Retina, Right F Retina, Left J Lens, Right K Lens, Left	3 Percutaneous	Z No Device	X Diagnostic Z No Qualifier
6 Sclera, Right 7 Sclera, Left 8 Cornea, Right 9 Cornea, Left S Conjunctiva, Right T Conjunctiva, Left	X External	Z No Device	X Diagnostic Z No Qualifier
A Choroid, Right B Choroid, Left L Extraocular Muscle, Right M Extraocular Muscle, Left V Lacrimal Gland, Right W Lacrimal Gland, Left	Ø Open 3 Percutaneous	Z No Device	X Diagnostic Z No Qualifier
X Lacrimal Duct, Right Y Lacrimal Duct, Left	Ø Open 3 Percutaneous 7 Via Natural or Artificial Opening 8 Via Natural or Artificial Opening Endoscopic	Z No Device	X Diagnostic Z No Qualifier

Ø Medical and Surgical
8 Eye
C Extirpation Taking or cutting out solid matter from a body part

Body Part Character 4	Approach Character 5	Device Character 6	Qualifier Character 7
Ø Eye, Right **1** Eye, Left **6** Sclera, Right **7** Sclera, Left **8** Cornea, Right **9** Cornea, Left **S** Conjunctiva, Right **T** Conjunctiva, Left	**X** External	**Z** No Device	**Z** No Qualifier
2 Anterior Chamber, Right **3** Anterior Chamber, Left **4** Vitreous, Right **5** Vitreous, Left **C** Iris, Right **D** Iris, Left **E** Retina, Right **F** Retina, Left **G** Retinal Vessel, Right **H** Retinal Vessel, Left **J** Lens, Right **K** Lens, Left	**3** Percutaneous **X** External	**Z** No Device	**Z** No Qualifier
A Choroid, Right **B** Choroid, Left **L** Extraocular Muscle, Right **M** Extraocular Muscle, Left **N** Upper Eyelid, Right **P** Upper Eyelid, Left **Q** Lower Eyelid, Right **R** Lower Eyelid, Left **V** Lacrimal Gland, Right **W** Lacrimal Gland, Left	**Ø** Open **3** Percutaneous **X** External	**Z** No Device	**Z** No Qualifier
X Lacrimal Duct, Right **Y** Lacrimal Duct, Left	**Ø** Open **3** Percutaneous **7** Via Natural or Artificial Opening **8** Via Natural or Artificial Opening Endoscopic	**Z** No Device	**Z** No Qualifier

Ø Medical and Surgical
8 Eye
D Extraction Pulling or stripping out or off all or a portion of a body part by the use of force

Body Part Character 4	Approach Character 5	Device Character 6	Qualifier Character 7
8 Cornea, Right **9** Cornea, Left	**X** External	**Z** No Device	**X** Diagnostic **Z** No Qualifier
J Lens, Right **K** Lens, Left	**3** Percutaneous	**Z** No Device	**Z** No Qualifier

Ø Medical and Surgical
8 Eye
F Fragmentation Breaking solid matter in a body part into pieces

Body Part Character 4	Approach Character 5	Device Character 6	Qualifier Character 7
4 Vitreous, Right **5** Vitreous, Left	**3** Percutaneous **X** External	**Z** No Device	**Z** No Qualifier

Ø Medical and Surgical
8 Eye
H Insertion Putting in a nonbiological appliance that monitors, assists, performs, or prevents a physiological function but does not physically take the place of a body part

Body Part Character 4	Approach Character 5	Device Character 6	Qualifier Character 7
Ø Eye, Right **1** Eye, Left	**3** Percutaneous **X** External	**1** Radioactive Element **3** Infusion Device	**Z** No Qualifier

0 Medical and Surgical
8 Eye
J Inspection Visually and/or manually exploring a body part

Body Part Character 4	Approach Character 5	Device Character 6	Qualifier Character 7
0 Eye, Right 1 Eye, Left J Lens, Right K Lens, Left	X External	Z No Device	Z No Qualifier
L Extraocular Muscle, Right M Extraocular Muscle, Left	0 Open X External	Z No Device	Z No Qualifier

0 Medical and Surgical
8 Eye
L Occlusion Completely closing an orifice or the lumen of a tubular body part

Body Part Character 4	Approach Character 5	Device Character 6	Qualifier Character 7
X Lacrimal Duct, Right Y Lacrimal Duct, Left	0 Open 3 Percutaneous	C Extraluminal Device D Intraluminal Device Z No Device	Z No Qualifier
X Lacrimal Duct, Right Y Lacrimal Duct, Left	7 Via Natural or Artificial Opening 8 Via Natural or Artificial Opening Endoscopic	D Intraluminal Device Z No Device	Z No Qualifier

0 Medical and Surgical
8 Eye
M Reattachment Putting back in or on all or a portion of a separated body part to its normal location or other suitable location

Body Part Character 4	Approach Character 5	Device Character 6	Qualifier Character 7
N Upper Eyelid, Right P Upper Eyelid, Left Q Lower Eyelid, Right R Lower Eyelid, Left	X External	Z No Device	Z No Qualifier

0 Medical and Surgical
8 Eye
N Release Freeing a body part from an abnormal physical constraint

Body Part Character 4	Approach Character 5	Device Character 6	Qualifier Character 7
0 Eye, Right 1 Eye, Left 6 Sclera, Right 7 Sclera, Left 8 Cornea, Right 9 Cornea, Left S Conjunctiva, Right T Conjunctiva, Left	X External	Z No Device	Z No Qualifier
2 Anterior Chamber, Right 3 Anterior Chamber, Left 4 Vitreous, Right 5 Vitreous, Left C Iris, Right D Iris, Left E Retina, Right F Retina, Left G Retinal Vessel, Right H Retinal Vessel, Left J Lens, Right K Lens, Left	3 Percutaneous	Z No Device	Z No Qualifier
A Choroid, Right B Choroid, Left L Extraocular Muscle, Right M Extraocular Muscle, Left V Lacrimal Gland, Right W Lacrimal Gland, Left	0 Open 3 Percutaneous	Z No Device	Z No Qualifier
N Upper Eyelid, Right P Upper Eyelid, Left Q Lower Eyelid, Right R Lower Eyelid, Left	0 Open 3 Percutaneous X External	Z No Device	Z No Qualifier

08N Continued on next page

Ø8N Continued

Ø Medical and Surgical
8 Eye
N Release Freeing a body part from an abnormal physical constraint

Body Part Character 4	Approach Character 5	Device Character 6	Qualifier Character 7
X Lacrimal Duct, Right **Y** Lacrimal Duct, Left	**Ø** Open **3** Percutaneous **7** Via Natural or Artificial Opening **8** Via Natural or Artificial Opening Endoscopic	**Z** No Device	**Z** No Qualifier

Ø Medical and Surgical
8 Eye
P Removal Taking out or off a device from a body part

Body Part Character 4	Approach Character 5	Device Character 6	Qualifier Character 7
Ø Eye, Right **1** Eye, Left	**Ø** Open **3** Percutaneous **7** Via Natural or Artificial Opening **8** Via Natural or Artificial Opening Endoscopic **X** External	**Ø** Drainage Device **1** Radioactive Element **3** Infusion Device **7** Autologous Tissue Substitute **C** Extraluminal Device **D** Intraluminal Device **J** Synthetic Substitute **K** Nonautologous Tissue Substitute	**Z** No Qualifier
J Lens, Right **K** Lens, Left	**3** Percutaneous	**J** Synthetic Substitute	**Z** No Qualifier
L Extraocular Muscle, Right **M** Extraocular Muscle, Left	**Ø** Open **3** Percutaneous	**Ø** Drainage Device **7** Autologous Tissue Substitute **J** Synthetic Substitute **K** Nonautologous Tissue Substitute	**Z** No Qualifier

Ø Medical and Surgical
8 Eye
Q Repair Restoring, to the extent possible, a body part to its normal anatomic structure and function

Body Part Character 4	Approach Character 5	Device Character 6	Qualifier Character 7
Ø Eye, Right **1** Eye, Left **6** Sclera, Right **7** Sclera, Left **8** Cornea, Right **9** Cornea, Left **S** Conjunctiva, Right **T** Conjunctiva, Left	**X** External	**Z** No Device	**Z** No Qualifier
2 Anterior Chamber, Right **3** Anterior Chamber, Left **4** Vitreous, Right **5** Vitreous, Left **C** Iris, Right **D** Iris, Left **E** Retina, Right **F** Retina, Left **G** Retinal Vessel, Right **H** Retinal Vessel, Left **J** Lens, Right **K** Lens, Left	**3** Percutaneous	**Z** No Device	**Z** No Qualifier
A Choroid, Right **B** Choroid, Left **L** Extraocular Muscle, Right **M** Extraocular Muscle, Left **V** Lacrimal Gland, Right **W** Lacrimal Gland, Left	**Ø** Open **3** Percutaneous	**Z** No Device	**Z** No Qualifier
N Upper Eyelid, Right **P** Upper Eyelid, Left **Q** Lower Eyelid, Right **R** Lower Eyelid, Left	**Ø** Open **3** Percutaneous **X** External	**Z** No Device	**Z** No Qualifier
X Lacrimal Duct, Right **Y** Lacrimal Duct, Left	**Ø** Open **3** Percutaneous **7** Via Natural or Artificial Opening **8** Via Natural or Artificial Opening Endoscopic	**Z** No Device	**Z** No Qualifier

Ø Medical and Surgical
8 Eye
R Replacement Putting in or on biological or synthetic material that physically takes the place and/or function of all or a portion of a body part

Body Part Character 4	Approach Character 5	Device Character 6	Qualifier Character 7
Ø Eye, Right **1** Eye, Left **A** Choroid, Right **B** Choroid, Left	**Ø** Open **3** Percutaneous	**7** Autologous Tissue Substitute **J** Synthetic Substitute **K** Nonautologous Tissue Substitute	**Z** No Qualifier
4 Vitreous, Right **5** Vitreous, Left **C** Iris, Right **D** Iris, Left **G** Retinal Vessel, Right **H** Retinal Vessel, Left	**3** Percutaneous	**7** Autologous Tissue Substitute **J** Synthetic Substitute **K** Nonautologous Tissue Substitute	**Z** No Qualifier
6 Sclera, Right **7** Sclera, Left **S** Conjunctiva, Right **T** Conjunctiva, Left	**X** External	**7** Autologous Tissue Substitute **J** Synthetic Substitute **K** Nonautologous Tissue Substitute	**Z** No Qualifier
8 Cornea, Right **9** Cornea, Left	**3** Percutaneous **X** External	**7** Autologous Tissue Substitute **J** Synthetic Substitute **K** Nonautologous Tissue Substitute	**Z** No Qualifier
J Lens, Right **K** Lens, Left	**3** Percutaneous	**Ø** **Synthetic Substitute, Intraocular Telescope** **7** Autologous Tissue Substitute **J** Synthetic Substitute **K** Nonautologous Tissue Substitute	**Z** No Qualifier
N Upper Eyelid, Right **P** Upper Eyelid, Left **Q** Lower Eyelid, Right **R** Lower Eyelid, Left	**Ø** Open **3** Percutaneous **X** External	**7** Autologous Tissue Substitute **J** Synthetic Substitute **K** Nonautologous Tissue Substitute	**Z** No Qualifier
X Lacrimal Duct, Right **Y** Lacrimal Duct, Left	**Ø** Open **3** Percutaneous **7** Via Natural or Artificial Opening **8** Via Natural or Artificial Opening Endoscopic	**7** Autologous Tissue Substitute **J** Synthetic Substitute **K** Nonautologous Tissue Substitute	**Z** No Qualifier

Ø Medical and Surgical
8 Eye
S Reposition Moving to its normal location or other suitable location all or a portion of a body part

Body Part Character 4	Approach Character 5	Device Character 6	Qualifier Character 7
C Iris, Right **D** Iris, Left **G** Retinal Vessel, Right **H** Retinal Vessel, Left **J** Lens, Right **K** Lens, Left	**3** Percutaneous	**Z** No Device	**Z** No Qualifier
L Extraocular Muscle, Right **M** Extraocular Muscle, Left **V** Lacrimal Gland, Right **W** Lacrimal Gland, Left	**Ø** Open **3** Percutaneous	**Z** No Device	**Z** No Qualifier
N Upper Eyelid, Right **P** Upper Eyelid, Left **Q** Lower Eyelid, Right **R** Lower Eyelid, Left	**Ø** Open **3** Percutaneous **X** External	**Z** No Device	**Z** No Qualifier
X Lacrimal Duct, Right **Y** Lacrimal Duct, Left	**Ø** Open **3** Percutaneous **7** Via Natural or Artificial Opening **8** Via Natural or Artificial Opening Endoscopic	**Z** No Device	**Z** No Qualifier

Ø Medical and Surgical
8 Eye
T Resection Cutting out or off, without replacement, all of a body part

Body Part Character 4	Approach Character 5	Device Character 6	Qualifier Character 7
Ø Eye, Right **1** Eye, Left **8** Cornea, Right **9** Cornea, Left	**X** External	**Z** No Device	**Z** No Qualifier
4 Vitreous, Right **5** Vitreous, Left **C** Iris, Right **D** Iris, Left **J** Lens, Right **K** Lens, Left	**3** Percutaneous	**Z** No Device	**Z** No Qualifier
L Extraocular Muscle, Right **M** Extraocular Muscle, Left **V** Lacrimal Gland, Right **W** Lacrimal Gland, Left	**Ø** Open **3** Percutaneous	**Z** No Device	**Z** No Qualifier
N Upper Eyelid, Right **P** Upper Eyelid, Left **Q** Lower Eyelid, Right **R** Lower Eyelid, Left	**Ø** Open **X** External	**Z** No Device	**Z** No Qualifier
X Lacrimal Duct, Right **Y** Lacrimal Duct, Left	**Ø** Open **3** Percutaneous **7** Via Natural or Artificial Opening **8** Via Natural or Artificial Opening Endoscopic	**Z** No Device	**Z** No Qualifier

Ø Medical and Surgical
8 Eye
U Supplement Putting in or on biological or synthetic material that physically reinforces and/or augments the function of a portion of a body part

Body Part Character 4	Approach Character 5	Device Character 6	Qualifier Character 7
Ø Eye, Right **1** Eye, Left **C** Iris, Right **D** Iris, Left **E** Retina, Right **F** Retina, Left **G** Retinal Vessel, Right **H** Retinal Vessel, Left **L** Extraocular Muscle, Right **M** Extraocular Muscle, Left	**Ø** Open **3** Percutaneous	**7** Autologous Tissue Substitute **J** Synthetic Substitute **K** Nonautologous Tissue Substitute	**Z** No Qualifier
8 Cornea, Right **9** Cornea, Left **N** Upper Eyelid, Right **P** Upper Eyelid, Left **Q** Lower Eyelid, Right **R** Lower Eyelid, Left	**Ø** Open **3** Percutaneous **X** External	**7** Autologous Tissue Substitute **J** Synthetic Substitute **K** Nonautologous Tissue Substitute	**Z** No Qualifier
X Lacrimal Duct, Right **Y** Lacrimal Duct, Left	**Ø** Open **3** Percutaneous **7** Via Natural or Artificial Opening **8** Via Natural or Artificial Opening Endoscopic	**7** Autologous Tissue Substitute **J** Synthetic Substitute **K** Nonautologous Tissue Substitute	**Z** No Qualifier

Ø Medical and Surgical
8 Eye
V Restriction Partially closing an orifice or the lumen of a tubular body part

Body Part Character 4	Approach Character 5	Device Character 6	Qualifier Character 7
X Lacrimal Duct, Right **Y** Lacrimal Duct, Left	**Ø** Open **3** Percutaneous	**C** Extraluminal Device **D** Intraluminal Device **Z** No Device	**Z** No Qualifier
X Lacrimal Duct, Right **Y** Lacrimal Duct, Left	**7** Via Natural or Artificial Opening **8** Via Natural or Artificial Opening Endoscopic	**D** Intraluminal Device **Z** No Device	**Z** No Qualifier

0 Medical and Surgical
8 Eye
W Revision Correcting, to the extent possible, a portion of a malfunctioning device or the position of a displaced device

Body Part Character 4	Approach Character 5	Device Character 6	Qualifier Character 7
0 Eye, Right **1** Eye, Left	**0** Open **3** Percutaneous **7** Via Natural or Artificial Opening **8** Via Natural or Artificial Opening Endoscopic **X** External	**0** Drainage Device **3** Infusion Device **7** Autologous Tissue Substitute **C** Extraluminal Device **D** Intraluminal Device **J** Synthetic Substitute **K** Nonautologous Tissue Substitute	**Z** No Qualifier
J Lens, Right **K** Lens, Left	**3** Percutaneous **X** External	**J** Synthetic Substitute	**Z** No Qualifier
L Extraocular Muscle, Right **M** Extraocular Muscle, Left	**0** Open **3** Percutaneous	**0** Drainage Device **7** Autologous Tissue Substitute **J** Synthetic Substitute **K** Nonautologous Tissue Substitute	**Z** No Qualifier

0 Medical and Surgical
8 Eye
X Transfer Moving, without taking out, all or a portion of a body part to another location to take over the function of all or a portion of a body part

Body Part Character 4	Approach Character 5	Device Character 6	Qualifier Character 7
L Extraocular Muscle, Right **M** Extraocular Muscle, Left	**0** Open **3** Percutaneous	**Z** No Device	**Z** No Qualifier

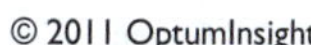

Ear, Nose, Sinus Ø9Ø–Ø9W

Ø Medical and Surgical
9 Ear, Nose, Sinus
Ø Alteration Modifying the anatomic structure of a body part without affecting the function of the body part

Body Part Character 4	Approach Character 5	Device Character 6	Qualifier Character 7
Ø External Ear, Right **1** External Ear, Left **2** External Ear, Bilateral **K** Nose	**Ø** Open **3** Percutaneous **4** Percutaneous Endoscopic **X** External	**7** Autologous Tissue Substitute **J** Synthetic Substitute **K** Nonautologous Tissue Substitute **Z** No Device	**Z** No Qualifier

Ø Medical and Surgical
9 Ear, Nose, Sinus
1 Bypass Altering the route of passage of the contents of a tubular body part

Body Part Character 4	Approach Character 5	Device Character 6	Qualifier Character 7
D Inner Ear, Right **E** Inner Ear, Left	**Ø** Open	**7** Autologous Tissue Substitute **J** Synthetic Substitute **K** Nonautologous Tissue Substitute **Z** No Device	**Ø** Endolymphatic

Ø Medical and Surgical
9 Ear, Nose, Sinus
2 Change Taking out or off a device from a body part and putting back an identical or similar device in or on the same body part without cutting or puncturing the skin or a mucous membrane

Body Part Character 4	Approach Character 5	Device Character 6	Qualifier Character 7
H Ear, Right **J** Ear, Left **K** Nose **Y** Sinus	**X** External	**Ø** Drainage Device **Y** Other Device	**Z** No Qualifier

Ø Medical and Surgical
9 Ear, Nose, Sinus
5 Destruction Physical eradication of all or a portion of a body part by the direct use of energy, force, or a destructive agent

Body Part Character 4	Approach Character 5	Device Character 6	Qualifier Character 7
Ø External Ear, Right **1** External Ear, Left **K** Nose	**Ø** Open **3** Percutaneous **4** Percutaneous Endoscopic **X** External	**Z** No Device	**Z** No Qualifier
3 External Auditory Canal, Right **4** External Auditory Canal, Left	**Ø** Open **3** Percutaneous **4** Percutaneous Endoscopic **7** Via Natural or Artificial Opening **8** Via Natural or Artificial Opening Endoscopic **X** External	**Z** No Device	**Z** No Qualifier
5 Middle Ear, Right **6** Middle Ear, Left **9** Auditory Ossicle, Right **A** Auditory Ossicle, Left **D** Inner Ear, Right **E** Inner Ear, Left	**Ø** Open	**Z** No Device	**Z** No Qualifier
7 Tympanic Membrane, Right **8** Tympanic Membrane, Left **F** Eustachian Tube, Right **G** Eustachian Tube, Left **L** Nasal Turbinate **N** Nasopharynx	**Ø** Open **3** Percutaneous **4** Percutaneous Endoscopic **7** Via Natural or Artificial Opening **8** Via Natural or Artificial Opening Endoscopic	**Z** No Device	**Z** No Qualifier

Ø95 Continued on next page

095 Continued

0 Medical and Surgical
9 Ear, Nose, Sinus
5 Destruction Physical eradication of all or a portion of a body part by the direct use of energy, force, or a destructive agent

Body Part Character 4	Approach Character 5	Device Character 6	Qualifier Character 7
B Mastoid Sinus, Right C Mastoid Sinus, Left M Nasal Septum P Accessory Sinus Q Maxillary Sinus, Right R Maxillary Sinus, Left S Frontal Sinus, Right T Frontal Sinus, Left U Ethmoid Sinus, Right V Ethmoid Sinus, Left W Sphenoid Sinus, Right X Sphenoid Sinus, Left	0 Open 3 Percutaneous 4 Percutaneous Endoscopic	Z No Device	Z No Qualifier

0 Medical and Surgical
9 Ear, Nose, Sinus
7 Dilation Expanding an orifice or the lumen of a tubular body part

Body Part Character 4	Approach Character 5	Device Character 6	Qualifier Character 7
F Eustachian Tube, Right G Eustachian Tube, Left	0 Open 7 Via Natural or Artificial Opening 8 Via Natural or Artificial Opening Endoscopic	D Intraluminal Device Z No Device	Z No Qualifier
F Eustachian Tube, Right G Eustachian Tube, Left	3 Percutaneous 4 Percutaneous Endoscopic	Z No Device	Z No Qualifier

0 Medical and Surgical
9 Ear, Nose, Sinus
8 Division Cutting into a body part without draining fluids and/or gases from the body part in order to separate or transect a body part

Body Part Character 4	Approach Character 5	Device Character 6	Qualifier Character 7
L Nasal Turbinate	0 Open 3 Percutaneous 4 Percutaneous Endoscopic 7 Via Natural or Artificial Opening 8 Via Natural or Artificial Opening Endoscopic	Z No Device	Z No Qualifier

0 Medical and Surgical
9 Ear, Nose, Sinus
9 Drainage Taking or letting out fluids and/or gases from a body part

Body Part Character 4	Approach Character 5	Device Character 6	Qualifier Character 7
0 External Ear, Right 1 External Ear, Left K Nose	0 Open 3 Percutaneous 4 Percutaneous Endoscopic X External	0 Drainage Device	Z No Qualifier
0 External Ear, Right 1 External Ear, Left K Nose	0 Open 3 Percutaneous 4 Percutaneous Endoscopic X External	Z No Device	X Diagnostic Z No Qualifier
3 External Auditory Canal, Right 4 External Auditory Canal, Left	0 Open 3 Percutaneous 4 Percutaneous Endoscopic 7 Via Natural or Artificial Opening 8 Via Natural or Artificial Opening Endoscopic X External	0 Drainage Device	Z No Qualifier
3 External Auditory Canal, Right 4 External Auditory Canal, Left	0 Open 3 Percutaneous 4 Percutaneous Endoscopic 7 Via Natural or Artificial Opening 8 Via Natural or Artificial Opening Endoscopic X External	Z No Device	X Diagnostic Z No Qualifier

099 Continued on next page

Ø Medical and Surgical
9 Ear, Nose, Sinus
9 Drainage Taking or letting out fluids and/or gases from a body part

Ø99 Continued

Body Part Character 4	Approach Character 5	Device Character 6	Qualifier Character 7
5 Middle Ear, Right **6** Middle Ear, Left **9** Auditory Ossicle, Right **A** Auditory Ossicle, Left **D** Inner Ear, Right **E** Inner Ear, Left	**Ø** Open	**Ø** Drainage Device	**Z** No Qualifier
5 Middle Ear, Right **6** Middle Ear, Left **9** Auditory Ossicle, Right **A** Auditory Ossicle, Left **D** Inner Ear, Right **E** Inner Ear, Left	**Ø** Open	**Z** No Device	**X** Diagnostic **Z** No Qualifier
7 Tympanic Membrane, Right **8** Tympanic Membrane, Left **F** Eustachian Tube, Right **G** Eustachian Tube, Left **L** Nasal Turbinate **N** Nasopharynx	**Ø** Open **3** Percutaneous **4** Percutaneous Endoscopic **7** Via Natural or Artificial Opening **8** Via Natural or Artificial Opening Endoscopic	**Ø** Drainage Device	**Z** No Qualifier
7 Tympanic Membrane, Right **8** Tympanic Membrane, Left **F** Eustachian Tube, Right **G** Eustachian Tube, Left **L** Nasal Turbinate **N** Nasopharynx	**Ø** Open **3** Percutaneous **4** Percutaneous Endoscopic **7** Via Natural or Artificial Opening **8** Via Natural or Artificial Opening Endoscopic	**Z** No Device	**X** Diagnostic **Z** No Qualifier
B Mastoid Sinus, Right **C** Mastoid Sinus, Left **M** Nasal Septum **P** Accessory Sinus **Q** Maxillary Sinus, Right **R** Maxillary Sinus, Left **S** Frontal Sinus, Right **T** Frontal Sinus, Left **U** Ethmoid Sinus, Right **V** Ethmoid Sinus, Left **W** Sphenoid Sinus, Right **X** Sphenoid Sinus, Left	**Ø** Open **3** Percutaneous **4** Percutaneous Endoscopic	**Ø** Drainage Device	**Z** No Qualifier
B Mastoid Sinus, Right **C** Mastoid Sinus, Left **M** Nasal Septum **P** Accessory Sinus **Q** Maxillary Sinus, Right **R** Maxillary Sinus, Left **S** Frontal Sinus, Right **T** Frontal Sinus, Left **U** Ethmoid Sinus, Right **V** Ethmoid Sinus, Left **W** Sphenoid Sinus, Right **X** Sphenoid Sinus, Left	**Ø** Open **3** Percutaneous **4** Percutaneous Endoscopic	**Z** No Device	**X** Diagnostic **Z** No Qualifier

Ø Medical and Surgical
9 Ear, Nose, Sinus
B Excision Cutting out or off, without replacement, a portion of a body part

Body Part Character 4	Approach Character 5	Device Character 6	Qualifier Character 7
Ø External Ear, Right **1** External Ear, Left **K** Nose	**Ø** Open **3** Percutaneous **4** Percutaneous Endoscopic **X** External	**Z** No Device	**X** Diagnostic **Z** No Qualifier
3 External Auditory Canal, Right **4** External Auditory Canal, Left	**Ø** Open **3** Percutaneous **4** Percutaneous Endoscopic **7** Via Natural or Artificial Opening **8** Via Natural or Artificial Opening Endoscopic **X** External	**Z** No Device	**X** Diagnostic **Z** No Qualifier
5 Middle Ear, Right **6** Middle Ear, Left **9** Auditory Ossicle, Right **A** Auditory Ossicle, Left **D** Inner Ear, Right **E** Inner Ear, Left	**Ø** Open	**Z** No Device	**X** Diagnostic **Z** No Qualifier

Ø9B Continued on next page

0 Medical and Surgical
9 Ear, Nose, Sinus
B Excision Cutting out or off, without replacement, a portion of a body part

09B Continued

Body Part Character 4	Approach Character 5	Device Character 6	Qualifier Character 7
7 Tympanic Membrane, Right **8** Tympanic Membrane, Left **F** Eustachian Tube, Right **G** Eustachian Tube, Left **L** Nasal Turbinate **N** Nasopharynx	**0** Open **3** Percutaneous **4** Percutaneous Endoscopic **7** Via Natural or Artificial Opening **8** Via Natural or Artificial Opening Endoscopic	**Z** No Device	**X** Diagnostic **Z** No Qualifier
B Mastoid Sinus, Right **C** Mastoid Sinus, Left **M** Nasal Septum **P** Accessory Sinus **Q** Maxillary Sinus, Right **R** Maxillary Sinus, Left **S** Frontal Sinus, Right **T** Frontal Sinus, Left **U** Ethmoid Sinus, Right **V** Ethmoid Sinus, Left **W** Sphenoid Sinus, Right **X** Sphenoid Sinus, Left	**0** Open **3** Percutaneous **4** Percutaneous Endoscopic	**Z** No Device	**X** Diagnostic **Z** No Qualifier

0 Medical and Surgical
9 Ear, Nose, Sinus
C Extirpation Taking or cutting out solid matter from a body part

Body Part Character 4	Approach Character 5	Device Character 6	Qualifier Character 7
0 External Ear, Right **1** External Ear, Left **K** Nose	**0** Open **3** Percutaneous **4** Percutaneous Endoscopic **X** External	**Z** No Device	**Z** No Qualifier
3 External Auditory Canal, Right **4** External Auditory Canal, Left	**0** Open **3** Percutaneous **4** Percutaneous Endoscopic **7** Via Natural or Artificial Opening **8** Via Natural or Artificial Opening Endoscopic **X** External	**Z** No Device	**Z** No Qualifier
5 Middle Ear, Right **6** Middle Ear, Left **9** Auditory Ossicle, Right **A** Auditory Ossicle, Left **D** Inner Ear, Right **E** Inner Ear, Left	**0** Open	**Z** No Device	**Z** No Qualifier
7 Tympanic Membrane, Right **8** Tympanic Membrane, Left **F** Eustachian Tube, Right **G** Eustachian Tube, Left **L** Nasal Turbinate **N** Nasopharynx	**0** Open **3** Percutaneous **4** Percutaneous Endoscopic **7** Via Natural or Artificial Opening **8** Via Natural or Artificial Opening Endoscopic	**Z** No Device	**Z** No Qualifier
B Mastoid Sinus, Right **C** Mastoid Sinus, Left **M** Nasal Septum **P** Accessory Sinus **Q** Maxillary Sinus, Right **R** Maxillary Sinus, Left **S** Frontal Sinus, Right **T** Frontal Sinus, Left **U** Ethmoid Sinus, Right **V** Ethmoid Sinus, Left **W** Sphenoid Sinus, Right **X** Sphenoid Sinus, Left	**0** Open **3** Percutaneous **4** Percutaneous Endoscopic	**Z** No Device	**Z** No Qualifier

Ø Medical and Surgical
9 Ear, Nose, Sinus
D Extraction Pulling or stripping out or off all or a portion of a body part by the use of force

Body Part Character 4	Approach Character 5	Device Character 6	Qualifier Character 7
7 Tympanic Membrane, Right 8 Tympanic Membrane, Left L Nasal Turbinate	Ø Open 3 Percutaneous 4 Percutaneous Endoscopic 7 Via Natural or Artificial Opening 8 Via Natural or Artificial Opening Endoscopic	Z No Device	Z No Qualifier
9 Auditory Ossicle, Right A Auditory Ossicle, Left	Ø Open	Z No Device	Z No Qualifier
B Mastoid Sinus, Right C Mastoid Sinus, Left M Nasal Septum P Accessory Sinus Q Maxillary Sinus, Right R Maxillary Sinus, Left S Frontal Sinus, Right T Frontal Sinus, Left U Ethmoid Sinus, Right V Ethmoid Sinus, Left W Sphenoid Sinus, Right X Sphenoid Sinus, Left	Ø Open 3 Percutaneous 4 Percutaneous Endoscopic	Z No Device	Z No Qualifier

Ø Medical and Surgical
9 Ear, Nose, Sinus
H Insertion Putting in a nonbiological appliance that monitors, assists, performs, or prevents a physiological function but does not physically take the place of a body part

Body Part Character 4	Approach Character 5	Device Character 6	Qualifier Character 7
D Inner Ear, Right E Inner Ear, Left	Ø Open 3 **Percutaneous** 4 **Percutaneous Endoscopic**	4 **Hearing Device, Bone Conduction** 5 **Hearing Device, Single Channel Cochlear Prosthesis** 6 **Hearing Device, Multiple Channel Cochlear Prosthesis** S **Hearing Device**	Z No Qualifier
N Nasopharynx	7 Via Natural or Artificial Opening 8 Via Natural or Artificial Opening Endoscopic	B **Intraluminal Device, Airway**	Z No Qualifier

Ø Medical and Surgical
9 Ear, Nose, Sinus
J Inspection Visually and/or manually exploring a body part

Body Part Character 4	Approach Character 5	Device Character 6	Qualifier Character 7
7 Tympanic Membrane, Right 8 Tympanic Membrane, Left H Ear, Right J Ear, Left	Ø Open 3 Percutaneous 4 Percutaneous Endoscopic 7 Via Natural or Artificial Opening 8 Via Natural or Artificial Opening Endoscopic X External	Z No Device	Z No Qualifier
D Inner Ear, Right E Inner Ear, Left K Nose Y Sinus	Ø Open 3 Percutaneous 4 Percutaneous Endoscopic X External	Z No Device	Z No Qualifier

Ø Medical and Surgical
9 Ear, Nose, Sinus
M Reattachment Putting back in or on all or a portion of a separated body part to its normal location or other suitable location

Body Part Character 4	Approach Character 5	Device Character 6	Qualifier Character 7
Ø External Ear, Right 1 External Ear, Left K Nose	X External	Z No Device	Z No Qualifier

0 Medical and Surgical
9 Ear, Nose, Sinus
N Release Freeing a body part from an abnormal physical constraint

Body Part Character 4	Approach Character 5	Device Character 6	Qualifier Character 7
0 External Ear, Right 1 External Ear, Left K Nose	0 Open 3 Percutaneous 4 Percutaneous Endoscopic X External	Z No Device	Z No Qualifier
3 External Auditory Canal, Right 4 External Auditory Canal, Left	0 Open 3 Percutaneous 4 Percutaneous Endoscopic 7 Via Natural or Artificial Opening 8 Via Natural or Artificial Opening Endoscopic X External	Z No Device	Z No Qualifier
5 Middle Ear, Right 6 Middle Ear, Left 9 Auditory Ossicle, Right A Auditory Ossicle, Left D Inner Ear, Right E Inner Ear, Left	0 Open	Z No Device	Z No Qualifier
7 Tympanic Membrane, Right 8 Tympanic Membrane, Left F Eustachian Tube, Right G Eustachian Tube, Left L Nasal Turbinate N Nasopharynx	0 Open 3 Percutaneous 4 Percutaneous Endoscopic 7 Via Natural or Artificial Opening 8 Via Natural or Artificial Opening Endoscopic	Z No Device	Z No Qualifier
B Mastoid Sinus, Right C Mastoid Sinus, Left M Nasal Septum P Accessory Sinus Q Maxillary Sinus, Right R Maxillary Sinus, Left S Frontal Sinus, Right T Frontal Sinus, Left U Ethmoid Sinus, Right V Ethmoid Sinus, Left W Sphenoid Sinus, Right X Sphenoid Sinus, Left	0 Open 3 Percutaneous 4 Percutaneous Endoscopic	Z No Device	Z No Qualifier

0 Medical and Surgical
9 Ear, Nose, Sinus
P Removal Taking out or off a device from a body part

Body Part Character 4	Approach Character 5	Device Character 6	Qualifier Character 7
7 Tympanic Membrane, Right 8 Tympanic Membrane, Left	0 Open 7 Via Natural or Artificial Opening 8 Via Natural or Artificial Opening Endoscopic X External	0 Drainage Device	Z No Qualifier
D Inner Ear, Right E Inner Ear, Left	0 Open 7 Via Natural or Artificial Opening 8 Via Natural or Artificial Opening Endoscopic	S Hearing Device	Z No Qualifier
H Ear, Right J Ear, Left K Nose	0 Open 3 Percutaneous 4 Percutaneous Endoscopic 7 Via Natural or Artificial Opening 8 Via Natural or Artificial Opening Endoscopic X External	0 Drainage Device 7 Autologous Tissue Substitute D Intraluminal Device J Synthetic Substitute K Nonautologous Tissue Substitute	Z No Qualifier
Y Sinus	0 Open 3 Percutaneous 4 Percutaneous Endoscopic X External	0 Drainage Device	Z No Qualifier

0 Medical and Surgical
9 Ear, Nose, Sinus
Q Repair Restoring, to the extent possible, a body part to its normal anatomic structure and function

Body Part Character 4	Approach Character 5	Device Character 6	Qualifier Character 7
0 External Ear, Right **1** External Ear, Left **2** External Ear, Bilateral **K** Nose	**0** Open **3** Percutaneous **4** Percutaneous Endoscopic **X** External	**Z** No Device	**Z** No Qualifier
3 External Auditory Canal, Right **4** External Auditory Canal, Left **F** Eustachian Tube, Right **G** Eustachian Tube, Left	**0** Open **3** Percutaneous **4** Percutaneous Endoscopic **7** Via Natural or Artificial Opening **8** Via Natural or Artificial Opening Endoscopic **X** External	**Z** No Device	**Z** No Qualifier
5 Middle Ear, Right **6** Middle Ear, Left **9** Auditory Ossicle, Right **A** Auditory Ossicle, Left **D** Inner Ear, Right **E** Inner Ear, Left	**0** Open	**Z** No Device	**Z** No Qualifier
7 Tympanic Membrane, Right **8** Tympanic Membrane, Left **L** Nasal Turbinate **N** Nasopharynx	**0** Open **3** Percutaneous **4** Percutaneous Endoscopic **7** Via Natural or Artificial Opening **8** Via Natural or Artificial Opening Endoscopic	**Z** No Device	**Z** No Qualifier
B Mastoid Sinus, Right **C** Mastoid Sinus, Left **M** Nasal Septum **P** Accessory Sinus **Q** Maxillary Sinus, Right **R** Maxillary Sinus, Left **S** Frontal Sinus, Right **T** Frontal Sinus, Left **U** Ethmoid Sinus, Right **V** Ethmoid Sinus, Left **W** Sphenoid Sinus, Right **X** Sphenoid Sinus, Left	**0** Open **3** Percutaneous **4** Percutaneous Endoscopic	**Z** No Device	**Z** No Qualifier

0 Medical and Surgical
9 Ear, Nose, Sinus
R Replacement Putting in or on biological or synthetic material that physically takes the place and/or function of all or a portion of a body part

Body Part Character 4	Approach Character 5	Device Character 6	Qualifier Character 7
0 External Ear, Right **1** External Ear, Left **2** External Ear, Bilateral **K** Nose	**0** Open **X** External	**7** Autologous Tissue Substitute **J** Synthetic Substitute **K** Nonautologous Tissue Substitute	**Z** No Qualifier
5 Middle Ear, Right **6** Middle Ear, Left **9** Auditory Ossicle, Right **A** Auditory Ossicle, Left **D** Inner Ear, Right **E** Inner Ear, Left	**0** Open	**7** Autologous Tissue Substitute **J** Synthetic Substitute **K** Nonautologous Tissue Substitute	**Z** No Qualifier
7 Tympanic Membrane, Right **8** Tympanic Membrane, Left **N** Nasopharynx	**0** Open **7** Via Natural or Artificial Opening **8** Via Natural or Artificial Opening Endoscopic	**7** Autologous Tissue Substitute **J** Synthetic Substitute **K** Nonautologous Tissue Substitute	**Z** No Qualifier
L Nasal Turbinate	**0** Open **3** Percutaneous **4** Percutaneous Endoscopic **7** Via Natural or Artificial Opening **8** Via Natural or Artificial Opening Endoscopic	**7** Autologous Tissue Substitute **J** Synthetic Substitute **K** Nonautologous Tissue Substitute	**Z** No Qualifier
M Nasal Septum	**0** Open **3** Percutaneous **4** Percutaneous Endoscopic	**7** Autologous Tissue Substitute **J** Synthetic Substitute **K** Nonautologous Tissue Substitute	**Z** No Qualifier

0 Medical and Surgical
9 Ear, Nose, Sinus
S Reposition Moving to its normal location or other suitable location all or a portion of a body part

Body Part Character 4	Approach Character 5	Device Character 6	Qualifier Character 7
0 External Ear, Right **1** External Ear, Left **2** External Ear, Bilateral **K** Nose	**0** Open **4** Percutaneous Endoscopic **X** External	**Z** No Device	**Z** No Qualifier
7 Tympanic Membrane, Right **8** Tympanic Membrane, Left **F** Eustachian Tube, Right **G** Eustachian Tube, Left **L** Nasal Turbinate	**0** Open **4** Percutaneous Endoscopic **7** Via Natural or Artificial Opening **8** Via Natural or Artificial Opening Endoscopic	**Z** No Device	**Z** No Qualifier
9 Auditory Ossicle, Right **A** Auditory Ossicle, Left **M** Nasal Septum	**0** Open **4** Percutaneous Endoscopic	**Z** No Device	**Z** No Qualifier

0 Medical and Surgical
9 Ear, Nose, Sinus
T Resection Cutting out or off, without replacement, all of a body part

Body Part Character 4	Approach Character 5	Device Character 6	Qualifier Character 7
0 External Ear, Right **1** External Ear, Left **K** Nose	**0** Open **4** Percutaneous Endoscopic **X** External	**Z** No Device	**Z** No Qualifier
5 Middle Ear, Right **6** Middle Ear, Left **9** Auditory Ossicle, Right **A** Auditory Ossicle, Left **D** Inner Ear, Right **E** Inner Ear, Left	**0** Open	**Z** No Device	**Z** No Qualifier
7 Tympanic Membrane, Right **8** Tympanic Membrane, Left **F** Eustachian Tube, Right **G** Eustachian Tube, Left **L** Nasal Turbinate **N** Nasopharynx	**0** Open **4** Percutaneous Endoscopic **7** Via Natural or Artificial Opening **8** Via Natural or Artificial Opening Endoscopic	**Z** No Device	**Z** No Qualifier
B Mastoid Sinus, Right **C** Mastoid Sinus, Left **M** Nasal Septum **P** Accessory Sinus **Q** Maxillary Sinus, Right **R** Maxillary Sinus, Left **S** Frontal Sinus, Right **T** Frontal Sinus, Left **U** Ethmoid Sinus, Right **V** Ethmoid Sinus, Left **W** Sphenoid Sinus, Right **X** Sphenoid Sinus, Left	**0** Open **4** Percutaneous Endoscopic	**Z** No Device	**Z** No Qualifier

Ø Medical and Surgical
9 Ear, Nose, Sinus
U Supplement Putting in or on biological or synthetic material that physically reinforces and/or augments the function of a portion of a body part

Body Part Character 4	Approach Character 5	Device Character 6	Qualifier Character 7
Ø External Ear, Right **1** External Ear, Left **2** External Ear, Bilateral **K** Nose	**Ø** Open **X** External	**7** Autologous Tissue Substitute **J** Synthetic Substitute **K** Nonautologous Tissue Substitute	**Z** No Qualifier
5 Middle Ear, Right **6** Middle Ear, Left **9** Auditory Ossicle, Right **A** Auditory Ossicle, Left **D** Inner Ear, Right **E** Inner Ear, Left	**Ø** Open	**7** Autologous Tissue Substitute **J** Synthetic Substitute **K** Nonautologous Tissue Substitute	**Z** No Qualifier
7 Tympanic Membrane, Right **8** Tympanic Membrane, Left **N** Nasopharynx	**Ø** Open **7** Via Natural or Artificial Opening **8** Via Natural or Artificial Opening Endoscopic	**7** Autologous Tissue Substitute **J** Synthetic Substitute **K** Nonautologous Tissue Substitute	**Z** No Qualifier
L Nasal Turbinate	**Ø** Open **3** Percutaneous **4** Percutaneous Endoscopic **7** Via Natural or Artificial Opening **8** Via Natural or Artificial Opening Endoscopic	**7** Autologous Tissue Substitute **J** Synthetic Substitute **K** Nonautologous Tissue Substitute	**Z** No Qualifier
M Nasal Septum	**Ø** Open **3** Percutaneous **4** Percutaneous Endoscopic	**7** Autologous Tissue Substitute **J** Synthetic Substitute **K** Nonautologous Tissue Substitute	**Z** No Qualifier

Ø Medical and Surgical
9 Ear, Nose, Sinus
W Revision Correcting, to the extent possible, a portion of a malfunctioning device or the position of a displaced device

Body Part Character 4	Approach Character 5	Device Character 6	Qualifier Character 7
7 Tympanic Membrane, Right **8** Tympanic Membrane, Left **9** Auditory Ossicle, Right **A** Auditory Ossicle, Left	**Ø** Open **7** Via Natural or Artificial Opening **8** Via Natural or Artificial Opening Endoscopic	**7** Autologous Tissue Substitute **J** Synthetic Substitute **K** Nonautologous Tissue Substitute	**Z** No Qualifier
D Inner Ear, Right **E** Inner Ear, Left	**Ø** Open **7** Via Natural or Artificial Opening **8** Via Natural or Artificial Opening Endoscopic	**S** Hearing Device	**Z** No Qualifier
H Ear, Right **J** Ear, Left **K** Nose	**Ø** Open **3** Percutaneous **4** Percutaneous Endoscopic **7** Via Natural or Artificial Opening **8** Via Natural or Artificial Opening Endoscopic **X** External	**Ø** Drainage Device **7** Autologous Tissue Substitute **D** Intraluminal Device **J** Synthetic Substitute **K** Nonautologous Tissue Substitute	**Z** No Qualifier
Y Sinus	**Ø** Open **3** Percutaneous **4** Percutaneous Endoscopic **X** External	**Ø** Drainage Device	**Z** No Qualifier

Respiratory System 0B1–0BY

0 Medical and Surgical
B Respiratory System
1 Bypass Altering the route of passage of the contents of a tubular body part

Body Part Character 4	Approach Character 5	Device Character 6	Qualifier Character 7
1 Trachea	**0** Open	**D** Intraluminal Device	**6** Esophagus
1 Trachea	**0** Open **3** Percutaneous **4** Percutaneous Endoscopic	**F** Tracheostomy Device **Z** No Device	**4** Cutaneous

0 Medical and Surgical
B Respiratory System
2 Change Taking out or off a device from a body part and putting back an identical or similar device in or on the same body part without cutting or puncturing the skin or a mucous membrane

Body Part Character 4	Approach Character 5	Device Character 6	Qualifier Character 7
0 Tracheobronchial Tree **K** Lung, Right **L** Lung, Left **Q** Pleura **T** Diaphragm	**X** External	**0** Drainage Device **Y** Other Device	**Z** No Qualifier
1 Trachea	**X** External	**0** Drainage Device **E** Intraluminal Device, Endotracheal Airway **F** Tracheostomy Device **Y** Other Device	**Z** No Qualifier

0 Medical and Surgical
B Respiratory System
5 Destruction Physical eradication of all or a portion of a body part by the direct use of energy, force, or a destructive agent

Body Part Character 4	Approach Character 5	Device Character 6	Qualifier Character 7
1 Trachea **2** Carina **3** Main Bronchus, Right **4** Upper Lobe Bronchus, Right **5** Middle Lobe Bronchus, Right **6** Lower Lobe Bronchus, Right **7** Main Bronchus, Left **8** Upper Lobe Bronchus, Left **9** Lingula Bronchus **B** Lower Lobe Bronchus, Left **C** Upper Lung Lobe, Right **D** Middle Lung Lobe, Right **F** Lower Lung Lobe, Right **G** Upper Lung Lobe, Left **H** Lung Lingula **J** Lower Lung Lobe, Left **K** Lung, Right **L** Lung, Left **M** Lungs, Bilateral	**0** Open **3** Percutaneous **4** Percutaneous Endoscopic **7** Via Natural or Artificial Opening **8** Via Natural or Artificial Opening Endoscopic	**Z** No Device	**Z** No Qualifier
N Pleura, Right **P** Pleura, Left **R** Diaphragm, Right **S** Diaphragm, Left	**0** Open **3** Percutaneous **4** Percutaneous Endoscopic	**Z** No Device	**Z** No Qualifier

Ø Medical and Surgical
B Respiratory System
7 Dilation Expanding an orifice or the lumen of a tubular body part

Body Part Character 4	Approach Character 5	Device Character 6	Qualifier Character 7
1 Trachea **2** Carina **3** Main Bronchus, Right **4** Upper Lobe Bronchus, Right **5** Middle Lobe Bronchus, Right **6** Lower Lobe Bronchus, Right **7** Main Bronchus, Left **8** Upper Lobe Bronchus, Left **9** Lingula Bronchus **B** Lower Lobe Bronchus, Left	**Ø** Open **3** Percutaneous **4** Percutaneous Endoscopic **7** Via Natural or Artificial Opening **8** Via Natural or Artificial Opening Endoscopic	**D** Intraluminal Device **Z** No Device	**Z** No Qualifier

Ø Medical and Surgical
B Respiratory System
9 Drainage Taking or letting out fluids and/or gases from a body part

Body Part Character 4	Approach Character 5	Device Character 6	Qualifier Character 7
1 Trachea **2** Carina **3** Main Bronchus, Right **4** Upper Lobe Bronchus, Right **5** Middle Lobe Bronchus, Right **6** Lower Lobe Bronchus, Right **7** Main Bronchus, Left **8** Upper Lobe Bronchus, Left **9** Lingula Bronchus **B** Lower Lobe Bronchus, Left **C** Upper Lung Lobe, Right **D** Middle Lung Lobe, Right **F** Lower Lung Lobe, Right **G** Upper Lung Lobe, Left **H** Lung Lingula **J** Lower Lung Lobe, Left **K** Lung, Right **L** Lung, Left **M** Lungs, Bilateral	**Ø** Open **3** Percutaneous **4** Percutaneous Endoscopic **7** Via Natural or Artificial Opening **8** Via Natural or Artificial Opening Endoscopic	**Ø** Drainage Device	**Z** No Qualifier
1 Trachea **2** Carina **3** Main Bronchus, Right **4** Upper Lobe Bronchus, Right **5** Middle Lobe Bronchus, Right **6** Lower Lobe Bronchus, Right **7** Main Bronchus, Left **8** Upper Lobe Bronchus, Left **9** Lingula Bronchus **B** Lower Lobe Bronchus, Left **C** Upper Lung Lobe, Right **D** Middle Lung Lobe, Right **F** Lower Lung Lobe, Right **G** Upper Lung Lobe, Left **H** Lung Lingula **J** Lower Lung Lobe, Left **K** Lung, Right **L** Lung, Left **M** Lungs, Bilateral	**Ø** Open **3** Percutaneous **4** Percutaneous Endoscopic **7** Via Natural or Artificial Opening **8** Via Natural or Artificial Opening Endoscopic	**Z** No Device	**X** Diagnostic **Z** No Qualifier
N Pleura, Right **P** Pleura, Left **R** Diaphragm, Right **S** Diaphragm, Left	**Ø** Open **3** Percutaneous **4** Percutaneous Endoscopic	**Ø** Drainage Device	**Z** No Qualifier
N Pleura, Right **P** Pleura, Left **R** Diaphragm, Right **S** Diaphragm, Left	**Ø** Open **3** Percutaneous **4** Percutaneous Endoscopic	**Z** No Device	**X** Diagnostic **Z** No Qualifier

0 Medical and Surgical
B Respiratory System
B Excision Cutting out or off, without replacement, a portion of a body part

Body Part Character 4	Approach Character 5	Device Character 6	Qualifier Character 7
1 Trachea 2 Carina 3 Main Bronchus, Right 4 Upper Lobe Bronchus, Right 5 Middle Lobe Bronchus, Right 6 Lower Lobe Bronchus, Right 7 Main Bronchus, Left 8 Upper Lobe Bronchus, Left 9 Lingula Bronchus B Lower Lobe Bronchus, Left C Upper Lung Lobe, Right D Middle Lung Lobe, Right F Lower Lung Lobe, Right G Upper Lung Lobe, Left H Lung Lingula J Lower Lung Lobe, Left K Lung, Right L Lung, Left M Lungs, Bilateral	0 Open 3 Percutaneous 4 Percutaneous Endoscopic 7 Via Natural or Artificial Opening 8 Via Natural or Artificial Opening Endoscopic	Z No Device	X Diagnostic Z No Qualifier
N Pleura, Right P Pleura, Left R Diaphragm, Right S Diaphragm, Left	0 Open 3 Percutaneous 4 Percutaneous Endoscopic	Z No Device	X Diagnostic Z No Qualifier

0 Medical and Surgical
B Respiratory System
C Extirpation Taking or cutting out solid matter from a body part

Body Part Character 4	Approach Character 5	Device Character 6	Qualifier Character 7
1 Trachea 2 Carina 3 Main Bronchus, Right 4 Upper Lobe Bronchus, Right 5 Middle Lobe Bronchus, Right 6 Lower Lobe Bronchus, Right 7 Main Bronchus, Left 8 Upper Lobe Bronchus, Left 9 Lingula Bronchus B Lower Lobe Bronchus, Left C Upper Lung Lobe, Right D Middle Lung Lobe, Right F Lower Lung Lobe, Right G Upper Lung Lobe, Left H Lung Lingula J Lower Lung Lobe, Left K Lung, Right L Lung, Left M Lungs, Bilateral	0 Open 3 Percutaneous 4 Percutaneous Endoscopic 7 Via Natural or Artificial Opening 8 Via Natural or Artificial Opening Endoscopic	Z No Device	Z No Qualifier
N Pleura, Right P Pleura, Left R Diaphragm, Right S Diaphragm, Left	0 Open 3 Percutaneous 4 Percutaneous Endoscopic	Z No Device	Z No Qualifier

0 Medical and Surgical
B Respiratory System
D Extraction Pulling or stripping out or off all or a portion of a body part by the use of force

Body Part Character 4	Approach Character 5	Device Character 6	Qualifier Character 7
N Pleura, Right P Pleura, Left	0 Open 3 Percutaneous 4 Percutaneous Endoscopic	Z No Device	X Diagnostic Z No Qualifier

Ø Medical and Surgical
B Respiratory System
F Fragmentation Breaking solid matter in a body part into pieces

Body Part Character 4	Approach Character 5	Device Character 6	Qualifier Character 7
1 Trachea 2 Carina 3 Main Bronchus, Right 4 Upper Lobe Bronchus, Right 5 Middle Lobe Bronchus, Right 6 Lower Lobe Bronchus, Right 7 Main Bronchus, Left 8 Upper Lobe Bronchus, Left 9 Lingula Bronchus B Lower Lobe Bronchus, Left	Ø Open 3 Percutaneous 4 Percutaneous Endoscopic 7 Via Natural or Artificial Opening 8 Via Natural or Artificial Opening Endoscopic X External	Z No Device	Z No Qualifier

Ø Medical and Surgical
B Respiratory System
H Insertion Putting in a nonbiological appliance that monitors, assists, performs, or prevents a physiological function but does not physically take the place of a body part

Body Part Character 4	Approach Character 5	Device Character 6	Qualifier Character 7
Ø Tracheobronchial Tree	Ø Open 3 Percutaneous 4 Percutaneous Endoscopic 7 Via Natural or Artificial Opening 8 Via Natural or Artificial Opening Endoscopic	1 Radioactive Element 2 Monitoring Device 3 Infusion Device D Intraluminal Device	Z No Qualifier
1 Trachea	Ø Open	2 Monitoring Device D Intraluminal Device	Z No Qualifier
1 Trachea	3 Percutaneous	D Intraluminal Device **E Intraluminal Device, Endotracheal Airway**	Z No Qualifier
1 Trachea	4 Percutaneous Endoscopic	D Intraluminal Device	Z No Qualifier
1 Trachea	7 Via Natural or Artificial Opening 8 Via Natural or Artificial Opening Endoscopic	2 Monitoring Device D Intraluminal Device **E Intraluminal Device, Endotracheal Airway**	Z No Qualifier
3 Main Bronchus, Right 4 Upper Lobe Bronchus, Right 5 Middle Lobe Bronchus, Right 6 Lower Lobe Bronchus, Right 7 Main Bronchus, Left 8 Upper Lobe Bronchus, Left 9 Lingula Bronchus B Lower Lobe Bronchus, Left	Ø Open 3 Percutaneous 4 Percutaneous Endoscopic 7 Via Natural or Artificial Opening 8 Via Natural or Artificial Opening Endoscopic	G Endobronchial Valve	Z No Qualifier
K Lung, Right L Lung, Left	Ø Open 3 Percutaneous 4 Percutaneous Endoscopic 7 Via Natural or Artificial Opening 8 Via Natural or Artificial Opening Endoscopic	1 Radioactive Element 2 Monitoring Device 3 Infusion Device	Z No Qualifier
R Diaphragm, Right S Diaphragm, Left	Ø Open 3 Percutaneous 4 Percutaneous Endoscopic	2 Monitoring Device M Diaphragmatic Pacemaker Lead	Z No Qualifier

Ø Medical and Surgical
B Respiratory System
J Inspection Visually and/or manually exploring a body part

Body Part Character 4	Approach Character 5	Device Character 6	Qualifier Character 7
Ø Tracheobronchial Tree 1 Trachea K Lung, Right L Lung, Left Q Pleura T Diaphragm	Ø Open 3 Percutaneous 4 Percutaneous Endoscopic 7 Via Natural or Artificial Opening 8 Via Natural or Artificial Opening Endoscopic X External	Z No Device	Z No Qualifier

Ø Medical and Surgical
B Respiratory System
L Occlusion Completely closing an orifice or the lumen of a tubular body part

Body Part Character 4	Approach Character 5	Device Character 6	Qualifier Character 7
1 Trachea 2 Carina 3 Main Bronchus, Right 4 Upper Lobe Bronchus, Right 5 Middle Lobe Bronchus, Right 6 Lower Lobe Bronchus, Right 7 Main Bronchus, Left 8 Upper Lobe Bronchus, Left 9 Lingula Bronchus B Lower Lobe Bronchus, Left	Ø Open 3 Percutaneous 4 Percutaneous Endoscopic	C Extraluminal Device D Intraluminal Device Z No Device	Z No Qualifier
1 Trachea 2 Carina 3 Main Bronchus, Right 4 Upper Lobe Bronchus, Right 5 Middle Lobe Bronchus, Right 6 Lower Lobe Bronchus, Right 7 Main Bronchus, Left 8 Upper Lobe Bronchus, Left 9 Lingula Bronchus B Lower Lobe Bronchus, Left	7 Via Natural or Artificial Opening 8 Via Natural or Artificial Opening Endoscopic	D Intraluminal Device Z No Device	Z No Qualifier

Ø Medical and Surgical
B Respiratory System
M Reattachment Putting back in or on all or a portion of a separated body part to its normal location or other suitable location

Body Part Character 4	Approach Character 5	Device Character 6	Qualifier Character 7
1 Trachea 2 Carina 3 Main Bronchus, Right 4 Upper Lobe Bronchus, Right 5 Middle Lobe Bronchus, Right 6 Lower Lobe Bronchus, Right 7 Main Bronchus, Left 8 Upper Lobe Bronchus, Left 9 Lingula Bronchus B Lower Lobe Bronchus, Left C Upper Lung Lobe, Right D Middle Lung Lobe, Right F Lower Lung Lobe, Right G Upper Lung Lobe, Left H Lung Lingula J Lower Lung Lobe, Left K Lung, Right L Lung, Left R Diaphragm, Right S Diaphragm, Left	Ø Open	Z No Device	Z No Qualifier

Ø Medical and Surgical
B Respiratory System
N Release Freeing a body part from an abnormal physical constraint

Body Part Character 4	Approach Character 5	Device Character 6	Qualifier Character 7
1 Trachea 2 Carina 3 Main Bronchus, Right 4 Upper Lobe Bronchus, Right 5 Middle Lobe Bronchus, Right 6 Lower Lobe Bronchus, Right 7 Main Bronchus, Left 8 Upper Lobe Bronchus, Left 9 Lingula Bronchus B Lower Lobe Bronchus, Left C Upper Lung Lobe, Right D Middle Lung Lobe, Right F Lower Lung Lobe, Right G Upper Lung Lobe, Left H Lung Lingula J Lower Lung Lobe, Left K Lung, Right L Lung, Left M Lungs, Bilateral	Ø Open 3 Percutaneous 4 Percutaneous Endoscopic 7 Via Natural or Artificial Opening 8 Via Natural or Artificial Opening Endoscopic	Z No Device	Z No Qualifier

ØBN Continued on next page

ØBN Continued

Ø Medical and Surgical
B Respiratory System
N Release Freeing a body part from an abnormal physical constraint

Body Part Character 4	Approach Character 5	Device Character 6	Qualifier Character 7
N Pleura, Right **P** Pleura, Left **R** Diaphragm, Right **S** Diaphragm, Left	**Ø** Open **3** Percutaneous **4** Percutaneous Endoscopic	**Z** No Device	**Z** No Qualifier

Ø Medical and Surgical
B Respiratory System
P Removal Taking out or off a device from a body part

Body Part Character 4	Approach Character 5	Device Character 6	Qualifier Character 7
Ø Tracheobronchial Tree	**Ø** Open **3** Percutaneous **4** Percutaneous Endoscopic **7** Via Natural or Artificial Opening **8** Via Natural or Artificial Opening Endoscopic	**Ø** Drainage Device **1** Radioactive Element **2** Monitoring Device **3** Infusion Device **7** Autologous Tissue Substitute **C** Extraluminal Device **D** Intraluminal Device **J** Synthetic Substitute **K** Nonautologous Tissue Substitute	**Z** No Qualifier
Ø Tracheobronchial Tree	**X** External	**Ø** Drainage Device **1** Radioactive Element **2** Monitoring Device **3** Infusion Device **D** Intraluminal Device	**Z** No Qualifier
1 Trachea	**Ø** Open **3** Percutaneous **4** Percutaneous Endoscopic **7** Via Natural or Artificial Opening **8** Via Natural or Artificial Opening Endoscopic	**Ø** Drainage Device **2** Monitoring Device **7** Autologous Tissue Substitute **C** Extraluminal Device **D** Intraluminal Device **F** Tracheostomy Device **J** Synthetic Substitute **K** Nonautologous Tissue Substitute	**Z** No Qualifier
1 Trachea	**X** External	**Ø** Drainage Device **2** Monitoring Device **D** Intraluminal Device **F** Tracheostomy Device	**Z** No Qualifier
K Lung, Right **L** Lung, Left	**Ø** Open **3** Percutaneous **4** Percutaneous Endoscopic **7** Via Natural or Artificial Opening **8** Via Natural or Artificial Opening Endoscopic **X** External	**Ø** Drainage Device **1** Radioactive Element **2** Monitoring Device **3** Infusion Device	**Z** No Qualifier
Q Pleura	**Ø** Open **3** Percutaneous **4** Percutaneous Endoscopic **7** Via Natural or Artificial Opening **8** Via Natural or Artificial Opening Endoscopic **X** External	**Ø** Drainage Device **1** Radioactive Element **2** Monitoring Device	**Z** No Qualifier
T Diaphragm	**Ø** Open **3** Percutaneous **4** Percutaneous Endoscopic **7** Via Natural or Artificial Opening **8** Via Natural or Artificial Opening Endoscopic	**Ø** Drainage Device **2** Monitoring Device **7** Autologous Tissue Substitute **J** Synthetic Substitute **K** Nonautologous Tissue Substitute **M** Diaphragmatic Pacemaker Lead	**Z** No Qualifier
T Diaphragm	**X** External	**Ø** Drainage Device **2** Monitoring Device **M** Diaphragmatic Pacemaker Lead	**Z** No Qualifier

0 Medical and Surgical
B Respiratory System
Q Repair Restoring, to the extent possible, a body part to its normal anatomic structure and function

Body Part Character 4	Approach Character 5	Device Character 6	Qualifier Character 7
1 Trachea **2** Carina **3** Main Bronchus, Right **4** Upper Lobe Bronchus, Right **5** Middle Lobe Bronchus, Right **6** Lower Lobe Bronchus, Right **7** Main Bronchus, Left **8** Upper Lobe Bronchus, Left **9** Lingula Bronchus **B** Lower Lobe Bronchus, Left **C** Upper Lung Lobe, Right **D** Middle Lung Lobe, Right **F** Lower Lung Lobe, Right **G** Upper Lung Lobe, Left **H** Lung Lingula **J** Lower Lung Lobe, Left **K** Lung, Right **L** Lung, Left **M** Lungs, Bilateral	**0** Open **3** Percutaneous **4** Percutaneous Endoscopic **7** Via Natural or Artificial Opening **8** Via Natural or Artificial Opening Endoscopic	**Z** No Device	**Z** No Qualifier
N Pleura, Right **P** Pleura, Left **R** Diaphragm, Right **S** Diaphragm, Left	**0** Open **3** Percutaneous **4** Percutaneous Endoscopic	**Z** No Device	**Z** No Qualifier

0 Medical and Surgical
B Respiratory System
S Reposition Moving to its normal location or other suitable location all or a portion of a body part

Body Part Character 4	Approach Character 5	Device Character 6	Qualifier Character 7
1 Trachea **2** Carina **3** Main Bronchus, Right **4** Upper Lobe Bronchus, Right **5** Middle Lobe Bronchus, Right **6** Lower Lobe Bronchus, Right **7** Main Bronchus, Left **8** Upper Lobe Bronchus, Left **9** Lingula Bronchus **B** Lower Lobe Bronchus, Left **C** Upper Lung Lobe, Right **D** Middle Lung Lobe, Right **F** Lower Lung Lobe, Right **G** Upper Lung Lobe, Left **H** Lung Lingula **J** Lower Lung Lobe, Left **K** Lung, Right **L** Lung, Left **R** Diaphragm, Right **S** Diaphragm, Left	**0** Open	**Z** No Device	**Z** No Qualifier

Ø Medical and Surgical
B Respiratory System
T Resection Cutting out or off, without replacement, all of a body part

Body Part Character 4	Approach Character 5	Device Character 6	Qualifier Character 7
1 Trachea 2 Carina 3 Main Bronchus, Right 4 Upper Lobe Bronchus, Right 5 Middle Lobe Bronchus, Right 6 Lower Lobe Bronchus, Right 7 Main Bronchus, Left 8 Upper Lobe Bronchus, Left 9 Lingula Bronchus B Lower Lobe Bronchus, Left C Upper Lung Lobe, Right D Middle Lung Lobe, Right F Lower Lung Lobe, Right G Upper Lung Lobe, Left H Lung Lingula J Lower Lung Lobe, Left K Lung, Right L Lung, Left M Lungs, Bilateral R Diaphragm, Right S Diaphragm, Left	Ø Open 4 Percutaneous Endoscopic	Z No Device	Z No Qualifier

Ø Medical and Surgical
B Respiratory System
U Supplement Putting in or on biological or synthetic material that physically reinforces and/or augments the function of a portion of a body part

Body Part Character 4	Approach Character 5	Device Character 6	Qualifier Character 7
1 Trachea 2 Carina 3 Main Bronchus, Right 4 Upper Lobe Bronchus, Right 5 Middle Lobe Bronchus, Right 6 Lower Lobe Bronchus, Right 7 Main Bronchus, Left 8 Upper Lobe Bronchus, Left 9 Lingula Bronchus B Lower Lobe Bronchus, Left R Diaphragm, Right S Diaphragm, Left	Ø Open 4 Percutaneous Endoscopic	7 Autologous Tissue Substitute J Synthetic Substitute K Nonautologous Tissue Substitute	Z No Qualifier

Ø Medical and Surgical
B Respiratory System
V Restriction Partially closing an orifice or the lumen of a tubular body part

Body Part Character 4	Approach Character 5	Device Character 6	Qualifier Character 7
1 Trachea 2 Carina 3 Main Bronchus, Right 4 Upper Lobe Bronchus, Right 5 Middle Lobe Bronchus, Right 6 Lower Lobe Bronchus, Right 7 Main Bronchus, Left 8 Upper Lobe Bronchus, Left 9 Lingula Bronchus B Lower Lobe Bronchus, Left	Ø Open 3 Percutaneous 4 Percutaneous Endoscopic	C Extraluminal Device D Intraluminal Device Z No Device	Z No Qualifier
1 Trachea 2 Carina 3 Main Bronchus, Right 4 Upper Lobe Bronchus, Right 5 Middle Lobe Bronchus, Right 6 Lower Lobe Bronchus, Right 7 Main Bronchus, Left 8 Upper Lobe Bronchus, Left 9 Lingula Bronchus B Lower Lobe Bronchus, Left	7 Via Natural or Artificial Opening 8 Via Natural or Artificial Opening Endoscopic	D Intraluminal Device Z No Device	Z No Qualifier

0 Medical and Surgical
B Respiratory System
W Revision Correcting, to the extent possible, a portion of a malfunctioning device or the position of a displaced device

Body Part Character 4	Approach Character 5	Device Character 6	Qualifier Character 7
0 Tracheobronchial Tree	**0** Open **3** Percutaneous **4** Percutaneous Endoscopic **7** Via Natural or Artificial Opening **8** Via Natural or Artificial Opening Endoscopic **X** External	**0** Drainage Device **2** Monitoring Device **3** Infusion Device **7** Autologous Tissue Substitute **C** Extraluminal Device **D** Intraluminal Device **J** Synthetic Substitute **K** Nonautologous Tissue Substitute	**Z** No Qualifier
1 Trachea	**0** Open **3** Percutaneous **4** Percutaneous Endoscopic **7** Via Natural or Artificial Opening **8** Via Natural or Artificial Opening Endoscopic **X** External	**0** Drainage Device **2** Monitoring Device **7** Autologous Tissue Substitute **C** Extraluminal Device **D** Intraluminal Device **F** Tracheostomy Device **J** Synthetic Substitute **K** Nonautologous Tissue Substitute	**Z** No Qualifier
K Lung, Right **L** Lung, Left	**0** Open **3** Percutaneous **4** Percutaneous Endoscopic **7** Via Natural or Artificial Opening **8** Via Natural or Artificial Opening Endoscopic **X** External	**0** Drainage Device **2** Monitoring Device **3** Infusion Device	**Z** No Qualifier
Q Pleura	**0** Open **3** Percutaneous **4** Percutaneous Endoscopic **7** Via Natural or Artificial Opening **8** Via Natural or Artificial Opening Endoscopic **X** External	**0** Drainage Device **2** Monitoring Device	**Z** No Qualifier
T Diaphragm	**0** Open **3** Percutaneous **4** Percutaneous Endoscopic **7** Via Natural or Artificial Opening **8** Via Natural or Artificial Opening Endoscopic **X** External	**0** Drainage Device **2** Monitoring Device **7** Autologous Tissue Substitute **J** Synthetic Substitute **K** Nonautologous Tissue Substitute **M** Diaphragmatic Pacemaker Lead	**Z** No Qualifier

0 Medical and Surgical
B Respiratory System
Y Transplantation Putting in or on all or a portion of a living body part taken from another individual or animal to physically take the place and/or function of all or a portion of a similar body part

Body Part Character 4	Approach Character 5	Device Character 6	Qualifier Character 7
C Upper Lung Lobe, Right **D** Middle Lung Lobe, Right **F** Lower Lung Lobe, Right **G** Upper Lung Lobe, Left **H** Lung Lingula **J** Lower Lung Lobe, Left **K** Lung, Right **L** Lung, Left **M** Lungs, Bilateral	**0** Open	**Z** No Device	**0** Allogeneic **1** Syngeneic **2** Zooplastic

Mouth and Throat ØCØ–ØCX

Ø Medical and Surgical
C Mouth and Throat
Ø Alteration Modifying the anatomic structure of a body part without affecting the function of the body part

Body Part Character 4	Approach Character 5	Device Character 6	Qualifier Character 7
Ø Upper Lip **1** Lower Lip	**X** External	**7** Autologous Tissue Substitute **J** Synthetic Substitute **K** Nonautologous Tissue Substitute **Z** No Device	**Z** No Qualifier

Ø Medical and Surgical
C Mouth and Throat
2 Change Taking out or off a device from a body part and putting back an identical or similar device in or on the same body part without cutting or puncturing the skin or a mucous membrane

Body Part Character 4	Approach Character 5	Device Character 6	Qualifier Character 7
A Salivary Gland **S** Larynx **Y** Mouth and Throat	**X** External	**Ø** Drainage Device **Y** Other Device	**Z** No Qualifier

Ø Medical and Surgical
C Mouth and Throat
5 Destruction Physical eradication of all or a portion of a body part by the direct use of energy, force, or a destructive agent

Body Part Character 4	Approach Character 5	Device Character 6	Qualifier Character 7
Ø Upper Lip **1** Lower Lip **2** Hard Palate **3** Soft Palate **4** Buccal Mucosa **5** Upper Gingiva **6** Lower Gingiva **7** Tongue **N** Uvula **P** Tonsils **Q** Adenoids	**Ø** Open **3** Percutaneous **X** External	**Z** No Device	**Z** No Qualifier
8 Parotid Gland, Right **9** Parotid Gland, Left **B** Parotid Duct, Right **C** Parotid Duct, Left **D** Sublingual Gland, Right **F** Sublingual Gland, Left **G** Submaxillary Gland, Right **H** Submaxillary Gland, Left **J** Minor Salivary Gland	**Ø** Open **3** Percutaneous	**Z** No Device	**Z** No Qualifier
M Pharynx **R** Epiglottis **S** Larynx **T** Vocal Cord, Right **V** Vocal Cord, Left	**Ø** Open **3** Percutaneous **4** Percutaneous Endoscopic **7** Via Natural or Artificial Opening **8** Via Natural or Artificial Opening Endoscopic	**Z** No Device	**Z** No Qualifier
W Upper Tooth **X** Lower Tooth	**Ø** Open **X** External	**Z** No Device	**Ø** Single **1** Multiple **2** All

0 Medical and Surgical
C Mouth and Throat
7 Dilation Expanding an orifice or the lumen of a tubular body part

Body Part Character 4	Approach Character 5	Device Character 6	Qualifier Character 7
B Parotid Duct, Right C Parotid Duct, Left	0 Open 3 Percutaneous 7 Via Natural or Artificial Opening	D Intraluminal Device Z No Device	Z No Qualifier
M Pharynx	7 Via Natural or Artificial Opening 8 Via Natural or Artificial Opening Endoscopic	D Intraluminal Device Z No Device	Z No Qualifier
S Larynx	0 Open 3 Percutaneous 4 Percutaneous Endoscopic 7 Via Natural or Artificial Opening 8 Via Natural or Artificial Opening Endoscopic	D Intraluminal Device Z No Device	Z No Qualifier

0 Medical and Surgical
C Mouth and Throat
9 Drainage Taking or letting out fluids and/or gases from a body part

Body Part Character 4	Approach Character 5	Device Character 6	Qualifier Character 7
0 Upper Lip 1 Lower Lip 2 Hard Palate 3 Soft Palate 4 Buccal Mucosa 5 Upper Gingiva 6 Lower Gingiva 7 Tongue N Uvula P Tonsils Q Adenoids	0 Open 3 Percutaneous X External	0 Drainage Device	Z No Qualifier
0 Upper Lip 1 Lower Lip 2 Hard Palate 3 Soft Palate 4 Buccal Mucosa 5 Upper Gingiva 6 Lower Gingiva 7 Tongue N Uvula P Tonsils Q Adenoids	0 Open 3 Percutaneous X External	Z No Device	X Diagnostic Z No Qualifier
8 Parotid Gland, Right 9 Parotid Gland, Left B Parotid Duct, Right C Parotid Duct, Left D Sublingual Gland, Right F Sublingual Gland, Left G Submaxillary Gland, Right H Submaxillary Gland, Left J Minor Salivary Gland	0 Open 3 Percutaneous	0 Drainage Device	Z No Qualifier
8 Parotid Gland, Right 9 Parotid Gland, Left B Parotid Duct, Right C Parotid Duct, Left D Sublingual Gland, Right F Sublingual Gland, Left G Submaxillary Gland, Right H Submaxillary Gland, Left J Minor Salivary Gland	0 Open 3 Percutaneous	Z No Device	X Diagnostic Z No Qualifier
M Pharynx R Epiglottis S Larynx T Vocal Cord, Right V Vocal Cord, Left	0 Open 3 Percutaneous 4 Percutaneous Endoscopic 7 Via Natural or Artificial Opening 8 Via Natural or Artificial Opening Endoscopic	0 Drainage Device	Z No Qualifier

0C9 Continued on next page

ØC9 Continued

Ø Medical and Surgical
C Mouth and Throat
9 Drainage Taking or letting out fluids and/or gases from a body part

Body Part Character 4	Approach Character 5	Device Character 6	Qualifier Character 7
M Pharynx **R** Epiglottis **S** Larynx **T** Vocal Cord, Right **V** Vocal Cord, Left	**Ø** Open **3** Percutaneous **4** Percutaneous Endoscopic **7** Via Natural or Artificial Opening **8** Via Natural or Artificial Opening Endoscopic	**Z** No Device	**X** Diagnostic **Z** No Qualifier
W Upper Tooth **X** Lower Tooth	**Ø** Open **X** External	**Ø** Drainage Device **Z** No Device	**Ø** Single **1** Multiple **2** All

Ø Medical and Surgical
C Mouth and Throat
B Excision Cutting out or off, without replacement, a portion of a body part

Body Part Character 4	Approach Character 5	Device Character 6	Qualifier Character 7
Ø Upper Lip **1** Lower Lip **2** Hard Palate **3** Soft Palate **4** Buccal Mucosa **5** Upper Gingiva **6** Lower Gingiva **7** Tongue **N** Uvula **P** Tonsils **Q** Adenoids	**Ø** Open **3** Percutaneous **X** External	**Z** No Device	**X** Diagnostic **Z** No Qualifier
8 Parotid Gland, Right **9** Parotid Gland, Left **B** Parotid Duct, Right **C** Parotid Duct, Left **D** Sublingual Gland, Right **F** Sublingual Gland, Left **G** Submaxillary Gland, Right **H** Submaxillary Gland, Left **J** Minor Salivary Gland	**Ø** Open **3** Percutaneous	**Z** No Device	**X** Diagnostic **Z** No Qualifier
M Pharynx **R** Epiglottis **S** Larynx **T** Vocal Cord, Right **V** Vocal Cord, Left	**Ø** Open **3** Percutaneous **4** Percutaneous Endoscopic **7** Via Natural or Artificial Opening **8** Via Natural or Artificial Opening Endoscopic	**Z** No Device	**X** Diagnostic **Z** No Qualifier
W Upper Tooth **X** Lower Tooth	**Ø** Open **X** External	**Z** No Device	**Ø** Single **1** Multiple **2** All

0 Medical and Surgical
C Mouth and Throat
C Extirpation Taking or cutting out solid matter from a body part

Body Part Character 4	Approach Character 5	Device Character 6	Qualifier Character 7
0 Upper Lip **1** Lower Lip **2** Hard Palate **3** Soft Palate **4** Buccal Mucosa **5** Upper Gingiva **6** Lower Gingiva **7** Tongue **N** Uvula **P** Tonsils **Q** Adenoids	**0** Open **3** Percutaneous **X** External	**Z** No Device	**Z** No Qualifier
8 Parotid Gland, Right **9** Parotid Gland, Left **B** Parotid Duct, Right **C** Parotid Duct, Left **D** Sublingual Gland, Right **F** Sublingual Gland, Left **G** Submaxillary Gland, Right **H** Submaxillary Gland, Left **J** Minor Salivary Gland	**0** Open **3** Percutaneous	**Z** No Device	**Z** No Qualifier
M Pharynx **R** Epiglottis **S** Larynx **T** Vocal Cord, Right **V** Vocal Cord, Left	**0** Open **3** Percutaneous **4** Percutaneous Endoscopic **7** Via Natural or Artificial Opening **8** Via Natural or Artificial Opening Endoscopic	**Z** No Device	**Z** No Qualifier
W Upper Tooth **X** Lower Tooth	**0** Open **X** External	**Z** No Device	**0** Single **1** Multiple **2** All

0 Medical and Surgical
C Mouth and Throat
D Extraction Pulling or stripping out or off all or a portion of a body part by the use of force

Body Part Character 4	Approach Character 5	Device Character 6	Qualifier Character 7
T Vocal Cord, Right **V** Vocal Cord, Left	**0** Open **3** Percutaneous **4** Percutaneous Endoscopic **7** Via Natural or Artificial Opening **8** Via Natural or Artificial Opening Endoscopic	**Z** No Device	**Z** No Qualifier
W Upper Tooth **X** Lower Tooth	**X** External	**Z** No Device	**0** Single **1** Multiple **2** All

0 Medical and Surgical
C Mouth and Throat
F Fragmentation Breaking solid matter in a body part into pieces

Body Part Character 4	Approach Character 5	Device Character 6	Qualifier Character 7
B Parotid Duct, Right **C** Parotid Duct, Left	**0** Open **3** Percutaneous **7** Via Natural or Artificial Opening **X** External	**Z** No Device	**Z** No Qualifier

0 Medical and Surgical
C Mouth and Throat
H Insertion Putting in a nonbiological appliance that monitors, assists, performs, or prevents a physiological function but does not physically take the place of a body part

Body Part Character 4	Approach Character 5	Device Character 6	Qualifier Character 7
7 Tongue	**0** Open **3** Percutaneous **X** External	**1** Radioactive Element	**Z** No Qualifier
Y Mouth and Throat	**7** Via Natural or Artificial Opening **8** Via Natural or Artificial Opening Endoscopic	**B** **Intraluminal Device, Airway**	**Z** No Qualifier

Ø Medical and Surgical
C Mouth and Throat
J Inspection Visually and/or manually exploring a body part

Body Part Character 4	Approach Character 5	Device Character 6	Qualifier Character 7
A Salivary Gland	**Ø** Open **3** Percutaneous **X** External	**Z** No Device	**Z** No Qualifier
S Larynx **Y** Mouth and Throat	**Ø** Open **3** Percutaneous **4** Percutaneous Endoscopic **7** Via Natural or Artificial Opening **8** Via Natural or Artificial Opening Endoscopic **X** External	**Z** No Device	**Z** No Qualifier

Ø Medical and Surgical
C Mouth and Throat
L Occlusion Completely closing an orifice or the lumen of a tubular body part

Body Part Character 4	Approach Character 5	Device Character 6	Qualifier Character 7
B Parotid Duct, Right **C** Parotid Duct, Left	**Ø** Open **3** Percutaneous **4** Percutaneous Endoscopic	**C** Extraluminal Device **D** Intraluminal Device **Z** No Device	**Z** No Qualifier
B Parotid Duct, Right **C** Parotid Duct, Left	**7** Via Natural or Artificial Opening **8** Via Natural or Artificial Opening Endoscopic	**D** Intraluminal Device **Z** No Device	**Z** No Qualifier

Ø Medical and Surgical
C Mouth and Throat
M Reattachment Putting back in or on all or a portion of a separated body part to its normal location or other suitable location

Body Part Character 4	Approach Character 5	Device Character 6	Qualifier Character 7
Ø Upper Lip **1** Lower Lip **3** Soft Palate **7** Tongue **N** Uvula	**Ø** Open	**Z** No Device	**Z** No Qualifier
W Upper Tooth **X** Lower Tooth	**Ø** Open **X** External	**Z** No Device	**Ø** Single **1** Multiple **2** All

Ø Medical and Surgical
C Mouth and Throat
N Release Freeing a body part from an abnormal physical constraint

Body Part Character 4	Approach Character 5	Device Character 6	Qualifier Character 7
Ø Upper Lip **1** Lower Lip **2** Hard Palate **3** Soft Palate **4** Buccal Mucosa **5** Upper Gingiva **6** Lower Gingiva **7** Tongue **N** Uvula **P** Tonsils **Q** Adenoids	**Ø** Open **3** Percutaneous **X** External	**Z** No Device	**Z** No Qualifier
8 Parotid Gland, Right **9** Parotid Gland, Left **B** Parotid Duct, Right **C** Parotid Duct, Left **D** Sublingual Gland, Right **F** Sublingual Gland, Left **G** Submaxillary Gland, Right **H** Submaxillary Gland, Left **J** Minor Salivary Gland	**Ø** Open **3** Percutaneous	**Z** No Device	**Z** No Qualifier

ØCN Continued on next page

0 Medical and Surgical
C Mouth and Throat
N Release Freeing a body part from an abnormal physical constraint

0CN Continued

Body Part Character 4	Approach Character 5	Device Character 6	Qualifier Character 7
W Upper Tooth X Lower Tooth	0 Open X External	Z No Device	0 Single 1 Multiple 2 All
M Pharynx R Epiglottis S Larynx T Vocal Cord, Right V Vocal Cord, Left	0 Open 3 Percutaneous 4 Percutaneous Endoscopic 7 Via Natural or Artificial Opening 8 Via Natural or Artificial Opening Endoscopic	Z No Device	Z No Qualifier

0 Medical and Surgical
C Mouth and Throat
P Removal Taking out or off a device from a body part

Body Part Character 4	Approach Character 5	Device Character 6	Qualifier Character 7
A Salivary Gland	0 Open 3 Percutaneous	0 Drainage Device C Extraluminal Device	Z No Qualifier
S Larynx	0 Open 3 Percutaneous 7 Via Natural or Artificial Opening 8 Via Natural or Artificial Opening Endoscopic X External	0 Drainage Device 7 Autologous Tissue Substitute D Intraluminal Device J Synthetic Substitute K Nonautologous Tissue Substitute	Z No Qualifier
Y Mouth and Throat	0 Open 3 Percutaneous 7 Via Natural or Artificial Opening 8 Via Natural or Artificial Opening Endoscopic X External	0 Drainage Device 1 Radioactive Element 7 Autologous Tissue Substitute D Intraluminal Device J Synthetic Substitute K Nonautologous Tissue Substitute	Z No Qualifier

0 Medical and Surgical
C Mouth and Throat
Q Repair Restoring, to the extent possible, a body part to its normal anatomic structure and function

Body Part Character 4	Approach Character 5	Device Character 6	Qualifier Character 7
0 Upper Lip 1 Lower Lip 2 Hard Palate 3 Soft Palate 4 Buccal Mucosa 5 Upper Gingiva 6 Lower Gingiva 7 Tongue N Uvula P Tonsils Q Adenoids	0 Open 3 Percutaneous X External	Z No Device	Z No Qualifier
8 Parotid Gland, Right 9 Parotid Gland, Left B Parotid Duct, Right C Parotid Duct, Left D Sublingual Gland, Right F Sublingual Gland, Left G Submaxillary Gland, Right H Submaxillary Gland, Left J Minor Salivary Gland	0 Open 3 Percutaneous	Z No Device	Z No Qualifier
M Pharynx R Epiglottis S Larynx T Vocal Cord, Right V Vocal Cord, Left	0 Open 3 Percutaneous 4 Percutaneous Endoscopic 7 Via Natural or Artificial Opening 8 Via Natural or Artificial Opening Endoscopic	Z No Device	Z No Qualifier
W Upper Tooth X Lower Tooth	0 Open X External	Z No Device	0 Single 1 Multiple 2 All

Ø Medical and Surgical
C Mouth and Throat
R Replacement Putting in or on biological or synthetic material that physically takes the place and/or function of all or a portion of a body part

Body Part Character 4	Approach Character 5	Device Character 6	Qualifier Character 7
Ø Upper Lip **1** Lower Lip **2** Hard Palate **3** Soft Palate **4** Buccal Mucosa **5** Upper Gingiva **6** Lower Gingiva **7** Tongue **N** Uvula	**Ø** Open **3** Percutaneous **X** External	**7** Autologous Tissue Substitute **J** Synthetic Substitute **K** Nonautologous Tissue Substitute	**Z** No Qualifier
B Parotid Duct, Right **C** Parotid Duct, Left	**Ø** Open **3** Percutaneous	**7** Autologous Tissue Substitute **J** Synthetic Substitute **K** Nonautologous Tissue Substitute	**Z** No Qualifier
M Pharynx **R** Epiglottis **S** Larynx **T** Vocal Cord, Right **V** Vocal Cord, Left	**Ø** Open **7** Via Natural or Artificial Opening **8** Via Natural or Artificial Opening Endoscopic	**7** Autologous Tissue Substitute **J** Synthetic Substitute **K** Nonautologous Tissue Substitute	**Z** No Qualifier
W Upper Tooth **X** Lower Tooth	**Ø** Open **X** External	**7** Autologous Tissue Substitute **J** Synthetic Substitute **K** Nonautologous Tissue Substitute	**Ø** Single **1** Multiple **2** All

Ø Medical and Surgical
C Mouth and Throat
S Reposition Moving to its normal location or other suitable location all or a portion of a body part

Body Part Character 4	Approach Character 5	Device Character 6	Qualifier Character 7
Ø Upper Lip **1** Lower Lip **2** Hard Palate **3** Soft Palate **7** Tongue **N** Uvula	**Ø** Open **X** External	**Z** No Device	**Z** No Qualifier
B Parotid Duct, Right **C** Parotid Duct, Left	**Ø** Open **3** Percutaneous	**Z** No Device	**Z** No Qualifier
R Epiglottis **T** Vocal Cord, Right **V** Vocal Cord, Left	**Ø** Open **7** Via Natural or Artificial Opening **8** Via Natural or Artificial Opening Endoscopic	**Z** No Device	**Z** No Qualifier
W Upper Tooth **X** Lower Tooth	**Ø** Open **X** External	**5** External Fixation Device **Z** No Device	**Ø** Single **1** Multiple **2** All

Ø Medical and Surgical
C Mouth and Throat
T Resection Cutting out or off, without replacement, all of a body part

Body Part Character 4	Approach Character 5	Device Character 6	Qualifier Character 7
Ø Upper Lip **1** Lower Lip **2** Hard Palate **3** Soft Palate **7** Tongue **N** Uvula **P** Tonsils **Q** Adenoids	**Ø** Open **X** External	**Z** No Device	**Z** No Qualifier
8 Parotid Gland, Right **9** Parotid Gland, Left **B** Parotid Duct, Right **C** Parotid Duct, Left **D** Sublingual Gland, Right **F** Sublingual Gland, Left **G** Submaxillary Gland, Right **H** Submaxillary Gland, Left **J** Minor Salivary Gland	**Ø** Open	**Z** No Device	**Z** No Qualifier

ØCT Continued on next page

0 Medical and Surgical
C Mouth and Throat
T Resection Cutting out or off, without replacement, all of a body part

0CT Continued

Body Part Character 4	Approach Character 5	Device Character 6	Qualifier Character 7
M Pharynx **R** Epiglottis **S** Larynx **T** Vocal Cord, Right **V** Vocal Cord, Left	**0** Open **4** Percutaneous Endoscopic **7** Via Natural or Artificial Opening **8** Via Natural or Artificial Opening Endoscopic	**Z** No Device	**Z** No Qualifier
W Upper Tooth **X** Lower Tooth	**0** Open	**Z** No Device	**0** Single **1** Multiple **2** All

0 Medical and Surgical
C Mouth and Throat
U Supplement Putting in or on biological or synthetic material that physically reinforces and/or augments the function of a portion of a body part

Body Part Character 4	Approach Character 5	Device Character 6	Qualifier Character 7
0 Upper Lip **1** Lower Lip **2** Hard Palate **3** Soft Palate **4** Buccal Mucosa **5** Upper Gingiva **6** Lower Gingiva **7** Tongue **N** Uvula	**0** Open **3** Percutaneous **X** External	**7** Autologous Tissue Substitute **J** Synthetic Substitute **K** Nonautologous Tissue Substitute	**Z** No Qualifier
M Pharynx **R** Epiglottis **S** Larynx **T** Vocal Cord, Right **V** Vocal Cord, Left	**0** Open **7** Via Natural or Artificial Opening **8** Via Natural or Artificial Opening Endoscopic	**7** Autologous Tissue Substitute **J** Synthetic Substitute **K** Nonautologous Tissue Substitute	**Z** No Qualifier

0 Medical and Surgical
C Mouth and Throat
V Restriction Partially closing an orifice or the lumen of a tubular body part

Body Part Character 4	Approach Character 5	Device Character 6	Qualifier Character 7
B Parotid Duct, Right **C** Parotid Duct, Left	**0** Open **3** Percutaneous	**C** Extraluminal Device **D** Intraluminal Device **Z** No Device	**Z** No Qualifier
B Parotid Duct, Right **C** Parotid Duct, Left	**7** Via Natural or Artificial Opening **8** Via Natural or Artificial Opening Endoscopic	**D** Intraluminal Device **Z** No Device	**Z** No Qualifier

Ø Medical and Surgical
C Mouth and Throat
W Revision Correcting, to the extent possible, a portion of a malfunctioning device or the position of a displaced device

Body Part Character 4	Approach Character 5	Device Character 6	Qualifier Character 7
A Salivary Gland	**Ø** Open **3** Percutaneous **X** External	**Ø** Drainage Device **C** Extraluminal Device	**Z** No Qualifier
S Larynx	**Ø** Open **3** Percutaneous **7** Via Natural or Artificial Opening **8** Via Natural or Artificial Opening Endoscopic **X** External	**Ø** Drainage Device **7** Autologous Tissue Substitute **D** Intraluminal Device **J** Synthetic Substitute **K** Nonautologous Tissue Substitute	**Z** No Qualifier
Y Mouth and Throat	**Ø** Open **3** Percutaneous **7** Via Natural or Artificial Opening **8** Via Natural or Artificial Opening Endoscopic **X** External	**Ø** Drainage Device **1** Radioactive Element **7** Autologous Tissue Substitute **D** Intraluminal Device **J** Synthetic Substitute **K** Nonautologous Tissue Substitute	**Z** No Qualifier

Ø Medical and Surgical
C Mouth and Throat
X Transfer Moving, without taking out, all or a portion of a body part to another location to take over the function of all or a portion of a body part

Body Part Character 4	Approach Character 5	Device Character 6	Qualifier Character 7
Ø Upper Lip **1** Lower Lip **3** Soft Palate **4** Buccal Mucosa **5** Upper Gingiva **6** Lower Gingiva **7** Tongue	**Ø** Open **X** External	**Z** No Device	**Z** No Qualifier

0D1- bypass

Gastrointestinal System ØD1–ØDY

Ø Medical and Surgical
D Gastrointestinal System
1 Bypass Altering the route of passage of the contents of a tubular body part

Body Part Character 4	Approach Character 5	Device Character 6	Qualifier Character 7
1 Esophagus, Upper 2 Esophagus, Middle 3 Esophagus, Lower 5 Esophagus	Ø Open 4 Percutaneous Endoscopic 8 Via Natural or Artificial Opening Endoscopic	7 Autologous Tissue Substitute J Synthetic Substitute K Nonautologous Tissue Substitute Z No Device	4 Cutaneous 6 Stomach 9 Duodenum A Jejunum B Ileum
1 Esophagus, Upper 2 Esophagus, Middle 3 Esophagus, Lower 5 Esophagus 6 Stomach 9 Duodenum A Jejunum B Ileum H Cecum K Ascending Colon L Transverse Colon M Descending Colon N Sigmoid Colon	3 Percutaneous	J Synthetic Substitute	4 Cutaneous
6 Stomach 9 Duodenum	Ø Open 4 Percutaneous Endoscopic 8 Via Natural or Artificial Opening Endoscopic	7 Autologous Tissue Substitute J Synthetic Substitute K Nonautologous Tissue Substitute Z No Device	4 Cutaneous 9 Duodenum A Jejunum B Ileum L Transverse Colon
A Jejunum	Ø Open 4 Percutaneous Endoscopic 8 Via Natural or Artificial Opening Endoscopic	7 Autologous Tissue Substitute J Synthetic Substitute K Nonautologous Tissue Substitute Z No Device	4 Cutaneous A Jejunum B Ileum H Cecum K Ascending Colon L Transverse Colon M Descending Colon N Sigmoid Colon P Rectum Q Anus
B Ileum	Ø Open 4 Percutaneous Endoscopic 8 Via Natural or Artificial Opening Endoscopic	7 Autologous Tissue Substitute J Synthetic Substitute K Nonautologous Tissue Substitute Z No Device	4 Cutaneous B Ileum H Cecum K Ascending Colon L Transverse Colon M Descending Colon N Sigmoid Colon P Rectum Q Anus
H Cecum	Ø Open 4 Percutaneous Endoscopic 8 Via Natural or Artificial Opening Endoscopic	7 Autologous Tissue Substitute J Synthetic Substitute K Nonautologous Tissue Substitute Z No Device	4 Cutaneous H Cecum K Ascending Colon L Transverse Colon M Descending Colon N Sigmoid Colon P Rectum
K Ascending Colon	Ø Open 4 Percutaneous Endoscopic 8 Via Natural or Artificial Opening Endoscopic	7 Autologous Tissue Substitute J Synthetic Substitute K Nonautologous Tissue Substitute Z No Device	4 Cutaneous K Ascending Colon L Transverse Colon M Descending Colon N Sigmoid Colon P Rectum
L Transverse Colon	Ø Open 4 Percutaneous Endoscopic 8 Via Natural or Artificial Opening Endoscopic	7 Autologous Tissue Substitute J Synthetic Substitute K Nonautologous Tissue Substitute Z No Device	4 Cutaneous L Transverse Colon M Descending Colon N Sigmoid Colon P Rectum
M Descending Colon	Ø Open 4 Percutaneous Endoscopic 8 Via Natural or Artificial Opening Endoscopic	7 Autologous Tissue Substitute J Synthetic Substitute K Nonautologous Tissue Substitute Z No Device	4 Cutaneous M Descending Colon N Sigmoid Colon P Rectum
N Sigmoid Colon	Ø Open 4 Percutaneous Endoscopic 8 Via Natural or Artificial Opening Endoscopic	7 Autologous Tissue Substitute J Synthetic Substitute K Nonautologous Tissue Substitute Z No Device	4 Cutaneous N Sigmoid Colon P Rectum

Ø Medical and Surgical
D Gastrointestinal System
2 Change Taking out or off a device from a body part and putting back an identical or similar device in or on the same body part without cutting or puncturing the skin or a mucous membrane

Body Part Character 4	Approach Character 5	Device Character 6	Qualifier Character 7
Ø Upper Intestinal Tract D Lower Intestinal Tract	X External	Ø Drainage Device U Feeding Device Y Other Device	Z No Qualifier
U Omentum V Mesentery W Peritoneum	X External	Ø Drainage Device Y Other Device	Z No Qualifier

Ø Medical and Surgical
D Gastrointestinal System
5 Destruction Physical eradication of all or a portion of a body part by the direct use of energy, force, or a destructive agent

Body Part Character 4	Approach Character 5	Device Character 6	Qualifier Character 7
1 Esophagus, Upper 2 Esophagus, Middle 3 Esophagus, Lower 4 Esophagogastric Junction 5 Esophagus 6 Stomach 7 Stomach, Pylorus 8 Small Intestine 9 Duodenum A Jejunum B Ileum C Ileocecal Valve E Large Intestine F Large Intestine, Right G Large Intestine, Left H Cecum J Appendix K Ascending Colon L Transverse Colon M Descending Colon N Sigmoid Colon P Rectum	Ø Open 3 Percutaneous 4 Percutaneous Endoscopic 7 Via Natural or Artificial Opening 8 Via Natural or Artificial Opening Endoscopic	Z No Device	Z No Qualifier
Q Anus	Ø Open 3 Percutaneous 4 Percutaneous Endoscopic 7 Via Natural or Artificial Opening 8 Via Natural or Artificial Opening Endoscopic X External	Z No Device	Z No Qualifier
R Anal Sphincter S Greater Omentum T Lesser Omentum V Mesentery W Peritoneum	Ø Open 3 Percutaneous 4 Percutaneous Endoscopic	Z No Device	Z No Qualifier

Ø Medical and Surgical
D Gastrointestinal System
7 Dilation Expanding an orifice or the lumen of a tubular body part

Body Part Character 4	Approach Character 5	Device Character 6	Qualifier Character 7
1 Esophagus, Upper **2** Esophagus, Middle **3** Esophagus, Lower **4** Esophagogastric Junction **5** Esophagus **6** Stomach **7** Stomach, Pylorus **8** Small Intestine **9** Duodenum **A** Jejunum **B** Ileum **C** Ileocecal Valve **E** Large Intestine **F** Large Intestine, Right **G** Large Intestine, Left **H** Cecum **K** Ascending Colon **L** Transverse Colon **M** Descending Colon **N** Sigmoid Colon **P** Rectum **Q** Anus	**Ø** Open **3** Percutaneous **4** Percutaneous Endoscopic **7** Via Natural or Artificial Opening **8** Via Natural or Artificial Opening Endoscopic	**D** Intraluminal Device **Z** No Device	**Z** No Qualifier

Ø Medical and Surgical
D Gastrointestinal System
8 Division Cutting into a body part without draining fluids and/or gases from the body part in order to separate or transect a body part

Body Part Character 4	Approach Character 5	Device Character 6	Qualifier Character 7
4 Esophagogastric Junction **7 Stomach, Pylorus**	**Ø** Open **3** Percutaneous **4** Percutaneous Endoscopic **7** Via Natural or Artificial Opening **8** Via Natural or Artificial Opening Endoscopic	**Z** No Device	**Z** No Qualifier
R Anal Sphincter	**Ø** Open **3** Percutaneous	**Z** No Device	**Z** No Qualifier

Ø Medical and Surgical
D Gastrointestinal System
9 Drainage Taking or letting out fluids and/or gases from a body part

Body Part Character 4	Approach Character 5	Device Character 6	Qualifier Character 7
1 Esophagus, Upper **2** Esophagus, Middle **3** Esophagus, Lower **4** Esophagogastric Junction **5** Esophagus **6** Stomach **7** Stomach, Pylorus **8** Small Intestine **9** Duodenum **A** Jejunum **B** Ileum **C** Ileocecal Valve **E** Large Intestine **F** Large Intestine, Right **G** Large Intestine, Left **H** Cecum **J** Appendix **K** Ascending Colon **L** Transverse Colon **M** Descending Colon **N** Sigmoid Colon **P** Rectum	**Ø** Open **3** Percutaneous **4** Percutaneous Endoscopic **7** Via Natural or Artificial Opening **8** Via Natural or Artificial Opening Endoscopic	**Ø** Drainage Device	**Z** No Qualifier

ØD9 Continued on next page

ØD9 Continued

Ø Medical and Surgical
D Gastrointestinal System
9 Drainage Taking or letting out fluids and/or gases from a body part

Body Part Character 4	Approach Character 5	Device Character 6	Qualifier Character 7
1 Esophagus, Upper **2** Esophagus, Middle **3** Esophagus, Lower **4** Esophagogastric Junction **5** Esophagus **6** Stomach **7** Stomach, Pylorus **8** Small Intestine **9** Duodenum **A** Jejunum **B** Ileum **C** Ileocecal Valve **E** Large Intestine **F** Large Intestine, Right **G** Large Intestine, Left **H** Cecum **J** Appendix **K** Ascending Colon **L** Transverse Colon **M** Descending Colon **N** Sigmoid Colon **P** Rectum	**Ø** Open **3** Percutaneous **4** Percutaneous Endoscopic **7** Via Natural or Artificial Opening **8** Via Natural or Artificial Opening Endoscopic	**Z** No Device	**X** Diagnostic **Z** No Qualifier
Q Anus	**Ø** Open **3** Percutaneous **4** Percutaneous Endoscopic **7** Via Natural or Artificial Opening **8** Via Natural or Artificial Opening Endoscopic **X** External	**Ø** Drainage Device	**Z** No Qualifier
Q Anus	**Ø** Open **3** Percutaneous **4** Percutaneous Endoscopic **7** Via Natural or Artificial Opening **8** Via Natural or Artificial Opening Endoscopic **X** External	**Z** No Device	**X** Diagnostic **Z** No Qualifier
R Anal Sphincter **S** Greater Omentum **T** Lesser Omentum **V** Mesentery **W** Peritoneum	**Ø** Open **3** Percutaneous **4** Percutaneous Endoscopic	**Ø** Drainage Device	**Z** No Qualifier
R Anal Sphincter **S** Greater Omentum **T** Lesser Omentum **V** Mesentery **W** Peritoneum	**Ø** Open **3** Percutaneous **4** Percutaneous Endoscopic	**Z** No Device	**X** Diagnostic **Z** No Qualifier

Ø Medical and Surgical
D Gastrointestinal System
B Excision Cutting out or off, without replacement, a portion of a body part

Body Part Character 4	Approach Character 5	Device Character 6	Qualifier Character 7
1 Esophagus, Upper **2** Esophagus, Middle **3** Esophagus, Lower **4** Esophagogastric Junction **5** Esophagus **7** Stomach, Pylorus **8** Small Intestine **9** Duodenum **A** Jejunum **B** Ileum **C** Ileocecal Valve **E** Large Intestine **F** Large Intestine, Right **G** Large Intestine, Left **H** Cecum **J** Appendix **K** Ascending Colon **L** Transverse Colon **M** Descending Colon **N** Sigmoid Colon **P** Rectum	**Ø** Open **3** Percutaneous **4** Percutaneous Endoscopic **7** Via Natural or Artificial Opening **8** Via Natural or Artificial Opening Endoscopic	**Z** No Device	**X** Diagnostic **Z** No Qualifier

ØDB Continued on next page

Ø Medical and Surgical
D Gastrointestinal System
B Excision Cutting out or off, without replacement, a portion of a body part

ØDB Continued

Body Part Character 4	Approach Character 5	Device Character 6	Qualifier Character 7
6 Stomach	Ø Open 3 Percutaneous 4 Percutaneous Endoscopic 7 Via Natural or Artificial Opening 8 Via Natural or Artificial Opening Endoscopic	Z No Device	3 Vertical X Diagnostic Z No Qualifier
Q Anus	Ø Open 3 Percutaneous 4 Percutaneous Endoscopic 7 Via Natural or Artificial Opening 8 Via Natural or Artificial Opening Endoscopic X External	Z No Device	X Diagnostic Z No Qualifier
R Anal Sphincter S Greater Omentum T Lesser Omentum V Mesentery W Peritoneum	Ø Open 3 Percutaneous 4 Percutaneous Endoscopic	Z No Device	X Diagnostic Z No Qualifier

Ø Medical and Surgical
D Gastrointestinal System
C Extirpation Taking or cutting out solid matter from a body part

Body Part Character 4	Approach Character 5	Device Character 6	Qualifier Character 7
1 Esophagus, Upper 2 Esophagus, Middle 3 Esophagus, Lower 4 Esophagogastric Junction 5 Esophagus 6 Stomach 7 Stomach, Pylorus 8 Small Intestine 9 Duodenum A Jejunum B Ileum C Ileocecal Valve E Large Intestine F Large Intestine, Right G Large Intestine, Left H Cecum J Appendix K Ascending Colon L Transverse Colon M Descending Colon N Sigmoid Colon P Rectum	Ø Open 3 Percutaneous 4 Percutaneous Endoscopic 7 Via Natural or Artificial Opening 8 Via Natural or Artificial Opening Endoscopic	Z No Device	Z No Qualifier
Q Anus	Ø Open 3 Percutaneous 4 Percutaneous Endoscopic 7 Via Natural or Artificial Opening 8 Via Natural or Artificial Opening Endoscopic X External	Z No Device	Z No Qualifier
R Anal Sphincter S Greater Omentum T Lesser Omentum V Mesentery W Peritoneum	Ø Open 3 Percutaneous 4 Percutaneous Endoscopic	Z No Device	Z No Qualifier

Ø Medical and Surgical
D Gastrointestinal System
F Fragmentation Breaking solid matter in a body part into pieces

Body Part Character 4	Approach Character 5	Device Character 6	Qualifier Character 7
5 Esophagus **6** Stomach **8** Small Intestine **9** Duodenum **A** Jejunum **B** Ileum **E** Large Intestine **F** Large Intestine, Right **G** Large Intestine, Left **H** Cecum **J** Appendix **K** Ascending Colon **L** Transverse Colon **M** Descending Colon **N** Sigmoid Colon **P** Rectum **Q** Anus	**Ø** Open **3** Percutaneous **4** Percutaneous Endoscopic **7** Via Natural or Artificial Opening **8** Via Natural or Artificial Opening Endoscopic **X** External	**Z** No Device	**Z** No Qualifier

Ø Medical and Surgical
D Gastrointestinal System
H Insertion Putting in a nonbiological appliance that monitors, assists, performs, or prevents a physiological function but does not physically take the place of a body part

Body Part Character 4	Approach Character 5	Device Character 6	Qualifier Character 7
5 Esophagus	**Ø** Open **3** Percutaneous **4** Percutaneous Endoscopic	**1** Radioactive Element **2** Monitoring Device **3** Infusion Device **D Intraluminal Device** **U** Feeding Device	**Z** No Qualifier
5 Esophagus	**7** Via Natural or Artificial Opening **8** Via Natural or Artificial Opening Endoscopic	**1** Radioactive Element **2** Monitoring Device **3** Infusion Device **B Intraluminal Device, Airway** **D Intraluminal Device** **U** Feeding Device	**Z** No Qualifier
6 Stomach	**Ø** Open **3** Percutaneous **4** Percutaneous Endoscopic	**2** Monitoring Device **3** Infusion Device **D Intraluminal Device** **M** Stimulator Lead **U** Feeding Device	**Z** No Qualifier
6 Stomach	**7** Via Natural or Artificial Opening **8** Via Natural or Artificial Opening Endoscopic	**2** Monitoring Device **3** Infusion Device **D Intraluminal Device** **U** Feeding Device	**Z** No Qualifier
8 Small Intestine **9** Duodenum **A** Jejunum **B** Ileum	**Ø** Open **3** Percutaneous **4** Percutaneous Endoscopic **7** Via Natural or Artificial Opening **8** Via Natural or Artificial Opening Endoscopic	**2** Monitoring Device **3** Infusion Device **D Intraluminal Device** **U** Feeding Device	**Z** No Qualifier
E Large Intestine	**Ø** Open **3** Percutaneous **4** Percutaneous Endoscopic **7** Via Natural or Artificial Opening **8** Via Natural or Artificial Opening Endoscopic	**D Intraluminal Device**	**Z** No Qualifier
P Rectum	**Ø** Open **3** Percutaneous **4** Percutaneous Endoscopic **7** Via Natural or Artificial Opening **8** Via Natural or Artificial Opening Endoscopic	**1** Radioactive Element **D Intraluminal Device**	**Z** No Qualifier
Q Anus	**Ø** Open **3** Percutaneous **4** Percutaneous Endoscopic	**D Intraluminal Device** **L** Artificial Sphincter	**Z** No Qualifier
Q Anus	**7** Via Natural or Artificial Opening **8** Via Natural or Artificial Opening Endoscopic	**D Intraluminal Device**	**Z** No Qualifier
R Anal Sphincter	**Ø** Open **3** Percutaneous **4** Percutaneous Endoscopic	**M** Stimulator Lead	**Z** No Qualifier

0 Medical and Surgical
D Gastrointestinal System
J Inspection Visually and/or manually exploring a body part

Body Part Character 4	Approach Character 5	Device Character 6	Qualifier Character 7
0 Upper Intestinal Tract **6** Stomach **D** Lower Intestinal Tract	**0** Open **3** Percutaneous **4** Percutaneous Endoscopic **7** Via Natural or Artificial Opening **8** Via Natural or Artificial Opening Endoscopic **X** External	**Z** No Device	**Z** No Qualifier
U Omentum **V** Mesentery **W** Peritoneum	**0** Open **3** Percutaneous **4** Percutaneous Endoscopic **X** External	**Z** No Device	**Z** No Qualifier

0 Medical and Surgical
D Gastrointestinal System
L Occlusion Completely closing an orifice or the lumen of a tubular body part

Body Part Character 4	Approach Character 5	Device Character 6	Qualifier Character 7
1 Esophagus, Upper **2** Esophagus, Middle **3** Esophagus, Lower **4** Esophagogastric Junction **5** Esophagus **6** Stomach **7** Stomach, Pylorus **8** Small Intestine **9** Duodenum **A** Jejunum **B** Ileum **C** Ileocecal Valve **E** Large Intestine **F** Large Intestine, Right **G** Large Intestine, Left **H** Cecum **K** Ascending Colon **L** Transverse Colon **M** Descending Colon **N** Sigmoid Colon **P** Rectum	**0** Open **3** Percutaneous **4** Percutaneous Endoscopic	**C** Extraluminal Device **D** Intraluminal Device **Z** No Device	**Z** No Qualifier
1 Esophagus, Upper **2** Esophagus, Middle **3** Esophagus, Lower **4** Esophagogastric Junction **5** Esophagus **6** Stomach **7** Stomach, Pylorus **8** Small Intestine **9** Duodenum **A** Jejunum **B** Ileum **C** Ileocecal Valve **E** Large Intestine **F** Large Intestine, Right **G** Large Intestine, Left **H** Cecum **K** Ascending Colon **L** Transverse Colon **M** Descending Colon **N** Sigmoid Colon **P** Rectum **Q** Anus	**7** Via Natural or Artificial Opening **8** Via Natural or Artificial Opening Endoscopic	**D** Intraluminal Device **Z** No Device	**Z** No Qualifier
Q Anus	**0** Open **3** Percutaneous **4** Percutaneous Endoscopic **X** External	**C** Extraluminal Device **D** Intraluminal Device **Z** No Device	**Z** No Qualifier

Ø Medical and Surgical
D Gastrointestinal System
M Reattachment Putting back in or on all or a portion of a separated body part to its normal location or other suitable location

Body Part Character 4	Approach Character 5	Device Character 6	Qualifier Character 7
5 Esophagus **6** Stomach **8** Small Intestine **9** Duodenum **A** Jejunum **B** Ileum **E** Large Intestine **F** Large Intestine, Right **G** Large Intestine, Left **H** Cecum **K** Ascending Colon **L** Transverse Colon **M** Descending Colon **N** Sigmoid Colon **P** Rectum	**Ø** Open **4** Percutaneous Endoscopic	**Z** No Device	**Z** No Qualifier

Ø Medical and Surgical
D Gastrointestinal System
N Release Freeing a body part from an abnormal physical constraint

Body Part Character 4	Approach Character 5	Device Character 6	Qualifier Character 7
1 Esophagus, Upper **2** Esophagus, Middle **3** Esophagus, Lower **4** Esophagogastric Junction **5** Esophagus **6** Stomach **7** Stomach, Pylorus **8** Small Intestine **9** Duodenum **A** Jejunum **B** Ileum **C** Ileocecal Valve **E** Large Intestine **F** Large Intestine, Right **G** Large Intestine, Left **H** Cecum **J** Appendix **K** Ascending Colon **L** Transverse Colon **M** Descending Colon **N** Sigmoid Colon **P** Rectum	**Ø** Open **3** Percutaneous **4** Percutaneous Endoscopic **7** Via Natural or Artificial Opening **8** Via Natural or Artificial Opening Endoscopic	**Z** No Device	**Z** No Qualifier
Q Anus	**Ø** Open **3** Percutaneous **4** Percutaneous Endoscopic **7** Via Natural or Artificial Opening **8** Via Natural or Artificial Opening Endoscopic **X** External	**Z** No Device	**Z** No Qualifier
R Anal Sphincter **S** Greater Omentum **T** Lesser Omentum **V** Mesentery **W** Peritoneum	**Ø** Open **3** Percutaneous **4** Percutaneous Endoscopic	**Z** No Device	**Z** No Qualifier

0 Medical and Surgical
D Gastrointestinal System
P Removal Taking out or off a device from a body part

Body Part Character 4	Approach Character 5	Device Character 6	Qualifier Character 7
0 Upper Intestinal Tract 6 Stomach D Lower Intestinal Tract	X External	0 Drainage Device 2 Monitoring Device 3 Infusion Device D Intraluminal Device U Feeding Device	Z No Qualifier
0 Upper Intestinal Tract D Lower Intestinal Tract	0 Open 3 Percutaneous 4 Percutaneous Endoscopic 7 Via Natural or Artificial Opening 8 Via Natural or Artificial Opening Endoscopic	0 Drainage Device 2 Monitoring Device 3 Infusion Device 7 Autologous Tissue Substitute C Extraluminal Device D Intraluminal Device J Synthetic Substitute K Nonautologous Tissue Substitute U Feeding Device	Z No Qualifier
5 Esophagus	0 Open 3 Percutaneous 4 Percutaneous Endoscopic	1 Radioactive Element 2 Monitoring Device 3 Infusion Device U Feeding Device	Z No Qualifier
5 Esophagus	7 Via Natural or Artificial Opening 8 Via Natural or Artificial Opening Endoscopic	1 Radioactive Element **D Intraluminal Device**	Z No Qualifier
5 Esophagus	X External	1 Radioactive Element 2 Monitoring Device 3 Infusion Device B Airway U Feeding Device	Z No Qualifier
6 Stomach	0 Open 3 Percutaneous 4 Percutaneous Endoscopic	0 Drainage Device 2 Monitoring Device 3 Infusion Device 7 Autologous Tissue Substitute C Extraluminal Device D Intraluminal Device J Synthetic Substitute K Nonautologous Tissue Substitute M Stimulator Lead U Feeding Device	Z No Qualifier
6 Stomach	7 Via Natural or Artificial Opening 8 Via Natural or Artificial Opening Endoscopic	0 Drainage Device 2 Monitoring Device 3 Infusion Device 7 Autologous Tissue Substitute C Extraluminal Device D Intraluminal Device J Synthetic Substitute K Nonautologous Tissue Substitute U Feeding Device	Z No Qualifier
P Rectum	0 Open 3 Percutaneous 4 Percutaneous Endoscopic 7 Via Natural or Artificial Opening 8 Via Natural or Artificial Opening Endoscopic X External	1 Radioactive Element	Z No Qualifier
Q Anus	0 Open 3 Percutaneous 4 Percutaneous Endoscopic 7 Via Natural or Artificial Opening 8 Via Natural or Artificial Opening Endoscopic	L Artificial Sphincter	Z No Qualifier
R Anal Sphincter	0 Open 3 Percutaneous 4 Percutaneous Endoscopic	M Stimulator Lead	Z No Qualifier
U Omentum V Mesentery W Peritoneum	0 Open 3 Percutaneous 4 Percutaneous Endoscopic	0 Drainage Device 1 Radioactive Element 7 Autologous Tissue Substitute J Synthetic Substitute K Nonautologous Tissue Substitute	Z No Qualifier

Ø Medical and Surgical
D Gastrointestinal System
Q Repair Restoring, to the extent possible, a body part to its normal anatomic structure and function

Body Part Character 4	Approach Character 5	Device Character 6	Qualifier Character 7
1 Esophagus, Upper 2 Esophagus, Middle 3 Esophagus, Lower 4 Esophagogastric Junction 5 Esophagus 6 Stomach 7 Stomach, Pylorus 8 Small Intestine 9 Duodenum A Jejunum B Ileum C Ileocecal Valve E Large Intestine F Large Intestine, Right G Large Intestine, Left H Cecum J Appendix K Ascending Colon L Transverse Colon M Descending Colon N Sigmoid Colon P Rectum	Ø Open 3 Percutaneous 4 Percutaneous Endoscopic 7 Via Natural or Artificial Opening 8 Via Natural or Artificial Opening Endoscopic	Z No Device	Z No Qualifier
Q Anus	Ø Open 3 Percutaneous 4 Percutaneous Endoscopic 7 Via Natural or Artificial Opening 8 Via Natural or Artificial Opening Endoscopic X External	Z No Device	Z No Qualifier
R Anal Sphincter S Greater Omentum T Lesser Omentum V Mesentery W Peritoneum	Ø Open 3 Percutaneous 4 Percutaneous Endoscopic	Z No Device	Z No Qualifier

Ø Medical and Surgical
D Gastrointestinal System
R Replacement Putting in or on biological or synthetic material that physically takes the place and/or function of all or a portion of a body part

Body Part Character 4	Approach Character 5	Device Character 6	Qualifier Character 7
5 Esophagus	Ø Open 4 Percutaneous Endoscopic 7 Via Natural or Artificial Opening 8 Via Natural or Artificial Opening Endoscopic	7 Autologous Tissue Substitute J Synthetic Substitute K Nonautologous Tissue Substitute	Z No Qualifier
R Anal Sphincter S Greater Omentum T Lesser Omentum V Mesentery W Peritoneum	Ø Open 4 Percutaneous Endoscopic	7 Autologous Tissue Substitute J Synthetic Substitute K Nonautologous Tissue Substitute	Z No Qualifier

Ø Medical and Surgical
D Gastrointestinal System
S Reposition Moving to its normal location or other suitable location all or a portion of a body part

Body Part Character 4	Approach Character 5	Device Character 6	Qualifier Character 7
5 Esophagus 6 Stomach 9 Duodenum A Jejunum B Ileum H Cecum K Ascending Colon L Transverse Colon M Descending Colon N Sigmoid Colon P Rectum Q Anus	Ø Open 4 Percutaneous Endoscopic 7 Via Natural or Artificial Opening 8 Via Natural or Artificial Opening Endoscopic X External	Z No Device	Z No Qualifier

0 Medical and Surgical
D Gastrointestinal System
T Resection Cutting out or off, without replacement, all of a body part

Body Part Character 4	Approach Character 5	Device Character 6	Qualifier Character 7
1 Esophagus, Upper **2** Esophagus, Middle **3** Esophagus, Lower **4** Esophagogastric Junction **5** Esophagus **6** Stomach **7** Stomach, Pylorus **8** Small Intestine **9** Duodenum **A** Jejunum **B** Ileum **C** Ileocecal Valve **E** Large Intestine **F** Large Intestine, Right **G** Large Intestine, Left **H** Cecum **J** Appendix **K** Ascending Colon **L** Transverse Colon **M** Descending Colon **N** Sigmoid Colon **P** Rectum **Q** Anus	**0** Open **4** Percutaneous Endoscopic **7** Via Natural or Artificial Opening **8** Via Natural or Artificial Opening Endoscopic	**Z** No Device	**Z** No Qualifier
R Anal Sphincter **S** Greater Omentum **T** Lesser Omentum	**0** Open **4** Percutaneous Endoscopic	**Z** No Device	**Z** No Qualifier

0 Medical and Surgical
D Gastrointestinal System
U Supplement Putting in or on biological or synthetic material that physically reinforces and/or augments the function of a portion of a body part

Body Part Character 4	Approach Character 5	Device Character 6	Qualifier Character 7
1 Esophagus, Upper **2** Esophagus, Middle **3** Esophagus, Lower **4** Esophagogastric Junction **5** Esophagus **6** Stomach **7** Stomach, Pylorus **8** Small Intestine **9** Duodenum **A** Jejunum **B** Ileum **C** Ileocecal Valve **E** Large Intestine **F** Large Intestine, Right **G** Large Intestine, Left **H** Cecum **K** Ascending Colon **L** Transverse Colon **M** Descending Colon **N** Sigmoid Colon **P** Rectum	**0** Open **4** Percutaneous Endoscopic **7** Via Natural or Artificial Opening **8** Via Natural or Artificial Opening Endoscopic	**7** Autologous Tissue Substitute **J** Synthetic Substitute **K** Nonautologous Tissue Substitute	**Z** No Qualifier
Q Anus	**0** Open **4** Percutaneous Endoscopic **7** Via Natural or Artificial Opening **8** Via Natural or Artificial Opening Endoscopic **X** External	**7** Autologous Tissue Substitute **J** Synthetic Substitute **K** Nonautologous Tissue Substitute	**Z** No Qualifier
R Anal Sphincter **S** Greater Omentum **T** Lesser Omentum **V** Mesentery **W** Peritoneum	**0** Open **4** Percutaneous Endoscopic	**7** Autologous Tissue Substitute **J** Synthetic Substitute **K** Nonautologous Tissue Substitute	**Z** No Qualifier

Ø Medical and Surgical
D Gastrointestinal System
V Restriction Partially closing an orifice or the lumen of a tubular body part

Body Part Character 4	Approach Character 5	Device Character 6	Qualifier Character 7
1 Esophagus, Upper **2** Esophagus, Middle **3** Esophagus, Lower **4** Esophagogastric Junction **5** Esophagus **6** Stomach **7** Stomach, Pylorus **8** Small Intestine **9** Duodenum **A** Jejunum **B** Ileum **C** Ileocecal Valve **E** Large Intestine **F** Large Intestine, Right **G** Large Intestine, Left **H** Cecum **K** Ascending Colon **L** Transverse Colon **M** Descending Colon **N** Sigmoid Colon **P** Rectum	**Ø** Open **3** Percutaneous **4** Percutaneous Endoscopic	**C** Extraluminal Device **D** Intraluminal Device **Z** No Device	**Z** No Qualifier
1 Esophagus, Upper **2** Esophagus, Middle **3** Esophagus, Lower **4** Esophagogastric Junction **5** Esophagus **6** Stomach **7** Stomach, Pylorus **8** Small Intestine **9** Duodenum **A** Jejunum **B** Ileum **C** Ileocecal Valve **E** Large Intestine **F** Large Intestine, Right **G** Large Intestine, Left **H** Cecum **K** Ascending Colon **L** Transverse Colon **M** Descending Colon **N** Sigmoid Colon **P** Rectum **Q** Anus	**7** Via Natural or Artificial Opening **8** Via Natural or Artificial Opening Endoscopic	**D** Intraluminal Device **Z** No Device	**Z** No Qualifier
Q Anus	**Ø** Open **3** Percutaneous **4** Percutaneous Endoscopic **X** External	**C** Extraluminal Device **D** Intraluminal Device **Z** No Device	**Z** No Qualifier

Ø Medical and Surgical
D Gastrointestinal System
W Revision Correcting, to the extent possible, a portion of a malfunctioning device or the position of a displaced device

Body Part Character 4	Approach Character 5	Device Character 6	Qualifier Character 7
Ø Upper Intestinal Tract **D** Lower Intestinal Tract	**Ø** Open **3** Percutaneous **4** Percutaneous Endoscopic **7** Via Natural or Artificial Opening **8** Via Natural or Artificial Opening Endoscopic **X** External	**Ø** Drainage Device **2** Monitoring Device **3** Infusion Device **7** Autologous Tissue Substitute **C** Extraluminal Device **D** Intraluminal Device **J** Synthetic Substitute **K** Nonautologous Tissue Substitute **U** Feeding Device	**Z** No Qualifier
5 Esophagus	**7** Via Natural or Artificial Opening **8** Via Natural or Artificial Opening Endoscopic **X** External	**D Intraluminal Device**	**Z** No Qualifier

ØDW Continued on next page

0 Medical and Surgical
D Gastrointestinal System
W Revision Correcting, to the extent possible, a portion of a malfunctioning device or the position of a displaced device

0DW Continued

Body Part Character 4	Approach Character 5	Device Character 6	Qualifier Character 7
6 Stomach	0 Open 3 Percutaneous 4 Percutaneous Endoscopic	0 Drainage Device 2 Monitoring Device 3 Infusion Device 7 Autologous Tissue Substitute C Extraluminal Device D Intraluminal Device J Synthetic Substitute K Nonautologous Tissue Substitute M Stimulator Lead U Feeding Device	Z No Qualifier
6 Stomach	7 Via Natural or Artificial Opening 8 Via Natural or Artificial Opening Endoscopic X External	0 Drainage Device 2 Monitoring Device 3 Infusion Device 7 Autologous Tissue Substitute C Extraluminal Device D Intraluminal Device J Synthetic Substitute K Nonautologous Tissue Substitute U Feeding Device	Z No Qualifier
8 Small Intestine E Large Intestine	0 Open 4 Percutaneous Endoscopic 7 Via Natural or Artificial Opening 8 Via Natural or Artificial Opening Endoscopic	7 Autologous Tissue Substitute J Synthetic Substitute K Nonautologous Tissue Substitute	Z No Qualifier
Q Anus	0 Open 3 Percutaneous 4 Percutaneous Endoscopic 7 Via Natural or Artificial Opening 8 Via Natural or Artificial Opening Endoscopic	L Artificial Sphincter	Z No Qualifier
R Anal Sphincter	0 Open 3 Percutaneous 4 Percutaneous Endoscopic	M Stimulator Lead	Z No Qualifier
U Omentum V Mesentery W Peritoneum	0 Open 3 Percutaneous 4 Percutaneous Endoscopic	0 Drainage Device 7 Autologous Tissue Substitute J Synthetic Substitute K Nonautologous Tissue Substitute	Z No Qualifier

0 Medical and Surgical
D Gastrointestinal System
X Transfer Moving, without taking out, all or a portion of a body part to another location to take over the function of all or a portion of a body part

Body Part Character 4	Approach Character 5	Device Character 6	Qualifier Character 7
6 Stomach 8 Small Intestine E Large Intestine	0 Open 4 Percutaneous Endoscopic	Z No Device	5 Esophagus

0 Medical and Surgical
D Gastrointestinal System
Y Transplantation Putting in or on all or a portion of a living body part taken from another individual or animal to physically take the place and/or function of all or a portion of a similar body part

Body Part Character 4	Approach Character 5	Device Character 6	Qualifier Character 7
5 Esophagus 6 Stomach 8 Small Intestine E Large Intestine	0 Open	Z No Device	0 Allogeneic 1 Syngeneic 2 Zooplastic

Hepatobiliary System and Pancreas ØF1–ØFY

Ø Medical and Surgical
F Hepatobiliary System and Pancreas
1 Bypass Altering the route of passage of the contents of a tubular body part

Body Part Character 4	Approach Character 5	Device Character 6	Qualifier Character 7
4 Gallbladder 5 Hepatic Duct, Right 6 Hepatic Duct, Left 8 Cystic Duct 9 Common Bile Duct	Ø Open 4 Percutaneous Endoscopic	D Intraluminal Device Z No Device	3 Duodenum 4 Stomach 5 Hepatic Duct, Right 6 Hepatic Duct, Left 7 Hepatic Duct, Caudate 8 Cystic Duct 9 Common Bile Duct B Small Intestine
D Pancreatic Duct F Pancreatic Duct, Accessory G Pancreas	Ø Open 4 Percutaneous Endoscopic	D Intraluminal Device Z No Device	3 Duodenum B Small Intestine C Large Intestine

Ø Medical and Surgical
F Hepatobiliary System and Pancreas
2 Change Taking out or off a device from a body part and putting back an identical or similar device in or on the same body part without cutting or puncturing the skin or a mucous membrane

Body Part Character 4	Approach Character 5	Device Character 6	Qualifier Character 7
Ø Liver 4 Gallbladder B Hepatobiliary Duct D Pancreatic Duct G Pancreas	X External	Ø Drainage Device Y Other Device	Z No Qualifier

Ø Medical and Surgical
F Hepatobiliary System and Pancreas
5 Destruction Physical eradication of all or a portion of a body part by the direct use of energy, force, or a destructive agent

Body Part Character 4	Approach Character 5	Device Character 6	Qualifier Character 7
Ø Liver 1 Liver, Right Lobe 2 Liver, Left Lobe 4 Gallbladder G Pancreas	Ø Open 3 Percutaneous 4 Percutaneous Endoscopic	Z No Device	Z No Qualifier
5 Hepatic Duct, Right 6 Hepatic Duct, Left 8 Cystic Duct 9 Common Bile Duct C Ampulla of Vater D Pancreatic Duct F Pancreatic Duct, Accessory	Ø Open 3 Percutaneous 4 Percutaneous Endoscopic 7 Via Natural or Artificial Opening 8 Via Natural or Artificial Opening Endoscopic	Z No Device	Z No Qualifier

Ø Medical and Surgical
F Hepatobiliary System and Pancreas
7 Dilation Expanding an orifice or the lumen of a tubular body part

Body Part Character 4	Approach Character 5	Device Character 6	Qualifier Character 7
5 Hepatic Duct, Right 6 Hepatic Duct, Left 8 Cystic Duct 9 Common Bile Duct C Ampulla of Vater D Pancreatic Duct F Pancreatic Duct, Accessory	Ø Open 3 Percutaneous 4 Percutaneous Endoscopic 7 Via Natural or Artificial Opening 8 Via Natural or Artificial Opening Endoscopic	D Intraluminal Device Z No Device	Z No Qualifier

0 Medical and Surgical
F Hepatobiliary System and Pancreas
8 Division Cutting into a body part without draining fluids and/or gases from the body part in order to separate or transect a body part

Body Part Character 4	Approach Character 5	Device Character 6	Qualifier Character 7
G Pancreas	0 Open 3 Percutaneous 4 Percutaneous Endoscopic	Z No Device	Z No Qualifier

0 Medical and Surgical
F Hepatobiliary System and Pancreas
9 Drainage Taking or letting out fluids and/or gases from a body part

Body Part Character 4	Approach Character 5	Device Character 6	Qualifier Character 7
0 Liver 1 Liver, Right Lobe 2 Liver, Left Lobe 4 Gallbladder G Pancreas	0 Open 3 Percutaneous 4 Percutaneous Endoscopic	0 Drainage Device	Z No Qualifier
0 Liver 1 Liver, Right Lobe 2 Liver, Left Lobe 4 Gallbladder G Pancreas	0 Open 3 Percutaneous 4 Percutaneous Endoscopic	Z No Device	X Diagnostic Z No Qualifier
5 Hepatic Duct, Right 6 Hepatic Duct, Left 8 Cystic Duct 9 Common Bile Duct C Ampulla of Vater D Pancreatic Duct F Pancreatic Duct, Accessory	0 Open 3 Percutaneous 4 Percutaneous Endoscopic 7 Via Natural or Artificial Opening 8 Via Natural or Artificial Opening Endoscopic	0 Drainage Device	Z No Qualifier
5 Hepatic Duct, Right 6 Hepatic Duct, Left 8 Cystic Duct 9 Common Bile Duct C Ampulla of Vater D Pancreatic Duct F Pancreatic Duct, Accessory	0 Open 3 Percutaneous 4 Percutaneous Endoscopic 7 Via Natural or Artificial Opening 8 Via Natural or Artificial Opening Endoscopic	Z No Device	X Diagnostic Z No Qualifier

0 Medical and Surgical
F Hepatobiliary System and Pancreas
B Excision Cutting out or off, without replacement, a portion of a body part

Body Part Character 4	Approach Character 5	Device Character 6	Qualifier Character 7
0 Liver 1 Liver, Right Lobe 2 Liver, Left Lobe 4 Gallbladder G Pancreas	0 Open 3 Percutaneous 4 Percutaneous Endoscopic	Z No Device	X Diagnostic Z No Qualifier
5 Hepatic Duct, Right 6 Hepatic Duct, Left 8 Cystic Duct 9 Common Bile Duct C Ampulla of Vater D Pancreatic Duct F Pancreatic Duct, Accessory	0 Open 3 Percutaneous 4 Percutaneous Endoscopic 7 Via Natural or Artificial Opening 8 Via Natural or Artificial Opening Endoscopic	Z No Device	X Diagnostic Z No Qualifier

Ø Medical and Surgical
F Hepatobiliary System and Pancreas
C Extirpation Taking or cutting out solid matter from a body part

Body Part Character 4	Approach Character 5	Device Character 6	Qualifier Character 7
Ø Liver 1 Liver, Right Lobe 2 Liver, Left Lobe 4 Gallbladder G Pancreas	Ø Open 3 Percutaneous 4 Percutaneous Endoscopic	Z No Device	Z No Qualifier
5 Hepatic Duct, Right 6 Hepatic Duct, Left 8 Cystic Duct 9 Common Bile Duct C Ampulla of Vater D Pancreatic Duct F Pancreatic Duct, Accessory	Ø Open 3 Percutaneous 4 Percutaneous Endoscopic 7 Via Natural or Artificial Opening 8 Via Natural or Artificial Opening Endoscopic	Z No Device	Z No Qualifier

Ø Medical and Surgical
F Hepatobiliary System and Pancreas
F Fragmentation Breaking solid matter in a body part into pieces

Body Part Character 4	Approach Character 5	Device Character 6	Qualifier Character 7
4 Gallbladder 5 Hepatic Duct, Right 6 Hepatic Duct, Left 8 Cystic Duct 9 Common Bile Duct C Ampulla of Vater D Pancreatic Duct F Pancreatic Duct, Accessory	Ø Open 3 Percutaneous 4 Percutaneous Endoscopic 7 Via Natural or Artificial Opening 8 Via Natural or Artificial Opening Endoscopic X External	Z No Device	Z No Qualifier

Ø Medical and Surgical
F Hepatobiliary System and Pancreas
H Insertion Putting in a nonbiological appliance that monitors, assists, performs, or prevents a physiological function but does not physically take the place of a body part

Body Part Character 4	Approach Character 5	Device Character 6	Qualifier Character 7
Ø Liver 1 Liver, Right Lobe 2 Liver, Left Lobe 4 Gallbladder G Pancreas	Ø Open 3 Percutaneous 4 Percutaneous Endoscopic	2 Monitoring Device 3 Infusion Device	Z No Qualifier
B Hepatobiliary Duct D Pancreatic Duct	Ø Open 3 Percutaneous 4 Percutaneous Endoscopic 7 Via Natural or Artificial Opening 8 Via Natural or Artificial Opening Endoscopic	1 Radioactive Element 2 Monitoring Device 3 Infusion Device **D Intraluminal Device**	Z No Qualifier

Ø Medical and Surgical
F Hepatobiliary System and Pancreas
J Inspection Visually and/or manually exploring a body part

Body Part Character 4	Approach Character 5	Device Character 6	Qualifier Character 7
Ø Liver 4 Gallbladder G Pancreas	Ø Open 3 Percutaneous 4 Percutaneous Endoscopic X External	Z No Device	Z No Qualifier
B Hepatobiliary Duct D Pancreatic Duct	Ø Open 3 Percutaneous 4 Percutaneous Endoscopic 7 Via Natural or Artificial Opening 8 Via Natural or Artificial Opening Endoscopic	Z No Device	Z No Qualifier

0 Medical and Surgical
F Hepatobiliary System and Pancreas
L Occlusion Completely closing an orifice or the lumen of a tubular body part

Body Part Character 4	Approach Character 5	Device Character 6	Qualifier Character 7
5 Hepatic Duct, Right **6** Hepatic Duct, Left **8** Cystic Duct **9** Common Bile Duct **C** Ampulla of Vater **D** Pancreatic Duct **F** Pancreatic Duct, Accessory	**0** Open **3** Percutaneous **4** Percutaneous Endoscopic	**C** Extraluminal Device **D** Intraluminal Device **Z** No Device	**Z** No Qualifier
5 Hepatic Duct, Right **6** Hepatic Duct, Left **8** Cystic Duct **9** Common Bile Duct **C** Ampulla of Vater **D** Pancreatic Duct **F** Pancreatic Duct, Accessory	**7** Via Natural or Artificial Opening **8** Via Natural or Artificial Opening Endoscopic	**D** Intraluminal Device **Z** No Device	**Z** No Qualifier

0 Medical and Surgical
F Hepatobiliary System and Pancreas
M Reattachment Putting back in or on all or a portion of a separated body part to its normal location or other suitable location

Body Part Character 4	Approach Character 5	Device Character 6	Qualifier Character 7
0 Liver **1** Liver, Right Lobe **2** Liver, Left Lobe **4** Gallbladder **5** Hepatic Duct, Right **6** Hepatic Duct, Left **8** Cystic Duct **9** Common Bile Duct **C** Ampulla of Vater **D** Pancreatic Duct **F** Pancreatic Duct, Accessory **G** Pancreas	**0** Open **4** Percutaneous Endoscopic	**Z** No Device	**Z** No Qualifier

0 Medical and Surgical
F Hepatobiliary System and Pancreas
N Release Freeing a body part from an abnormal physical constraint

Body Part Character 4	Approach Character 5	Device Character 6	Qualifier Character 7
0 Liver **1** Liver, Right Lobe **2** Liver, Left Lobe **4** Gallbladder **G** Pancreas	**0** Open **3** Percutaneous **4** Percutaneous Endoscopic	**Z** No Device	**Z** No Qualifier
5 Hepatic Duct, Right **6** Hepatic Duct, Left **8** Cystic Duct **9** Common Bile Duct **C** Ampulla of Vater **D** Pancreatic Duct **F** Pancreatic Duct, Accessory	**0** Open **3** Percutaneous **4** Percutaneous Endoscopic **7** Via Natural or Artificial Opening **8** Via Natural or Artificial Opening Endoscopic	**Z** No Device	**Z** No Qualifier

Ø Medical and Surgical
F Hepatobiliary System and Pancreas
P Removal Taking out or off a device from a body part

Body Part Character 4	Approach Character 5	Device Character 6	Qualifier Character 7
Ø Liver	**Ø** Open **3** Percutaneous **4** Percutaneous Endoscopic **X** External	**Ø** Drainage Device **2** Monitoring Device **3** Infusion Device	**Z** No Qualifier
4 Gallbladder **G** Pancreas	**Ø** Open **3** Percutaneous **4** Percutaneous Endoscopic **X** External	**Ø** Drainage Device **2** Monitoring Device **3** Infusion Device **D** Intraluminal Device	**Z** No Qualifier
B Hepatobiliary Duct **D** Pancreatic Duct	**Ø** Open **3** Percutaneous **4** Percutaneous Endoscopic **7** Via Natural or Artificial Opening **8** Via Natural or Artificial Opening Endoscopic	**Ø** Drainage Device **1** Radioactive Element **2** Monitoring Device **3** Infusion Device **7** Autologous Tissue Substitute **C** Extraluminal Device **D** Intraluminal Device **J** Synthetic Substitute **K** Nonautologous Tissue Substitute	**Z** No Qualifier
B Hepatobiliary Duct **D** Pancreatic Duct	**X** External	**Ø** Drainage Device **1** Radioactive Element **2** Monitoring Device **3** Infusion Device **D** Intraluminal Device	**Z** No Qualifier

Ø Medical and Surgical
F Hepatobiliary System and Pancreas
Q Repair Restoring, to the extent possible, a body part to its normal anatomic structure and function

Body Part Character 4	Approach Character 5	Device Character 6	Qualifier Character 7
Ø Liver **1** Liver, Right Lobe **2** Liver, Left Lobe **4** Gallbladder **G** Pancreas	**Ø** Open **3** Percutaneous **4** Percutaneous Endoscopic	**Z** No Device	**Z** No Qualifier
5 Hepatic Duct, Right **6** Hepatic Duct, Left **8** Cystic Duct **9** Common Bile Duct **C** Ampulla of Vater **D** Pancreatic Duct **F** Pancreatic Duct, Accessory	**Ø** Open **3** Percutaneous **4** Percutaneous Endoscopic **7** Via Natural or Artificial Opening **8** Via Natural or Artificial Opening Endoscopic	**Z** No Device	**Z** No Qualifier

Ø Medical and Surgical
F Hepatobiliary System and Pancreas
R Replacement Putting in or on biological or synthetic material that physically takes the place and/or function of all or a portion of a body part

Body Part Character 4	Approach Character 5	Device Character 6	Qualifier Character 7
5 Hepatic Duct, Right **6** Hepatic Duct, Left **8** Cystic Duct **9** Common Bile Duct **C** Ampulla of Vater **D** Pancreatic Duct **F** Pancreatic Duct, Accessory	**Ø** Open **4** Percutaneous Endoscopic	**7** Autologous Tissue Substitute **J** Synthetic Substitute **K** Nonautologous Tissue Substitute	**Z** No Qualifier

0 Medical and Surgical
F Hepatobiliary System and Pancreas
S Reposition Moving to its normal location or other suitable location all or a portion of a body part

Body Part Character 4	Approach Character 5	Device Character 6	Qualifier Character 7
0 Liver 4 Gallbladder 5 Hepatic Duct, Right 6 Hepatic Duct, Left 8 Cystic Duct 9 Common Bile Duct C Ampulla of Vater D Pancreatic Duct F Pancreatic Duct, Accessory G Pancreas	0 Open 4 Percutaneous Endoscopic	Z No Device	Z No Qualifier

0 Medical and Surgical
F Hepatobiliary System and Pancreas
T Resection Cutting out or off, without replacement, all of a body part

Body Part Character 4	Approach Character 5	Device Character 6	Qualifier Character 7
0 Liver 1 Liver, Right Lobe 2 Liver, Left Lobe 4 Gallbladder G Pancreas	0 Open 4 Percutaneous Endoscopic	Z No Device	Z No Qualifier
5 Hepatic Duct, Right 6 Hepatic Duct, Left 8 Cystic Duct 9 Common Bile Duct C Ampulla of Vater D Pancreatic Duct F Pancreatic Duct, Accessory	0 Open 4 Percutaneous Endoscopic 7 Via Natural or Artificial Opening 8 Via Natural or Artificial Opening Endoscopic	Z No Device	Z No Qualifier

0 Medical and Surgical
F Hepatobiliary System and Pancreas
U Supplement Putting in or on biological or synthetic material that physically reinforces and/or augments the function of a portion of a body part

Body Part Character 4	Approach Character 5	Device Character 6	Qualifier Character 7
5 Hepatic Duct, Right 6 Hepatic Duct, Left 8 Cystic Duct 9 Common Bile Duct C Ampulla of Vater D Pancreatic Duct F Pancreatic Duct, Accessory	0 Open 3 Percutaneous 4 Percutaneous Endoscopic	7 Autologous Tissue Substitute J Synthetic Substitute K Nonautologous Tissue Substitute	Z No Qualifier

0 Medical and Surgical
F Hepatobiliary System and Pancreas
V Restriction Partially closing an orifice or the lumen of a tubular body part

Body Part Character 4	Approach Character 5	Device Character 6	Qualifier Character 7
5 Hepatic Duct, Right 6 Hepatic Duct, Left 8 Cystic Duct 9 Common Bile Duct C Ampulla of Vater D Pancreatic Duct F Pancreatic Duct, Accessory	0 Open 3 Percutaneous 4 Percutaneous Endoscopic	C Extraluminal Device D Intraluminal Device Z No Device	Z No Qualifier
5 Hepatic Duct, Right 6 Hepatic Duct, Left 8 Cystic Duct 9 Common Bile Duct C Ampulla of Vater D Pancreatic Duct F Pancreatic Duct, Accessory	7 Via Natural or Artificial Opening 8 Via Natural or Artificial Opening Endoscopic	D Intraluminal Device Z No Device	Z No Qualifier

Ø Medical and Surgical
F Hepatobiliary System and Pancreas
W Revision Correcting, to the extent possible, a portion of a malfunctioning device or the position of a displaced device

Body Part Character 4	Approach Character 5	Device Character 6	Qualifier Character 7
Ø Liver	**Ø** Open **3** Percutaneous **4** Percutaneous Endoscopic **X** External	**Ø** Drainage Device **2** Monitoring Device **3** Infusion Device	**Z** No Qualifier
4 Gallbladder **G** Pancreas	**Ø** Open **3** Percutaneous **4** Percutaneous Endoscopic **X** External	**Ø** Drainage Device **2** Monitoring Device **3** Infusion Device **D** Intraluminal Device	**Z** No Qualifier
B Hepatobiliary Duct **D** Pancreatic Duct	**Ø** Open **3** Percutaneous **4** Percutaneous Endoscopic **7** Via Natural or Artificial Opening **8** Via Natural or Artificial Opening Endoscopic **X** External	**Ø** Drainage Device **2** Monitoring Device **3** Infusion Device **7** Autologous Tissue Substitute **C** Extraluminal Device **D** Intraluminal Device **J** Synthetic Substitute **K** Nonautologous Tissue Substitute	**Z** No Qualifier

Ø Medical and Surgical
F Hepatobiliary System and Pancreas
Y Transplantation Putting in or on all or a portion of a living body part taken from another individual or animal to physically take the place and/or function of all or a portion of a similar body part

Body Part Character 4	Approach Character 5	Device Character 6	Qualifier Character 7
Ø Liver **G** Pancreas	**Ø** Open	**Z** No Device	**Ø** Allogeneic **1** Syngeneic **2** Zooplastic

Endocrine System 0G2–0GW

0 Medical and Surgical
G Endocrine System
2 Change Taking out or off a device from a body part and putting back an identical or similar device in or on the same body part without cutting or puncturing the skin or a mucous membrane

Body Part Character 4	Approach Character 5	Device Character 6	Qualifier Character 7
0 Pituitary Gland 1 Pineal Body 5 Adrenal Gland K Thyroid Gland R Parathyroid Gland S Endocrine Gland	X External	0 Drainage Device Y Other Device	Z No Qualifier

0 Medical and Surgical
G Endocrine System
5 Destruction Physical eradication of all or a portion of a body part by the direct use of energy, force, or a destructive agent

Body Part Character 4	Approach Character 5	Device Character 6	Qualifier Character 7
0 Pituitary Gland 1 Pineal Body 2 Adrenal Gland, Left 3 Adrenal Gland, Right 4 Adrenal Glands, Bilateral 6 Carotid Body, Left 7 Carotid Body, Right 8 Carotid Bodies, Bilateral 9 Para-aortic Body B Coccygeal Glomus C Glomus Jugulare D Aortic Body F Paraganglion Extremity G Thyroid Gland Lobe, Left H Thyroid Gland Lobe, Right K Thyroid Gland L Superior Parathyroid Gland, Right M Superior Parathyroid Gland, Left N Inferior Parathyroid Gland, Right P Inferior Parathyroid Gland, Left Q Parathyroid Glands, Multiple R Parathyroid Gland	0 Open 3 Percutaneous 4 Percutaneous Endoscopic	Z No Device	Z No Qualifier

0 Medical and Surgical
G Endocrine System
8 Division Cutting into a body part without draining fluids and/or gases from the body part in order to separate or transect a body part

Body Part Character 4	Approach Character 5	Device Character 6	Qualifier Character 7
0 Pituitary Gland J Thyroid Gland Isthmus	0 Open 3 Percutaneous 4 Percutaneous Endoscopic	Z No Device	Z No Qualifier

Ø Medical and Surgical
G Endocrine System
9 Drainage Taking or letting out fluids and/or gases from a body part

Body Part Character 4	Approach Character 5	Device Character 6	Qualifier Character 7
Ø Pituitary Gland **1** Pineal Body **2** Adrenal Gland, Left **3** Adrenal Gland, Right **4** Adrenal Glands, Bilateral **6** Carotid Body, Left **7** Carotid Body, Right **8** Carotid Bodies, Bilateral **9** Para-aortic Body **B** Coccygeal Glomus **C** Glomus Jugulare **D** Aortic Body **F** Paraganglion Extremity **G** Thyroid Gland Lobe, Left **H** Thyroid Gland Lobe, Right **K** Thyroid Gland **L** Superior Parathyroid Gland, Right **M** Superior Parathyroid Gland, Left **N** Inferior Parathyroid Gland, Right **P** Inferior Parathyroid Gland, Left **Q** Parathyroid Glands, Multiple **R** Parathyroid Gland	**Ø** Open **3** Percutaneous **4** Percutaneous Endoscopic	**Ø** Drainage Device	**Z** No Qualifier
Ø Pituitary Gland **1** Pineal Body **2** Adrenal Gland, Left **3** Adrenal Gland, Right **4** Adrenal Glands, Bilateral **6** Carotid Body, Left **7** Carotid Body, Right **8** Carotid Bodies, Bilateral **9** Para-aortic Body **B** Coccygeal Glomus **C** Glomus Jugulare **D** Aortic Body **F** Paraganglion Extremity **G** Thyroid Gland Lobe, Left **H** Thyroid Gland Lobe, Right **K** Thyroid Gland **L** Superior Parathyroid Gland, Right **M** Superior Parathyroid Gland, Left **N** Inferior Parathyroid Gland, Right **P** Inferior Parathyroid Gland, Left **Q** Parathyroid Glands, Multiple **R** Parathyroid Gland	**Ø** Open **3** Percutaneous **4** Percutaneous Endoscopic	**Z** No Device	**X** Diagnostic **Z** No Qualifier

Ø Medical and Surgical
G Endocrine System
B Excision Cutting out or off, without replacement, a portion of a body part

Body Part Character 4	Approach Character 5	Device Character 6	Qualifier Character 7
Ø Pituitary Gland **1** Pineal Body **2** Adrenal Gland, Left **3** Adrenal Gland, Right **4** Adrenal Glands, Bilateral **6** Carotid Body, Left **7** Carotid Body, Right **8** Carotid Bodies, Bilateral **9** Para-aortic Body **B** Coccygeal Glomus **C** Glomus Jugulare **D** Aortic Body **F** Paraganglion Extremity **G** Thyroid Gland Lobe, Left **H** Thyroid Gland Lobe, Right **L** Superior Parathyroid Gland, Right **M** Superior Parathyroid Gland, Left **N** Inferior Parathyroid Gland, Right **P** Inferior Parathyroid Gland, Left **Q** Parathyroid Glands, Multiple **R** Parathyroid Gland	**Ø** Open **3** Percutaneous **4** Percutaneous Endoscopic	**Z** No Device	**X** Diagnostic **Z** No Qualifier

Ø Medical and Surgical
G Endocrine System
C Extirpation Taking or cutting out solid matter from a body part

Body Part Character 4	Approach Character 5	Device Character 6	Qualifier Character 7
Ø Pituitary Gland **1** Pineal Body **2** Adrenal Gland, Left **3** Adrenal Gland, Right **4** Adrenal Glands, Bilateral **6** Carotid Body, Left **7** Carotid Body, Right **8** Carotid Bodies, Bilateral **9** Para-aortic Body **B** Coccygeal Glomus **C** Glomus Jugulare **D** Aortic Body **F** Paraganglion Extremity **G** Thyroid Gland Lobe, Left **H** Thyroid Gland Lobe, Right **K** Thyroid Gland **L** Superior Parathyroid Gland, Right **M** Superior Parathyroid Gland, Left **N** Inferior Parathyroid Gland, Right **P** Inferior Parathyroid Gland, Left **Q** Parathyroid Glands, Multiple **R** Parathyroid Gland	**Ø** Open **3** Percutaneous **4** Percutaneous Endoscopic	**Z** No Device	**Z** No Qualifier

Ø Medical and Surgical
G Endocrine System
H Insertion Putting in a nonbiological appliance that monitors, assists, performs, or prevents a physiological function but does not physically take the place of a body part

Body Part Character 4	Approach Character 5	Device Character 6	Qualifier Character 7
S Endocrine Gland	**Ø** Open **3** Percutaneous **4** Percutaneous Endoscopic	**2** Monitoring Device **3** Infusion Device	**Z** No Qualifier

Ø Medical and Surgical
G Endocrine System
J Inspection Visually and/or manually exploring a body part

Body Part Character 4	Approach Character 5	Device Character 6	Qualifier Character 7
Ø Pituitary Gland **1** Pineal Body **5** Adrenal Gland **K** Thyroid Gland **R** Parathyroid Gland **S** Endocrine Gland	**Ø** Open **3** Percutaneous **4** Percutaneous Endoscopic	**Z** No Device	**Z** No Qualifier

Ø Medical and Surgical
G Endocrine System
M Reattachment Putting back in or on all or a portion of a separated body part to its normal location or other suitable location

Body Part Character 4	Approach Character 5	Device Character 6	Qualifier Character 7
2 Adrenal Gland, Left **3** Adrenal Gland, Right **G** Thyroid Gland Lobe, Left **H** Thyroid Gland Lobe, Right **L** Superior Parathyroid Gland, Right **M** Superior Parathyroid Gland, Left **N** Inferior Parathyroid Gland, Right **P** Inferior Parathyroid Gland, Left **Q** Parathyroid Glands, Multiple **R** Parathyroid Gland	**Ø** Open **4** Percutaneous Endoscopic	**Z** No Device	**Z** No Qualifier

Ø Medical and Surgical
G Endocrine System
N Release Freeing a body part from an abnormal physical constraint

Body Part Character 4	Approach Character 5	Device Character 6	Qualifier Character 7
Ø Pituitary Gland **1** Pineal Body **2** Adrenal Gland, Left **3** Adrenal Gland, Right **4** Adrenal Glands, Bilateral **6** Carotid Body, Left **7** Carotid Body, Right **8** Carotid Bodies, Bilateral **9** Para-aortic Body **B** Coccygeal Glomus **C** Glomus Jugulare **D** Aortic Body **F** Paraganglion Extremity **G** Thyroid Gland Lobe, Left **H** Thyroid Gland Lobe, Right **K** Thyroid Gland **L** Superior Parathyroid Gland, Right **M** Superior Parathyroid Gland, Left **N** Inferior Parathyroid Gland, Right **P** Inferior Parathyroid Gland, Left **Q** Parathyroid Glands, Multiple **R** Parathyroid Gland	**Ø** Open **3** Percutaneous **4** Percutaneous Endoscopic	**Z** No Device	**Z** No Qualifier

Ø Medical and Surgical
G Endocrine System
P Removal Taking out or off a device from a body part

Body Part Character 4	Approach Character 5	Device Character 6	Qualifier Character 7
Ø Pituitary Gland **1** Pineal Body **5** Adrenal Gland **K** Thyroid Gland **R** Parathyroid Gland	**Ø** Open **3** Percutaneous **4** Percutaneous Endoscopic **X** External	**Ø** Drainage Device	**Z** No Qualifier
S Endocrine Gland	**Ø** Open **3** Percutaneous **4** Percutaneous Endoscopic **X** External	**Ø** Drainage Device **2** Monitoring Device **3** Infusion Device	**Z** No Qualifier

Ø Medical and Surgical
G Endocrine System
Q Repair Restoring, to the extent possible, a body part to its normal anatomic structure and function

Body Part Character 4	Approach Character 5	Device Character 6	Qualifier Character 7
Ø Pituitary Gland **1** Pineal Body **2** Adrenal Gland, Left **3** Adrenal Gland, Right **4** Adrenal Glands, Bilateral **6** Carotid Body, Left **7** Carotid Body, Right **8** Carotid Bodies, Bilateral **9** Para-aortic Body **B** Coccygeal Glomus **C** Glomus Jugulare **D** Aortic Body **F** Paraganglion Extremity **G** Thyroid Gland Lobe, Left **H** Thyroid Gland Lobe, Right **J** Thyroid Gland Isthmus **K** Thyroid Gland **L** Superior Parathyroid Gland, Right **M** Superior Parathyroid Gland, Left **N** Inferior Parathyroid Gland, Right **P** Inferior Parathyroid Gland, Left **Q** Parathyroid Glands, Multiple **R** Parathyroid Gland	**Ø** Open **3** Percutaneous **4** Percutaneous Endoscopic	**Z** No Device	**Z** No Qualifier

0 Medical and Surgical
G Endocrine System
S Reposition Moving to its normal location or other suitable location all or a portion of a body part

Body Part Character 4	Approach Character 5	Device Character 6	Qualifier Character 7
2 Adrenal Gland, Left **3** Adrenal Gland, Right **G** Thyroid Gland Lobe, Left **H** Thyroid Gland Lobe, Right **L** Superior Parathyroid Gland, Right **M** Superior Parathyroid Gland, Left **N** Inferior Parathyroid Gland, Right **P** Inferior Parathyroid Gland, Left **Q** Parathyroid Glands, Multiple **R** Parathyroid Gland	**0** Open **4** Percutaneous Endoscopic	**Z** No Device	**Z** No Qualifier

0 Medical and Surgical
G Endocrine System
T Resection Cutting out or off, without replacement, all of a body part

Body Part Character 4	Approach Character 5	Device Character 6	Qualifier Character 7
0 Pituitary Gland **1** Pineal Body **2** Adrenal Gland, Left **3** Adrenal Gland, Right **4** Adrenal Glands, Bilateral **6** Carotid Body, Left **7** Carotid Body, Right **8** Carotid Bodies, Bilateral **9** Para-aortic Body **B** Coccygeal Glomus **C** Glomus Jugulare **D** Aortic Body **F** Paraganglion Extremity **G** Thyroid Gland Lobe, Left **H** Thyroid Gland Lobe, Right **K** Thyroid Gland **L** Superior Parathyroid Gland, Right **M** Superior Parathyroid Gland, Left **N** Inferior Parathyroid Gland, Right **P** Inferior Parathyroid Gland, Left **Q** Parathyroid Glands, Multiple **R** Parathyroid Gland	**0** Open **4** Percutaneous Endoscopic	**Z** No Device	**Z** No Qualifier

0 Medical and Surgical
G Endocrine System
W Revision Correcting, to the extent possible, a portion of a malfunctioning device or the position of a displaced device

Body Part Character 4	Approach Character 5	Device Character 6	Qualifier Character 7
0 Pituitary Gland **1** Pineal Body **5** Adrenal Gland **K** Thyroid Gland **R** Parathyroid Gland	**0** Open **3** Percutaneous **4** Percutaneous Endoscopic **X** External	**0** Drainage Device	**Z** No Qualifier
S Endocrine Gland	**0** Open **3** Percutaneous **4** Percutaneous Endoscopic **X** External	**0** Drainage Device **2** Monitoring Device **3** Infusion Device	**Z** No Qualifier

Skin and Breast ØHØ–ØHX

Ø Medical and Surgical
H Skin and Breast
Ø Alteration Modifying the anatomic structure of a body part without affecting the function of the body part

Body Part Character 4	Approach Character 5	Device Character 6	Qualifier Character 7
T Breast, Right **U** Breast, Left **V** Breast, Bilateral	**Ø** Open **3** Percutaneous **X** External	**7** Autologous Tissue Substitute **J** Synthetic Substitute **K** Nonautologous Tissue Substitute **Z** No Device	**Z** No Qualifier

Ø Medical and Surgical
H Skin and Breast
2 Change Taking out or off a device from a body part and putting back an identical or similar device in or on the same body part without cutting or puncturing the skin or a mucous membrane

Body Part Character 4	Approach Character 5	Device Character 6	Qualifier Character 7
P Skin **T** Breast, Right **U** Breast, Left	**X** External	**Ø** Drainage Device **Y** Other Device	**Z** No Qualifier

Ø Medical and Surgical
H Skin and Breast
5 Destruction Physical eradication of all or a portion of a body part by the direct use of energy, force, or a destructive agent

Body Part Character 4	Approach Character 5	Device Character 6	Qualifier Character 7
Ø Skin, Scalp **1** Skin, Face **2** Skin, Right Ear **3** Skin, Left Ear **4** Skin, Neck **5** Skin, Chest **6** Skin, Back **7** Skin, Abdomen **8** Skin, Buttock **9** Skin, Perineum **A** Skin, Genitalia **B** Skin, Right Upper Arm **C** Skin, Left Upper Arm **D** Skin, Right Lower Arm **E** Skin, Left Lower Arm **F** Skin, Right Hand **G** Skin, Left Hand **H** Skin, Right Upper Leg **J** Skin, Left Upper Leg **K** Skin, Right Lower Leg **L** Skin, Left Lower Leg **M** Skin, Right Foot **N** Skin, Left Foot	**X** External	**Z** No Device	**D** Multiple **Z** No Qualifier
Q Finger Nail **R** Toe Nail	**X** External	**Z** No Device	**Z** No Qualifier
T Breast, Right **U** Breast, Left **V** Breast, Bilateral **W** Nipple, Right **X** Nipple, Left	**Ø** Open **3** Percutaneous **7** Via Natural or Artificial Opening **8** Via Natural or Artificial Opening Endoscopic **X** External	**Z** No Device	**Z** No Qualifier

0 Medical and Surgical
H Skin and Breast
8 Division Cutting into a body part without draining fluids and/or gases from the body part in order to separate or transect a body part

Body Part Character 4	Approach Character 5	Device Character 6	Qualifier Character 7
0 Skin, Scalp **1** Skin, Face **2** Skin, Right Ear **3** Skin, Left Ear **4** Skin, Neck **5** Skin, Chest **6** Skin, Back **7** Skin, Abdomen **8** Skin, Buttock **9** Skin, Perineum **A** Skin, Genitalia **B** Skin, Right Upper Arm **C** Skin, Left Upper Arm **D** Skin, Right Lower Arm **E** Skin, Left Lower Arm **F** Skin, Right Hand **G** Skin, Left Hand **H** Skin, Right Upper Leg **J** Skin, Left Upper Leg **K** Skin, Right Lower Leg **L** Skin, Left Lower Leg **M** Skin, Right Foot **N** Skin, Left Foot	**X** External	**Z** No Device	**Z** No Qualifier

0 Medical and Surgical
H Skin and Breast
9 Drainage Taking or letting out fluids and/or gases from a body part

Body Part Character 4	Approach Character 5	Device Character 6	Qualifier Character 7
0 Skin, Scalp **1** Skin, Face **2** Skin, Right Ear **3** Skin, Left Ear **4** Skin, Neck **5** Skin, Chest **6** Skin, Back **7** Skin, Abdomen **8** Skin, Buttock **9** Skin, Perineum **A** Skin, Genitalia **B** Skin, Right Upper Arm **C** Skin, Left Upper Arm **D** Skin, Right Lower Arm **E** Skin, Left Lower Arm **F** Skin, Right Hand **G** Skin, Left Hand **H** Skin, Right Upper Leg **J** Skin, Left Upper Leg **K** Skin, Right Lower Leg **L** Skin, Left Lower Leg **M** Skin, Right Foot **N** Skin, Left Foot **Q** Finger Nail **R** Toe Nail	**X** External	**0** Drainage Device	**Z** No Qualifier

0H9 Continued on next page

ØH9 Continued

Ø Medical and Surgical
H Skin and Breast
9 Drainage Taking or letting out fluids and/or gases from a body part

Body Part Character 4	Approach Character 5	Device Character 6	Qualifier Character 7
Ø Skin, Scalp **1** Skin, Face **2** Skin, Right Ear **3** Skin, Left Ear **4** Skin, Neck **5** Skin, Chest **6** Skin, Back **7** Skin, Abdomen **8** Skin, Buttock **9** Skin, Perineum **A** Skin, Genitalia **B** Skin, Right Upper Arm **C** Skin, Left Upper Arm **D** Skin, Right Lower Arm **E** Skin, Left Lower Arm **F** Skin, Right Hand **G** Skin, Left Hand **H** Skin, Right Upper Leg **J** Skin, Left Upper Leg **K** Skin, Right Lower Leg **L** Skin, Left Lower Leg **M** Skin, Right Foot **N** Skin, Left Foot **Q** Finger Nail **R** Toe Nail	**X** External	**Z** No Device	**X** Diagnostic **Z** No Qualifier
T Breast, Right **U** Breast, Left **V** Breast, Bilateral **W** Nipple, Right **X** Nipple, Left	**Ø** Open **3** Percutaneous **7** Via Natural or Artificial Opening **8** Via Natural or Artificial Opening Endoscopic **X** External	**Ø** Drainage Device	**Z** No Qualifier
T Breast, Right **U** Breast, Left **V** Breast, Bilateral **W** Nipple, Right **X** Nipple, Left	**Ø** Open **3** Percutaneous **7** Via Natural or Artificial Opening **8** Via Natural or Artificial Opening Endoscopic **X** External	**Z** No Device	**X** Diagnostic **Z** No Qualifier

Ø Medical and Surgical
H Skin and Breast
B Excision Cutting out or off, without replacement, a portion of a body part

Body Part Character 4	Approach Character 5	Device Character 6	Qualifier Character 7
Ø Skin, Scalp **1** Skin, Face **2** Skin, Right Ear **3** Skin, Left Ear **4** Skin, Neck **5** Skin, Chest **6** Skin, Back **7** Skin, Abdomen **8** Skin, Buttock **9** Skin, Perineum **A** Skin, Genitalia **B** Skin, Right Upper Arm **C** Skin, Left Upper Arm **D** Skin, Right Lower Arm **E** Skin, Left Lower Arm **F** Skin, Right Hand **G** Skin, Left Hand **H** Skin, Right Upper Leg **J** Skin, Left Upper Leg **K** Skin, Right Lower Leg **L** Skin, Left Lower Leg **M** Skin, Right Foot **N** Skin, Left Foot **Q** Finger Nail **R** Toe Nail	**X** External	**Z** No Device	**X** Diagnostic **Z** No Qualifier
T Breast, Right **U** Breast, Left **V** Breast, Bilateral **W** Nipple, Right **X** Nipple, Left **Y** Supernumerary Breast	**Ø** Open **3** Percutaneous **7** Via Natural or Artificial Opening **8** Via Natural or Artificial Opening Endoscopic **X** External	**Z** No Device	**X** Diagnostic **Z** No Qualifier

0 Medical and Surgical
H Skin and Breast
C Extirpation Taking or cutting out solid matter from a body part

Body Part Character 4	Approach Character 5	Device Character 6	Qualifier Character 7
0 Skin, Scalp 1 Skin, Face 2 Skin, Right Ear 3 Skin, Left Ear 4 Skin, Neck 5 Skin, Chest 6 Skin, Back 7 Skin, Abdomen 8 Skin, Buttock 9 Skin, Perineum A Skin, Genitalia B Skin, Right Upper Arm C Skin, Left Upper Arm D Skin, Right Lower Arm E Skin, Left Lower Arm F Skin, Right Hand G Skin, Left Hand H Skin, Right Upper Leg J Skin, Left Upper Leg K Skin, Right Lower Leg L Skin, Left Lower Leg M Skin, Right Foot N Skin, Left Foot Q Finger Nail R Toe Nail	X External	Z No Device	Z No Qualifier
T Breast, Right U Breast, Left V Breast, Bilateral W Nipple, Right X Nipple, Left	0 Open 3 Percutaneous 7 Via Natural or Artificial Opening 8 Via Natural or Artificial Opening Endoscopic X External	Z No Device	Z No Qualifier

0 Medical and Surgical
H Skin and Breast
D Extraction Pulling or stripping out or off all or a portion of a body part by the use of force

Body Part Character 4	Approach Character 5	Device Character 6	Qualifier Character 7
0 Skin, Scalp 1 Skin, Face 2 Skin, Right Ear 3 Skin, Left Ear 4 Skin, Neck 5 Skin, Chest 6 Skin, Back 7 Skin, Abdomen 8 Skin, Buttock 9 Skin, Perineum A Skin, Genitalia B Skin, Right Upper Arm C Skin, Left Upper Arm D Skin, Right Lower Arm E Skin, Left Lower Arm F Skin, Right Hand G Skin, Left Hand H Skin, Right Upper Leg J Skin, Left Upper Leg K Skin, Right Lower Leg L Skin, Left Lower Leg M Skin, Right Foot N Skin, Left Foot Q Finger Nail R Toe Nail S Hair	X External	Z No Device	Z No Qualifier

Ø Medical and Surgical
H Skin and Breast
H Insertion Putting in a nonbiological appliance that monitors, assists, performs, or prevents a physiological function but does not physically take the place of a body part

Body Part Character 4	Approach Character 5	Device Character 6	Qualifier Character 7
T Breast, Right **U** Breast, Left **V** Breast, Bilateral **W** Nipple, Right **X** Nipple, Left	**Ø** Open **3** Percutaneous **7** Via Natural or Artificial Opening **8** Via Natural or Artificial Opening Endoscopic	**1** Radioactive Element **N** Tissue Expander	**Z** No Qualifier
T Breast, Right **U** Breast, Left **V** Breast, Bilateral **W** Nipple, Right **X** Nipple, Left	**X** External	**1** Radioactive Element	**Z** No Qualifier

Ø Medical and Surgical
H Skin and Breast
J Inspection Visually and/or manually exploring a body part

Body Part Character 4	Approach Character 5	Device Character 6	Qualifier Character 7
P Skin **Q** Finger Nail **R** Toe Nail	**X** External	**Z** No Device	**Z** No Qualifier
T Breast, Right **U** Breast, Left	**Ø** Open **3** Percutaneous **7** Via Natural or Artificial Opening **8** Via Natural or Artificial Opening Endoscopic **X** External	**Z** No Device	**Z** No Qualifier

Ø Medical and Surgical
H Skin and Breast
M Reattachment Putting back in or on all or a portion of a separated body part to its normal location or other suitable location

Body Part Character 4	Approach Character 5	Device Character 6	Qualifier Character 7
Ø Skin, Scalp **1** Skin, Face **2** Skin, Right Ear **3** Skin, Left Ear **4** Skin, Neck **5** Skin, Chest **6** Skin, Back **7** Skin, Abdomen **8** Skin, Buttock **9** Skin, Perineum **A** Skin, Genitalia **B** Skin, Right Upper Arm **C** Skin, Left Upper Arm **D** Skin, Right Lower Arm **E** Skin, Left Lower Arm **F** Skin, Right Hand **G** Skin, Left Hand **H** Skin, Right Upper Leg **J** Skin, Left Upper Leg **K** Skin, Right Lower Leg **L** Skin, Left Lower Leg **M** Skin, Right Foot **N** Skin, Left Foot **T** Breast, Right **U** Breast, Left **V** Breast, Bilateral **W** Nipple, Right **X** Nipple, Left	**X** External	**Z** No Device	**Z** No Qualifier

0 Medical and Surgical
H Skin and Breast
N Release Freeing a body part from an abnormal physical constraint

Body Part Character 4	Approach Character 5	Device Character 6	Qualifier Character 7
0 Skin, Scalp **1** Skin, Face **2** Skin, Right Ear **3** Skin, Left Ear **4** Skin, Neck **5** Skin, Chest **6** Skin, Back **7** Skin, Abdomen **8** Skin, Buttock **9** Skin, Perineum **A** Skin, Genitalia **B** Skin, Right Upper Arm **C** Skin, Left Upper Arm **D** Skin, Right Lower Arm **E** Skin, Left Lower Arm **F** Skin, Right Hand **G** Skin, Left Hand **H** Skin, Right Upper Leg **J** Skin, Left Upper Leg **K** Skin, Right Lower Leg **L** Skin, Left Lower Leg **M** Skin, Right Foot **N** Skin, Left Foot **Q** Finger Nail **R** Toe Nail	**X** External	**Z** No Device	**Z** No Qualifier
T Breast, Right **U** Breast, Left **V** Breast, Bilateral **W** Nipple, Right **X** Nipple, Left	**0** Open **3** Percutaneous **7** Via Natural or Artificial Opening **8** Via Natural or Artificial Opening Endoscopic **X** External	**Z** No Device	**Z** No Qualifier

0 Medical and Surgical
H Skin and Breast
P Removal Taking out or off a device from a body part

Body Part Character 4	Approach Character 5	Device Character 6	Qualifier Character 7
P Skin **Q** Finger Nail **R** Toe Nail	**X** External	**0** Drainage Device **7** Autologous Tissue Substitute **J** Synthetic Substitute **K** Nonautologous Tissue Substitute	**Z** No Qualifier
S Hair	**X** External	**7** Autologous Tissue Substitute **J** Synthetic Substitute **K** Nonautologous Tissue Substitute	**Z** No Qualifier
T Breast, Right **U** Breast, Left	**0** Open **3** Percutaneous **7** Via Natural or Artificial Opening **8** Via Natural or Artificial Opening Endoscopic	**0** Drainage Device **1** Radioactive Element **7** Autologous Tissue Substitute **J** Synthetic Substitute **K** Nonautologous Tissue Substitute **N** Tissue Expander	**Z** No Qualifier
T Breast, Right **U** Breast, Left	**X** External	**0** Drainage Device **1** Radioactive Element **7** Autologous Tissue Substitute **J** Synthetic Substitute **K** Nonautologous Tissue Substitute	**Z** No Qualifier

Ø Medical and Surgical
H Skin and Breast
Q Repair Restoring, to the extent possible, a body part to its normal anatomic structure and function

Body Part Character 4	Approach Character 5	Device Character 6	Qualifier Character 7
Ø Skin, Scalp **1** Skin, Face **2** Skin, Right Ear **3** Skin, Left Ear **4** Skin, Neck **5** Skin, Chest **6** Skin, Back **7** Skin, Abdomen **8** Skin, Buttock **9** Skin, Perineum **A** Skin, Genitalia **B** Skin, Right Upper Arm **C** Skin, Left Upper Arm **D** Skin, Right Lower Arm **E** Skin, Left Lower Arm **F** Skin, Right Hand **G** Skin, Left Hand **H** Skin, Right Upper Leg **J** Skin, Left Upper Leg **K** Skin, Right Lower Leg **L** Skin, Left Lower Leg **M** Skin, Right Foot **N** Skin, Left Foot **Q** Finger Nail **R** Toe Nail	**X** External	**Z** No Device	**Z** No Qualifier
T Breast, Right **U** Breast, Left **V** Breast, Bilateral **W** Nipple, Right **X** Nipple, Left **Y** Supernumerary Breast	**Ø** Open **3** Percutaneous **7** Via Natural or Artificial Opening **8** Via Natural or Artificial Opening Endoscopic **X** External	**Z** No Device	**Z** No Qualifier

Ø Medical and Surgical
H Skin and Breast
R Replacement Putting in or on biological or synthetic material that physically takes the place and/or function of all or a portion of a body part

Body Part Character 4	Approach Character 5	Device Character 6	Qualifier Character 7
Ø Skin, Scalp **1** Skin, Face **2** Skin, Right Ear **3** Skin, Left Ear **4** Skin, Neck **5** Skin, Chest **6** Skin, Back **7** Skin, Abdomen **8** Skin, Buttock **9** Skin, Perineum **A** Skin, Genitalia **B** Skin, Right Upper Arm **C** Skin, Left Upper Arm **D** Skin, Right Lower Arm **E** Skin, Left Lower Arm **F** Skin, Right Hand **G** Skin, Left Hand **H** Skin, Right Upper Leg **J** Skin, Left Upper Leg **K** Skin, Right Lower Leg **L** Skin, Left Lower Leg **M** Skin, Right Foot **N** Skin, Left Foot	**X** External	**7** Autologous Tissue Substitute **K** Nonautologous Tissue Substitute	**3** Full Thickness **4** Partial Thickness

ØHR Continued on next page

0 Medical and Surgical
H Skin and Breast
R Replacement Putting in or on biological or synthetic material that physically takes the place and/or function of all or a portion of a body part

0HR Continued

Body Part Character 4	Approach Character 5	Device Character 6	Qualifier Character 7
0 Skin, Scalp **1** Skin, Face **2** Skin, Right Ear **3** Skin, Left Ear **4** Skin, Neck **5** Skin, Chest **6** Skin, Back **7** Skin, Abdomen **8** Skin, Buttock **9** Skin, Perineum **A** Skin, Genitalia **B** Skin, Right Upper Arm **C** Skin, Left Upper Arm **D** Skin, Right Lower Arm **E** Skin, Left Lower Arm **F** Skin, Right Hand **G** Skin, Left Hand **H** Skin, Right Upper Leg **J** Skin, Left Upper Leg **K** Skin, Right Lower Leg **L** Skin, Left Lower Leg **M** Skin, Right Foot **N** Skin, Left Foot	**X** External	**J** Synthetic Substitute	**3** Full Thickness **4** Partial Thickness **Z** No Qualifier
Q Finger Nail **R** Toe Nail **S** Hair	**X** External	**7** Autologous Tissue Substitute **J** Synthetic Substitute **K** Nonautologous Tissue Substitute	**Z** No Qualifier
T Breast, Right **U** Breast, Left **V** Breast, Bilateral	**0** Open	**7** Autologous Tissue Substitute	**5** Latissimus Dorsi Myocutaneous Flap **6** Transverse Rectus Abdominis Myocutaneous Flap **7** Deep Inferior Epigastric Artery Perforator Flap **8** Superficial Inferior Epigastric Artery Flap **9** Gluteal Artery Perforator Flap **Z** No Qualifier
T Breast, Right **U** Breast, Left **V** Breast, Bilateral	**0** Open	**J** Synthetic Substitute **K** Nonautologous Tissue Substitute	**Z** No Qualifier
T Breast, Right **U** Breast, Left **V** Breast, Bilateral	**3** Percutaneous **X** External	**7** Autologous Tissue Substitute **J** Synthetic Substitute **K** Nonautologous Tissue Substitute	**Z** No Qualifier
W Nipple, Right **X** Nipple, Left	**0** Open **3** Percutaneous **X** External	**7** Autologous Tissue Substitute **J** Synthetic Substitute **K** Nonautologous Tissue Substitute	**Z** No Qualifier

0 Medical and Surgical
H Skin and Breast
S Reposition Moving to its normal location or other suitable location all or a portion of a body part

Body Part Character 4	Approach Character 5	Device Character 6	Qualifier Character 7
S Hair **W** Nipple, Right **X** Nipple, Left	**X** External	**Z** No Device	**Z** No Qualifier
T Breast, Right **U** Breast, Left **V** Breast, Bilateral	**0** Open	**Z** No Device	**Z** No Qualifier

Ø Medical and Surgical
H Skin and Breast
T Resection Cutting out or off, without replacement, all of a body part

Body Part Character 4	Approach Character 5	Device Character 6	Qualifier Character 7
Q Finger Nail R Toe Nail W Nipple, Right X Nipple, Left	X External	Z No Device	Z No Qualifier
T Breast, Right U Breast, Left V Breast, Bilateral Y Supernumerary Breast	Ø Open	Z No Device	Z No Qualifier

Ø Medical and Surgical
H Skin and Breast
U Supplement Putting in or on biological or synthetic material that physically reinforces and/or augments the function of a portion of a body part

Body Part Character 4	Approach Character 5	Device Character 6	Qualifier Character 7
T Breast, Right U Breast, Left V Breast, Bilateral W Nipple, Right X Nipple, Left	Ø Open 3 Percutaneous 7 Via Natural or Artificial Opening 8 Via Natural or Artificial Opening Endoscopic X External	7 Autologous Tissue Substitute J Synthetic Substitute K Nonautologous Tissue Substitute	Z No Qualifier

Ø Medical and Surgical
H Skin and Breast
W Revision Correcting, to the extent possible, a portion of a malfunctioning device or the position of a displaced device

Body Part Character 4	Approach Character 5	Device Character 6	Qualifier Character 7
P Skin Q Finger Nail R Toe Nail T Breast, Right U Breast, Left	X External	Ø Drainage Device 7 Autologous Tissue Substitute J Synthetic Substitute K Nonautologous Tissue Substitute	Z No Qualifier
S Hair	X External	7 Autologous Tissue Substitute J Synthetic Substitute K Nonautologous Tissue Substitute	Z No Qualifier
T Breast, Right U Breast, Left	Ø Open 3 Percutaneous 7 Via Natural or Artificial Opening 8 Via Natural or Artificial Opening Endoscopic	Ø Drainage Device 7 Autologous Tissue Substitute J Synthetic Substitute K Nonautologous Tissue Substitute N Tissue Expander	Z No Qualifier

Ø Medical and Surgical
H Skin and Breast
X Transfer Moving, without taking out, all or a portion of a body part to another location to take over the function of all or a portion of a body part

Body Part Character 4	Approach Character 5	Device Character 6	Qualifier Character 7
Ø Skin, Scalp 1 Skin, Face 2 Skin, Right Ear 3 Skin, Left Ear 4 Skin, Neck 5 Skin, Chest 6 Skin, Back 7 Skin, Abdomen 8 Skin, Buttock 9 Skin, Perineum A Skin, Genitalia B Skin, Right Upper Arm C Skin, Left Upper Arm D Skin, Right Lower Arm E Skin, Left Lower Arm F Skin, Right Hand G Skin, Left Hand H Skin, Right Upper Leg J Skin, Left Upper Leg K Skin, Right Lower Leg L Skin, Left Lower Leg M Skin, Right Foot N Skin, Left Foot	X External	Z No Device	Z No Qualifier

Subcutaneous Tissue and Fascia 0J0–0JX

0 Medical and Surgical
J Subcutaneous Tissue and Fascia
0 Alteration Modifying the anatomic structure of a body part without affecting the function of the body part

Body Part Character 4	Approach Character 5	Device Character 6	Qualifier Character 7
1 Subcutaneous Tissue and Fascia, Face 4 Subcutaneous Tissue and Fascia, Anterior Neck 5 Subcutaneous Tissue and Fascia, Posterior Neck 6 Subcutaneous Tissue and Fascia, Chest 7 Subcutaneous Tissue and Fascia, Back 8 Subcutaneous Tissue and Fascia, Abdomen 9 Subcutaneous Tissue and Fascia, Buttock D Subcutaneous Tissue and Fascia, Right Upper Arm F Subcutaneous Tissue and Fascia, Left Upper Arm G Subcutaneous Tissue and Fascia, Right Lower Arm H Subcutaneous Tissue and Fascia, Left Lower Arm L Subcutaneous Tissue and Fascia, Right Upper Leg M Subcutaneous Tissue and Fascia, Left Upper Leg N Subcutaneous Tissue and Fascia, Right Lower Leg P Subcutaneous Tissue and Fascia, Left Lower Leg	0 Open 3 Percutaneous	Z No Device	Z No Qualifier

0 Medical and Surgical
J Subcutaneous Tissue and Fascia
2 Change Taking out or off a device from a body part and putting back an identical or similar device in or on the same body part without cutting or puncturing the skin or a mucous membrane

Body Part Character 4	Approach Character 5	Device Character 6	Qualifier Character 7
S Subcutaneous Tissue and Fascia, Head and Neck T Subcutaneous Tissue and Fascia, Trunk V Subcutaneous Tissue and Fascia, Upper Extremity W Subcutaneous Tissue and Fascia, Lower Extremity	X External	0 Drainage Device Y Other Device	Z No Qualifier

0 Medical and Surgical
J Subcutaneous Tissue and Fascia
5 Destruction Physical eradication of all or a portion of a body part by the direct use of energy, force, or a destructive agent

Body Part Character 4	Approach Character 5	Device Character 6	Qualifier Character 7
0 Subcutaneous Tissue and Fascia, Scalp 1 Subcutaneous Tissue and Fascia, Face 4 Subcutaneous Tissue and Fascia, Anterior Neck 5 Subcutaneous Tissue and Fascia, Posterior Neck 6 Subcutaneous Tissue and Fascia, Chest 7 Subcutaneous Tissue and Fascia, Back 8 Subcutaneous Tissue and Fascia, Abdomen 9 Subcutaneous Tissue and Fascia, Buttock B Subcutaneous Tissue and Fascia, Perineum C Subcutaneous Tissue and Fascia, Pelvic Region D Subcutaneous Tissue and Fascia, Right Upper Arm F Subcutaneous Tissue and Fascia, Left Upper Arm G Subcutaneous Tissue and Fascia, Right Lower Arm H Subcutaneous Tissue and Fascia, Left Lower Arm J Subcutaneous Tissue and Fascia, Right Hand K Subcutaneous Tissue and Fascia, Left Hand L Subcutaneous Tissue and Fascia, Right Upper Leg M Subcutaneous Tissue and Fascia, Left Upper Leg N Subcutaneous Tissue and Fascia, Right Lower Leg P Subcutaneous Tissue and Fascia, Left Lower Leg Q Subcutaneous Tissue and Fascia, Right Foot R Subcutaneous Tissue and Fascia, Left Foot	0 Open 3 Percutaneous	Z No Device	Z No Qualifier

Ø Medical and Surgical
J Subcutaneous Tissue and Fascia
8 Division Cutting into a body part without draining fluids and/or gases from the body part in order to separate or transect a body part

Body Part Character 4	Approach Character 5	Device Character 6	Qualifier Character 7
Ø Subcutaneous Tissue and Fascia, Scalp **1** Subcutaneous Tissue and Fascia, Face **4** Subcutaneous Tissue and Fascia, Anterior Neck **5** Subcutaneous Tissue and Fascia, Posterior Neck **6** Subcutaneous Tissue and Fascia, Chest **7** Subcutaneous Tissue and Fascia, Back **8** Subcutaneous Tissue and Fascia, Abdomen **9** Subcutaneous Tissue and Fascia, Buttock **B** Subcutaneous Tissue and Fascia, Perineum **C** Subcutaneous Tissue and Fascia, Pelvic Region **D** Subcutaneous Tissue and Fascia, Right Upper Arm **F** Subcutaneous Tissue and Fascia, Left Upper Arm **G** Subcutaneous Tissue and Fascia, Right Lower Arm **H** Subcutaneous Tissue and Fascia, Left Lower Arm **J** Subcutaneous Tissue and Fascia, Right Hand **K** Subcutaneous Tissue and Fascia, Left Hand **L** Subcutaneous Tissue and Fascia, Right Upper Leg **M** Subcutaneous Tissue and Fascia, Left Upper Leg **N** Subcutaneous Tissue and Fascia, Right Lower Leg **P** Subcutaneous Tissue and Fascia, Left Lower Leg **Q** Subcutaneous Tissue and Fascia, Right Foot **R** Subcutaneous Tissue and Fascia, Left Foot **S** Subcutaneous Tissue and Fascia, Head and Neck **T** Subcutaneous Tissue and Fascia, Trunk **V** Subcutaneous Tissue and Fascia, Upper Extremity **W** Subcutaneous Tissue and Fascia, Lower Extremity	**Ø** Open **3** Percutaneous	**Z** No Device	**Z** No Qualifier

Ø Medical and Surgical
J Subcutaneous Tissue and Fascia
9 Drainage Taking or letting out fluids and/or gases from a body part

Body Part Character 4	Approach Character 5	Device Character 6	Qualifier Character 7
Ø Subcutaneous Tissue and Fascia, Scalp **1** Subcutaneous Tissue and Fascia, Face **4** Subcutaneous Tissue and Fascia, Anterior Neck **5** Subcutaneous Tissue and Fascia, Posterior Neck **6** Subcutaneous Tissue and Fascia, Chest **7** Subcutaneous Tissue and Fascia, Back **8** Subcutaneous Tissue and Fascia, Abdomen **9** Subcutaneous Tissue and Fascia, Buttock **B** Subcutaneous Tissue and Fascia, Perineum **C** Subcutaneous Tissue and Fascia, Pelvic Region **D** Subcutaneous Tissue and Fascia, Right Upper Arm **F** Subcutaneous Tissue and Fascia, Left Upper Arm **G** Subcutaneous Tissue and Fascia, Right Lower Arm **H** Subcutaneous Tissue and Fascia, Left Lower Arm **J** Subcutaneous Tissue and Fascia, Right Hand **K** Subcutaneous Tissue and Fascia, Left Hand **L** Subcutaneous Tissue and Fascia, Right Upper Leg **M** Subcutaneous Tissue and Fascia, Left Upper Leg **N** Subcutaneous Tissue and Fascia, Right Lower Leg **P** Subcutaneous Tissue and Fascia, Left Lower Leg **Q** Subcutaneous Tissue and Fascia, Right Foot **R** Subcutaneous Tissue and Fascia, Left Foot	**Ø** Open **3** Percutaneous	**Ø** Drainage Device	**Z** No Qualifier

ØJ9 Continued on next page

Ø Medical and Surgical
J Subcutaneous Tissue and Fascia
9 Drainage Taking or letting out fluids and/or gases from a body part

ØJ9 Continued

Body Part Character 4	Approach Character 5	Device Character 6	Qualifier Character 7
Ø Subcutaneous Tissue and Fascia, Scalp **1** Subcutaneous Tissue and Fascia, Face **4** Subcutaneous Tissue and Fascia, Anterior Neck **5** Subcutaneous Tissue and Fascia, Posterior Neck **6** Subcutaneous Tissue and Fascia, Chest **7** Subcutaneous Tissue and Fascia, Back **8** Subcutaneous Tissue and Fascia, Abdomen **9** Subcutaneous Tissue and Fascia, Buttock **B** Subcutaneous Tissue and Fascia, Perineum **C** Subcutaneous Tissue and Fascia, Pelvic Region **D** Subcutaneous Tissue and Fascia, Right Upper Arm **F** Subcutaneous Tissue and Fascia, Left Upper Arm **G** Subcutaneous Tissue and Fascia, Right Lower Arm **H** Subcutaneous Tissue and Fascia, Left Lower Arm **J** Subcutaneous Tissue and Fascia, Right Hand **K** Subcutaneous Tissue and Fascia, Left Hand **L** Subcutaneous Tissue and Fascia, Right Upper Leg **M** Subcutaneous Tissue and Fascia, Left Upper Leg **N** Subcutaneous Tissue and Fascia, Right Lower Leg **P** Subcutaneous Tissue and Fascia, Left Lower Leg **Q** Subcutaneous Tissue and Fascia, Right Foot **R** Subcutaneous Tissue and Fascia, Left Foot	**Ø** Open **3** Percutaneous	**Z** No Device	**X** Diagnostic **Z** No Qualifier

Ø Medical and Surgical
J Subcutaneous Tissue and Fascia
B Excision Cutting out or off, without replacement, a portion of a body part

Body Part Character 4	Approach Character 5	Device Character 6	Qualifier Character 7
Ø Subcutaneous Tissue and Fascia, Scalp **1** Subcutaneous Tissue and Fascia, Face **4** Subcutaneous Tissue and Fascia, Anterior Neck **5** Subcutaneous Tissue and Fascia, Posterior Neck **6** Subcutaneous Tissue and Fascia, Chest **7** Subcutaneous Tissue and Fascia, Back **8** Subcutaneous Tissue and Fascia, Abdomen **9** Subcutaneous Tissue and Fascia, Buttock **B** Subcutaneous Tissue and Fascia, Perineum **C** Subcutaneous Tissue and Fascia, Pelvic Region **D** Subcutaneous Tissue and Fascia, Right Upper Arm **F** Subcutaneous Tissue and Fascia, Left Upper Arm **G** Subcutaneous Tissue and Fascia, Right Lower Arm **H** Subcutaneous Tissue and Fascia, Left Lower Arm **J** Subcutaneous Tissue and Fascia, Right Hand **K** Subcutaneous Tissue and Fascia, Left Hand **L** Subcutaneous Tissue and Fascia, Right Upper Leg **M** Subcutaneous Tissue and Fascia, Left Upper Leg **N** Subcutaneous Tissue and Fascia, Right Lower Leg **P** Subcutaneous Tissue and Fascia, Left Lower Leg **Q** Subcutaneous Tissue and Fascia, Right Foot **R** Subcutaneous Tissue and Fascia, Left Foot	**Ø** Open **3** Percutaneous	**Z** No Device	**X** Diagnostic **Z** No Qualifier

Ø Medical and Surgical
J Subcutaneous Tissue and Fascia
C Extirpation Taking or cutting out solid matter from a body part

Body Part Character 4	Approach Character 5	Device Character 6	Qualifier Character 7
Ø Subcutaneous Tissue and Fascia, Scalp **1** Subcutaneous Tissue and Fascia, Face **4** Subcutaneous Tissue and Fascia, Anterior Neck **5** Subcutaneous Tissue and Fascia, Posterior Neck **6** Subcutaneous Tissue and Fascia, Chest **7** Subcutaneous Tissue and Fascia, Back **8** Subcutaneous Tissue and Fascia, Abdomen **9** Subcutaneous Tissue and Fascia, Buttock **B** Subcutaneous Tissue and Fascia, Perineum **C** Subcutaneous Tissue and Fascia, Pelvic Region **D** Subcutaneous Tissue and Fascia, Right Upper Arm **F** Subcutaneous Tissue and Fascia, Left Upper Arm **G** Subcutaneous Tissue and Fascia, Right Lower Arm **H** Subcutaneous Tissue and Fascia, Left Lower Arm **J** Subcutaneous Tissue and Fascia, Right Hand **K** Subcutaneous Tissue and Fascia, Left Hand **L** Subcutaneous Tissue and Fascia, Right Upper Leg **M** Subcutaneous Tissue and Fascia, Left Upper Leg **N** Subcutaneous Tissue and Fascia, Right Lower Leg **P** Subcutaneous Tissue and Fascia, Left Lower Leg **Q** Subcutaneous Tissue and Fascia, Right Foot **R** Subcutaneous Tissue and Fascia, Left Foot	**Ø** Open **3** Percutaneous	**Z** No Device	**Z** No Qualifier

Ø Medical and Surgical
J Subcutaneous Tissue and Fascia
D Extraction Pulling or stripping out or off all or a portion of a body part by the use of force

Body Part Character 4	Approach Character 5	Device Character 6	Qualifier Character 7
Ø Subcutaneous Tissue and Fascia, Scalp **1** Subcutaneous Tissue and Fascia, Face **4** Subcutaneous Tissue and Fascia, Anterior Neck **5** Subcutaneous Tissue and Fascia, Posterior Neck **6** Subcutaneous Tissue and Fascia, Chest **7** Subcutaneous Tissue and Fascia, Back **8** Subcutaneous Tissue and Fascia, Abdomen **9** Subcutaneous Tissue and Fascia, Buttock **B** Subcutaneous Tissue and Fascia, Perineum **C** Subcutaneous Tissue and Fascia, Pelvic Region **D** Subcutaneous Tissue and Fascia, Right Upper Arm **F** Subcutaneous Tissue and Fascia, Left Upper Arm **G** Subcutaneous Tissue and Fascia, Right Lower Arm **H** Subcutaneous Tissue and Fascia, Left Lower Arm **J** Subcutaneous Tissue and Fascia, Right Hand **K** Subcutaneous Tissue and Fascia, Left Hand **L** Subcutaneous Tissue and Fascia, Right Upper Leg **M** Subcutaneous Tissue and Fascia, Left Upper Leg **N** Subcutaneous Tissue and Fascia, Right Lower Leg **P** Subcutaneous Tissue and Fascia, Left Lower Leg **Q** Subcutaneous Tissue and Fascia, Right Foot **R** Subcutaneous Tissue and Fascia, Left Foot	**Ø** Open **3** Percutaneous	**Z** No Device	**Z** No Qualifier

Ø Medical and Surgical
J Subcutaneous Tissue and Fascia
H Insertion Putting in a nonbiological appliance that monitors, assists, performs, or prevents a physiological function but does not physically take the place of a body part

Body Part Character 4	Approach Character 5	Device Character 6	Qualifier Character 7
Ø Subcutaneous Tissue and Fascia, Scalp **1** Subcutaneous Tissue and Fascia, Face **4** Subcutaneous Tissue and Fascia, Anterior Neck **5** Subcutaneous Tissue and Fascia, Posterior Neck **9** Subcutaneous Tissue and Fascia, Buttock **B** Subcutaneous Tissue and Fascia, Perineum **C** Subcutaneous Tissue and Fascia, Pelvic Region **J** Subcutaneous Tissue and Fascia, Right Hand **K** Subcutaneous Tissue and Fascia, Left Hand **Q** Subcutaneous Tissue and Fascia, Right Foot **R** Subcutaneous Tissue and Fascia, Left Foot	**Ø** Open **3** Percutaneous	**N** Tissue Expander	**Z** No Qualifier
6 Subcutaneous Tissue and Fascia, Chest **8** Subcutaneous Tissue and Fascia, Abdomen	**Ø** Open **3** Percutaneous	**Ø Monitoring Device, Hemodynamic** **2 Monitoring Device** **4 Pacemaker, Single Chamber** **5 Pacemaker, Single Chamber Rate Responsive** **6 Pacemaker, Dual Chamber** **7 Cardiac Resynchronization Pacemaker Pulse Generator** **8 Defibrillator Generator** **9 Cardiac Resynchronization Defibrillator Pulse Generator** **A Contractility Modulation Device** **B Stimulator Generator, Single Array** **C Stimulator Generator, Single Array Rechargeable** **D Stimulator Generator, Multiple Array** **E Stimulator Generator, Multiple Array Rechargeable** **H Contraceptive Device** **M Stimulator Generator** **N Tissue Expander** **P Cardiac Rhythm Related Device** **V Infusion Device, Pump** **W Vascular Access Device, Reservoir** **X Vascular Access Device**	**Z** No Qualifier
7 Subcutaneous Tissue and Fascia, Back	**Ø** Open **3** Percutaneous	**B Stimulator Generator, Single Array** **C Stimulator Generator, Single Array Rechargeable** **D Stimulator Generator, Multiple Array** **E Stimulator Generator, Multiple Array Rechargeable** **M Stimulator Generator** **N Tissue Expander** **V Infusion Device, Pump**	**Z** No Qualifier

ØJH Continued on next page

ØJH Continued

Ø Medical and Surgical
J Subcutaneous Tissue and Fascia
H Insertion Putting in a nonbiological appliance that monitors, assists, performs, or prevents a physiological function but does not physically take the place of a body part

Body Part Character 4	Approach Character 5	Device Character 6	Qualifier Character 7
D Subcutaneous Tissue and Fascia, Right Upper Arm **F** Subcutaneous Tissue and Fascia, Left Upper Arm **G** Subcutaneous Tissue and Fascia, Right Lower Arm **H** Subcutaneous Tissue and Fascia, Left Lower Arm **L** Subcutaneous Tissue and Fascia, Right Upper Leg **M** Subcutaneous Tissue and Fascia, Left Upper Leg **N** Subcutaneous Tissue and Fascia, Right Lower Leg **P** Subcutaneous Tissue and Fascia, Left Lower Leg	**Ø** Open **3** Percutaneous	**H** Contraceptive Device **N** Tissue Expander **V** Infusion Pump **W** Reservoir **X** Vascular Access Device	**Z** No Qualifier
S Subcutaneous Tissue and Fascia, Head and Neck **V** Subcutaneous Tissue and Fascia, Upper Extremity **W** Subcutaneous Tissue and Fascia, Lower Extremity	**Ø** Open **3** Percutaneous	**1** Radioactive Element **3** Infusion Device	**Z** No Qualifier
T Subcutaneous Tissue and Fascia, Trunk	**Ø** Open **3** Percutaneous	**1** Radioactive Element **3** Infusion Device **V** Infusion Pump	**Z** No Qualifier

Ø Medical and Surgical
J Subcutaneous Tissue and Fascia
J Inspection Visually and/or manually exploring a body part

Body Part Character 4	Approach Character 5	Device Character 6	Qualifier Character 7
S Subcutaneous Tissue and Fascia, Head and Neck **T** Subcutaneous Tissue and Fascia, Trunk **V** Subcutaneous Tissue and Fascia, Upper Extremity **W** Subcutaneous Tissue and Fascia, Lower Extremity	**Ø** Open **3** Percutaneous **X** External	**Z** No Device	**Z** No Qualifier

Ø Medical and Surgical
J Subcutaneous Tissue and Fascia
N Release Freeing a body part from an abnormal physical constraint

Body Part Character 4	Approach Character 5	Device Character 6	Qualifier Character 7
Ø Subcutaneous Tissue and Fascia, Scalp **1** Subcutaneous Tissue and Fascia, Face **4** Subcutaneous Tissue and Fascia, Anterior Neck **5** Subcutaneous Tissue and Fascia, Posterior Neck **6** Subcutaneous Tissue and Fascia, Chest **7** Subcutaneous Tissue and Fascia, Back **8** Subcutaneous Tissue and Fascia, Abdomen **9** Subcutaneous Tissue and Fascia, Buttock **B** Subcutaneous Tissue and Fascia, Perineum **C** Subcutaneous Tissue and Fascia, Pelvic Region **D** Subcutaneous Tissue and Fascia, Right Upper Arm **F** Subcutaneous Tissue and Fascia, Left Upper Arm **G** Subcutaneous Tissue and Fascia, Right Lower Arm **H** Subcutaneous Tissue and Fascia, Left Lower Arm **J** Subcutaneous Tissue and Fascia, Right Hand **K** Subcutaneous Tissue and Fascia, Left Hand **L** Subcutaneous Tissue and Fascia, Right Upper Leg **M** Subcutaneous Tissue and Fascia, Left Upper Leg **N** Subcutaneous Tissue and Fascia, Right Lower Leg **P** Subcutaneous Tissue and Fascia, Left Lower Leg **Q** Subcutaneous Tissue and Fascia, Right Foot **R** Subcutaneous Tissue and Fascia, Left Foot	**Ø** Open **3** Percutaneous **X** External	**Z** No Device	**Z** No Qualifier

0 Medical and Surgical
J Subcutaneous Tissue and Fascia
P Removal Taking out or off a device from a body part

Body Part Character 4	Approach Character 5	Device Character 6	Qualifier Character 7
S Subcutaneous Tissue and Fascia, Head and Neck	**0** Open **3** Percutaneous	**0** Drainage Device **1** Radioactive Element **3** Infusion Device **7** Autologous Tissue Substitute **J** Synthetic Substitute **K** Nonautologous Tissue Substitute **N** Tissue Expander	**Z** No Qualifier
S Subcutaneous Tissue and Fascia, Head and Neck	**X** External	**0** Drainage Device **1** Radioactive Element **3** Infusion Device	**Z** No Qualifier
T Subcutaneous Tissue and Fascia, Trunk	**0** Open **3** Percutaneous	**0** Drainage Device **1** Radioactive Element **2** Monitoring Device **3** Infusion Device **7** Autologous Tissue Substitute **H** Contraceptive Device **J** Synthetic Substitute **K** Nonautologous Tissue Substitute **M** Stimulator Generator **N** Tissue Expander **P** Cardiac Rhythm Related Device **V** Infusion Pump **W** Reservoir **X** Vascular Access Device	**Z** No Qualifier
T Subcutaneous Tissue and Fascia, Trunk	**X** External	**0** Drainage Device **1** Radioactive Element **2** Monitoring Device **3** Infusion Device **H** Contraceptive Device **V** Infusion Pump **X** Vascular Access Device	**Z** No Qualifier
V Subcutaneous Tissue and Fascia, Upper Extremity **W** Subcutaneous Tissue and Fascia, Lower Extremity	**0** Open **3** Percutaneous	**0** Drainage Device **1** Radioactive Element **3** Infusion Device **7** Autologous Tissue Substitute **H** Contraceptive Device **J** Synthetic Substitute **K** Nonautologous Tissue Substitute **N** Tissue Expander **V** Infusion Pump **W** Reservoir **X** Vascular Access Device	**Z** No Qualifier
V Subcutaneous Tissue and Fascia, Upper Extremity **W** Subcutaneous Tissue and Fascia, Lower Extremity	**X** External	**0** Drainage Device **1** Radioactive Element **3** Infusion Device **H** Contraceptive Device **V** Infusion Pump **X** Vascular Access Device	**Z** No Qualifier

Ø Medical and Surgical
J Subcutaneous Tissue and Fascia
Q Repair Restoring, to the extent possible, a body part to its normal anatomic structure and function

Body Part Character 4	Approach Character 5	Device Character 6	Qualifier Character 7
Ø Subcutaneous Tissue and Fascia, Scalp **1** Subcutaneous Tissue and Fascia, Face **4** Subcutaneous Tissue and Fascia, Anterior Neck **5** Subcutaneous Tissue and Fascia, Posterior Neck **6** Subcutaneous Tissue and Fascia, Chest **7** Subcutaneous Tissue and Fascia, Back **8** Subcutaneous Tissue and Fascia, Abdomen **9** Subcutaneous Tissue and Fascia, Buttock **B** Subcutaneous Tissue and Fascia, Perineum **C** Subcutaneous Tissue and Fascia, Pelvic Region **D** Subcutaneous Tissue and Fascia, Right Upper Arm **F** Subcutaneous Tissue and Fascia, Left Upper Arm **G** Subcutaneous Tissue and Fascia, Right Lower Arm **H** Subcutaneous Tissue and Fascia, Left Lower Arm **J** Subcutaneous Tissue and Fascia, Right Hand **K** Subcutaneous Tissue and Fascia, Left Hand **L** Subcutaneous Tissue and Fascia, Right Upper Leg **M** Subcutaneous Tissue and Fascia, Left Upper Leg **N** Subcutaneous Tissue and Fascia, Right Lower Leg **P** Subcutaneous Tissue and Fascia, Left Lower Leg **Q** Subcutaneous Tissue and Fascia, Right Foot **R** Subcutaneous Tissue and Fascia, Left Foot	**Ø** Open **3** Percutaneous	**Z** No Device	**Z** No Qualifier

Ø Medical and Surgical
J Subcutaneous Tissue and Fascia
R Replacement Putting in or on biological or synthetic material that physically takes the place and/or function of all or a portion of a body part

Body Part Character 4	Approach Character 5	Device Character 6	Qualifier Character 7
Ø Subcutaneous Tissue and Fascia, Scalp **1** Subcutaneous Tissue and Fascia, Face **4** Subcutaneous Tissue and Fascia, Anterior Neck **5** Subcutaneous Tissue and Fascia, Posterior Neck **6** Subcutaneous Tissue and Fascia, Chest **7** Subcutaneous Tissue and Fascia, Back **8** Subcutaneous Tissue and Fascia, Abdomen **9** Subcutaneous Tissue and Fascia, Buttock **B** Subcutaneous Tissue and Fascia, Perineum **C** Subcutaneous Tissue and Fascia, Pelvic Region **D** Subcutaneous Tissue and Fascia, Right Upper Arm **F** Subcutaneous Tissue and Fascia, Left Upper Arm **G** Subcutaneous Tissue and Fascia, Right Lower Arm **H** Subcutaneous Tissue and Fascia, Left Lower Arm **J** Subcutaneous Tissue and Fascia, Right Hand **K** Subcutaneous Tissue and Fascia, Left Hand **L** Subcutaneous Tissue and Fascia, Right Upper Leg **M** Subcutaneous Tissue and Fascia, Left Upper Leg **N** Subcutaneous Tissue and Fascia, Right Lower Leg **P** Subcutaneous Tissue and Fascia, Left Lower Leg **Q** Subcutaneous Tissue and Fascia, Right Foot **R** Subcutaneous Tissue and Fascia, Left Foot	**Ø** Open **3** Percutaneous	**7** Autologous Tissue Substitute **J** Synthetic Substitute **K** Nonautologous Tissue Substitute	**Z** No Qualifier

0 Medical and Surgical
J Subcutaneous Tissue and Fascia
U Supplement: Putting in or on biological or synthetic material that physically reinforces and/or augments the function of a portion of a body part

Body Part Character 4	Approach Character 5	Device Character 6	Qualifier Character 7
0 Subcutaneous Tissue and Fascia, Scalp **1** Subcutaneous Tissue and Fascia, Face **4** Subcutaneous Tissue and Fascia, Anterior Neck **5** Subcutaneous Tissue and Fascia, Posterior Neck **6** Subcutaneous Tissue and Fascia, Chest **7** Subcutaneous Tissue and Fascia, Back **8** Subcutaneous Tissue and Fascia, Abdomen **9** Subcutaneous Tissue and Fascia, Buttock **B** Subcutaneous Tissue and Fascia, Perineum **C** Subcutaneous Tissue and Fascia, Pelvic Region **D** Subcutaneous Tissue and Fascia, Right Upper Arm **F** Subcutaneous Tissue and Fascia, Left Upper Arm **G** Subcutaneous Tissue and Fascia, Right Lower Arm **H** Subcutaneous Tissue and Fascia, Left Lower Arm **J** Subcutaneous Tissue and Fascia, Right Hand **K** Subcutaneous Tissue and Fascia, Left Hand **L** Subcutaneous Tissue and Fascia, Right Upper Leg **M** Subcutaneous Tissue and Fascia, Left Upper Leg **N** Subcutaneous Tissue and Fascia, Right Lower Leg **P** Subcutaneous Tissue and Fascia, Left Lower Leg **Q** Subcutaneous Tissue and Fascia, Right Foot **R** Subcutaneous Tissue and Fascia, Left Foot	**0** Open **3** Percutaneous	**7** Autologous Tissue Substitute **J** Synthetic Substitute **K** Nonautologous Tissue Substitute	**Z** No Qualifier

Ø Medical and Surgical
J Subcutaneous Tissue and Fascia
W Revision Correcting, to the extent possible, a portion of a malfunctioning device or the position of a displaced device

Body Part Character 4	Approach Character 5	Device Character 6	Qualifier Character 7
S Subcutaneous Tissue and Fascia, Head and Neck	**Ø** Open **3** Percutaneous **X** External	**Ø** Drainage Device **3** Infusion Device **7** Autologous Tissue Substitute **J** Synthetic Substitute **K** Nonautologous Tissue Substitute **N** Tissue Expander	**Z** No Qualifier
T Subcutaneous Tissue and Fascia, Trunk	**Ø** Open **3** Percutaneous **X** External	**Ø** Drainage Device **2** Monitoring Device **3** Infusion Device **7** Autologous Tissue Substitute **H** Contraceptive Device **J** Synthetic Substitute **K** Nonautologous Tissue Substitute **M** Stimulator Generator **N** Tissue Expander **P** Cardiac Rhythm Related Device **V** Infusion Pump **W** Reservoir **X** Vascular Access Device	**Z** No Qualifier
V Subcutaneous Tissue and Fascia, Upper Extremity **W** Subcutaneous Tissue and Fascia, Lower Extremity	**Ø** Open **3** Percutaneous **X** External	**Ø** Drainage Device **3** Infusion Device **7** Autologous Tissue Substitute **H** Contraceptive Device **J** Synthetic Substitute **K** Nonautologous Tissue Substitute **N** Tissue Expander **V** Infusion Pump **W** Reservoir **X** Vascular Access Device	**Z** No Qualifier

Ø Medical and Surgical
J Subcutaneous Tissue and Fascia
X Transfer Moving, without taking out, all or a portion of a body part to another location to take over the function of all or a portion of a body part

Body Part Character 4	Approach Character 5	Device Character 6	Qualifier Character 7
Ø Subcutaneous Tissue and Fascia, Scalp **1** Subcutaneous Tissue and Fascia, Face **4** Subcutaneous Tissue and Fascia, Anterior Neck **5** Subcutaneous Tissue and Fascia, Posterior Neck **6** Subcutaneous Tissue and Fascia, Chest **7** Subcutaneous Tissue and Fascia, Back **8** Subcutaneous Tissue and Fascia, Abdomen **9** Subcutaneous Tissue and Fascia, Buttock **B** Subcutaneous Tissue and Fascia, Perineum **C** Subcutaneous Tissue and Fascia, Pelvic Region **D** Subcutaneous Tissue and Fascia, Right Upper Arm **F** Subcutaneous Tissue and Fascia, Left Upper Arm **G** Subcutaneous Tissue and Fascia, Right Lower Arm **H** Subcutaneous Tissue and Fascia, Left Lower Arm **J** Subcutaneous Tissue and Fascia, Right Hand **K** Subcutaneous Tissue and Fascia, Left Hand **L** Subcutaneous Tissue and Fascia, Right Upper Leg **M** Subcutaneous Tissue and Fascia, Left Upper Leg **N** Subcutaneous Tissue and Fascia, Right Lower Leg **P** Subcutaneous Tissue and Fascia, Left Lower Leg **Q** Subcutaneous Tissue and Fascia, Right Foot **R** Subcutaneous Tissue and Fascia, Left Foot	**Ø** Open **3** Percutaneous	**Z** No Device	**B** Skin and Subcutaneous Tissue **C** Skin, Subcutaneous Tissue and Fascia **Z** No Qualifier

Muscles ØK2–ØKX

Ø Medical and Surgical
K Muscles
2 Change Taking out or off a device from a body part and putting back an identical or similar device in or on the same body part without cutting or puncturing the skin or a mucous membrane

Body Part Character 4	Approach Character 5	Device Character 6	Qualifier Character 7
X Upper Muscle Y Lower Muscle	X External	Ø Drainage Device Y Other Device	Z No Qualifier

Ø Medical and Surgical
K Muscles
5 Destruction Physical eradication of all or a portion of a body part by the direct use of energy, force, or a destructive agent

Body Part Character 4	Approach Character 5	Device Character 6	Qualifier Character 7
Ø Head Muscle 1 Facial Muscle 2 Neck Muscle, Right 3 Neck Muscle, Left 4 Tongue, Palate, Pharynx Muscle 5 Shoulder Muscle, Right 6 Shoulder Muscle, Left 7 Upper Arm Muscle, Right 8 Upper Arm Muscle, Left 9 Lower Arm and Wrist Muscle, Right B Lower Arm and Wrist Muscle, Left C Hand Muscle, Right D Hand Muscle, Left F Trunk Muscle, Right G Trunk Muscle, Left H Thorax Muscle, Right J Thorax Muscle, Left K Abdomen Muscle, Right L Abdomen Muscle, Left M Perineum Muscle N Hip Muscle, Right P Hip Muscle, Left Q Upper Leg Muscle, Right R Upper Leg Muscle, Left S Lower Leg Muscle, Right T Lower Leg Muscle, Left V Foot Muscle, Right W Foot Muscle, Left	Ø Open 3 Percutaneous 4 Percutaneous Endoscopic	Z No Device	Z No Qualifier

Ø Medical and Surgical
K Muscles
8 Division Cutting into a body part without draining fluids and/or gases from the body part in order to separate or transect a body part

Body Part Character 4	Approach Character 5	Device Character 6	Qualifier Character 7
Ø Head Muscle 1 Facial Muscle 2 Neck Muscle, Right 3 Neck Muscle, Left 4 Tongue, Palate, Pharynx Muscle 5 Shoulder Muscle, Right 6 Shoulder Muscle, Left 7 Upper Arm Muscle, Right 8 Upper Arm Muscle, Left 9 Lower Arm and Wrist Muscle, Right B Lower Arm and Wrist Muscle, Left C Hand Muscle, Right D Hand Muscle, Left F Trunk Muscle, Right G Trunk Muscle, Left H Thorax Muscle, Right J Thorax Muscle, Left K Abdomen Muscle, Right L Abdomen Muscle, Left M Perineum Muscle N Hip Muscle, Right P Hip Muscle, Left Q Upper Leg Muscle, Right R Upper Leg Muscle, Left S Lower Leg Muscle, Right T Lower Leg Muscle, Left V Foot Muscle, Right W Foot Muscle, Left	Ø Open 3 Percutaneous 4 Percutaneous Endoscopic	Z No Device	Z No Qualifier

Ø Medical and Surgical
K Muscles
9 Drainage Taking or letting out fluids and/or gases from a body part

Body Part Character 4	Approach Character 5	Device Character 6	Qualifier Character 7
Ø Head Muscle 1 Facial Muscle 2 Neck Muscle, Right 3 Neck Muscle, Left 4 Tongue, Palate, Pharynx Muscle 5 Shoulder Muscle, Right 6 Shoulder Muscle, Left 7 Upper Arm Muscle, Right 8 Upper Arm Muscle, Left 9 Lower Arm and Wrist Muscle, Right B Lower Arm and Wrist Muscle, Left C Hand Muscle, Right D Hand Muscle, Left F Trunk Muscle, Right G Trunk Muscle, Left H Thorax Muscle, Right J Thorax Muscle, Left K Abdomen Muscle, Right L Abdomen Muscle, Left M Perineum Muscle N Hip Muscle, Right P Hip Muscle, Left Q Upper Leg Muscle, Right R Upper Leg Muscle, Left S Lower Leg Muscle, Right T Lower Leg Muscle, Left V Foot Muscle, Right W Foot Muscle, Left	Ø Open 3 Percutaneous 4 Percutaneous Endoscopic	Ø Drainage Device	Z No Qualifier

ØK9 Continued on next page

Ø Medical and Surgical
K Muscles
9 Drainage Taking or letting out fluids and/or gases from a body part

ØK9 Continued

Body Part Character 4	Approach Character 5	Device Character 6	Qualifier Character 7
Ø Head Muscle **1** Facial Muscle **2** Neck Muscle, Right **3** Neck Muscle, Left **4** Tongue, Palate, Pharynx Muscle **5** Shoulder Muscle, Right **6** Shoulder Muscle, Left **7** Upper Arm Muscle, Right **8** Upper Arm Muscle, Left **9** Lower Arm and Wrist Muscle, Right **B** Lower Arm and Wrist Muscle, Left **C** Hand Muscle, Right **D** Hand Muscle, Left **F** Trunk Muscle, Right **G** Trunk Muscle, Left **H** Thorax Muscle, Right **J** Thorax Muscle, Left **K** Abdomen Muscle, Right **L** Abdomen Muscle, Left **M** Perineum Muscle **N** Hip Muscle, Right **P** Hip Muscle, Left **Q** Upper Leg Muscle, Right **R** Upper Leg Muscle, Left **S** Lower Leg Muscle, Right **T** Lower Leg Muscle, Left **V** Foot Muscle, Right **W** Foot Muscle, Left	**Ø** Open **3** Percutaneous **4** Percutaneous Endoscopic	**Z** No Device	**X** Diagnostic **Z** No Qualifier

Ø Medical and Surgical
K Muscles
B Excision Cutting out or off, without replacement, a portion of a body part

Body Part Character 4	Approach Character 5	Device Character 6	Qualifier Character 7
Ø Head Muscle **1** Facial Muscle **2** Neck Muscle, Right **3** Neck Muscle, Left **4** Tongue, Palate, Pharynx Muscle **5** Shoulder Muscle, Right **6** Shoulder Muscle, Left **7** Upper Arm Muscle, Right **8** Upper Arm Muscle, Left **9** Lower Arm and Wrist Muscle, Right **B** Lower Arm and Wrist Muscle, Left **C** Hand Muscle, Right **D** Hand Muscle, Left **F** Trunk Muscle, Right **G** Trunk Muscle, Left **H** Thorax Muscle, Right **J** Thorax Muscle, Left **K** Abdomen Muscle, Right **L** Abdomen Muscle, Left **M** Perineum Muscle **N** Hip Muscle, Right **P** Hip Muscle, Left **Q** Upper Leg Muscle, Right **R** Upper Leg Muscle, Left **S** Lower Leg Muscle, Right **T** Lower Leg Muscle, Left **V** Foot Muscle, Right **W** Foot Muscle, Left	**Ø** Open **3** Percutaneous **4** Percutaneous Endoscopic	**Z** No Device	**X** Diagnostic **Z** No Qualifier

Ø Medical and Surgical
K Muscles
C Extirpation Taking or cutting out solid matter from a body part

Body Part Character 4	Approach Character 5	Device Character 6	Qualifier Character 7
Ø Head Muscle **1** Facial Muscle **2** Neck Muscle, Right **3** Neck Muscle, Left **4** Tongue, Palate, Pharynx Muscle **5** Shoulder Muscle, Right **6** Shoulder Muscle, Left **7** Upper Arm Muscle, Right **8** Upper Arm Muscle, Left **9** Lower Arm and Wrist Muscle, Right **B** Lower Arm and Wrist Muscle, Left **C** Hand Muscle, Right **D** Hand Muscle, Left **F** Trunk Muscle, Right **G** Trunk Muscle, Left **H** Thorax Muscle, Right **J** Thorax Muscle, Left **K** Abdomen Muscle, Right **L** Abdomen Muscle, Left **M** Perineum Muscle **N** Hip Muscle, Right **P** Hip Muscle, Left **Q** Upper Leg Muscle, Right **R** Upper Leg Muscle, Left **S** Lower Leg Muscle, Right **T** Lower Leg Muscle, Left **V** Foot Muscle, Right **W** Foot Muscle, Left	**Ø** Open **3** Percutaneous **4** Percutaneous Endoscopic	**Z** No Device	**Z** No Qualifier

Ø Medical and Surgical
K Muscles
H Insertion Putting in a nonbiological appliance that monitors, assists, performs, or prevents a physiological function but does not physically take the place of a body part

Body Part Character 4	Approach Character 5	Device Character 6	Qualifier Character 7
X Upper Muscle **Y** Lower Muscle	**Ø** Open **3** Percutaneous **4** Percutaneous Endoscopic	**M** Stimulator Lead	**Z** No Qualifier

Ø Medical and Surgical
K Muscles
J Inspection Visually and/or manually exploring a body part

Body Part Character 4	Approach Character 5	Device Character 6	Qualifier Character 7
X Upper Muscle **Y** Lower Muscle	**Ø** Open **3** Percutaneous **4** Percutaneous Endoscopic **X** External	**Z** No Device	**Z** No Qualifier

0 Medical and Surgical
K Muscles
M Reattachment Putting back in or on all or a portion of a separated body part to its normal location or other suitable location

Body Part Character 4	Approach Character 5	Device Character 6	Qualifier Character 7
0 Head Muscle 1 Facial Muscle 2 Neck Muscle, Right 3 Neck Muscle, Left 4 Tongue, Palate, Pharynx Muscle 5 Shoulder Muscle, Right 6 Shoulder Muscle, Left 7 Upper Arm Muscle, Right 8 Upper Arm Muscle, Left 9 Lower Arm and Wrist Muscle, Right B Lower Arm and Wrist Muscle, Left C Hand Muscle, Right D Hand Muscle, Left F Trunk Muscle, Right G Trunk Muscle, Left H Thorax Muscle, Right J Thorax Muscle, Left K Abdomen Muscle, Right L Abdomen Muscle, Left M Perineum Muscle N Hip Muscle, Right P Hip Muscle, Left Q Upper Leg Muscle, Right R Upper Leg Muscle, Left S Lower Leg Muscle, Right T Lower Leg Muscle, Left V Foot Muscle, Right W Foot Muscle, Left	0 Open 4 Percutaneous Endoscopic	Z No Device	Z No Qualifier

0 Medical and Surgical
K Muscles
N Release Freeing a body part from an abnormal physical constraint

Body Part Character 4	Approach Character 5	Device Character 6	Qualifier Character 7
0 Head Muscle 1 Facial Muscle 2 Neck Muscle, Right 3 Neck Muscle, Left 4 Tongue, Palate, Pharynx Muscle 5 Shoulder Muscle, Right 6 Shoulder Muscle, Left 7 Upper Arm Muscle, Right 8 Upper Arm Muscle, Left 9 Lower Arm and Wrist Muscle, Right B Lower Arm and Wrist Muscle, Left C Hand Muscle, Right D Hand Muscle, Left F Trunk Muscle, Right G Trunk Muscle, Left H Thorax Muscle, Right J Thorax Muscle, Left K Abdomen Muscle, Right L Abdomen Muscle, Left M Perineum Muscle N Hip Muscle, Right P Hip Muscle, Left Q Upper Leg Muscle, Right R Upper Leg Muscle, Left S Lower Leg Muscle, Right T Lower Leg Muscle, Left V Foot Muscle, Right W Foot Muscle, Left	0 Open 3 Percutaneous 4 Percutaneous Endoscopic X External	Z No Device	Z No Qualifier

Ø Medical and Surgical
K Muscles
P Removal Taking out or off a device from a body part

Body Part Character 4	Approach Character 5	Device Character 6	Qualifier Character 7
X Upper Muscle **Y** Lower Muscle	**Ø** Open **3** Percutaneous **4** Percutaneous Endoscopic	**Ø** Drainage Device **7** Autologous Tissue Substitute **J** Synthetic Substitute **K** Nonautologous Tissue Substitute **M** Stimulator Lead	**Z** No Qualifier
X Upper Muscle **Y** Lower Muscle	**X** External	**Ø** Drainage Device **M** Stimulator Lead	**Z** No Qualifier

Ø Medical and Surgical
K Muscles
Q Repair Restoring, to the extent possible, a body part to its normal anatomic structure and function

Body Part Character 4	Approach Character 5	Device Character 6	Qualifier Character 7
Ø Head Muscle **1** Facial Muscle **2** Neck Muscle, Right **3** Neck Muscle, Left **4** Tongue, Palate, Pharynx Muscle **5** Shoulder Muscle, Right **6** Shoulder Muscle, Left **7** Upper Arm Muscle, Right **8** Upper Arm Muscle, Left **9** Lower Arm and Wrist Muscle, Right **B** Lower Arm and Wrist Muscle, Left **C** Hand Muscle, Right **D** Hand Muscle, Left **F** Trunk Muscle, Right **G** Trunk Muscle, Left **H** Thorax Muscle, Right **J** Thorax Muscle, Left **K** Abdomen Muscle, Right **L** Abdomen Muscle, Left **M** Perineum Muscle **N** Hip Muscle, Right **P** Hip Muscle, Left **Q** Upper Leg Muscle, Right **R** Upper Leg Muscle, Left **S** Lower Leg Muscle, Right **T** Lower Leg Muscle, Left **V** Foot Muscle, Right **W** Foot Muscle, Left	**Ø** Open **3** Percutaneous **4** Percutaneous Endoscopic	**Z** No Device	**Z** No Qualifier

0 Medical and Surgical
K Muscles
S Reposition Moving to its normal location or other suitable location all or a portion of a body part

Body Part Character 4	Approach Character 5	Device Character 6	Qualifier Character 7
0 Head Muscle 1 Facial Muscle 2 Neck Muscle, Right 3 Neck Muscle, Left 4 Tongue, Palate, Pharynx Muscle 5 Shoulder Muscle, Right 6 Shoulder Muscle, Left 7 Upper Arm Muscle, Right 8 Upper Arm Muscle, Left 9 Lower Arm and Wrist Muscle, Right B Lower Arm and Wrist Muscle, Left C Hand Muscle, Right D Hand Muscle, Left F Trunk Muscle, Right G Trunk Muscle, Left H Thorax Muscle, Right J Thorax Muscle, Left K Abdomen Muscle, Right L Abdomen Muscle, Left M Perineum Muscle N Hip Muscle, Right P Hip Muscle, Left Q Upper Leg Muscle, Right R Upper Leg Muscle, Left S Lower Leg Muscle, Right T Lower Leg Muscle, Left V Foot Muscle, Right W Foot Muscle, Left	0 Open 4 Percutaneous Endoscopic	Z No Device	Z No Qualifier

0 Medical and Surgical
K Muscles
T Resection Cutting out or off, without replacement, all of a body part

Body Part Character 4	Approach Character 5	Device Character 6	Qualifier Character 7
0 Head Muscle 1 Facial Muscle 2 Neck Muscle, Right 3 Neck Muscle, Left 4 Tongue, Palate, Pharynx Muscle 5 Shoulder Muscle, Right 6 Shoulder Muscle, Left 7 Upper Arm Muscle, Right 8 Upper Arm Muscle, Left 9 Lower Arm and Wrist Muscle, Right B Lower Arm and Wrist Muscle, Left C Hand Muscle, Right D Hand Muscle, Left F Trunk Muscle, Right G Trunk Muscle, Left H Thorax Muscle, Right J Thorax Muscle, Left K Abdomen Muscle, Right L Abdomen Muscle, Left M Perineum Muscle N Hip Muscle, Right P Hip Muscle, Left Q Upper Leg Muscle, Right R Upper Leg Muscle, Left S Lower Leg Muscle, Right T Lower Leg Muscle, Left V Foot Muscle, Right W Foot Muscle, Left	0 Open 4 Percutaneous Endoscopic	Z No Device	Z No Qualifier

Ø Medical and Surgical
K Muscles
U Supplement Putting in or on biological or synthetic material that physically reinforces and/or augments the function of a portion of a body part

Body Part Character 4	Approach Character 5	Device Character 6	Qualifier Character 7
Ø Head Muscle **1** Facial Muscle **2** Neck Muscle, Right **3** Neck Muscle, Left **4** Tongue, Palate, Pharynx Muscle **5** Shoulder Muscle, Right **6** Shoulder Muscle, Left **7** Upper Arm Muscle, Right **8** Upper Arm Muscle, Left **9** Lower Arm and Wrist Muscle, Right **B** Lower Arm and Wrist Muscle, Left **C** Hand Muscle, Right **D** Hand Muscle, Left **F** Trunk Muscle, Right **G** Trunk Muscle, Left **H** Thorax Muscle, Right **J** Thorax Muscle, Left **K** Abdomen Muscle, Right **L** Abdomen Muscle, Left **M** Perineum Muscle **N** Hip Muscle, Right **P** Hip Muscle, Left **Q** Upper Leg Muscle, Right **R** Upper Leg Muscle, Left **S** Lower Leg Muscle, Right **T** Lower Leg Muscle, Left **V** Foot Muscle, Right **W** Foot Muscle, Left	**Ø** Open **4** Percutaneous Endoscopic	**7** Autologous Tissue Substitute **J** Synthetic Substitute **K** Nonautologous Tissue Substitute	**Z** No Qualifier

Ø Medical and Surgical
K Muscles
W Revision Correcting, to the extent possible, a portion of a malfunctioning device or the position of a displaced device

Body Part Character 4	Approach Character 5	Device Character 6	Qualifier Character 7
X Upper Muscle **Y** Lower Muscle	**Ø** Open **3** Percutaneous **4** Percutaneous Endoscopic **X** External	**Ø** Drainage Device **7** Autologous Tissue Substitute **J** Synthetic Substitute **K** Nonautologous Tissue Substitute **M** Stimulator Lead	**Z** No Qualifier

0 Medical and Surgical
K Muscles
X Transfer Moving, without taking out, all or a portion of a body part to another location to take over the function of all or a portion of a body part

Body Part Character 4	Approach Character 5	Device Character 6	Qualifier Character 7
0 Head Muscle **1** Facial Muscle **2** Neck Muscle, Right **3** Neck Muscle, Left **4** Tongue, Palate, Pharynx Muscle **5** Shoulder Muscle, Right **6** Shoulder Muscle, Left **7** Upper Arm Muscle, Right **8** Upper Arm Muscle, Left **9** Lower Arm and Wrist Muscle, Right **B** Lower Arm and Wrist Muscle, Left **C** Hand Muscle, Right **D** Hand Muscle, Left **F** Trunk Muscle, Right **G** Trunk Muscle, Left **H** Thorax Muscle, Right **J** Thorax Muscle, Left **M** Perineum Muscle **N** Hip Muscle, Right **P** Hip Muscle, Left **Q** Upper Leg Muscle, Right **R** Upper Leg Muscle, Left **S** Lower Leg Muscle, Right **T** Lower Leg Muscle, Left **V** Foot Muscle, Right **W** Foot Muscle, Left	**0** Open **4** Percutaneous Endoscopic	**Z** No Device	**0** Skin **1** Subcutaneous Tissue **2** Skin and Subcutaneous Tissue **Z** No Qualifier
K Abdomen Muscle, Right **L** Abdomen Muscle, Left	**0** Open **4** Percutaneous Endoscopic	**Z** No Device	**0** Skin **1** Subcutaneous Tissue **2** Skin and Subcutaneous Tissue **6** Transverse Rectus Abdominis Myocutaneous Flap **Z** No Qualifier

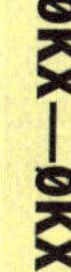

Tendons ØL2–ØLX

Ø Medical and Surgical
L Tendons
2 Change Taking out or off a device from a body part and putting back an identical or similar device in or on the same body part without cutting or puncturing the skin or a mucous membrane

Body Part Character 4	Approach Character 5	Device Character 6	Qualifier Character 7
X Upper Tendon Y Lower Tendon	X External	Ø Drainage Device Y Other Device	Z No Qualifier

Ø Medical and Surgical
L Tendons
5 Destruction Physical eradication of all or a portion of a body part by the direct use of energy, force, or a destructive agent

Body Part Character 4	Approach Character 5	Device Character 6	Qualifier Character 7
Ø Head and Neck Tendon 1 Shoulder Tendon, Right 2 Shoulder Tendon, Left 3 Upper Arm Tendon, Right 4 Upper Arm Tendon, Left 5 Lower Arm and Wrist Tendon, Right 6 Lower Arm and Wrist Tendon, Left 7 Hand Tendon, Right 8 Hand Tendon, Left 9 Trunk Tendon, Right B Trunk Tendon, Left C Thorax Tendon, Right D Thorax Tendon, Left F Abdomen Tendon, Right G Abdomen Tendon, Left H Perineum Tendon J Hip Tendon, Right K Hip Tendon, Left L Upper Leg Tendon, Right M Upper Leg Tendon, Left N Lower Leg Tendon, Right P Lower Leg Tendon, Left Q Knee Tendon, Right R Knee Tendon, Left S Ankle Tendon, Right T Ankle Tendon, Left V Foot Tendon, Right W Foot Tendon, Left	Ø Open 3 Percutaneous 4 Percutaneous Endoscopic	Z No Device	Z No Qualifier

0 Medical and Surgical
L Tendons
8 Division Cutting into a body part without draining fluids and/or gases from the body part in order to separate or transect a body part

Body Part Character 4	Approach Character 5	Device Character 6	Qualifier Character 7
0 Head and Neck Tendon 1 Shoulder Tendon, Right 2 Shoulder Tendon, Left 3 Upper Arm Tendon, Right 4 Upper Arm Tendon, Left 5 Lower Arm and Wrist Tendon, Right 6 Lower Arm and Wrist Tendon, Left 7 Hand Tendon, Right 8 Hand Tendon, Left 9 Trunk Tendon, Right B Trunk Tendon, Left C Thorax Tendon, Right D Thorax Tendon, Left F Abdomen Tendon, Right G Abdomen Tendon, Left H Perineum Tendon J Hip Tendon, Right K Hip Tendon, Left L Upper Leg Tendon, Right M Upper Leg Tendon, Left N Lower Leg Tendon, Right P Lower Leg Tendon, Left Q Knee Tendon, Right R Knee Tendon, Left S Ankle Tendon, Right T Ankle Tendon, Left V Foot Tendon, Right W Foot Tendon, Left	0 Open 3 Percutaneous 4 Percutaneous Endoscopic	Z No Device	Z No Qualifier

0 Medical and Surgical
L Tendons
9 Drainage Taking or letting out fluids and/or gases from a body part

Body Part Character 4	Approach Character 5	Device Character 6	Qualifier Character 7
0 Head and Neck Tendon 1 Shoulder Tendon, Right 2 Shoulder Tendon, Left 3 Upper Arm Tendon, Right 4 Upper Arm Tendon, Left 5 Lower Arm and Wrist Tendon, Right 6 Lower Arm and Wrist Tendon, Left 7 Hand Tendon, Right 8 Hand Tendon, Left 9 Trunk Tendon, Right B Trunk Tendon, Left C Thorax Tendon, Right D Thorax Tendon, Left F Abdomen Tendon, Right G Abdomen Tendon, Left H Perineum Tendon J Hip Tendon, Right K Hip Tendon, Left L Upper Leg Tendon, Right M Upper Leg Tendon, Left N Lower Leg Tendon, Right P Lower Leg Tendon, Left Q Knee Tendon, Right R Knee Tendon, Left S Ankle Tendon, Right T Ankle Tendon, Left V Foot Tendon, Right W Foot Tendon, Left	0 Open 3 Percutaneous 4 Percutaneous Endoscopic	0 Drainage Device	Z No Qualifier

0L9 Continued on next page

ØL9 Continued

Ø Medical and Surgical
L Tendons
9 Drainage Taking or letting out fluids and/or gases from a body part

Body Part Character 4	Approach Character 5	Device Character 6	Qualifier Character 7
Ø Head and Neck Tendon 1 Shoulder Tendon, Right 2 Shoulder Tendon, Left 3 Upper Arm Tendon, Right 4 Upper Arm Tendon, Left 5 Lower Arm and Wrist Tendon, Right 6 Lower Arm and Wrist Tendon, Left 7 Hand Tendon, Right 8 Hand Tendon, Left 9 Trunk Tendon, Right B Trunk Tendon, Left C Thorax Tendon, Right D Thorax Tendon, Left F Abdomen Tendon, Right G Abdomen Tendon, Left H Perineum Tendon J Hip Tendon, Right K Hip Tendon, Left L Upper Leg Tendon, Right M Upper Leg Tendon, Left N Lower Leg Tendon, Right P Lower Leg Tendon, Left Q Knee Tendon, Right R Knee Tendon, Left S Ankle Tendon, Right T Ankle Tendon, Left V Foot Tendon, Right W Foot Tendon, Left	Ø Open 3 Percutaneous 4 Percutaneous Endoscopic	Z No Device	X Diagnostic Z No Qualifier

Ø Medical and Surgical
L Tendons
B Excision Cutting out or off, without replacement, a portion of a body part

Body Part Character 4	Approach Character 5	Device Character 6	Qualifier Character 7
Ø Head and Neck Tendon 1 Shoulder Tendon, Right 2 Shoulder Tendon, Left 3 Upper Arm Tendon, Right 4 Upper Arm Tendon, Left 5 Lower Arm and Wrist Tendon, Right 6 Lower Arm and Wrist Tendon, Left 7 Hand Tendon, Right 8 Hand Tendon, Left 9 Trunk Tendon, Right B Trunk Tendon, Left C Thorax Tendon, Right D Thorax Tendon, Left F Abdomen Tendon, Right G Abdomen Tendon, Left H Perineum Tendon J Hip Tendon, Right K Hip Tendon, Left L Upper Leg Tendon, Right M Upper Leg Tendon, Left N Lower Leg Tendon, Right P Lower Leg Tendon, Left Q Knee Tendon, Right R Knee Tendon, Left S Ankle Tendon, Right T Ankle Tendon, Left V Foot Tendon, Right W Foot Tendon, Left	Ø Open 3 Percutaneous 4 Percutaneous Endoscopic	Z No Device	X Diagnostic Z No Qualifier

Ø Medical and Surgical
L Tendons
C Extirpation Taking or cutting out solid matter from a body part

Body Part Character 4	Approach Character 5	Device Character 6	Qualifier Character 7
Ø Head and Neck Tendon **1** Shoulder Tendon, Right **2** Shoulder Tendon, Left **3** Upper Arm Tendon, Right **4** Upper Arm Tendon, Left **5** Lower Arm and Wrist Tendon, Right **6** Lower Arm and Wrist Tendon, Left **7** Hand Tendon, Right **8** Hand Tendon, Left **9** Trunk Tendon, Right **B** Trunk Tendon, Left **C** Thorax Tendon, Right **D** Thorax Tendon, Left **F** Abdomen Tendon, Right **G** Abdomen Tendon, Left **H** Perineum Tendon **J** Hip Tendon, Right **K** Hip Tendon, Left **L** Upper Leg Tendon, Right **M** Upper Leg Tendon, Left **N** Lower Leg Tendon, Right **P** Lower Leg Tendon, Left **Q** Knee Tendon, Right **R** Knee Tendon, Left **S** Ankle Tendon, Right **T** Ankle Tendon, Left **V** Foot Tendon, Right **W** Foot Tendon, Left	**Ø** Open **3** Percutaneous **4** Percutaneous Endoscopic	**Z** No Device	**Z** No Qualifier

Ø Medical and Surgical
L Tendons
J Inspection Visually and/or manually exploring a body part

Body Part Character 4	Approach Character 5	Device Character 6	Qualifier Character 7
X Upper Tendon **Y** Lower Tendon	**Ø** Open **3** Percutaneous **4** Percutaneous Endoscopic **X** External	**Z** No Device	**Z** No Qualifier

Ø Medical and Surgical
L Tendons
M Reattachment Putting back in or on all or a portion of a separated body part to its normal location or other suitable location

Body Part Character 4	Approach Character 5	Device Character 6	Qualifier Character 7
Ø Head and Neck Tendon **1** Shoulder Tendon, Right **2** Shoulder Tendon, Left **3** Upper Arm Tendon, Right **4** Upper Arm Tendon, Left **5** Lower Arm and Wrist Tendon, Right **6** Lower Arm and Wrist Tendon, Left **7** Hand Tendon, Right **8** Hand Tendon, Left **9** Trunk Tendon, Right **B** Trunk Tendon, Left **C** Thorax Tendon, Right **D** Thorax Tendon, Left **F** Abdomen Tendon, Right **G** Abdomen Tendon, Left **H** Perineum Tendon **J** Hip Tendon, Right **K** Hip Tendon, Left **L** Upper Leg Tendon, Right **M** Upper Leg Tendon, Left **N** Lower Leg Tendon, Right **P** Lower Leg Tendon, Left **Q** Knee Tendon, Right **R** Knee Tendon, Left **S** Ankle Tendon, Right **T** Ankle Tendon, Left **V** Foot Tendon, Right **W** Foot Tendon, Left	**Ø** Open **4** Percutaneous Endoscopic	**Z** No Device	**Z** No Qualifier

Ø Medical and Surgical
L Tendons
N Release Freeing a body part from an abnormal physical constraint

Body Part Character 4	Approach Character 5	Device Character 6	Qualifier Character 7
Ø Head and Neck Tendon **1** Shoulder Tendon, Right **2** Shoulder Tendon, Left **3** Upper Arm Tendon, Right **4** Upper Arm Tendon, Left **5** Lower Arm and Wrist Tendon, Right **6** Lower Arm and Wrist Tendon, Left **7** Hand Tendon, Right **8** Hand Tendon, Left **9** Trunk Tendon, Right **B** Trunk Tendon, Left **C** Thorax Tendon, Right **D** Thorax Tendon, Left **F** Abdomen Tendon, Right **G** Abdomen Tendon, Left **H** Perineum Tendon **J** Hip Tendon, Right **K** Hip Tendon, Left **L** Upper Leg Tendon, Right **M** Upper Leg Tendon, Left **N** Lower Leg Tendon, Right **P** Lower Leg Tendon, Left **Q** Knee Tendon, Right **R** Knee Tendon, Left **S** Ankle Tendon, Right **T** Ankle Tendon, Left **V** Foot Tendon, Right **W** Foot Tendon, Left	**Ø** Open **3** Percutaneous **4** Percutaneous Endoscopic **X** External	**Z** No Device	**Z** No Qualifier

Ø Medical and Surgical
L Tendons
P Removal Taking out or off a device from a body part

Body Part Character 4	Approach Character 5	Device Character 6	Qualifier Character 7
X Upper Tendon **Y** Lower Tendon	**Ø** Open **3** Percutaneous **4** Percutaneous Endoscopic	**Ø** Drainage Device **7** Autologous Tissue Substitute **J** Synthetic Substitute **K** Nonautologous Tissue Substitute	**Z** No Qualifier
X Upper Tendon **Y** Lower Tendon	**X** External	**Ø** Drainage Device	**Z** No Qualifier

0 Medical and Surgical
L Tendons
Q Repair Restoring, to the extent possible, a body part to its normal anatomic structure and function

Body Part Character 4	Approach Character 5	Device Character 6	Qualifier Character 7
0 Head and Neck Tendon 1 Shoulder Tendon, Right 2 Shoulder Tendon, Left 3 Upper Arm Tendon, Right 4 Upper Arm Tendon, Left 5 Lower Arm and Wrist Tendon, Right 6 Lower Arm and Wrist Tendon, Left 7 Hand Tendon, Right 8 Hand Tendon, Left 9 Trunk Tendon, Right B Trunk Tendon, Left C Thorax Tendon, Right D Thorax Tendon, Left F Abdomen Tendon, Right G Abdomen Tendon, Left H Perineum Tendon J Hip Tendon, Right K Hip Tendon, Left L Upper Leg Tendon, Right M Upper Leg Tendon, Left N Lower Leg Tendon, Right P Lower Leg Tendon, Left Q Knee Tendon, Right R Knee Tendon, Left S Ankle Tendon, Right T Ankle Tendon, Left V Foot Tendon, Right W Foot Tendon, Left	0 Open 3 Percutaneous 4 Percutaneous Endoscopic	Z No Device	Z No Qualifier

0 Medical and Surgical
L Tendons
R Replacement Putting in or on biological or synthetic material that physically takes the place and/or function of all or a portion of a body part

Body Part Character 4	Approach Character 5	Device Character 6	Qualifier Character 7
0 Head and Neck Tendon 1 Shoulder Tendon, Right 2 Shoulder Tendon, Left 3 Upper Arm Tendon, Right 4 Upper Arm Tendon, Left 5 Lower Arm and Wrist Tendon, Right 6 Lower Arm and Wrist Tendon, Left 7 Hand Tendon, Right 8 Hand Tendon, Left 9 Trunk Tendon, Right B Trunk Tendon, Left C Thorax Tendon, Right D Thorax Tendon, Left F Abdomen Tendon, Right G Abdomen Tendon, Left H Perineum Tendon J Hip Tendon, Right K Hip Tendon, Left L Upper Leg Tendon, Right M Upper Leg Tendon, Left N Lower Leg Tendon, Right P Lower Leg Tendon, Left Q Knee Tendon, Right R Knee Tendon, Left S Ankle Tendon, Right T Ankle Tendon, Left V Foot Tendon, Right W Foot Tendon, Left	0 Open 4 Percutaneous Endoscopic	7 Autologous Tissue Substitute J Synthetic Substitute K Nonautologous Tissue Substitute	Z No Qualifier

Ø Medical and Surgical
L Tendons
S Reposition Moving to its normal location or other suitable location all or a portion of a body part

Body Part Character 4	Approach Character 5	Device Character 6	Qualifier Character 7
Ø Head and Neck Tendon **1** Shoulder Tendon, Right **2** Shoulder Tendon, Left **3** Upper Arm Tendon, Right **4** Upper Arm Tendon, Left **5** Lower Arm and Wrist Tendon, Right **6** Lower Arm and Wrist Tendon, Left **7** Hand Tendon, Right **8** Hand Tendon, Left **9** Trunk Tendon, Right **B** Trunk Tendon, Left **C** Thorax Tendon, Right **D** Thorax Tendon, Left **F** Abdomen Tendon, Right **G** Abdomen Tendon, Left **H** Perineum Tendon **J** Hip Tendon, Right **K** Hip Tendon, Left **L** Upper Leg Tendon, Right **M** Upper Leg Tendon, Left **N** Lower Leg Tendon, Right **P** Lower Leg Tendon, Left **Q** Knee Tendon, Right **R** Knee Tendon, Left **S** Ankle Tendon, Right **T** Ankle Tendon, Left **V** Foot Tendon, Right **W** Foot Tendon, Left	**Ø** Open **4** Percutaneous Endoscopic	**Z** No Device	**Z** No Qualifier

Ø Medical and Surgical
L Tendons
T Resection Cutting out or off, without replacement, all of a body part

Body Part Character 4	Approach Character 5	Device Character 6	Qualifier Character 7
Ø Head and Neck Tendon **1** Shoulder Tendon, Right **2** Shoulder Tendon, Left **3** Upper Arm Tendon, Right **4** Upper Arm Tendon, Left **5** Lower Arm and Wrist Tendon, Right **6** Lower Arm and Wrist Tendon, Left **7** Hand Tendon, Right **8** Hand Tendon, Left **9** Trunk Tendon, Right **B** Trunk Tendon, Left **C** Thorax Tendon, Right **D** Thorax Tendon, Left **F** Abdomen Tendon, Right **G** Abdomen Tendon, Left **H** Perineum Tendon **J** Hip Tendon, Right **K** Hip Tendon, Left **L** Upper Leg Tendon, Right **M** Upper Leg Tendon, Left **N** Lower Leg Tendon, Right **P** Lower Leg Tendon, Left **Q** Knee Tendon, Right **R** Knee Tendon, Left **S** Ankle Tendon, Right **T** Ankle Tendon, Left **V** Foot Tendon, Right **W** Foot Tendon, Left	**Ø** Open **4** Percutaneous Endoscopic	**Z** No Device	**Z** No Qualifier

0 Medical and Surgical
L Tendons
U Supplement Putting in or on biological or synthetic material that physically reinforces and/or augments the function of a portion of a body part

Body Part Character 4	Approach Character 5	Device Character 6	Qualifier Character 7
0 Head and Neck Tendon 1 Shoulder Tendon, Right 2 Shoulder Tendon, Left 3 Upper Arm Tendon, Right 4 Upper Arm Tendon, Left 5 Lower Arm and Wrist Tendon, Right 6 Lower Arm and Wrist Tendon, Left 7 Hand Tendon, Right 8 Hand Tendon, Left 9 Trunk Tendon, Right B Trunk Tendon, Left C Thorax Tendon, Right D Thorax Tendon, Left F Abdomen Tendon, Right G Abdomen Tendon, Left H Perineum Tendon J Hip Tendon, Right K Hip Tendon, Left L Upper Leg Tendon, Right M Upper Leg Tendon, Left N Lower Leg Tendon, Right P Lower Leg Tendon, Left Q Knee Tendon, Right R Knee Tendon, Left S Ankle Tendon, Right T Ankle Tendon, Left V Foot Tendon, Right W Foot Tendon, Left	0 Open 4 Percutaneous Endoscopic	7 Autologous Tissue Substitute J Synthetic Substitute K Nonautologous Tissue Substitute	Z No Qualifier

0 Medical and Surgical
L Tendons
W Revision Correcting, to the extent possible, a portion of a malfunctioning device or the position of a displaced device

Body Part Character 4	Approach Character 5	Device Character 6	Qualifier Character 7
X Upper Tendon Y Lower Tendon	0 Open 3 Percutaneous 4 Percutaneous Endoscopic X External	0 Drainage Device 7 Autologous Tissue Substitute J Synthetic Substitute K Nonautologous Tissue Substitute	Z No Qualifier

0 Medical and Surgical
L Tendons
X Transfer Moving, without taking out, all or a portion of a body part to another location to take over the function of all or a portion of a body part

Body Part Character 4	Approach Character 5	Device Character 6	Qualifier Character 7
0 Head and Neck Tendon 1 Shoulder Tendon, Right 2 Shoulder Tendon, Left 3 Upper Arm Tendon, Right 4 Upper Arm Tendon, Left 5 Lower Arm and Wrist Tendon, Right 6 Lower Arm and Wrist Tendon, Left 7 Hand Tendon, Right 8 Hand Tendon, Left 9 Trunk Tendon, Right B Trunk Tendon, Left C Thorax Tendon, Right D Thorax Tendon, Left F Abdomen Tendon, Right G Abdomen Tendon, Left H Perineum Tendon J Hip Tendon, Right K Hip Tendon, Left L Upper Leg Tendon, Right M Upper Leg Tendon, Left N Lower Leg Tendon, Right P Lower Leg Tendon, Left Q Knee Tendon, Right R Knee Tendon, Left S Ankle Tendon, Right T Ankle Tendon, Left V Foot Tendon, Right W Foot Tendon, Left	0 Open 4 Percutaneous Endoscopic	Z No Device	Z No Qualifier

Bursae and Ligaments ØM2–ØMX

Ø Medical and Surgical
M Bursae and Ligaments
2 Change Taking out or off a device from a body part and putting back an identical or similar device in or on the same body part without cutting or puncturing the skin or a mucous membrane

Body Part Character 4	Approach Character 5	Device Character 6	Qualifier Character 7
X Upper Bursa and Ligament **Y** Lower Bursa and Ligament	**X** External	**Ø** Drainage Device **Y** Other Device	**Z** No Qualifier

Ø Medical and Surgical
M Bursae and Ligaments
5 Destruction Physical eradication of all or a portion of a body part by the direct use of energy, force, or a destructive agent

Body Part Character 4	Approach Character 5	Device Character 6	Qualifier Character 7
Ø Head and Neck Bursa and Ligament **1** Shoulder Bursa and Ligament, Right **2** Shoulder Bursa and Ligament, Left **3** Elbow Bursa and Ligament, Right **4** Elbow Bursa and Ligament, Left **5** Wrist Bursa and Ligament, Right **6** Wrist Bursa and Ligament, Left **7** Hand Bursa and Ligament, Right **8** Hand Bursa and Ligament, Left **9** Upper Extremity Bursa and Ligament, Right **B** Upper Extremity Bursa and Ligament, Left **C** Trunk Bursa and Ligament, Right **D** Trunk Bursa and Ligament, Left **F** Thorax Bursa and Ligament, Right **G** Thorax Bursa and Ligament, Left **H** Abdomen Bursa and Ligament, Right **J** Abdomen Bursa and Ligament, Left **K** Perineum Bursa and Ligament **L** Hip Bursa and Ligament, Right **M** Hip Bursa and Ligament, Left **N** Knee Bursa and Ligament, Right **P** Knee Bursa and Ligament, Left **Q** Ankle Bursa and Ligament, Right **R** Ankle Bursa and Ligament, Left **S** Foot Bursa and Ligament, Right **T** Foot Bursa and Ligament, Left **V** Lower Extremity Bursa and Ligament, Right **W** Lower Extremity Bursa and Ligament, Left	**Ø** Open **3** Percutaneous **4** Percutaneous Endoscopic	**Z** No Device	**Z** No Qualifier

Ø Medical and Surgical
M Bursae and Ligaments
8 Division Cutting into a body part without draining fluids and/or gases from the body part in order to separate or transect a body part

Body Part Character 4	Approach Character 5	Device Character 6	Qualifier Character 7
Ø Head and Neck Bursa and Ligament 1 Shoulder Bursa and Ligament, Right 2 Shoulder Bursa and Ligament, Left 3 Elbow Bursa and Ligament, Right 4 Elbow Bursa and Ligament, Left 5 Wrist Bursa and Ligament, Right 6 Wrist Bursa and Ligament, Left 7 Hand Bursa and Ligament, Right 8 Hand Bursa and Ligament, Left 9 Upper Extremity Bursa and Ligament, Right B Upper Extremity Bursa and Ligament, Left C Trunk Bursa and Ligament, Right D Trunk Bursa and Ligament, Left F Thorax Bursa and Ligament, Right G Thorax Bursa and Ligament, Left H Abdomen Bursa and Ligament, Right J Abdomen Bursa and Ligament, Left K Perineum Bursa and Ligament L Hip Bursa and Ligament, Right M Hip Bursa and Ligament, Left N Knee Bursa and Ligament, Right P Knee Bursa and Ligament, Left Q Ankle Bursa and Ligament, Right R Ankle Bursa and Ligament, Left S Foot Bursa and Ligament, Right T Foot Bursa and Ligament, Left V Lower Extremity Bursa and Ligament, Right W Lower Extremity Bursa and Ligament, Left	Ø Open 3 Percutaneous 4 Percutaneous Endoscopic	Z No Device	Z No Qualifier

Ø Medical and Surgical
M Bursae and Ligaments
9 Drainage Taking or letting out fluids and/or gases from a body part

Body Part Character 4	Approach Character 5	Device Character 6	Qualifier Character 7
Ø Head and Neck Bursa and Ligament 1 Shoulder Bursa and Ligament, Right 2 Shoulder Bursa and Ligament, Left 3 Elbow Bursa and Ligament, Right 4 Elbow Bursa and Ligament, Left 5 Wrist Bursa and Ligament, Right 6 Wrist Bursa and Ligament, Left 7 Hand Bursa and Ligament, Right 8 Hand Bursa and Ligament, Left 9 Upper Extremity Bursa and Ligament, Right B Upper Extremity Bursa and Ligament, Left C Trunk Bursa and Ligament, Right D Trunk Bursa and Ligament, Left F Thorax Bursa and Ligament, Right G Thorax Bursa and Ligament, Left H Abdomen Bursa and Ligament, Right J Abdomen Bursa and Ligament, Left K Perineum Bursa and Ligament L Hip Bursa and Ligament, Right M Hip Bursa and Ligament, Left N Knee Bursa and Ligament, Right P Knee Bursa and Ligament, Left Q Ankle Bursa and Ligament, Right R Ankle Bursa and Ligament, Left S Foot Bursa and Ligament, Right T Foot Bursa and Ligament, Left V Lower Extremity Bursa and Ligament, Right W Lower Extremity Bursa and Ligament, Left	Ø Open 3 Percutaneous 4 Percutaneous Endoscopic	Ø Drainage Device	Z No Qualifier

ØM9 Continued on next page

ØM9 Continued

Ø Medical and Surgical
M Bursae and Ligaments
9 Drainage Taking or letting out fluids and/or gases from a body part

Body Part Character 4	Approach Character 5	Device Character 6	Qualifier Character 7
Ø Head and Neck Bursa and Ligament **1** Shoulder Bursa and Ligament, Right **2** Shoulder Bursa and Ligament, Left **3** Elbow Bursa and Ligament, Right **4** Elbow Bursa and Ligament, Left **5** Wrist Bursa and Ligament, Right **6** Wrist Bursa and Ligament, Left **7** Hand Bursa and Ligament, Right **8** Hand Bursa and Ligament, Left **9** Upper Extremity Bursa and Ligament, Right **B** Upper Extremity Bursa and Ligament, Left **C** Trunk Bursa and Ligament, Right **D** Trunk Bursa and Ligament, Left **F** Thorax Bursa and Ligament, Right **G** Thorax Bursa and Ligament, Left **H** Abdomen Bursa and Ligament, Right **J** Abdomen Bursa and Ligament, Left **K** Perineum Bursa and Ligament **L** Hip Bursa and Ligament, Right **M** Hip Bursa and Ligament, Left **N** Knee Bursa and Ligament, Right **P** Knee Bursa and Ligament, Left **Q** Ankle Bursa and Ligament, Right **R** Ankle Bursa and Ligament, Left **S** Foot Bursa and Ligament, Right **T** Foot Bursa and Ligament, Left **V** Lower Extremity Bursa and Ligament, Right **W** Lower Extremity Bursa and Ligament, Left	**Ø** Open **3** Percutaneous **4** Percutaneous Endoscopic	**Z** No Device	**X** Diagnostic **Z** No Qualifier

Ø Medical and Surgical
M Bursae and Ligaments
B Excision Cutting out or off, without replacement, a portion of a body part

Body Part Character 4	Approach Character 5	Device Character 6	Qualifier Character 7
Ø Head and Neck Bursa and Ligament **1** Shoulder Bursa and Ligament, Right **2** Shoulder Bursa and Ligament, Left **3** Elbow Bursa and Ligament, Right **4** Elbow Bursa and Ligament, Left **5** Wrist Bursa and Ligament, Right **6** Wrist Bursa and Ligament, Left **7** Hand Bursa and Ligament, Right **8** Hand Bursa and Ligament, Left **9** Upper Extremity Bursa and Ligament, Right **B** Upper Extremity Bursa and Ligament, Left **C** Trunk Bursa and Ligament, Right **D** Trunk Bursa and Ligament, Left **F** Thorax Bursa and Ligament, Right **G** Thorax Bursa and Ligament, Left **H** Abdomen Bursa and Ligament, Right **J** Abdomen Bursa and Ligament, Left **K** Perineum Bursa and Ligament **L** Hip Bursa and Ligament, Right **M** Hip Bursa and Ligament, Left **N** Knee Bursa and Ligament, Right **P** Knee Bursa and Ligament, Left **Q** Ankle Bursa and Ligament, Right **R** Ankle Bursa and Ligament, Left **S** Foot Bursa and Ligament, Right **T** Foot Bursa and Ligament, Left **V** Lower Extremity Bursa and Ligament, Right **W** Lower Extremity Bursa and Ligament, Left	**Ø** Open **3** Percutaneous **4** Percutaneous Endoscopic	**Z** No Device	**X** Diagnostic **Z** No Qualifier

0 Medical and Surgical
M Bursae and Ligaments
C Extirpation Taking or cutting out solid matter from a body part

Body Part Character 4	Approach Character 5	Device Character 6	Qualifier Character 7
0 Head and Neck Bursa and Ligament 1 Shoulder Bursa and Ligament, Right 2 Shoulder Bursa and Ligament, Left 3 Elbow Bursa and Ligament, Right 4 Elbow Bursa and Ligament, Left 5 Wrist Bursa and Ligament, Right 6 Wrist Bursa and Ligament, Left 7 Hand Bursa and Ligament, Right 8 Hand Bursa and Ligament, Left 9 Upper Extremity Bursa and Ligament, Right B Upper Extremity Bursa and Ligament, Left C Trunk Bursa and Ligament, Right D Trunk Bursa and Ligament, Left F Thorax Bursa and Ligament, Right G Thorax Bursa and Ligament, Left H Abdomen Bursa and Ligament, Right J Abdomen Bursa and Ligament, Left K Perineum Bursa and Ligament L Hip Bursa and Ligament, Right M Hip Bursa and Ligament, Left N Knee Bursa and Ligament, Right P Knee Bursa and Ligament, Left Q Ankle Bursa and Ligament, Right R Ankle Bursa and Ligament, Left S Foot Bursa and Ligament, Right T Foot Bursa and Ligament, Left V Lower Extremity Bursa and Ligament, Right W Lower Extremity Bursa and Ligament, Left	0 Open 3 Percutaneous 4 Percutaneous Endoscopic	Z No Device	Z No Qualifier

0 Medical and Surgical
M Bursae and Ligaments
D Extraction Pulling or stripping out or off all or a portion of a body part by the use of force

Body Part Character 4	Approach Character 5	Device Character 6	Qualifier Character 7
0 Head and Neck Bursa and Ligament 1 Shoulder Bursa and Ligament, Right 2 Shoulder Bursa and Ligament, Left 3 Elbow Bursa and Ligament, Right 4 Elbow Bursa and Ligament, Left 5 Wrist Bursa and Ligament, Right 6 Wrist Bursa and Ligament, Left 7 Hand Bursa and Ligament, Right 8 Hand Bursa and Ligament, Left 9 Upper Extremity Bursa and Ligament, Right B Upper Extremity Bursa and Ligament, Left C Trunk Bursa and Ligament, Right D Trunk Bursa and Ligament, Left F Thorax Bursa and Ligament, Right G Thorax Bursa and Ligament, Left H Abdomen Bursa and Ligament, Right J Abdomen Bursa and Ligament, Left K Perineum Bursa and Ligament L Hip Bursa and Ligament, Right M Hip Bursa and Ligament, Left N Knee Bursa and Ligament, Right P Knee Bursa and Ligament, Left Q Ankle Bursa and Ligament, Right R Ankle Bursa and Ligament, Left S Foot Bursa and Ligament, Right T Foot Bursa and Ligament, Left V Lower Extremity Bursa and Ligament, Right W Lower Extremity Bursa and Ligament, Left	0 Open 3 Percutaneous 4 Percutaneous Endoscopic	Z No Device	Z No Qualifier

Ø Medical and Surgical
M Bursae and Ligaments
J Inspection Visually and/or manually exploring a body part

Body Part Character 4	Approach Character 5	Device Character 6	Qualifier Character 7
X Upper Bursa and Ligament **Y** Lower Bursa and Ligament	**Ø** Open **3** Percutaneous **4** Percutaneous Endoscopic **X** External	**Z** No Device	**Z** No Qualifier

Ø Medical and Surgical
M Bursae and Ligaments
M Reattachment Putting back in or on all or a portion of a separated body part to its normal location or other suitable location

Body Part Character 4	Approach Character 5	Device Character 6	Qualifier Character 7
Ø Head and Neck Bursa and Ligament **1** Shoulder Bursa and Ligament, Rightv **2** Shoulder Bursa and Ligament, Left **3** Elbow Bursa and Ligament, Right **4** Elbow Bursa and Ligament, Left **5** Wrist Bursa and Ligament, Right **6** Wrist Bursa and Ligament, Left **7** Hand Bursa and Ligament, Right **8** Hand Bursa and Ligament, Left **9** Upper Extremity Bursa and Ligament, Right **B** Upper Extremity Bursa and Ligament, Left **C** Trunk Bursa and Ligament, Right **D** Trunk Bursa and Ligament, Left **F** Thorax Bursa and Ligament, Right **G** Thorax Bursa and Ligament, Left **H** Abdomen Bursa and Ligament, Right **J** Abdomen Bursa and Ligament, Left **K** Perineum Bursa and Ligament **L** Hip Bursa and Ligament, Right **M** Hip Bursa and Ligament, Left **N** Knee Bursa and Ligament, Right **P** Knee Bursa and Ligament, Left **Q** Ankle Bursa and Ligament, Right **R** Ankle Bursa and Ligament, Left **S** Foot Bursa and Ligament, Right **T** Foot Bursa and Ligament, Left **V** Lower Extremity Bursa and Ligament, Right **W** Lower Extremity Bursa and Ligament, Left	**Ø** Open **4** Percutaneous Endoscopic	**Z** No Device	**Z** No Qualifier

0 Medical and Surgical
M Bursae and Ligaments
N Release Freeing a body part from an abnormal physical constraint

Body Part Character 4	Approach Character 5	Device Character 6	Qualifier Character 7
0 Head and Neck Bursa and Ligament **1** Shoulder Bursa and Ligament, Right **2** Shoulder Bursa and Ligament, Left **3** Elbow Bursa and Ligament, Right **4** Elbow Bursa and Ligament, Left **5** Wrist Bursa and Ligament, Right **6** Wrist Bursa and Ligament, Left **7** Hand Bursa and Ligament, Right **8** Hand Bursa and Ligament, Left **9** Upper Extremity Bursa and Ligament, Right **B** Upper Extremity Bursa and Ligament, Left **C** Trunk Bursa and Ligament, Right **D** Trunk Bursa and Ligament, Left **F** Thorax Bursa and Ligament, Right **G** Thorax Bursa and Ligament, Left **H** Abdomen Bursa and Ligament, Right **J** Abdomen Bursa and Ligament, Left **K** Perineum Bursa and Ligament **L** Hip Bursa and Ligament, Right **M** Hip Bursa and Ligament, Left **N** Knee Bursa and Ligament, Right **P** Knee Bursa and Ligament, Left **Q** Ankle Bursa and Ligament, Right **R** Ankle Bursa and Ligament, Left **S** Foot Bursa and Ligament, Right **T** Foot Bursa and Ligament, Left **V** Lower Extremity Bursa and Ligament, Right **W** Lower Extremity Bursa and Ligament, Left	**0** Open **3** Percutaneous **4** Percutaneous Endoscopic **X** External	**Z** No Device	**Z** No Qualifier

0 Medical and Surgical
M Bursae and Ligaments
P Removal Taking out or off a device from a body part

Body Part Character 4	Approach Character 5	Device Character 6	Qualifier Character 7
X Upper Bursa and Ligament **Y** Lower Bursa and Ligament	**0** Open **3** Percutaneous **4** Percutaneous Endoscopic	**0** Drainage Device **7** Autologous Tissue Substitute **J** Synthetic Substitute **K** Nonautologous Tissue Substitute	**Z** No Qualifier
X Upper Bursa and Ligament **Y** Lower Bursa and Ligament	**X** External	**0** Drainage Device	**Z** No Qualifier

Ø Medical and Surgical
M Bursae and Ligaments
Q Repair Restoring, to the extent possible, a body part to its normal anatomic structure and function

Body Part Character 4	Approach Character 5	Device Character 6	Qualifier Character 7
Ø Head and Neck Bursa and Ligament 1 Shoulder Bursa and Ligament, Right 2 Shoulder Bursa and Ligament, Left 3 Elbow Bursa and Ligament, Right 4 Elbow Bursa and Ligament, Left 5 Wrist Bursa and Ligament, Right 6 Wrist Bursa and Ligament, Left 7 Hand Bursa and Ligament, Right 8 Hand Bursa and Ligament, Left 9 Upper Extremity Bursa and Ligament, Right B Upper Extremity Bursa and Ligament, Left C Trunk Bursa and Ligament, Right D Trunk Bursa and Ligament, Left F Thorax Bursa and Ligament, Right G Thorax Bursa and Ligament, Left H Abdomen Bursa and Ligament, Right J Abdomen Bursa and Ligament, Left K Perineum Bursa and Ligament L Hip Bursa and Ligament, Right M Hip Bursa and Ligament, Left N Knee Bursa and Ligament, Right P Knee Bursa and Ligament, Left Q Ankle Bursa and Ligament, Right R Ankle Bursa and Ligament, Left S Foot Bursa and Ligament, Right T Foot Bursa and Ligament, Left V Lower Extremity Bursa and Ligament, Right W Lower Extremity Bursa and Ligament, Left	Ø Open 3 Percutaneous 4 Percutaneous Endoscopic	Z No Device	Z No Qualifier

Ø Medical and Surgical
M Bursae and Ligaments
S Reposition Moving to its normal location or other suitable location all or a portion of a body part

Body Part Character 4	Approach Character 5	Device Character 6	Qualifier Character 7
Ø Head and Neck Bursa and Ligament 1 Shoulder Bursa and Ligament, Right 2 Shoulder Bursa and Ligament, Left 3 Elbow Bursa and Ligament, Right 4 Elbow Bursa and Ligament, Left 5 Wrist Bursa and Ligament, Right 6 Wrist Bursa and Ligament, Left 7 Hand Bursa and Ligament, Right 8 Hand Bursa and Ligament, Left 9 Upper Extremity Bursa and Ligament, Right B Upper Extremity Bursa and Ligament, Left C Trunk Bursa and Ligament, Right D Trunk Bursa and Ligament, Left F Thorax Bursa and Ligament, Right G Thorax Bursa and Ligament, Left H Abdomen Bursa and Ligament, Right J Abdomen Bursa and Ligament, Left K Perineum Bursa and Ligament L Hip Bursa and Ligament, Right M Hip Bursa and Ligament, Left N Knee Bursa and Ligament, Right P Knee Bursa and Ligament, Left Q Ankle Bursa and Ligament, Right R Ankle Bursa and Ligament, Left S Foot Bursa and Ligament, Right T Foot Bursa and Ligament, Left V Lower Extremity Bursa and Ligament, Right W Lower Extremity Bursa and Ligament, Left	Ø Open 4 Percutaneous Endoscopic	Z No Device	Z No Qualifier

Ø Medical and Surgical
M Bursae and Ligaments
T Resection Cutting out or off, without replacement, all of a body part

Body Part Character 4	Approach Character 5	Device Character 6	Qualifier Character 7
Ø Head and Neck Bursa and Ligament 1 Shoulder Bursa and Ligament, Right 2 Shoulder Bursa and Ligament, Left 3 Elbow Bursa and Ligament, Right 4 Elbow Bursa and Ligament, Left 5 Wrist Bursa and Ligament, Right 6 Wrist Bursa and Ligament, Left 7 Hand Bursa and Ligament, Right 8 Hand Bursa and Ligament, Left 9 Upper Extremity Bursa and Ligament, Right B Upper Extremity Bursa and Ligament, Left C Trunk Bursa and Ligament, Right D Trunk Bursa and Ligament, Left F Thorax Bursa and Ligament, Right G Thorax Bursa and Ligament, Left H Abdomen Bursa and Ligament, Right J Abdomen Bursa and Ligament, Left K Perineum Bursa and Ligament L Hip Bursa and Ligament, Right M Hip Bursa and Ligament, Left N Knee Bursa and Ligament, Right P Knee Bursa and Ligament, Left Q Ankle Bursa and Ligament, Right R Ankle Bursa and Ligament, Left S Foot Bursa and Ligament, Right T Foot Bursa and Ligament, Left V Lower Extremity Bursa and Ligament, Right W Lower Extremity Bursa and Ligament, Left	Ø Open 4 Percutaneous Endoscopic	Z No Device	Z No Qualifier

Ø Medical and Surgical
M Bursae and Ligaments
U Supplement Putting in or on biological or synthetic material that physically reinforces and/or augments the function of a portion of a body part

Body Part Character 4	Approach Character 5	Device Character 6	Qualifier Character 7
Ø Head and Neck Bursa and Ligament 1 Shoulder Bursa and Ligament, Right 2 Shoulder Bursa and Ligament, Left 3 Elbow Bursa and Ligament, Right 4 Elbow Bursa and Ligament, Left 5 Wrist Bursa and Ligament, Right 6 Wrist Bursa and Ligament, Left 7 Hand Bursa and Ligament, Right 8 Hand Bursa and Ligament, Left 9 Upper Extremity Bursa and Ligament, Right B Upper Extremity Bursa and Ligament, Left C Trunk Bursa and Ligament, Right D Trunk Bursa and Ligament, Left F Thorax Bursa and Ligament, Right G Thorax Bursa and Ligament, Left H Abdomen Bursa and Ligament, Right J Abdomen Bursa and Ligament, Left K Perineum Bursa and Ligament L Hip Bursa and Ligament, Right M Hip Bursa and Ligament, Left N Knee Bursa and Ligament, Right P Knee Bursa and Ligament, Left Q Ankle Bursa and Ligament, Right R Ankle Bursa and Ligament, Left S Foot Bursa and Ligament, Right T Foot Bursa and Ligament, Left V Lower Extremity Bursa and Ligament, Right W Lower Extremity Bursa and Ligament, Left	Ø Open 4 Percutaneous Endoscopic	7 Autologous Tissue Substitute J Synthetic Substitute K Nonautologous Tissue Substitute	Z No Qualifier

Ø Medical and Surgical
M Bursae and Ligaments
W Revision Correcting, to the extent possible, a portion of a malfunctioning device or the position of a displaced device

Body Part Character 4	Approach Character 5	Device Character 6	Qualifier Character 7
X Upper Bursa and Ligament **Y** Lower Bursa and Ligament	**Ø** Open **3** Percutaneous **4** Percutaneous Endoscopic **X** External	**Ø** Drainage Device **7** Autologous Tissue Substitute **J** Synthetic Substitute **K** Nonautologous Tissue Substitute	**Z** No Qualifier

Ø Medical and Surgical
M Bursae and Ligaments
X Transfer Moving, without taking out, all or a portion of a body part to another location to take over the function of all or a portion of a body part

Body Part Character 4	Approach Character 5	Device Character 6	Qualifier Character 7
Ø Head and Neck Bursa and Ligament **1** Shoulder Bursa and Ligament, Right **2** Shoulder Bursa and Ligament, Left **3** Elbow Bursa and Ligament, Right **4** Elbow Bursa and Ligament, Left **5** Wrist Bursa and Ligament, Right **6** Wrist Bursa and Ligament, Left **7** Hand Bursa and Ligament, Right **8** Hand Bursa and Ligament, Left **9** Upper Extremity Bursa and Ligament, Right **B** Upper Extremity Bursa and Ligament, Left **C** Trunk Bursa and Ligament, Right **D** Trunk Bursa and Ligament, Left **F** Thorax Bursa and Ligament, Right **G** Thorax Bursa and Ligament, Left **H** Abdomen Bursa and Ligament, Right **J** Abdomen Bursa and Ligament, Left **K** Perineum Bursa and Ligament **L** Hip Bursa and Ligament, Right **M** Hip Bursa and Ligament, Left **N** Knee Bursa and Ligament, Right **P** Knee Bursa and Ligament, Left **Q** Ankle Bursa and Ligament, Right **R** Ankle Bursa and Ligament, Left **S** Foot Bursa and Ligament, Right **T** Foot Bursa and Ligament, Left **V** Lower Extremity Bursa and Ligament, Right **W** Lower Extremity Bursa and Ligament, Left	**Ø** Open **4** Percutaneous Endoscopic	**Z** No Device	**Z** No Qualifier

Head and Facial Bones ØN2–ØNW

Ø Medical and Surgical
N Head and Facial Bones
2 Change Taking out or off a device from a body part and putting back an identical or similar device in or on the same body part without cutting or puncturing the skin or a mucous membrane

Body Part Character 4	Approach Character 5	Device Character 6	Qualifier Character 7
Ø Skull **B** Nasal Bone **W** Facial Bone	**X** External	**Ø** Drainage Device **Y** Other Device	**Z** No Qualifier

Ø Medical and Surgical
N Head and Facial Bones
5 Destruction Physical eradication of all or a portion of a body part by the direct use of energy, force, or a destructive agent

Body Part Character 4	Approach Character 5	Device Character 6	Qualifier Character 7
Ø Skull **1** Frontal Bone, Right **2** Frontal Bone, Left **3** Parietal Bone, Right **4** Parietal Bone, Left **5** Temporal Bone, Right **6** Temporal Bone, Left **7** Occipital Bone, Right **8** Occipital Bone, Left **B** Nasal Bone **C** Sphenoid Bone, Right **D** Sphenoid Bone, Left **F** Ethmoid Bone, Right **G** Ethmoid Bone, Left **H** Lacrimal Bone, Right **J** Lacrimal Bone, Left **K** Palatine Bone, Right **L** Palatine Bone, Left **M** Zygomatic Bone, Right **N** Zygomatic Bone, Left **P** Orbit, Right **Q** Orbit, Left **R** Maxilla, Right **S** Maxilla, Left **T** Mandible, Right **V** Mandible, Left **X** Hyoid Bone	**Ø** Open **3** Percutaneous **4** Percutaneous Endoscopic	**Z** No Device	**Z** No Qualifier

Ø Medical and Surgical
N Head and Facial Bones
8 Division Cutting into a body part without draining fluids and/or gases from the body part in order to separate or transect a body part

Body Part Character 4	Approach Character 5	Device Character 6	Qualifier Character 7
Ø Skull **1** Frontal Bone, Right **2** Frontal Bone, Left **3** Parietal Bone, Right **4** Parietal Bone, Left **5** Temporal Bone, Right **6** Temporal Bone, Left **7** Occipital Bone, Right **8** Occipital Bone, Left **B** Nasal Bone **C** Sphenoid Bone, Right **D** Sphenoid Bone, Left **F** Ethmoid Bone, Right **G** Ethmoid Bone, Left **H** Lacrimal Bone, Right **J** Lacrimal Bone, Left **K** Palatine Bone, Right **L** Palatine Bone, Left **M** Zygomatic Bone, Right **N** Zygomatic Bone, Left **P** Orbit, Right **Q** Orbit, Left **R** Maxilla, Right **S** Maxilla, Left **T** Mandible, Right **V** Mandible, Left **X** Hyoid Bone	**Ø** Open **3** Percutaneous **4** Percutaneous Endoscopic	**Z** No Device	**Z** No Qualifier

Ø Medical and Surgical
N Head and Facial Bones
9 Drainage Taking or letting out fluids and/or gases from a body part

Body Part Character 4	Approach Character 5	Device Character 6	Qualifier Character 7
Ø Skull **1** Frontal Bone, Right **2** Frontal Bone, Left **3** Parietal Bone, Right **4** Parietal Bone, Left **5** Temporal Bone, Right **6** Temporal Bone, Left **7** Occipital Bone, Right **8** Occipital Bone, Left **B** Nasal Bone **C** Sphenoid Bone, Right **D** Sphenoid Bone, Left **F** Ethmoid Bone, Right **G** Ethmoid Bone, Left **H** Lacrimal Bone, Right **J** Lacrimal Bone, Left **K** Palatine Bone, Right **L** Palatine Bone, Left **M** Zygomatic Bone, Right **N** Zygomatic Bone, Left **P** Orbit, Right **Q** Orbit, Left **R** Maxilla, Right **S** Maxilla, Left **T** Mandible, Right **V** Mandible, Left **X** Hyoid Bone	**Ø** Open **3** Percutaneous **4** Percutaneous Endoscopic	**Ø** Drainage Device	**Z** No Qualifier

ØN9 Continued on next page

ØN9 Continued

Ø Medical and Surgical
N Head and Facial Bones
9 Drainage Taking or letting out fluids and/or gases from a body part

Body Part Character 4	Approach Character 5	Device Character 6	Qualifier Character 7
Ø Skull **1** Frontal Bone, Right **2** Frontal Bone, Left **3** Parietal Bone, Right **4** Parietal Bone, Left **5** Temporal Bone, Right **6** Temporal Bone, Left **7** Occipital Bone, Right **8** Occipital Bone, Left **B** Nasal Bone **C** Sphenoid Bone, Right **D** Sphenoid Bone, Left **F** Ethmoid Bone, Right **G** Ethmoid Bone, Left **H** Lacrimal Bone, Right **J** Lacrimal Bone, Left **K** Palatine Bone, Right **L** Palatine Bone, Left **M** Zygomatic Bone, Right **N** Zygomatic Bone, Left **P** Orbit, Right **Q** Orbit, Left **R** Maxilla, Right **S** Maxilla, Left **T** Mandible, Right **V** Mandible, Left **X** Hyoid Bone	**Ø** Open **3** Percutaneous **4** Percutaneous Endoscopic	**Z** No Device	**X** Diagnostic **Z** No Qualifier

Ø Medical and Surgical
N Head and Facial Bones
B Excision Cutting out or off, without replacement, a portion of a body part

Body Part Character 4	Approach Character 5	Device Character 6	Qualifier Character 7
Ø Skull **1** Frontal Bone, Right **2** Frontal Bone, Left **3** Parietal Bone, Right **4** Parietal Bone, Left **5** Temporal Bone, Right **6** Temporal Bone, Left **7** Occipital Bone, Right **8** Occipital Bone, Left **B** Nasal Bone **C** Sphenoid Bone, Right **D** Sphenoid Bone, Left **F** Ethmoid Bone, Right **G** Ethmoid Bone, Left **H** Lacrimal Bone, Right **J** Lacrimal Bone, Left **K** Palatine Bone, Right **L** Palatine Bone, Left **M** Zygomatic Bone, Right **N** Zygomatic Bone, Left **P** Orbit, Right **Q** Orbit, Left **R** Maxilla, Right **S** Maxilla, Left **T** Mandible, Right **V** Mandible, Left **X** Hyoid Bone	**Ø** Open **3** Percutaneous **4** Percutaneous Endoscopic	**Z** No Device	**X** Diagnostic **Z** No Qualifier

Ø Medical and Surgical
N Head and Facial Bones
C Extirpation Taking or cutting out solid matter from a body part

Body Part Character 4	Approach Character 5	Device Character 6	Qualifier Character 7
1 Frontal Bone, Right **2** Frontal Bone, Left **3** Parietal Bone, Right **4** Parietal Bone, Left **5** Temporal Bone, Right **6** Temporal Bone, Left **7** Occipital Bone, Right **8** Occipital Bone, Left **B** Nasal Bone **C** Sphenoid Bone, Right **D** Sphenoid Bone, Left **F** Ethmoid Bone, Right **G** Ethmoid Bone, Left **H** Lacrimal Bone, Right **J** Lacrimal Bone, Left **K** Palatine Bone, Right **L** Palatine Bone, Left **M** Zygomatic Bone, Right **N** Zygomatic Bone, Left **P** Orbit, Right **Q** Orbit, Left **R** Maxilla, Right **S** Maxilla, Left **T** Mandible, Right **V** Mandible, Left **X** Hyoid Bone	**Ø** Open **3** Percutaneous **4** Percutaneous Endoscopic	**Z** No Device	**Z** No Qualifier

Ø Medical and Surgical
N Head and Facial Bones
H Insertion Putting in a nonbiological appliance that monitors, assists, performs, or prevents a physiological function but does not physically take the place of a body part

Body Part Character 4	Approach Character 5	Device Character 6	Qualifier Character 7
Ø Skull	**Ø** Open	**4** Internal Fixation Device **5** External Fixation Device **M** Bone Growth Stimulator **N** Neurostimulator Generator	**Z** No Qualifier
Ø Skull	**3** Percutaneous **4** Percutaneous Endoscopic	**4** Internal Fixation Device **5** External Fixation Device **M** Bone Growth Stimulator	**Z** No Qualifier
1 Frontal Bone, Right **2** Frontal Bone, Left **3** Parietal Bone, Right **4** Parietal Bone, Left **7** Occipital Bone, Right **8** Occipital Bone, Left **C** Sphenoid Bone, Right **D** Sphenoid Bone, Left **F** Ethmoid Bone, Right **G** Ethmoid Bone, Left **H** Lacrimal Bone, Right **J** Lacrimal Bone, Left **K** Palatine Bone, Right **L** Palatine Bone, Left **M** Zygomatic Bone, Right **N** Zygomatic Bone, Left **P** Orbit, Right **Q** Orbit, Left **X** Hyoid Bone	**Ø** Open **3** Percutaneous **4** Percutaneous Endoscopic	**4** Internal Fixation Device	**Z** No Qualifier
5 Temporal Bone, Right **6** Temporal Bone, Left	**Ø** Open **3** Percutaneous **4** Percutaneous Endoscopic	**4** Internal Fixation Device **S Hearing Device, Bone Conduction**	**Z** No Qualifier
B Nasal Bone	**Ø** Open **3** Percutaneous **4** Percutaneous Endoscopic	**4** Internal Fixation Device **M** Bone Growth Stimulator	**Z** No Qualifier
R Maxilla, Right **S** Maxilla, Left **T** Mandible, Right **V** Mandible, Left	**Ø** Open **3** Percutaneous **4** Percutaneous Endoscopic	**4** Internal Fixation Device **5** External Fixation Device	**Z** No Qualifier
W Facial Bone	**Ø** Open **3** Percutaneous **4** Percutaneous Endoscopic	**M** Bone Growth Stimulator	**Z** No Qualifier

Ø Medical and Surgical
N Head and Facial Bones
J Inspection Visually and/or manually exploring a body part

Body Part Character 4	Approach Character 5	Device Character 6	Qualifier Character 7
Ø Skull **B** Nasal Bone **W** Facial Bone	**Ø** Open **3** Percutaneous **4** Percutaneous Endoscopic **X** External	**Z** No Device	**Z** No Qualifier

Ø Medical and Surgical
N Head and Facial Bones
N Release Freeing a body part from an abnormal physical constraint

Body Part Character 4	Approach Character 5	Device Character 6	Qualifier Character 7
1 Frontal Bone, Right **2** Frontal Bone, Left **3** Parietal Bone, Right **4** Parietal Bone, Left **5** Temporal Bone, Right **6** Temporal Bone, Left **7** Occipital Bone, Right **8** Occipital Bone, Left **B** Nasal Bone **C** Sphenoid Bone, Right **D** Sphenoid Bone, Left **F** Ethmoid Bone, Right **G** Ethmoid Bone, Left **H** Lacrimal Bone, Right **J** Lacrimal Bone, Left **K** Palatine Bone, Right **L** Palatine Bone, Left **M** Zygomatic Bone, Right **N** Zygomatic Bone, Left **P** Orbit, Right **Q** Orbit, Left **R** Maxilla, Right **S** Maxilla, Left **T** Mandible, Right **V** Mandible, Left **X** Hyoid Bone	**Ø** Open **3** Percutaneous **4** Percutaneous Endoscopic	**Z** No Device	**Z** No Qualifier

Ø Medical and Surgical
N Head and Facial Bones
P Removal Taking out or off a device from a body part

Body Part Character 4	Approach Character 5	Device Character 6	Qualifier Character 7
Ø Skull	**Ø** Open	**Ø** Drainage Device **4** Internal Fixation Device **5** External Fixation Device **7** Autologous Tissue Substitute **J** Synthetic Substitute **K** Nonautologous Tissue Substitute **M** Bone Growth Stimulator **N** Neurostimulator Generator **S** **Hearing Device, Bone Conduction**	**Z** No Qualifier
Ø Skull	**3** Percutaneous **4** Percutaneous Endoscopic	**Ø** Drainage Device **4** Internal Fixation Device **5** External Fixation Device **7** Autologous Tissue Substitute **J** Synthetic Substitute **K** Nonautologous Tissue Substitute **M** Bone Growth Stimulator **S** **Hearing Device, Bone Conduction**	**Z** No Qualifier
Ø Skull	**X** External	**Ø** Drainage Device **4** Internal Fixation Device **5** External Fixation Device **M** Bone Growth Stimulator **S** **Hearing Device, Bone Conduction**	**Z** No Qualifier
B Nasal Bone **W** Facial Bone	**Ø** Open **3** Percutaneous **4** Percutaneous Endoscopic	**Ø** Drainage Device **4** Internal Fixation Device **7** Autologous Tissue Substitute **J** Synthetic Substitute **K** Nonautologous Tissue Substitute **M** Bone Growth Stimulator	**Z** No Qualifier

ØNP Continued on next page

ØNP Continued

Ø Medical and Surgical
N Head and Facial Bones
P Removal Taking out or off a device from a body part

Body Part Character 4	Approach Character 5	Device Character 6	Qualifier Character 7
B Nasal Bone W Facial Bone	X External	Ø Drainage Device 4 Internal Fixation Device M Bone Growth Stimulator	Z No Qualifier

Ø Medical and Surgical
N Head and Facial Bones
Q Repair Restoring, to the extent possible, a body part to its normal anatomic structure and function

Body Part Character 4	Approach Character 5	Device Character 6	Qualifier Character 7
Ø Skull 1 Frontal Bone, Right 2 Frontal Bone, Left 3 Parietal Bone, Right 4 Parietal Bone, Left 5 Temporal Bone, Right 6 Temporal Bone, Left 7 Occipital Bone, Right 8 Occipital Bone, Left B Nasal Bone C Sphenoid Bone, Right D Sphenoid Bone, Left F Ethmoid Bone, Right G Ethmoid Bone, Left H Lacrimal Bone, Right J Lacrimal Bone, Left K Palatine Bone, Right L Palatine Bone, Left M Zygomatic Bone, Right N Zygomatic Bone, Left P Orbit, Right Q Orbit, Left R Maxilla, Right S Maxilla, Left T Mandible, Right V Mandible, Left X Hyoid Bone	Ø Open 3 Percutaneous 4 Percutaneous Endoscopic X External	Z No Device	Z No Qualifier

Ø Medical and Surgical
N Head and Facial Bones
R Replacement Putting in or on biological or synthetic material that physically takes the place and/or function of all or a portion of a body part

Body Part Character 4	Approach Character 5	Device Character 6	Qualifier Character 7
Ø Skull 1 Frontal Bone, Right 2 Frontal Bone, Left 3 Parietal Bone, Right 4 Parietal Bone, Left 5 Temporal Bone, Right 6 Temporal Bone, Left 7 Occipital Bone, Right 8 Occipital Bone, Left B Nasal Bone C Sphenoid Bone, Right D Sphenoid Bone, Left F Ethmoid Bone, Right G Ethmoid Bone, Left H Lacrimal Bone, Right J Lacrimal Bone, Left K Palatine Bone, Right L Palatine Bone, Left M Zygomatic Bone, Right N Zygomatic Bone, Left P Orbit, Right Q Orbit, Left R Maxilla, Right S Maxilla, Left T Mandible, Right V Mandible, Left X Hyoid Bone	Ø Open 3 Percutaneous 4 Percutaneous Endoscopic	7 Autologous Tissue Substitute J Synthetic Substitute K Nonautologous Tissue Substitute	Z No Qualifier

0 Medical and Surgical
N Head and Facial Bones
S Reposition Moving to its normal location or other suitable location all or a portion of a body part

Body Part Character 4	Approach Character 5	Device Character 6	Qualifier Character 7
0 Skull 1 Frontal Bone, Right 2 Frontal Bone, Left 3 Parietal Bone, Right 4 Parietal Bone, Left 5 Temporal Bone, Right 6 Temporal Bone, Left 7 Occipital Bone, Right 8 Occipital Bone, Left B Nasal Bone C Sphenoid Bone, Right D Sphenoid Bone, Left F Ethmoid Bone, Right G Ethmoid Bone, Left H Lacrimal Bone, Right J Lacrimal Bone, Left K Palatine Bone, Right L Palatine Bone, Left M Zygomatic Bone, Right N Zygomatic Bone, Left P Orbit, Right Q Orbit, Left R Maxilla, Right S Maxilla, Left T Mandible, Right V Mandible, Left X Hyoid Bone	X External	Z No Device	Z No Qualifier
0 Skull R Maxilla, Right S Maxilla, Left T Mandible, Right V Mandible, Left	0 Open 3 Percutaneous 4 Percutaneous Endoscopic	4 Internal Fixation Device 5 External Fixation Device Z No Device	Z No Qualifier
1 Frontal Bone, Right 2 Frontal Bone, Left 3 Parietal Bone, Right 4 Parietal Bone, Left 5 Temporal Bone, Right 6 Temporal Bone, Left 7 Occipital Bone, Right 8 Occipital Bone, Left B Nasal Bone C Sphenoid Bone, Right D Sphenoid Bone, Left F Ethmoid Bone, Right G Ethmoid Bone, Left H Lacrimal Bone, Right J Lacrimal Bone, Left K Palatine Bone, Right L Palatine Bone, Left M Zygomatic Bone, Right N Zygomatic Bone, Left P Orbit, Right Q Orbit, Left X Hyoid Bone	0 Open 3 Percutaneous 4 Percutaneous Endoscopic	4 Internal Fixation Device Z No Device	Z No Qualifier

Ø Medical and Surgical
N Head and Facial Bones
T Resection Cutting out or off, without replacement, all of a body part

Body Part Character 4	Approach Character 5	Device Character 6	Qualifier Character 7
1 Frontal Bone, Right **2** Frontal Bone, Left **3** Parietal Bone, Right **4** Parietal Bone, Left **5** Temporal Bone, Right **6** Temporal Bone, Left **7** Occipital Bone, Right **8** Occipital Bone, Left **B** Nasal Bone **C** Sphenoid Bone, Right **D** Sphenoid Bone, Left **F** Ethmoid Bone, Right **G** Ethmoid Bone, Left **H** Lacrimal Bone, Right **J** Lacrimal Bone, Left **K** Palatine Bone, Right **L** Palatine Bone, Left **M** Zygomatic Bone, Right **N** Zygomatic Bone, Left **P** Orbit, Right **Q** Orbit, Left **R** Maxilla, Right **S** Maxilla, Left **T** Mandible, Right **V** Mandible, Left **X** Hyoid Bone	**Ø** Open	**Z** No Device	**Z** No Qualifier

Ø Medical and Surgical
N Head and Facial Bones
U Supplement Putting in or on biological or synthetic material that physically reinforces and/or augments the function of a portion of a body part

Body Part Character 4	Approach Character 5	Device Character 6	Qualifier Character 7
Ø Skull **1** Frontal Bone, Right **2** Frontal Bone, Left **3** Parietal Bone, Right **4** Parietal Bone, Left **5** Temporal Bone, Right **6** Temporal Bone, Left **7** Occipital Bone, Right **8** Occipital Bone, Left **B** Nasal Bone **C** Sphenoid Bone, Right **D** Sphenoid Bone, Left **F** Ethmoid Bone, Right **G** Ethmoid Bone, Left **H** Lacrimal Bone, Right **J** Lacrimal Bone, Left **K** Palatine Bone, Right **L** Palatine Bone, Left **M** Zygomatic Bone, Right **N** Zygomatic Bone, Left **P** Orbit, Right **Q** Orbit, Left **R** Maxilla, Right **S** Maxilla, Left **T** Mandible, Right **V** Mandible, Left **X** Hyoid Bone	**Ø** Open **3** Percutaneous **4** Percutaneous Endoscopic	**7** Autologous Tissue Substitute **J** Synthetic Substitute **K** Nonautologous Tissue Substitute	**Z** No Qualifier

Ø Medical and Surgical
N Head and Facial Bones
W Revision Correcting, to the extent possible, a portion of a malfunctioning device or the position of a displaced device

Body Part Character 4	Approach Character 5	Device Character 6	Qualifier Character 7
Ø Skull	**Ø** Open	**Ø** Drainage Device **4** Internal Fixation Device **5** External Fixation Device **7** Autologous Tissue Substitute **J** Synthetic Substitute **K** Nonautologous Tissue Substitute **M** Bone Growth Stimulator **N** Neurostimulator Generator **S** **Hearing Device, Bone Conduction**	**Z** No Qualifier
Ø Skull	**3** Percutaneous **4** Percutaneous Endoscopic **X** External	**Ø** Drainage Device **4** Internal Fixation Device **5** External Fixation Device **7** Autologous Tissue Substitute **J** Synthetic Substitute **K** Nonautologous Tissue Substitute **M** Bone Growth Stimulator **S** **Hearing Device, Bone Conduction**	**Z** No Qualifier
B Nasal Bone **W** Facial Bone	**Ø** Open **3** Percutaneous **4** Percutaneous Endoscopic **X** External	**Ø** Drainage Device **4** Internal Fixation Device **7** Autologous Tissue Substitute **J** Synthetic Substitute **K** Nonautologous Tissue Substitute **M** Bone Growth Stimulator	**Z** No Qualifier

Upper Bones ØP2–ØPW

Ø Medical and Surgical
P Upper Bones
2 Change Taking out or off a device from a body part and putting back an identical or similar device in or on the same body part without cutting or puncturing the skin or a mucous membrane

Body Part Character 4	Approach Character 5	Device Character 6	Qualifier Character 7
Y Upper Bone	**X** External	**Ø** Drainage Device **Y** Other Device	**Z** No Qualifier

Ø Medical and Surgical
P Upper Bones
5 Destruction Physical eradication of all or a portion of a body part by the direct use of energy, force, or a destructive agent

Body Part Character 4	Approach Character 5	Device Character 6	Qualifier Character 7
Ø Sternum **1** Rib, Right **2** Rib, Left **3** Cervical Vertebra **4** Thoracic Vertebra **5** Scapula, Right **6** Scapula, Left **7** Glenoid Cavity, Right **8** Glenoid Cavity, Left **9** Clavicle, Right **B** Clavicle, Left **C** Humeral Head, Right **D** Humeral Head, Left **F** Humeral Shaft, Right **G** Humeral Shaft, Left **H** Radius, Right **J** Radius, Left **K** Ulna, Right **L** Ulna, Left **M** Carpal, Right **N** Carpal, Left **P** Metacarpal, Right **Q** Metacarpal, Left **R** Thumb Phalanx, Right **S** Thumb Phalanx, Left **T** Finger Phalanx, Right **V** Finger Phalanx, Left	**Ø** Open **3** Percutaneous **4** Percutaneous Endoscopic	**Z** No Device	**Z** No Qualifier

Ø Medical and Surgical
P Upper Bones
8 Division Cutting into a body part without draining fluids and/or gases from the body part in order to separate or transect a body part

Body Part Character 4	Approach Character 5	Device Character 6	Qualifier Character 7
Ø Sternum **1** Rib, Right **2** Rib, Left **3** Cervical Vertebra **4** Thoracic Vertebra **5** Scapula, Right **6** Scapula, Left **7** Glenoid Cavity, Right **8** Glenoid Cavity, Left **9** Clavicle, Right **B** Clavicle, Left **C** Humeral Head, Right **D** Humeral Head, Left **F** Humeral Shaft, Right **G** Humeral Shaft, Left **H** Radius, Right **J** Radius, Left **K** Ulna, Right **L** Ulna, Left **M** Carpal, Right **N** Carpal, Left **P** Metacarpal, Right **Q** Metacarpal, Left **R** Thumb Phalanx, Right **S** Thumb Phalanx, Left **T** Finger Phalanx, Right **V** Finger Phalanx, Left	**Ø** Open **3** Percutaneous **4** Percutaneous Endoscopic	**Z** No Device	**Z** No Qualifier

0 Medical and Surgical
P Upper Bones
9 Drainage Taking or letting out fluids and/or gases from a body part

Body Part Character 4	Approach Character 5	Device Character 6	Qualifier Character 7
0 Sternum **1** Rib, Right **2** Rib, Left **3** Cervical Vertebra **4** Thoracic Vertebra **5** Scapula, Right **6** Scapula, Left **7** Glenoid Cavity, Right **8** Glenoid Cavity, Left **9** Clavicle, Right **B** Clavicle, Left **C** Humeral Head, Right **D** Humeral Head, Left **F** Humeral Shaft, Right **G** Humeral Shaft, Left **H** Radius, Right **J** Radius, Left **K** Ulna, Right **L** Ulna, Left **M** Carpal, Right **N** Carpal, Left **P** Metacarpal, Right **Q** Metacarpal, Left **R** Thumb Phalanx, Right **S** Thumb Phalanx, Left **T** Finger Phalanx, Right **V** Finger Phalanx, Left	**0** Open **3** Percutaneous **4** Percutaneous Endoscopic	**0** Drainage Device	**Z** No Qualifier
0 Sternum **1** Rib, Right **2** Rib, Left **3** Cervical Vertebra **4** Thoracic Vertebra **5** Scapula, Right **6** Scapula, Left **7** Glenoid Cavity, Right **8** Glenoid Cavity, Left **9** Clavicle, Right **B** Clavicle, Left **C** Humeral Head, Right **D** Humeral Head, Left **F** Humeral Shaft, Right **G** Humeral Shaft, Left **H** Radius, Right **J** Radius, Left **K** Ulna, Right **L** Ulna, Left **M** Carpal, Right **N** Carpal, Left **P** Metacarpal, Right **Q** Metacarpal, Left **R** Thumb Phalanx, Right **S** Thumb Phalanx, Left **T** Finger Phalanx, Right **V** Finger Phalanx, Left	**0** Open **3** Percutaneous **4** Percutaneous Endoscopic	**Z** No Device	**X** Diagnostic **Z** No Qualifier

Ø Medical and Surgical
P Upper Bones
B Excision Cutting out or off, without replacement, a portion of a body part

Body Part Character 4	Approach Character 5	Device Character 6	Qualifier Character 7
Ø Sternum **1** Rib, Right **2** Rib, Left **3** Cervical Vertebra **4** Thoracic Vertebra **5** Scapula, Right **6** Scapula, Left **7** Glenoid Cavity, Right **8** Glenoid Cavity, Left **9** Clavicle, Right **B** Clavicle, Left **C** Humeral Head, Right **D** Humeral Head, Left **F** Humeral Shaft, Right **G** Humeral Shaft, Left **H** Radius, Right **J** Radius, Left **K** Ulna, Right **L** Ulna, Left **M** Carpal, Right **N** Carpal, Left **P** Metacarpal, Right **Q** Metacarpal, Left **R** Thumb Phalanx, Right **S** Thumb Phalanx, Left **T** Finger Phalanx, Right **V** Finger Phalanx, Left	**Ø** Open **3** Percutaneous **4** Percutaneous Endoscopic	**Z** No Device	**X** Diagnostic **Z** No Qualifier

Ø Medical and Surgical
P Upper Bones
C Extirpation Taking or cutting out solid matter from a body part

Body Part Character 4	Approach Character 5	Device Character 6	Qualifier Character 7
Ø Sternum **1** Rib, Right **2** Rib, Left **3** Cervical Vertebra **4** Thoracic Vertebra **5** Scapula, Right **6** Scapula, Left **7** Glenoid Cavity, Right **8** Glenoid Cavity, Left **9** Clavicle, Right **B** Clavicle, Left **C** Humeral Head, Right **D** Humeral Head, Left **F** Humeral Shaft, Right **G** Humeral Shaft, Left **H** Radius, Right **J** Radius, Left **K** Ulna, Right **L** Ulna, Left **M** Carpal, Right **N** Carpal, Left **P** Metacarpal, Right **Q** Metacarpal, Left **R** Thumb Phalanx, Right **S** Thumb Phalanx, Left **T** Finger Phalanx, Right **V** Finger Phalanx, Left	**Ø** Open **3** Percutaneous **4** Percutaneous Endoscopic	**Z** No Device	**Z** No Qualifier

0 Medical and Surgical
P Upper Bones
H Insertion Putting in a nonbiological appliance that monitors, assists, performs, or prevents a physiological function but does not physically take the place of a body part

Body Part Character 4	Approach Character 5	Device Character 6	Qualifier Character 7
0 Sternum	0 Open 3 Percutaneous 4 Percutaneous Endoscopic	**0 Internal Fixation Device, Rigid Plate** 4 Internal Fixation Device	Z No Qualifier
1 Rib, Right 2 Rib, Left 3 Cervical Vertebra 4 Thoracic Vertebra 5 Scapula, Right 6 Scapula, Left 7 Glenoid Cavity, Right 8 Glenoid Cavity, Left 9 Clavicle, Right B Clavicle, Left	0 Open 3 Percutaneous 4 Percutaneous Endoscopic	4 Internal Fixation Device	Z No Qualifier
C Humeral Head, Right D Humeral Head, Left F Humeral Shaft, Right G Humeral Shaft, Left H Radius, Right J Radius, Left K Ulna, Right L Ulna, Left	0 Open 3 Percutaneous 4 Percutaneous Endoscopic	4 Internal Fixation Device **5 External Fixation Device** **6 Internal Fixation Device, Intramedullary** **8 External Fixation Device, Limb Lengthening** **B External Fixation Device, Monoplanar** **C External Fixation Device, Ring** **D External Fixation Device, Hybrid**	Z No Qualifier
M Carpal, Right N Carpal, Left P Metacarpal, Right Q Metacarpal, Left R Thumb Phalanx, Right S Thumb Phalanx, Left T Finger Phalanx, Right V Finger Phalanx, Left	0 Open 3 Percutaneous 4 Percutaneous Endoscopic	4 Internal Fixation Device 5 External Fixation Device	Z No Qualifier
Y Upper Bone	0 Open 3 Percutaneous 4 Percutaneous Endoscopic	M Bone Growth Stimulator	Z No Qualifier

0 Medical and Surgical
P Upper Bones
J Inspection Visually and/or manually exploring a body part

Body Part Character 4	Approach Character 5	Device Character 6	Qualifier Character 7
Y Upper Bone	0 Open 3 Percutaneous 4 Percutaneous Endoscopic X External	Z No Device	Z No Qualifier

Ø Medical and Surgical
P Upper Bones
N Release Freeing a body part from an abnormal physical constraint

Body Part Character 4	Approach Character 5	Device Character 6	Qualifier Character 7
Ø Sternum **1** Rib, Right **2** Rib, Left **3** Cervical Vertebra **4** Thoracic Vertebra **5** Scapula, Right **6** Scapula, Left **7** Glenoid Cavity, Right **8** Glenoid Cavity, Left **9** Clavicle, Right **B** Clavicle, Left **C** Humeral Head, Right **D** Humeral Head, Left **F** Humeral Shaft, Right **G** Humeral Shaft, Left **H** Radius, Right **J** Radius, Left **K** Ulna, Right **L** Ulna, Left **M** Carpal, Right **N** Carpal, Left **P** Metacarpal, Right **Q** Metacarpal, Left **R** Thumb Phalanx, Right **S** Thumb Phalanx, Left **T** Finger Phalanx, Right **V** Finger Phalanx, Left	**Ø** Open **3** Percutaneous **4** Percutaneous Endoscopic	**Z** No Device	**Z** No Qualifier

Ø Medical and Surgical
P Upper Bones
P Removal Taking out or off a device from a body part

Body Part Character 4	Approach Character 5	Device Character 6	Qualifier Character 7
Ø Sternum **1** Rib, Right **2** Rib, Left **3** Cervical Vertebra **4** Thoracic Vertebra **5** Scapula, Right **6** Scapula, Left **7** Glenoid Cavity, Right **8** Glenoid Cavity, Left **9** Clavicle, Right **B** Clavicle, Left	**Ø** Open **3** Percutaneous **4** Percutaneous Endoscopic	**4** Internal Fixation Device **7** Autologous Tissue Substitute **J** Synthetic Substitute **K** Nonautologous Tissue Substitute	**Z** No Qualifier
Ø Sternum **1** Rib, Right **2** Rib, Left **3** Cervical Vertebra **4** Thoracic Vertebra **5** Scapula, Right **6** Scapula, Left **7** Glenoid Cavity, Right **8** Glenoid Cavity, Left **9** Clavicle, Right **B** Clavicle, Left	**X** External	**4** Internal Fixation Device	**Z** No Qualifier
C Humeral Head, Right **D** Humeral Head, Left **F** Humeral Shaft, Right **G** Humeral Shaft, Left **H** Radius, Right **J** Radius, Left **K** Ulna, Right **L** Ulna, Left **M** Carpal, Right **N** Carpal, Left **P** Metacarpal, Right **Q** Metacarpal, Left **R** Thumb Phalanx, Right **S** Thumb Phalanx, Left **T** Finger Phalanx, Right **V** Finger Phalanx, Left	**Ø** Open **3** Percutaneous **4** Percutaneous Endoscopic	**4** Internal Fixation Device **5** External Fixation Device **7** Autologous Tissue Substitute **J** Synthetic Substitute **K** Nonautologous Tissue Substitute	**Z** No Qualifier

ØPP Continued on next page

0 Medical and Surgical
P Upper Bones
P Removal Taking out or off a device from a body part

0PP Continued

Body Part Character 4	Approach Character 5	Device Character 6	Qualifier Character 7
C Humeral Head, Right **D** Humeral Head, Left **F** Humeral Shaft, Right **G** Humeral Shaft, Left **H** Radius, Right **J** Radius, Left **K** Ulna, Right **L** Ulna, Left **M** Carpal, Right **N** Carpal, Left **P** Metacarpal, Right **Q** Metacarpal, Left **R** Thumb Phalanx, Right **S** Thumb Phalanx, Left **T** Finger Phalanx, Right **V** Finger Phalanx, Left	**X** External	**4** Internal Fixation Device **5** External Fixation Device	**Z** No Qualifier
Y Upper Bone	**0** Open **3** Percutaneous **4** Percutaneous Endoscopic **X** External	**0** Drainage Device **M** Bone Growth Stimulator	**Z** No Qualifier

0 Medical and Surgical
P Upper Bones
Q Repair Restoring, to the extent possible, a body part to its normal anatomic structure and function

Body Part Character 4	Approach Character 5	Device Character 6	Qualifier Character 7
0 Sternum **1** Rib, Right **2** Rib, Left **3** Cervical Vertebra **4** Thoracic Vertebra **5** Scapula, Right **6** Scapula, Left **7** Glenoid Cavity, Right **8** Glenoid Cavity, Left **9** Clavicle, Right **B** Clavicle, Left **C** Humeral Head, Right **D** Humeral Head, Left **F** Humeral Shaft, Right **G** Humeral Shaft, Left **H** Radius, Right **J** Radius, Left **K** Ulna, Right **L** Ulna, Left **M** Carpal, Right **N** Carpal, Left **P** Metacarpal, Right **Q** Metacarpal, Left **R** Thumb Phalanx, Right **S** Thumb Phalanx, Left **T** Finger Phalanx, Right **V** Finger Phalanx, Left	**0** Open **3** Percutaneous **4** Percutaneous Endoscopic **X** External	**Z** No Device	**Z** No Qualifier

Ø Medical and Surgical
P Upper Bones
R Replacement Putting in or on biological or synthetic material that physically takes the place and/or function of all or a portion of a body part

Body Part Character 4	Approach Character 5	Device Character 6	Qualifier Character 7
Ø Sternum 1 Rib, Right 2 Rib, Left 3 Cervical Vertebra 4 Thoracic Vertebra 5 Scapula, Right 6 Scapula, Left 7 Glenoid Cavity, Right 8 Glenoid Cavity, Left 9 Clavicle, Right B Clavicle, Left C Humeral Head, Right D Humeral Head, Left F Humeral Shaft, Right G Humeral Shaft, Left H Radius, Right J Radius, Left K Ulna, Right L Ulna, Left M Carpal, Right N Carpal, Left P Metacarpal, Right Q Metacarpal, Left R Thumb Phalanx, Right S Thumb Phalanx, Left T Finger Phalanx, Right V Finger Phalanx, Left	Ø Open 3 Percutaneous 4 Percutaneous Endoscopic	7 Autologous Tissue Substitute J Synthetic Substitute K Nonautologous Tissue Substitute	Z No Qualifier

Ø Medical and Surgical
P Upper Bones
S Reposition Moving to its normal location or other suitable location all or a portion of a body part

Body Part Character 4	Approach Character 5	Device Character 6	Qualifier Character 7
Ø Sternum	Ø Open 3 Percutaneous 4 Percutaneous Endoscopic	**Ø Internal Fixation Device, Rigid Plate** 4 Internal Fixation Device Z No Device	Z No Qualifier
1 Rib, Right 2 Rib, Left 3 Cervical Vertebra 4 Thoracic Vertebra 5 Scapula, Right 6 Scapula, Left 7 Glenoid Cavity, Right 8 Glenoid Cavity, Left 9 Clavicle, Right B Clavicle, Left	Ø Open 3 Percutaneous 4 Percutaneous Endoscopic	4 Internal Fixation Device Z No Device	Z No Qualifier
Ø Sternum 1 Rib, Right 2 Rib, Left 3 Cervical Vertebra 4 Thoracic Vertebra 5 Scapula, Right 6 Scapula, Left 7 Glenoid Cavity, Right 8 Glenoid Cavity, Left 9 Clavicle, Right B Clavicle, Left	X External	Z No Device	Z No Qualifier
C Humeral Head, Right D Humeral Head, Left F Humeral Shaft, Right G Humeral Shaft, Left H Radius, Right J Radius, Left K Ulna, Right L Ulna, Left	Ø Open 3 Percutaneous 4 Percutaneous Endoscopic	4 Internal Fixation Device 5 External Fixation Device **6 Internal Fixation Device, Intramedullary** **B External Fixation Device, Monoplanar** **C External Fixation Device, Ring** **D External Fixation Device, Hybrid** Z No Device	Z No Qualifier

ØPS Continued on next page

Ø Medical and Surgical
P Upper Bones
S Reposition Moving to its normal location or other suitable location all or a portion of a body part

ØPS Continued

Body Part Character 4	Approach Character 5	Device Character 6	Qualifier Character 7
C Humeral Head, Right **D** Humeral Head, Left **F** Humeral Shaft, Right **G** Humeral Shaft, Left **H** Radius, Right **J** Radius, Left **K** Ulna, Right **L** Ulna, Left	**X** External	**Z** No Device	**Z** No Qualifier
M Carpal, Right **N** Carpal, Left **P** Metacarpal, Right **Q** Metacarpal, Left **R** Thumb Phalanx, Right **S** Thumb Phalanx, Left **T** Finger Phalanx, Right **V** Finger Phalanx, Left	**Ø** Open **3** Percutaneous **4** Percutaneous Endoscopic	**4** Internal Fixation Device **5** External Fixation Device **Z** No Device	**Z** No Qualifier
M Carpal, Right **N** Carpal, Left **P** Metacarpal, Right **Q** Metacarpal, Left **R** Thumb Phalanx, Right **S** Thumb Phalanx, Left **T** Finger Phalanx, Right **V** Finger Phalanx, Left	**X** External	**Z** No Device	**Z** No Qualifier

Ø Medical and Surgical
P Upper Bones
T Resection Cutting out or off, without replacement, all of a body part

Body Part Character 4	Approach Character 5	Device Character 6	Qualifier Character 7
Ø Sternum **1** Rib, Right **2** Rib, Left **5** Scapula, Right **6** Scapula, Left **7** Glenoid Cavity, Right **8** Glenoid Cavity, Left **9** Clavicle, Right **B** Clavicle, Left **C** Humeral Head, Right **D** Humeral Head, Left **F** Humeral Shaft, Right **G** Humeral Shaft, Left **H** Radius, Right **J** Radius, Left **K** Ulna, Right **L** Ulna, Left **M** Carpal, Right **N** Carpal, Left **P** Metacarpal, Right **Q** Metacarpal, Left **R** Thumb Phalanx, Right **S** Thumb Phalanx, Left **T** Finger Phalanx, Right **V** Finger Phalanx, Left	**Ø** Open	**Z** No Device	**Z** No Qualifier

Ø Medical and Surgical
P Upper Bones
U Supplement Putting in or on biological or synthetic material that physically reinforces and/or augments the function of a portion of a body part

Body Part Character 4	Approach Character 5	Device Character 6	Qualifier Character 7
Ø Sternum **1** Rib, Right **2** Rib, Left **3** Cervical Vertebra **4** Thoracic Vertebra **5** Scapula, Right **6** Scapula, Left **7** Glenoid Cavity, Right **8** Glenoid Cavity, Left **9** Clavicle, Right **B** Clavicle, Left **C** Humeral Head, Right **D** Humeral Head, Left **F** Humeral Shaft, Right **G** Humeral Shaft, Left **H** Radius, Right **J** Radius, Left **K** Ulna, Right **L** Ulna, Left **M** Carpal, Right **N** Carpal, Left **P** Metacarpal, Right **Q** Metacarpal, Left **R** Thumb Phalanx, Right **S** Thumb Phalanx, Left **T** Finger Phalanx, Right **V** Finger Phalanx, Left	**Ø** Open **3** Percutaneous **4** Percutaneous Endoscopic	**7** Autologous Tissue Substitute **J** Synthetic Substitute **K** Nonautologous Tissue Substitute	**Z** No Qualifier

Ø Medical and Surgical
P Upper Bones
W Revision Correcting, to the extent possible, a portion of a malfunctioning device or the position of a displaced device

Body Part Character 4	Approach Character 5	Device Character 6	Qualifier Character 7
Ø Sternum **1** Rib, Right **2** Rib, Left **3** Cervical Vertebra **4** Thoracic Vertebra **5** Scapula, Right **6** Scapula, Left **7** Glenoid Cavity, Right **8** Glenoid Cavity, Left **9** Clavicle, Right **B** Clavicle, Left	**Ø** Open **3** Percutaneous **4** Percutaneous Endoscopic **X** External	**4** Internal Fixation Device **7** Autologous Tissue Substitute **J** Synthetic Substitute **K** Nonautologous Tissue Substitute	**Z** No Qualifier
C Humeral Head, Right **D** Humeral Head, Left **F** Humeral Shaft, Right **G** Humeral Shaft, Left **H** Radius, Right **J** Radius, Left **K** Ulna, Right **L** Ulna, Left **M** Carpal, Right **N** Carpal, Left **P** Metacarpal, Right **Q** Metacarpal, Left **R** Thumb Phalanx, Right **S** Thumb Phalanx, Left **T** Finger Phalanx, Right **V** Finger Phalanx, Left	**Ø** Open **3** Percutaneous **4** Percutaneous Endoscopic **X** External	**4** Internal Fixation Device **5** External Fixation Device **7** Autologous Tissue Substitute **J** Synthetic Substitute **K** Nonautologous Tissue Substitute	**Z** No Qualifier
Y Upper Bone	**Ø** Open **3** Percutaneous **4** Percutaneous Endoscopic **X** External	**Ø** Drainage Device **M** Bone Growth Stimulator	**Z** No Qualifier

Lower Bones 0Q2–0QW

0 Medical and Surgical
Q Lower Bones
2 Change Taking out or off a device from a body part and putting back an identical or similar device in or on the same body part without cutting or puncturing the skin or a mucous membrane

Body Part Character 4	Approach Character 5	Device Character 6	Qualifier Character 7
Y Lower Bone	**X** External	**0** Drainage Device **Y** Other Device	**Z** No Qualifier

0 Medical and Surgical
Q Lower Bones
5 Destruction Physical eradication of all or a portion of a body part by the direct use of energy, force, or a destructive agent

Body Part Character 4	Approach Character 5	Device Character 6	Qualifier Character 7
0 Lumbar Vertebra **1** Sacrum **2** Pelvic Bone, Right **3** Pelvic Bone, Left **4** Acetabulum, Right **5** Acetabulum, Left **6** Upper Femur, Right **7** Upper Femur, Left **8** Femoral Shaft, Right **9** Femoral Shaft, Left **B** Lower Femur, Right **C** Lower Femur, Left **D** Patella, Right **F** Patella, Left **G** Tibia, Right **H** Tibia, Left **J** Fibula, Right **K** Fibula, Left **L** Tarsal, Right **M** Tarsal, Left **N** Metatarsal, Right **P** Metatarsal, Left **Q** Toe Phalanx, Right **R** Toe Phalanx, Left **S** Coccyx	**0** Open **3** Percutaneous **4** Percutaneous Endoscopic	**Z** No Device	**Z** No Qualifier

0 Medical and Surgical
Q Lower Bones
8 Division Cutting into a body part without draining fluids and/or gases from the body part in order to separate or transect a body part

Body Part Character 4	Approach Character 5	Device Character 6	Qualifier Character 7
0 Lumbar Vertebra **1** Sacrum **2** Pelvic Bone, Right **3** Pelvic Bone, Left **4** Acetabulum, Right **5** Acetabulum, Left **6** Upper Femur, Right **7** Upper Femur, Left **8** Femoral Shaft, Right **9** Femoral Shaft, Left **B** Lower Femur, Right **C** Lower Femur, Left **D** Patella, Right **F** Patella, Left **G** Tibia, Right **H** Tibia, Left **J** Fibula, Right **K** Fibula, Left **L** Tarsal, Right **M** Tarsal, Left **N** Metatarsal, Right **P** Metatarsal, Left **Q** Toe Phalanx, Right **R** Toe Phalanx, Left **S** Coccyx	**0** Open **3** Percutaneous **4** Percutaneous Endoscopic	**Z** No Device	**Z** No Qualifier

Ø Medical and Surgical
Q Lower Bones
9 Drainage Taking or letting out fluids and/or gases from a body part

Body Part Character 4	Approach Character 5	Device Character 6	Qualifier Character 7
Ø Lumbar Vertebra **1** Sacrum **2** Pelvic Bone, Right **3** Pelvic Bone, Left **4** Acetabulum, Right **5** Acetabulum, Left **6** Upper Femur, Right **7** Upper Femur, Left **8** Femoral Shaft, Right **9** Femoral Shaft, Left **B** Lower Femur, Right **C** Lower Femur, Left **D** Patella, Right **F** Patella, Left **G** Tibia, Right **H** Tibia, Left **J** Fibula, Right **K** Fibula, Left **L** Tarsal, Right **M** Tarsal, Left **N** Metatarsal, Right **P** Metatarsal, Left **Q** Toe Phalanx, Right **R** Toe Phalanx, Left **S** Coccyx	**Ø** Open **3** Percutaneous **4** Percutaneous Endoscopic	**Ø** Drainage Device	**Z** No Qualifier
Ø Lumbar Vertebra **1** Sacrum **2** Pelvic Bone, Right **3** Pelvic Bone, Left **4** Acetabulum, Right **5** Acetabulum, Left **6** Upper Femur, Right **7** Upper Femur, Left **8** Femoral Shaft, Right **9** Femoral Shaft, Left **B** Lower Femur, Right **C** Lower Femur, Left **D** Patella, Right **F** Patella, Left **G** Tibia, Right **H** Tibia, Left **J** Fibula, Right **K** Fibula, Left **L** Tarsal, Right **M** Tarsal, Left **N** Metatarsal, Right **P** Metatarsal, Left **Q** Toe Phalanx, Right **R** Toe Phalanx, Left **S** Coccyx	**Ø** Open **3** Percutaneous **4** Percutaneous Endoscopic	**Z** No Device	**X** Diagnostic **Z** No Qualifier

0 Medical and Surgical
Q Lower Bones
B Excision Cutting out or off, without replacement, a portion of a body part

Body Part Character 4	Approach Character 5	Device Character 6	Qualifier Character 7
0 Lumbar Vertebra 1 Sacrum 2 Pelvic Bone, Right 3 Pelvic Bone, Left 4 Acetabulum, Right 5 Acetabulum, Left 6 Upper Femur, Right 7 Upper Femur, Left 8 Femoral Shaft, Right 9 Femoral Shaft, Left B Lower Femur, Right C Lower Femur, Left D Patella, Right F Patella, Left G Tibia, Right H Tibia, Left J Fibula, Right K Fibula, Left L Tarsal, Right M Tarsal, Left N Metatarsal, Right P Metatarsal, Left Q Toe Phalanx, Right R Toe Phalanx, Left S Coccyx	0 Open 3 Percutaneous 4 Percutaneous Endoscopic	Z No Device	X Diagnostic Z No Qualifier

0 Medical and Surgical
Q Lower Bones
C Extirpation Taking or cutting out solid matter from a body part

Body Part Character 4	Approach Character 5	Device Character 6	Qualifier Character 7
0 Lumbar Vertebra 1 Sacrum 2 Pelvic Bone, Right 3 Pelvic Bone, Left 4 Acetabulum, Right 5 Acetabulum, Left 6 Upper Femur, Right 7 Upper Femur, Left 8 Femoral Shaft, Right 9 Femoral Shaft, Left B Lower Femur, Right C Lower Femur, Left D Patella, Right F Patella, Left G Tibia, Right H Tibia, Left J Fibula, Right K Fibula, Left L Tarsal, Right M Tarsal, Left N Metatarsal, Right P Metatarsal, Left Q Toe Phalanx, Right R Toe Phalanx, Left S Coccyx	0 Open 3 Percutaneous 4 Percutaneous Endoscopic	Z No Device	Z No Qualifier

Ø Medical and Surgical
Q Lower Bones
H Insertion Putting in a nonbiological appliance that monitors, assists, performs, or prevents a physiological function but does not physically take the place of a body part

Body Part Character 4	Approach Character 5	Device Character 6	Qualifier Character 7
Ø Lumbar Vertebra **1** Sacrum **2** Pelvic Bone, Right **3** Pelvic Bone, Left **4** Acetabulum, Right **5** Acetabulum, Left **D** Patella, Right **F** Patella, Left **L** Tarsal, Right **M** Tarsal, Left **N** Metatarsal, Right **P** Metatarsal, Left **Q** Toe Phalanx, Right **R** Toe Phalanx, Left **S** Coccyx	**Ø** Open **3** Percutaneous **4** Percutaneous Endoscopic	**4** Internal Fixation Device **5** External Fixation Device	**Z** No Qualifier
6 Upper Femur, Right **7** Upper Femur, Left **8** Femoral Shaft, Right **9** Femoral Shaft, Left **B** Lower Femur, Right **C** Lower Femur, Left **G** Tibia, Right **H** Tibia, Left **J** Fibula, Right **K** Fibula, Left	**Ø** Open **3** Percutaneous **4** Percutaneous Endoscopic	**4** Internal Fixation Device **5** External Fixation Device **6** Internal Fixation Device, Intramedullary **8 External Fixation Device, Limb Lengthening** **B External Fixation Device, Monoplanar** **C External Fixation Device, Ring** **D External Fixation Device, Hybrid**	**Z** No Qualifier
Y Lower Bone	**Ø** Open **3** Percutaneous **4** Percutaneous Endoscopic	**M** Bone Growth Stimulator	**Z** No Qualifier

Ø Medical and Surgical
Q Lower Bones
J Inspection Visually and/or manually exploring a body part

Body Part Character 4	Approach Character 5	Device Character 6	Qualifier Character 7
Y Lower Bone	**Ø** Open **3** Percutaneous **4** Percutaneous Endoscopic **X** External	**Z** No Device	**Z** No Qualifier

Ø Medical and Surgical
Q Lower Bones
N Release Freeing a body part from an abnormal physical constraint

Body Part Character 4	Approach Character 5	Device Character 6	Qualifier Character 7
Ø Lumbar Vertebra **1** Sacrum **2** Pelvic Bone, Right **3** Pelvic Bone, Left **4** Acetabulum, Right **5** Acetabulum, Left **6** Upper Femur, Right **7** Upper Femur, Left **8** Femoral Shaft, Right **9** Femoral Shaft, Left **B** Lower Femur, Right **C** Lower Femur, Left **D** Patella, Right **F** Patella, Left **G** Tibia, Right **H** Tibia, Left **J** Fibula, Right **K** Fibula, Left **L** Tarsal, Right **M** Tarsal, Left **N** Metatarsal, Right **P** Metatarsal, Left **Q** Toe Phalanx, Right **R** Toe Phalanx, Left **S** Coccyx	**Ø** Open **3** Percutaneous **4** Percutaneous Endoscopic	**Z** No Device	**Z** No Qualifier

0 Medical and Surgical
Q Lower Bones
P Removal Taking out or off a device from a body part

Body Part Character 4	Approach Character 5	Device Character 6	Qualifier Character 7
0 Lumbar Vertebra **1** Sacrum **4** Acetabulum, Right **5** Acetabulum, Left **S** Coccyx	**0** Open **3** Percutaneous **4** Percutaneous Endoscopic	**4** Internal Fixation Device **7** Autologous Tissue Substitute **J** Synthetic Substitute **K** Nonautologous Tissue Substitute	**Z** No Qualifier
0 Lumbar Vertebra **1** Sacrum **4** Acetabulum, Right **5** Acetabulum, Left **S** Coccyx	**X** External	**4** Internal Fixation Device	**Z** No Qualifier
2 Pelvic Bone, Right **3** Pelvic Bone, Left **6** Upper Femur, Right **7** Upper Femur, Left **8** Femoral Shaft, Right **9** Femoral Shaft, Left **B** Lower Femur, Right **C** Lower Femur, Left **D** Patella, Right **F** Patella, Left **G** Tibia, Right **H** Tibia, Left **J** Fibula, Right **K** Fibula, Left **L** Tarsal, Right **M** Tarsal, Left **N** Metatarsal, Right **P** Metatarsal, Left **Q** Toe Phalanx, Right **R** Toe Phalanx, Left	**X** External	**4** Internal Fixation Device **5** External Fixation Device	**Z** No Qualifier

0QP Continued on next page

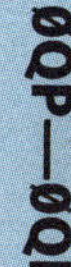

ØQP Continued

Ø Medical and Surgical
Q Lower Bones
P Removal Taking out or off a device from a body part

Body Part Character 4	Approach Character 5	Device Character 6	Qualifier Character 7
2 Pelvic Bone, Right **3** Pelvic Bone, Left **6** Upper Femur, Right **7** Upper Femur, Left **8** Femoral Shaft, Right **9** Femoral Shaft, Left **B** Lower Femur, Right **C** Lower Femur, Left **D** Patella, Right **F** Patella, Left **G** Tibia, Right **H** Tibia, Left **J** Fibula, Right **K** Fibula, Left **L** Tarsal, Right **M** Tarsal, Left **N** Metatarsal, Right **P** Metatarsal, Left **Q** Toe Phalanx, Right **R** Toe Phalanx, Left	**Ø** Open **3** Percutaneous **4** Percutaneous Endoscopic	**4** Internal Fixation Device **5** External Fixation Device **7** Autologous Tissue Substitute **J** Synthetic Substitute **K** Nonautologous Tissue Substitute	**Z** No Qualifier
Y Lower Bone	**Ø** Open **3** Percutaneous **4** Percutaneous Endoscopic **X** External	**Ø** Drainage Device **M** Bone Growth Stimulator	**Z** No Qualifier

Ø Medical and Surgical
Q Lower Bones
Q Repair Restoring, to the extent possible, a body part to its normal anatomic structure and function

Body Part Character 4	Approach Character 5	Device Character 6	Qualifier Character 7
Ø Lumbar Vertebra **1** Sacrum **2** Pelvic Bone, Right **3** Pelvic Bone, Left **4** Acetabulum, Right **5** Acetabulum, Left **6** Upper Femur, Right **7** Upper Femur, Left **8** Femoral Shaft, Right **9** Femoral Shaft, Left **B** Lower Femur, Right **C** Lower Femur, Left **D** Patella, Right **F** Patella, Left **G** Tibia, Right **H** Tibia, Left **J** Fibula, Right **K** Fibula, Left **L** Tarsal, Right **M** Tarsal, Left **N** Metatarsal, Right **P** Metatarsal, Left **Q** Toe Phalanx, Right **R** Toe Phalanx, Left **S** Coccyx	**Ø** Open **3** Percutaneous **4** Percutaneous Endoscopic **X** External	**Z** No Device	**Z** No Qualifier

0 Medical and Surgical
Q Lower Bones
R Replacement Putting in or on biological or synthetic material that physically takes the place and/or function of all or a portion of a body part

Body Part Character 4	Approach Character 5	Device Character 6	Qualifier Character 7
0 Lumbar Vertebra **1** Sacrum **2** Pelvic Bone, Right **3** Pelvic Bone, Left **4** Acetabulum, Right **5** Acetabulum, Left **6** Upper Femur, Right **7** Upper Femur, Left **8** Femoral Shaft, Right **9** Femoral Shaft, Left **B** Lower Femur, Right **C** Lower Femur, Left **D** Patella, Right **F** Patella, Left **G** Tibia, Right **H** Tibia, Left **J** Fibula, Right **K** Fibula, Left **L** Tarsal, Right **M** Tarsal, Left **N** Metatarsal, Right **P** Metatarsal, Left **Q** Toe Phalanx, Right **R** Toe Phalanx, Left **S** Coccyx	**0** Open **3** Percutaneous **4** Percutaneous Endoscopic	**7** Autologous Tissue Substitute **J** Synthetic Substitute **K** Nonautologous Tissue Substitute	**Z** No Qualifier

0 Medical and Surgical
Q Lower Bones
S Reposition Moving to its normal location or other suitable location all or a portion of a body part

Body Part Character 4	Approach Character 5	Device Character 6	Qualifier Character 7
0 Lumbar Vertebra **1** Sacrum **4** Acetabulum, Right **5** Acetabulum, Left **S** Coccyx	**0** Open **3** Percutaneous **4** Percutaneous Endoscopic	**4** Internal Fixation Device **Z** No Device	**Z** No Qualifier
0 Lumbar Vertebra **1** Sacrum **4** Acetabulum, Right **5** Acetabulum, Left **S** Coccyx	**X** External	**Z** No Device	**Z** No Qualifier
2 Pelvic Bone, Right **3** Pelvic Bone, Left **D** Patella, Right **F** Patella, Left **L** Tarsal, Right **M** Tarsal, Left **N** Metatarsal, Right **P** Metatarsal, Left **Q** Toe Phalanx, Right **R** Toe Phalanx, Left	**0** Open **3** Percutaneous **4** Percutaneous Endoscopic	**4** Internal Fixation Device **5** External Fixation Device **Z** No Device	**Z** No Qualifier
2 Pelvic Bone, Right **3** Pelvic Bone, Left **D** Patella, Right **F** Patella, Left **L** Tarsal, Right **M** Tarsal, Left **N** Metatarsal, Right **P** Metatarsal, Left **Q** Toe Phalanx, Right **R** Toe Phalanx, Left	**X** External	**Z** No Device	**Z** No Qualifier
6 Upper Femur, Right **7** Upper Femur, Left **8** Femoral Shaft, Right 9 Femoral Shaft, Left **B** Lower Femur, Right C Lower Femur, Left **G** Tibia, Right **H** Tibia, Left **J** Fibula, Right **K** Fibula, Left	**0** Open **3** Percutaneous **4** Percutaneous Endoscopic	**4** Internal Fixation Device **5** External Fixation Device **6** **Internal Fixation Device, Intramedullary** **B** **External Fixation Device, Monoplanar** **C** **External Fixation Device, Ring** **D** **External Fixation Device, Hybrid** **Z** No Device	**Z** No Qualifier

0QS Continued on next page

ØQS Continued

Ø Medical and Surgical
Q Lower Bones
S Reposition Moving to its normal location or other suitable location all or a portion of a body part

Body Part Character 4	Approach Character 5	Device Character 6	Qualifier Character 7
6 Upper Femur, Right 7 Upper Femur, Left 8 Femoral Shaft, Right 9 Femoral Shaft, Left B Lower Femur, Right C Lower Femur, Left G Tibia, Right H Tibia, Left J Fibula, Right K Fibula, Left	X External	Z No Device	Z No Qualifier

Ø Medical and Surgical
Q Lower Bones
T Resection Cutting out or off, without replacement, all of a body part

Body Part Character 4	Approach Character 5	Device Character 6	Qualifier Character 7
2 Pelvic Bone, Right 3 Pelvic Bone, Left 4 Acetabulum, Right 5 Acetabulum, Left 6 Upper Femur, Right 7 Upper Femur, Left 8 Femoral Shaft, Right 9 Femoral Shaft, Left B Lower Femur, Right C Lower Femur, Left D Patella, Right F Patella, Left G Tibia, Right H Tibia, Left J Fibula, Right K Fibula, Left L Tarsal, Right M Tarsal, Left N Metatarsal, Right P Metatarsal, Left Q Toe Phalanx, Right R Toe Phalanx, Left S Coccyx	Ø Open	Z No Device	Z No Qualifier

Ø Medical and Surgical
Q Lower Bones
U Supplement Putting in or on biological or synthetic material that physically reinforces and/or augments the function of a portion of a body part

Body Part Character 4	Approach Character 5	Device Character 6	Qualifier Character 7
Ø Lumbar Vertebra 1 Sacrum 2 Pelvic Bone, Right 3 Pelvic Bone, Left 4 Acetabulum, Right 5 Acetabulum, Left 6 Upper Femur, Right 7 Upper Femur, Left 8 Femoral Shaft, Right 9 Femoral Shaft, Left B Lower Femur, Right C Lower Femur, Left D Patella, Right F Patella, Left G Tibia, Right H Tibia, Left J Fibula, Right K Fibula, Left L Tarsal, Right M Tarsal, Left N Metatarsal, Right P Metatarsal, Left Q Toe Phalanx, Right R Toe Phalanx, Left S Coccyx	Ø Open 3 Percutaneous 4 Percutaneous Endoscopic	7 Autologous Tissue Substitute J Synthetic Substitute K Nonautologous Tissue Substitute	Z No Qualifier

Ø Medical and Surgical
Q Lower Bones
W Revision Correcting, to the extent possible, a portion of a malfunctioning device or the position of a displaced device

Body Part Character 4	Approach Character 5	Device Character 6	Qualifier Character 7
Ø Lumbar Vertebra **1** Sacrum **4** Acetabulum, Right **5** Acetabulum, Left **S** Coccyx	**Ø** Open **3** Percutaneous **4** Percutaneous Endoscopic **X** External	**4** Internal Fixation Device **7** Autologous Tissue Substitute **J** Synthetic Substitute **K** Nonautologous Tissue Substitute	**Z** No Qualifier
2 Pelvic Bone, Right **3** Pelvic Bone, Left **6** Upper Femur, Right **7** Upper Femur, Left **8** Femoral Shaft, Right **9** Femoral Shaft, Left **B** Lower Femur, Right **C** Lower Femur, Left **D** Patella, Right **F** Patella, Left **G** Tibia, Right **H** Tibia, Left **J** Fibula, Right **K** Fibula, Left **L** Tarsal, Right **M** Tarsal, Left **N** Metatarsal, Right **P** Metatarsal, Left **Q** Toe Phalanx, Right **R** Toe Phalanx, Left	**Ø** Open **3** Percutaneous **4** Percutaneous Endoscopic **X** External	**4** Internal Fixation Device **5** External Fixation Device **7** Autologous Tissue Substitute **J** Synthetic Substitute **K** Nonautologous Tissue Substitute	**Z** No Qualifier
Y Lower Bone	**Ø** Open **3** Percutaneous **4** Percutaneous Endoscopic **X** External	**Ø** Drainage Device **M** Bone Growth Stimulator	**Z** No Qualifier

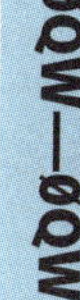

Upper Joints ØR2–ØRW

Ø Medical and Surgical
R Upper Joints
2 Change Taking out or off a device from a body part and putting back an identical or similar device in or on the same body part without cutting or puncturing the skin or a mucous membrane

Body Part Character 4	Approach Character 5	Device Character 6	Qualifier Character 7
Y Upper Joint	**X** External	**Ø** Drainage Device **Y** Other Device	**Z** No Qualifier

Ø Medical and Surgical
R Upper Joints
5 Destruction Physical eradication of all or a portion of a body part by the direct use of energy, force, or a destructive agent

Body Part Character 4	Approach Character 5	Device Character 6	Qualifier Character 7
Ø Occipital-cervical Joint **1** Cervical Vertebral Joint **3** Cervical Vertebral Disc **4** Cervicothoracic Vertebral Joint **5** Cervicothoracic Vertebral Disc **6** Thoracic Vertebral Joint **9** Thoracic Vertebral Disc **A** Thoracolumbar Vertebral Joint **B** Thoracolumbar Vertebral Disc **C** Temporomandibular Joint, Right **D** Temporomandibular Joint, Left **E** Sternoclavicular Joint, Right **F** Sternoclavicular Joint, Left **G** Acromioclavicular Joint, Right **H** Acromioclavicular Joint, Left **J** Shoulder Joint, Right **K** Shoulder Joint, Left **L** Elbow Joint, Right **M** Elbow Joint, Left **N** Wrist Joint, Right **P** Wrist Joint, Left **Q** Carpal Joint, Right **R** Carpal Joint, Left **S** Metacarpocarpal Joint, Right **T** Metacarpocarpal Joint, Left **U** Metacarpophalangeal Joint, Right **V** Metacarpophalangeal Joint, Left **W** Finger Phalangeal Joint, Right **X** Finger Phalangeal Joint, Left	**Ø** Open **3** Percutaneous **4** Percutaneous Endoscopic	**Z** No Device	**Z** No Qualifier

Ø Medical and Surgical
R Upper Joints
9 Drainage Taking or letting out fluids and/or gases from a body part

Body Part Character 4	Approach Character 5	Device Character 6	Qualifier Character 7
Ø Occipital-cervical Joint **1** Cervical Vertebral Joint **3** Cervical Vertebral Disc **4** Cervicothoracic Vertebral Joint **5** Cervicothoracic Vertebral Disc **6** Thoracic Vertebral Joint **9** Thoracic Vertebral Disc **A** Thoracolumbar Vertebral Joint **B** Thoracolumbar Vertebral Disc **C** Temporomandibular Joint, Right **D** Temporomandibular Joint, Left **E** Sternoclavicular Joint, Right **F** Sternoclavicular Joint, Left **G** Acromioclavicular Joint, Right **H** Acromioclavicular Joint, Left **J** Shoulder Joint, Right **K** Shoulder Joint, Left **L** Elbow Joint, Right **M** Elbow Joint, Left **N** Wrist Joint, Right **P** Wrist Joint, Left **Q** Carpal Joint, Right **R** Carpal Joint, Left **S** Metacarpocarpal Joint, Right **T** Metacarpocarpal Joint, Left **U** Metacarpophalangeal Joint, Right **V** Metacarpophalangeal Joint, Left **W** Finger Phalangeal Joint, Right **X** Finger Phalangeal Joint, Left	**Ø** Open **3** Percutaneous **4** Percutaneous Endoscopic	**Ø** Drainage Device	**Z** No Qualifier
Ø Occipital-cervical Joint **1** Cervical Vertebral Joint **3** Cervical Vertebral Disc **4** Cervicothoracic Vertebral Joint **5** Cervicothoracic Vertebral Disc **6** Thoracic Vertebral Joint **9** Thoracic Vertebral Disc **A** Thoracolumbar Vertebral Joint **B** Thoracolumbar Vertebral Disc **C** Temporomandibular Joint, Right **D** Temporomandibular Joint, Left **E** Sternoclavicular Joint, Right **F** Sternoclavicular Joint, Left **G** Acromioclavicular Joint, Right **H** Acromioclavicular Joint, Left **J** Shoulder Joint, Right **K** Shoulder Joint, Left **L** Elbow Joint, Right **M** Elbow Joint, Left **N** Wrist Joint, Right **P** Wrist Joint, Left **Q** Carpal Joint, Right **R** Carpal Joint, Left **S** Metacarpocarpal Joint, Right **T** Metacarpocarpal Joint, Left **U** Metacarpophalangeal Joint, Right **V** Metacarpophalangeal Joint, Left **W** Finger Phalangeal Joint, Right **X** Finger Phalangeal Joint, Left	**Ø** Open **3** Percutaneous **4** Percutaneous Endoscopic	**Z** No Device	**X** Diagnostic **Z** No Qualifier

Ø Medical and Surgical
R Upper Joints
B Excision Cutting out or off, without replacement, a portion of a body part

Body Part Character 4	Approach Character 5	Device Character 6	Qualifier Character 7
Ø Occipital-cervical Joint	**Ø** Open	**Z** No Device	**X** Diagnostic
1 Cervical Vertebral Joint	**3** Percutaneous		**Z** No Qualifier
3 Cervical Vertebral Disc	**4** Percutaneous Endoscopic		
4 Cervicothoracic Vertebral Joint			
5 Cervicothoracic Vertebral Disc			
6 Thoracic Vertebral Joint			
9 Thoracic Vertebral Disc			
A Thoracolumbar Vertebral Joint			
B Thoracolumbar Vertebral Disc			
C Temporomandibular Joint, Right			
D Temporomandibular Joint, Left			
E Sternoclavicular Joint, Right			
F Sternoclavicular Joint, Left			
G Acromioclavicular Joint, Right			
H Acromioclavicular Joint, Left			
J Shoulder Joint, Right			
K Shoulder Joint, Left			
L Elbow Joint, Right			
M Elbow Joint, Left			
N Wrist Joint, Right			
P Wrist Joint, Left			
Q Carpal Joint, Right			
R Carpal Joint, Left			
S Metacarpocarpal Joint, Right			
T Metacarpocarpal Joint, Left			
U Metacarpophalangeal Joint, Right			
V Metacarpophalangeal Joint, Left			
W Finger Phalangeal Joint, Right			
X Finger Phalangeal Joint, Left			

Ø Medical and Surgical
R Upper Joints
C Extirpation Taking or cutting out solid matter from a body part

Body Part Character 4	Approach Character 5	Device Character 6	Qualifier Character 7
Ø Occipital-cervical Joint	**Ø** Open	**Z** No Device	**Z** No Qualifier
1 Cervical Vertebral Joint	**3** Percutaneous		
3 Cervical Vertebral Disc	**4** Percutaneous Endoscopic		
4 Cervicothoracic Vertebral Joint			
5 Cervicothoracic Vertebral Disc			
6 Thoracic Vertebral Joint			
9 Thoracic Vertebral Disc			
A Thoracolumbar Vertebral Joint			
B Thoracolumbar Vertebral Disc			
C Temporomandibular Joint, Right			
D Temporomandibular Joint, Left			
E Sternoclavicular Joint, Right			
F Sternoclavicular Joint, Left			
G Acromioclavicular Joint, Right			
H Acromioclavicular Joint, Left			
J Shoulder Joint, Right			
K Shoulder Joint, Left			
L Elbow Joint, Right			
M Elbow Joint, Left			
N Wrist Joint, Right			
P Wrist Joint, Left			
Q Carpal Joint, Right			
R Carpal Joint, Left			
S Metacarpocarpal Joint, Right			
T Metacarpocarpal Joint, Left			
U Metacarpophalangeal Joint, Right			
V Metacarpophalangeal Joint, Left			
W Finger Phalangeal Joint, Right			
X Finger Phalangeal Joint, Left			

0 Medical and Surgical
R Upper Joints
G Fusion Joining together portions of an articular body part rendering the articular body part immobile

Body Part Character 4	Approach Character 5	Device Character 6	Qualifier Character 7
0 Occipital-cervical Joint 1 Cervical Vertebral Joint 2 Cervical Vertebral Joints, 2 or more 4 Cervicothoracic Vertebral Joint 6 Thoracic Vertebral Joint 7 Thoracic Vertebral Joints, 2 to 7 8 Thoracic Vertebral Joints, 8 or more A Thoracolumbar Vertebral Joint	0 Open 3 Percutaneous 4 Percutaneous Endoscopic	7 Autologous Tissue Substitute **A Interbody Fusion Device** J Synthetic Substitute K Nonautologous Tissue Substitute Z No Device	0 Anterior Approach, Anterior Column 1 Posterior Approach, Posterior Column J Posterior Approach, Anterior Column
C Temporomandibular Joint, Right D Temporomandibular Joint, Left E Sternoclavicular Joint, Right F Sternoclavicular Joint, Left G Acromioclavicular Joint, Right H Acromioclavicular Joint, Left J Shoulder Joint, Right K Shoulder Joint, Left	0 Open 3 Percutaneous 4 Percutaneous Endoscopic	4 Internal Fixation Device 7 Autologous Tissue Substitute J Synthetic Substitute K Nonautologous Tissue Substitute Z No Device	Z No Qualifier
L Elbow Joint, Right M Elbow Joint, Left N Wrist Joint, Right P Wrist Joint, Left Q Carpal Joint, Right R Carpal Joint, Left S Metacarpocarpal Joint, Right T Metacarpocarpal Joint, Left U Metacarpophalangeal Joint, Right V Metacarpophalangeal Joint, Left W Finger Phalangeal Joint, Right X Finger Phalangeal Joint, Left	0 Open 3 Percutaneous 4 Percutaneous Endoscopic	4 Internal Fixation Device 5 External Fixation Device 7 Autologous Tissue Substitute J Synthetic Substitute K Nonautologous Tissue Substitute Z No Device	Z No Qualifier

0 Medical and Surgical
R Upper Joints
H Insertion Putting in a nonbiological appliance that monitors, assists, performs, or prevents a physiological function but does not physically take the place of a body part

Body Part Character 4	Approach Character 5	Device Character 6	Qualifier Character 7
0 Occipital-cervical Joint 1 Cervical Vertebral Joint 4 Cervicothoracic Vertebral Joint 6 Thoracic Vertebral Joint A Thoracolumbar Vertebral Joint	0 Open 3 Percutaneous 4 Percutaneous Endoscopic	3 Infusion Device 4 Internal Fixation Device 8 Spacer **B Spinal Stabilization Device, Interspinous Process** **C Spinal Stabilization Device, Pedicle-Based** **D Spinal Stabilization Device, Facet Replacement**	Z No Qualifier
3 Cervical Vertebral Disc 5 Cervicothoracic Vertebral Disc 9 Thoracic Vertebral Disc B Thoracolumbar Vertebral Disc	0 Open 3 Percutaneous 4 Percutaneous Endoscopic	3 Infusion Device	Z No Qualifier
C Temporomandibular Joint, Right D Temporomandibular Joint, Left E Sternoclavicular Joint, Right F Sternoclavicular Joint, Left G Acromioclavicular Joint, Right H Acromioclavicular Joint, Left J Shoulder Joint, Right K Shoulder Joint, Left	0 Open 3 Percutaneous 4 Percutaneous Endoscopic	3 Infusion Device 4 Internal Fixation Device 8 Spacer	Z No Qualifier
L Elbow Joint, Right M Elbow Joint, Left N Wrist Joint, Right P Wrist Joint, Left Q Carpal Joint, Right R Carpal Joint, Left S Metacarpocarpal Joint, Right T Metacarpocarpal Joint, Left U Metacarpophalangeal Joint, Right V Metacarpophalangeal Joint, Left W Finger Phalangeal Joint, Right X Finger Phalangeal Joint, Left	0 Open 3 Percutaneous 4 Percutaneous Endoscopic	3 Infusion Device 4 Internal Fixation Device 5 External Fixation Device 8 Spacer	Z No Qualifier

Ø Medical and Surgical
R Upper Joints
J Inspection Visually and/or manually exploring a body part

Body Part Character 4	Approach Character 5	Device Character 6	Qualifier Character 7
Ø Occipital-cervical Joint **1** Cervical Vertebral Joint **3** Cervical Vertebral Disc **4** Cervicothoracic Vertebral Joint **5** Cervicothoracic Vertebral Disc **6** Thoracic Vertebral Joint **9** Thoracic Vertebral Disc **A** Thoracolumbar Vertebral Joint **B** Thoracolumbar Vertebral Disc **C** Temporomandibular Joint, Right **D** Temporomandibular Joint, Left **E** Sternoclavicular Joint, Right **F** Sternoclavicular Joint, Left **G** Acromioclavicular Joint, Right **H** Acromioclavicular Joint, Left **J** Shoulder Joint, Right **K** Shoulder Joint, Left **L** Elbow Joint, Right **M** Elbow Joint, Left **N** Wrist Joint, Right **P** Wrist Joint, Left **Q** Carpal Joint, Right **R** Carpal Joint, Left **S** Metacarpocarpal Joint, Right **T** Metacarpocarpal Joint, Left **U** Metacarpophalangeal Joint, Right **V** Metacarpophalangeal Joint, Left **W** Finger Phalangeal Joint, Right **X** Finger Phalangeal Joint, Left	**Ø** Open **3** Percutaneous **4** Percutaneous Endoscopic **X** External	**Z** No Device	**Z** No Qualifier

Ø Medical and Surgical
R Upper Joints
N Release Freeing a body part from an abnormal physical constraint

Body Part Character 4	Approach Character 5	Device Character 6	Qualifier Character 7
Ø Occipital-cervical Joint **1** Cervical Vertebral Joint **3** Cervical Vertebral Disc **4** Cervicothoracic Vertebral Joint **5** Cervicothoracic Vertebral Disc **6** Thoracic Vertebral Joint **9** Thoracic Vertebral Disc **A** Thoracolumbar Vertebral Joint **B** Thoracolumbar Vertebral Disc **C** Temporomandibular Joint, Right **D** Temporomandibular Joint, Left **E** Sternoclavicular Joint, Right **F** Sternoclavicular Joint, Left **G** Acromioclavicular Joint, Right **H** Acromioclavicular Joint, Left **J** Shoulder Joint, Right **K** Shoulder Joint, Left **L** Elbow Joint, Right **M** Elbow Joint, Left **N** Wrist Joint, Right **P** Wrist Joint, Left **Q** Carpal Joint, Right **R** Carpal Joint, Left **S** Metacarpocarpal Joint, Right **T** Metacarpocarpal Joint, Left **U** Metacarpophalangeal Joint, Right **V** Metacarpophalangeal Joint, Left **W** Finger Phalangeal Joint, Right **X** Finger Phalangeal Joint, Left	**Ø** Open **3** Percutaneous **4** Percutaneous Endoscopic **X** External	**Z** No Device	**Z** No Qualifier

Ø Medical and Surgical
R Upper Joints
P Removal Taking out or off a device from a body part

Body Part Character 4	Approach Character 5	Device Character 6	Qualifier Character 7
Ø Occipital-cervical Joint **1** Cervical Vertebral Joint **4** Cervicothoracic Vertebral Joint **6** Thoracic Vertebral Joint **A** Thoracolumbar Vertebral Joint **C** Temporomandibular Joint, Right **D** Temporomandibular Joint, Left **E** Sternoclavicular Joint, Right **F** Sternoclavicular Joint, Left **G** Acromioclavicular Joint, Right **H** Acromioclavicular Joint, Left **J** Shoulder Joint, Right **K** Shoulder Joint, Left	**Ø** Open **3** Percutaneous **4** Percutaneous Endoscopic	**Ø** Drainage Device **3** Infusion Device **4** Internal Fixation Device **7** Autologous Tissue Substitute **8** Spacer **A Interbody Fusion Device** **J** Synthetic Substitute **K** Nonautologous Tissue Substitute	**Z** No Qualifier
Ø Occipital-cervical Joint **1** Cervical Vertebral Joint **4** Cervicothoracic Vertebral Joint **6** Thoracic Vertebral Joint **A** Thoracolumbar Vertebral Joint **C** Temporomandibular Joint, Right **D** Temporomandibular Joint, Left **E** Sternoclavicular Joint, Right **F** Sternoclavicular Joint, Left **G** Acromioclavicular Joint, Right **H** Acromioclavicular Joint, Left **J** Shoulder Joint, Right **K** Shoulder Joint, Left	**X** External	**Ø** Drainage Device **3** Infusion Device **4** Internal Fixation Device	**Z** No Qualifier
3 Cervical Vertebral Disc **5** Cervicothoracic Vertebral Disc **9** Thoracic Vertebral Disc **B** Thoracolumbar Vertebral Disc	**Ø** Open **3** Percutaneous **4** Percutaneous Endoscopic	**Ø** Drainage Device **3** Infusion Device **7** Autologous Tissue Substitute **J** Synthetic Substitute **K** Nonautologous Tissue Substitute	**Z** No Qualifier
3 Cervical Vertebral Disc **5** Cervicothoracic Vertebral Disc **9** Thoracic Vertebral Disc **B** Thoracolumbar Vertebral Disc	**X** External	**Ø** Drainage Device **3** Infusion Device	**Z** No Qualifier
L Elbow Joint, Right **M** Elbow Joint, Left **N** Wrist Joint, Right **P** Wrist Joint, Left **Q** Carpal Joint, Right **R** Carpal Joint, Left **S** Metacarpocarpal Joint, Right **T** Metacarpocarpal Joint, Left **U** Metacarpophalangeal Joint, Right **V** Metacarpophalangeal Joint, Left **W** Finger Phalangeal Joint, Right **X** Finger Phalangeal Joint, Left	**Ø** Open **3** Percutaneous **4** Percutaneous Endoscopic	**Ø** Drainage Device **3** Infusion Device **4** Internal Fixation Device **5** External Fixation Device **7** Autologous Tissue Substitute **8** Spacer **J** Synthetic Substitute **K** Nonautologous Tissue Substitute	**Z** No Qualifier
L Elbow Joint, Right **M** Elbow Joint, Left **N** Wrist Joint, Right **P** Wrist Joint, Left **Q** Carpal Joint, Right **R** Carpal Joint, Left **S** Metacarpocarpal Joint, Right **T** Metacarpocarpal Joint, Left **U** Metacarpophalangeal Joint, Right **V** Metacarpophalangeal Joint, Left **W** Finger Phalangeal Joint, Right **X** Finger Phalangeal Joint, Left	**X** External	**Ø** Drainage Device **3** Infusion Device **4** Internal Fixation Device **5** External Fixation Device	**Z** No Qualifier

Ø Medical and Surgical
R Upper Joints
Q Repair Restoring, to the extent possible, a body part to its normal anatomic structure and function

Body Part Character 4	Approach Character 5	Device Character 6	Qualifier Character 7
Ø Occipital-cervical Joint **1** Cervical Vertebral Joint **3** Cervical Vertebral Disc **4** Cervicothoracic Vertebral Joint **5** Cervicothoracic Vertebral Disc **6** Thoracic Vertebral Joint **9** Thoracic Vertebral Disc **A** Thoracolumbar Vertebral Joint **B** Thoracolumbar Vertebral Disc **C** Temporomandibular Joint, Right **D** Temporomandibular Joint, Left **E** Sternoclavicular Joint, Right **F** Sternoclavicular Joint, Left **G** Acromioclavicular Joint, Right **H** Acromioclavicular Joint, Left **J** Shoulder Joint, Right **K** Shoulder Joint, Left **L** Elbow Joint, Right **M** Elbow Joint, Left **N** Wrist Joint, Right **P** Wrist Joint, Left **Q** Carpal Joint, Right **R** Carpal Joint, Left **S** Metacarpocarpal Joint, Right **T** Metacarpocarpal Joint, Left **U** Metacarpophalangeal Joint, Right **V** Metacarpophalangeal Joint, Left **W** Finger Phalangeal Joint, Right **X** Finger Phalangeal Joint, Left	**Ø** Open **3** Percutaneous **4** Percutaneous Endoscopic **X** External	**Z** No Device	**Z** No Qualifier

Ø Medical and Surgical
R Upper Joints
R Replacement Putting in or on biological or synthetic material that physically takes the place and/or function of all or a portion of a body part

Body Part Character 4	Approach Character 5	Device Character 6	Qualifier Character 7
Ø Occipital-cervical Joint **1** Cervical Vertebral Joint **3** Cervical Vertebral Disc **4** Cervicothoracic Vertebral Joint **5** Cervicothoracic Vertebral Disc **6** Thoracic Vertebral Joint **9** Thoracic Vertebral Disc **A** Thoracolumbar Vertebral Joint **B** Thoracolumbar Vertebral Disc **C** Temporomandibular Joint, Right **D** Temporomandibular Joint, Left **E** Sternoclavicular Joint, Right **F** Sternoclavicular Joint, Left **G** Acromioclavicular Joint, Right **H** Acromioclavicular Joint, Left **L** Elbow Joint, Right **M** Elbow Joint, Left **N** Wrist Joint, Right **P** Wrist Joint, Left **Q** Carpal Joint, Right **R** Carpal Joint, Left **S** Metacarpocarpal Joint, Right **T** Metacarpocarpal Joint, Left **U** Metacarpophalangeal Joint, Right **V** Metacarpophalangeal Joint, Left **W** Finger Phalangeal Joint, Right **X** Finger Phalangeal Joint, Left	**Ø** Open	**7** Autologous Tissue Substitute **J** Synthetic Substitute **K** Nonautologous Tissue Substitute	**Z** No Qualifier
J Shoulder Joint, Right **K** Shoulder Joint, Left	**Ø** Open	**Ø** **Synthetic Substitute, Reverse Ball and Socket** **7** Autologous Tissue Substitute **K** Nonautologous Tissue Substitute	**Z** No Qualifier

ØRR Continued on next page

0 Medical and Surgical
R Upper Joints
R Replacement Putting in or on biological or synthetic material that physically takes the place and/or function of all or a portion of a body part

0RR Continued

Body Part Character 4	Approach Character 5	Device Character 6	Qualifier Character 7
J Shoulder Joint, Right K Shoulder Joint, Left	0 Open	J Synthetic Substitute	6 Humeral Surface 7 Glenoid Surface Z No Qualifier

0 Medical and Surgical
R Upper Joints
S Reposition Moving to its normal location or other suitable location all or a portion of a body part

Body Part Character 4	Approach Character 5	Device Character 6	Qualifier Character 7
0 Occipital-cervical Joint 1 Cervical Vertebral Joint 4 Cervicothoracic Vertebral Joint 6 Thoracic Vertebral Joint A Thoracolumbar Vertebral Joint C Temporomandibular Joint, Right D Temporomandibular Joint, Left E Sternoclavicular Joint, Right F Sternoclavicular Joint, Left G Acromioclavicular Joint, Right H Acromioclavicular Joint, Left J Shoulder Joint, Right K Shoulder Joint, Left	0 Open 3 Percutaneous 4 Percutaneous Endoscopic X External	4 Internal Fixation Device Z No Device	Z No Qualifier
L Elbow Joint, Right M Elbow Joint, Left N Wrist Joint, Right P Wrist Joint, Left Q Carpal Joint, Right R Carpal Joint, Left S Metacarpocarpal Joint, Right T Metacarpocarpal Joint, Left U Metacarpophalangeal Joint, Right V Metacarpophalangeal Joint, Left W Finger Phalangeal Joint, Right X Finger Phalangeal Joint, Left	0 Open 3 Percutaneous 4 Percutaneous Endoscopic X External	4 Internal Fixation Device 5 External Fixation Device Z No Device	Z No Qualifier

0 Medical and Surgical
R Upper Joints
T Resection Cutting out or off, without replacement, all of a body part

Body Part Character 4	Approach Character 5	Device Character 6	Qualifier Character 7
3 Cervical Vertebral Disc 4 Cervicothoracic Vertebral Joint 5 Cervicothoracic Vertebral Disc 9 Thoracic Vertebral Disc B Thoracolumbar Vertebral Disc C Temporomandibular Joint, Right D Temporomandibular Joint, Left E Sternoclavicular Joint, Right F Sternoclavicular Joint, Left G Acromioclavicular Joint, Right H Acromioclavicular Joint, Left J Shoulder Joint, Right K Shoulder Joint, Left L Elbow Joint, Right M Elbow Joint, Left N Wrist Joint, Right P Wrist Joint, Left Q Carpal Joint, Right R Carpal Joint, Left S Metacarpocarpal Joint, Right T Metacarpocarpal Joint, Left U Metacarpophalangeal Joint, Right V Metacarpophalangeal Joint, Left W Finger Phalangeal Joint, Right X Finger Phalangeal Joint, Left	0 Open	Z No Device	Z No Qualifier

Ø Medical and Surgical
R Upper Joints
U Supplement Putting in or on biological or synthetic material that physically reinforces and/or augments the function of a portion of a body part

Body Part Character 4	Approach Character 5	Device Character 6	Qualifier Character 7
Ø Occipital-cervical Joint 1 Cervical Vertebral Joint 3 Cervical Vertebral Disc 4 Cervicothoracic Vertebral Joint 5 Cervicothoracic Vertebral Disc 6 Thoracic Vertebral Joint 9 Thoracic Vertebral Disc A Thoracolumbar Vertebral Joint B Thoracolumbar Vertebral Disc C Temporomandibular Joint, Right D Temporomandibular Joint, Left E Sternoclavicular Joint, Right F Sternoclavicular Joint, Left G Acromioclavicular Joint, Right H Acromioclavicular Joint, Left J Shoulder Joint, Right K Shoulder Joint, Left L Elbow Joint, Right M Elbow Joint, Left N Wrist Joint, Right P Wrist Joint, Left Q Carpal Joint, Right R Carpal Joint, Left S Metacarpocarpal Joint, Right T Metacarpocarpal Joint, Left U Metacarpophalangeal Joint, Right V Metacarpophalangeal Joint, Left W Finger Phalangeal X Finger Phalangeal Joint, Left	Ø Open 3 Percutaneous 4 Percutaneous Endoscopic	7 Autologous Tissue Substitute J Synthetic Substitute K Nonautologous Tissue Substitute	Z No Qualifier

Ø Medical and Surgical
R Upper Joints
W Revision Correcting, to the extent possible, a portion of a malfunctioning device or the position of a displaced device

Body Part Character 4	Approach Character 5	Device Character 6	Qualifier Character 7
Ø Occipital-cervical Joint 1 Cervical Vertebral Joint 4 Cervicothoracic Vertebral Joint 6 Thoracic Vertebral Joint A Thoracolumbar Vertebral Joint	Ø Open 3 Percutaneous 4 Percutaneous Endoscopic X External	Ø Drainage Device 3 Infusion Device 4 Internal Fixation Device 7 Autologous Tissue Substitute 8 Spacer **A Interbody Fusion Device** J Synthetic Substitute K Nonautologous Tissue Substitute	Z No Qualifier
3 Cervical Vertebral Disc 5 Cervicothoracic Vertebral Disc 9 Thoracic Vertebral Disc B Thoracolumbar Vertebral Disc	Ø Open 3 Percutaneous 4 Percutaneous Endoscopic X External	Ø Drainage Device 3 Infusion Device 7 Autologous Tissue Substitute J Synthetic Substitute K Nonautologous Tissue Substitute	Z No Qualifier
C Temporomandibular Joint, Right D Temporomandibular Joint, Left E Sternoclavicular Joint, Right F Sternoclavicular Joint, Left G Acromioclavicular Joint, Right H Acromioclavicular Joint, Left J Shoulder Joint, Right K Shoulder Joint, Left	Ø Open 3 Percutaneous 4 Percutaneous Endoscopic X External	Ø Drainage Device 3 Infusion Device 4 Internal Fixation Device 5 External Fixation Device 7 Autologous Tissue Substitute 8 Spacer J Synthetic Substitute K Nonautologous Tissue Substitute	Z No Qualifier
L Elbow Joint, Right M Elbow Joint, Left N Wrist Joint, Right P Wrist Joint, Left Q Carpal Joint, Right R Carpal Joint, Left S Metacarpocarpal Joint, Right T Metacarpocarpal Joint, Left U Metacarpophalangeal Joint, Right V Metacarpophalangeal Joint, Left W Finger Phalangeal Joint, Right X Finger Phalangeal Joint, Left	Ø Open 3 Percutaneous 4 Percutaneous Endoscopic X External	Ø Drainage Device 3 Infusion Device 4 Internal Fixation Device 5 External Fixation Device 7 Autologous Tissue Substitute 8 Spacer J Synthetic Substitute K Nonautologous Tissue Substitute	Z No Qualifier

Lower Joints ØS2–ØSW

Ø Medical and Surgical
S Lower Joints
2 Change Taking out or off a device from a body part and putting back an identical or similar device in or on the same body part without cutting or puncturing the skin or a mucous membrane

Body Part Character 4	Approach Character 5	Device Character 6	Qualifier Character 7
Y Lower Joint	X External	Ø Drainage Device Y Other Device	Z No Qualifier

Ø Medical and Surgical
S Lower Joints
5 Destruction Physical eradication of all or a portion of a body part by the direct use of energy, force, or a destructive agent

Body Part Character 4	Approach Character 5	Device Character 6	Qualifier Character 7
Ø Lumbar Vertebral Joint 2 Lumbar Vertebral Disc 3 Lumbosacral Joint 4 Lumbosacral Disc 5 Sacrococcygeal Joint 6 Coccygeal Joint 7 Sacroiliac Joint, Right 8 Sacroiliac Joint, Left 9 Hip Joint, Right B Hip Joint, Left C Knee Joint, Right D Knee Joint, Left F Ankle Joint, Right G Ankle Joint, Left H Tarsal Joint, Right J Tarsal Joint, Left K Metatarsal-Tarsal Joint, Right L Metatarsal-Tarsal Joint, Left M Metatarsal-Phalangeal Joint, Right N Metatarsal-Phalangeal Joint, Left P Toe Phalangeal Joint, Right Q Toe Phalangeal Joint, Left	Ø Open 3 Percutaneous 4 Percutaneous Endoscopic	Z No Device	Z No Qualifier

Ø Medical and Surgical
S Lower Joints
9 Drainage Taking or letting out fluids and/or gases from a body part

Body Part Character 4	Approach Character 5	Device Character 6	Qualifier Character 7
Ø Lumbar Vertebral Joint 2 Lumbar Vertebral Disc 3 Lumbosacral Joint 4 Lumbosacral Disc 5 Sacrococcygeal Joint 6 Coccygeal Joint 7 Sacroiliac Joint, Right 8 Sacroiliac Joint, Left 9 Hip Joint, Right B Hip Joint, Left C Knee Joint, Right D Knee Joint, Left F Ankle Joint, Right G Ankle Joint, Left H Tarsal Joint, Right J Tarsal Joint, Left K Metatarsal-Tarsal Joint, Right L Metatarsal-Tarsal Joint, Left M Metatarsal-Phalangeal Joint, Right N Metatarsal-Phalangeal Joint, Left P Toe Phalangeal Joint, Right Q Toe Phalangeal Joint, Left	Ø Open 3 Percutaneous 4 Percutaneous Endoscopic	Ø Drainage Device	Z No Qualifier

ØS9 Continued on next page

ØS9 Continued

Ø Medical and Surgical
S Lower Joints
9 Drainage Taking or letting out fluids and/or gases from a body part

Body Part Character 4	Approach Character 5	Device Character 6	Qualifier Character 7
Ø Lumbar Vertebral Joint **2** Lumbar Vertebral Disc **3** Lumbosacral Joint **4** Lumbosacral Disc **5** Sacrococcygeal Joint **6** Coccygeal Joint **7** Sacroiliac Joint, Right **8** Sacroiliac Joint, Left **9** Hip Joint, Right **B** Hip Joint, Left **C** Knee Joint, Right **D** Knee Joint, Left **F** Ankle Joint, Right **G** Ankle Joint, Left **H** Tarsal Joint, Right **J** Tarsal Joint, Left **K** Metatarsal-Tarsal Joint, Right **L** Metatarsal-Tarsal Joint, Left **M** Metatarsal-Phalangeal Joint, Right **N** Metatarsal-Phalangeal Joint, Left **P** Toe Phalangeal Joint, Right **Q** Toe Phalangeal Joint, Left	**Ø** Open **3** Percutaneous **4** Percutaneous Endoscopic	**Z** No Device	**X** Diagnostic **Z** No Qualifier

Ø Medical and Surgical
S Lower Joints
B Excision Cutting out or off, without replacement, a portion of a body part

Body Part Character 4	Approach Character 5	Device Character 6	Qualifier Character 7
Ø Lumbar Vertebral Joint **2** Lumbar Vertebral Disc **3** Lumbosacral Joint **4** Lumbosacral Disc **5** Sacrococcygeal Joint **6** Coccygeal Joint **7** Sacroiliac Joint, Right **8** Sacroiliac Joint, Left **9** Hip Joint, Right **B** Hip Joint, Left **C** Knee Joint, Right **D** Knee Joint, Left **F** Ankle Joint, Right **G** Ankle Joint, Left **H** Tarsal Joint, Right **J** Tarsal Joint, Left **K** Metatarsal-Tarsal Joint, Right **L** Metatarsal-Tarsal Joint, Left **M** Metatarsal-Phalangeal Joint, Right **N** Metatarsal-Phalangeal Joint, Left **P** Toe Phalangeal Joint, Right **Q** Toe Phalangeal Joint, Left	**Ø** Open **3** Percutaneous **4** Percutaneous Endoscopic	**Z** No Device	**X** Diagnostic **Z** No Qualifier

0 Medical and Surgical
S Lower Joints
C Extirpation Taking or cutting out solid matter from a body part

Body Part Character 4	Approach Character 5	Device Character 6	Qualifier Character 7
0 Lumbar Vertebral Joint 2 Lumbar Vertebral Disc 3 Lumbosacral Joint 4 Lumbosacral Disc 5 Sacrococcygeal Joint 6 Coccygeal Joint 7 Sacroiliac Joint, Right 8 Sacroiliac Joint, Left 9 Hip Joint, Right B Hip Joint, Left C Knee Joint, Right D Knee Joint, Left F Ankle Joint, Right G Ankle Joint, Left H Tarsal Joint, Right J Tarsal Joint, Left K Metatarsal-Tarsal Joint, Right L Metatarsal-Tarsal Joint, Left M Metatarsal-Phalangeal Joint, Right N Metatarsal-Phalangeal Joint, Left P Toe Phalangeal Joint, Right Q Toe Phalangeal Joint, Left	0 Open 3 Percutaneous 4 Percutaneous Endoscopic	Z No Device	Z No Qualifier

0 Medical and Surgical
S Lower Joints
G Fusion Joining together portions of an articular body part rendering the articular body part immobile

Body Part Character 4	Approach Character 5	Device Character 6	Qualifier Character 7
0 Lumbar Vertebral Joint 1 Lumbar Vertebral Joints, 2 or more 3 Lumbosacral Joint	0 Open 3 Percutaneous 4 Percutaneous Endoscopic	7 Autologous Tissue Substitute **A Interbody Fusion Device** J Synthetic Substitute K Nonautologous Tissue Substitute Z No Device	0 Anterior Approach, Anterior Column 1 Posterior Approach, Posterior Column J Posterior Approach, Anterior Column
5 Sacrococcygeal Joint 6 Coccygeal Joint 7 Sacroiliac Joint, Right 8 Sacroiliac Joint, Left	0 Open 3 Percutaneous 4 Percutaneous Endoscopic	4 Internal Fixation Device 7 Autologous Tissue Substitute J Synthetic Substitute K Nonautologous Tissue Substitute Z No Device	Z No Qualifier
9 Hip Joint, Right B Hip Joint, Left C Knee Joint, Right D Knee Joint, Left F Ankle Joint, Right G Ankle Joint, Left H Tarsal Joint, Right J Tarsal Joint, Left K Metatarsal-Tarsal Joint, Right L Metatarsal-Tarsal Joint, Left M Metatarsal-Phalangeal Joint, Right N Metatarsal-Phalangeal Joint, Left P Toe Phalangeal Joint, Right Q Toe Phalangeal Joint, Left	0 Open 3 Percutaneous 4 Percutaneous Endoscopic	4 Internal Fixation Device 5 External Fixation Device 7 Autologous Tissue Substitute J Synthetic Substitute K Nonautologous Tissue Substitute Z No Device	Z No Qualifier

Ø Medical and Surgical
S Lower Joints
H Insertion Putting in a nonbiological appliance that monitors, assists, performs, or prevents a physiological function but does not physically take the place of a body part

Body Part Character 4	Approach Character 5	Device Character 6	Qualifier Character 7
Ø Lumbar Vertebral Joint 3 Lumbosacral Joint	Ø Open 3 Percutaneous 4 Percutaneous Endoscopic	3 Infusion Device 4 Internal Fixation Device 8 Spacer **B Spinal Stabilization Device, Interspinous Process** **C Spinal Stabilization Device, Pedicle-Based** **D Spinal Stabilization Device, Facet Replacement**	Z No Qualifier
2 Lumbar Vertebral Disc 4 Lumbosacral Disc	Ø Open 3 Percutaneous 4 Percutaneous Endoscopic	3 Infusion Device 8 Spacer	Z No Qualifier
5 Sacrococcygeal Joint 6 Coccygeal Joint 7 Sacroiliac Joint, Right 8 Sacroiliac Joint, Left	Ø Open 3 Percutaneous 4 Percutaneous Endoscopic	3 Infusion Device 4 Internal Fixation Device 8 Spacer	Z No Qualifier
9 Hip Joint, Right B Hip Joint, Left C Knee Joint, Right D Knee Joint, Left F Ankle Joint, Right G Ankle Joint, Left H Tarsal Joint, Right J Tarsal Joint, Left K Metatarsal-Tarsal Joint, Right L Metatarsal-Tarsal Joint, Left M Metatarsal-Phalangeal Joint, Right N Metatarsal-Phalangeal Joint, Left P Toe Phalangeal Joint, Right Q Toe Phalangeal Joint, Left	Ø Open 3 Percutaneous 4 Percutaneous Endoscopic	3 Infusion Device 4 Internal Fixation Device 5 External Fixation Device 8 Spacer	Z No Qualifier

Ø Medical and Surgical
S Lower Joints
J Inspection Visually and/or manually exploring a body part

Body Part Character 4	Approach Character 5	Device Character 6	Qualifier Character 7
Ø Lumbar Vertebral Joint 2 Lumbar Vertebral Disc 3 Lumbosacral Joint 4 Lumbosacral Disc 5 Sacrococcygeal Joint 6 Coccygeal Joint 7 Sacroiliac Joint, Right 8 Sacroiliac Joint, Left 9 Hip Joint, Right B Hip Joint, Left C Knee Joint, Right D Knee Joint, Left F Ankle Joint, Right G Ankle Joint, Left H Tarsal Joint, Right J Tarsal Joint, Left K Metatarsal-Tarsal Joint, Right L Metatarsal-Tarsal Joint, Left M Metatarsal-Phalangeal Joint, Right N Metatarsal-Phalangeal Joint, Left P Toe Phalangeal Joint, Right Q Toe Phalangeal Joint, Left	Ø Open 3 Percutaneous 4 Percutaneous Endoscopic X External	Z No Device	Z No Qualifier

0 Medical and Surgical
S Lower Joints
N Release Freeing a body part from an abnormal physical constraint

Body Part Character 4	Approach Character 5	Device Character 6	Qualifier Character 7
0 Lumbar Vertebral Joint 2 Lumbar Vertebral Disc 3 Lumbosacral Joint 4 Lumbosacral Disc 5 Sacrococcygeal Joint 6 Coccygeal Joint 7 Sacroiliac Joint, Right 8 Sacroiliac Joint, Left 9 Hip Joint, Right B Hip Joint, Left C Knee Joint, Right D Knee Joint, Left F Ankle Joint, Right G Ankle Joint, Left H Tarsal Joint, Right J Tarsal Joint, Left K Metatarsal-Tarsal Joint, Right L Metatarsal-Tarsal Joint, Left M Metatarsal-Phalangeal Joint, Right N Metatarsal-Phalangeal Joint, Left P Toe Phalangeal Joint, Right Q Toe Phalangeal Joint, Left	0 Open 3 Percutaneous 4 Percutaneous Endoscopic X External	Z No Device	Z No Qualifier

0 Medical and Surgical
S Lower Joints
P Removal Taking out or off a device from a body part

Body Part Character 4	Approach Character 5	Device Character 6	Qualifier Character 7
0 Lumbar Vertebral Joint 3 Lumbosacral Joint	0 Open 3 Percutaneous 4 Percutaneous Endoscopic	0 Drainage Device 3 Infusion Device 4 Internal Fixation Device 7 Autologous Tissue Substitute 8 Spacer **A Interbody Fusion Device** J Synthetic Substitute K Nonautologous Tissue Substitute	Z No Qualifier
0 Lumbar Vertebral Joint 3 Lumbosacral Joint	X External	0 Drainage Device 3 Infusion Device 4 Internal Fixation Device	Z No Qualifier
5 Sacrococcygeal Joint 6 Coccygeal Joint 7 Sacroiliac Joint, Right 8 Sacroiliac Joint, Left	0 Open 3 Percutaneous 4 Percutaneous Endoscopic	0 Drainage Device 3 Infusion Device 4 Internal Fixation Device 7 Autologous Tissue Substitute 8 Spacer J Synthetic Substitute K Nonautologous Tissue Substitute	Z No Qualifier
5 Sacrococcygeal Joint 6 Coccygeal Joint 7 Sacroiliac Joint, Right 8 Sacroiliac Joint, Left	X External	0 Drainage Device 3 Infusion Device 4 Internal Fixation Device	Z No Qualifier
2 Lumbar Vertebral Disc 4 Lumbosacral Disc	0 Open 3 Percutaneous 4 Percutaneous Endoscopic	0 Drainage Device 3 Infusion Device 7 Autologous Tissue Substitute J Synthetic Substitute K Nonautologous Tissue Substitute	Z No Qualifier
2 Lumbar Vertebral Disc 4 Lumbosacral Disc	X External	0 Drainage Device 3 Infusion Device	Z No Qualifier
9 Hip Joint, Right B Hip Joint, Left	0 Open	0 Drainage Device 3 Infusion Device 4 Internal Fixation Device 5 External Fixation Device 7 Autologous Tissue Substitute 8 Spacer 9 Liner B Resurfacing Device J Synthetic Substitute K Nonautologous Tissue Substitute	Z No Qualifier

0SP Continued on next page

ØSP Continued

Ø Medical and Surgical
S Lower Joints
P Removal Taking out or off a device from a body part

Body Part Character 4	Approach Character 5	Device Character 6	Qualifier Character 7
9 Hip Joint, Right B Hip Joint, Left C Knee Joint, Right D Knee Joint, Left	3 Percutaneous 4 Percutaneous Endoscopic	Ø Drainage Device 3 Infusion Device 4 Internal Fixation Device 5 External Fixation Device 7 Autologous Tissue Substitute 8 Spacer J Synthetic Substitute K Nonautologous Tissue Substitute	Z No Qualifier
9 Hip Joint, Right B Hip Joint, Left C Knee Joint, Right D Knee Joint, Left F Ankle Joint, Right G Ankle Joint, Left H Tarsal Joint, Right J Tarsal Joint, Left K Metatarsal-Tarsal Joint, Right L Metatarsal-Tarsal Joint, Left M Metatarsal-Phalangeal Joint, Right N Metatarsal-Phalangeal Joint, Left P Toe Phalangeal Joint, Right Q Toe Phalangeal Joint, Left	X External	Ø Drainage Device 3 Infusion Device 4 Internal Fixation Device 5 External Fixation Device	Z No Qualifier
C Knee Joint, Right D Knee Joint, Left	Ø Open	Ø Drainage Device 3 Infusion Device 4 Internal Fixation Device 5 External Fixation Device 7 Autologous Tissue Substitute 8 Spacer 9 Liner J Synthetic Substitute K Nonautologous Tissue Substitute	Z No Qualifier
F Ankle Joint, Right G Ankle Joint, Left H Tarsal Joint, Right J Tarsal Joint, Left K Metatarsal-Tarsal Joint, Right L Metatarsal-Tarsal Joint, Left M Metatarsal-Phalangeal Joint, Right N Metatarsal-Phalangeal Joint, Left P Toe Phalangeal Joint, Right Q Toe Phalangeal Joint, Left	Ø Open 3 Percutaneous 4 Percutaneous Endoscopic	Ø Drainage Device 3 Infusion Device 4 Internal Fixation Device 5 External Fixation Device 7 Autologous Tissue Substitute 8 Spacer J Synthetic Substitute K Nonautologous Tissue Substitute	Z No Qualifier

Ø Medical and Surgical
S Lower Joints
Q Repair Restoring, to the extent possible, a body part to its normal anatomic structure and function

Body Part Character 4	Approach Character 5	Device Character 6	Qualifier Character 7
Ø Lumbar Vertebral Joint 2 Lumbar Vertebral Disc 3 Lumbosacral Joint 4 Lumbosacral Disc 5 Sacrococcygeal Joint 6 Coccygeal Joint 7 Sacroiliac Joint, Right 8 Sacroiliac Joint, Left 9 Hip Joint, Right B Hip Joint, Left C Knee Joint, Right D Knee Joint, Left F Ankle Joint, Right G Ankle Joint, Left H Tarsal Joint, Right J Tarsal Joint, Left K Metatarsal-Tarsal Joint, Right L Metatarsal-Tarsal Joint, Left M Metatarsal-Phalangeal Joint, Right N Metatarsal-Phalangeal Joint, Left P Toe Phalangeal Joint, Right Q Toe Phalangeal Joint, Left	Ø Open 3 Percutaneous 4 Percutaneous Endoscopic X External	Z No Device	Z No Qualifier

Ø Medical and Surgical
S Lower Joints
R Replacement Putting in or on biological or synthetic material that physically takes the place and/or function of all or a portion of a body part

Body Part Character 4	Approach Character 5	Device Character 6	Qualifier Character 7
Ø Lumbar Vertebral Joint 2 Lumbar Vertebral Disc 3 Lumbosacral Joint 4 Lumbosacral Disc 5 Sacrococcygeal Joint 6 Coccygeal Joint 7 Sacroiliac Joint, Right 8 Sacroiliac Joint, Left H Tarsal Joint, Right J Tarsal Joint, Left K Metatarsal-Tarsal Joint, Right L Metatarsal-Tarsal Joint, Left M Metatarsal-Phalangeal Joint, Right N Metatarsal-Phalangeal Joint, Left P Toe Phalangeal Joint, Right Q Toe Phalangeal Joint, Left	Ø Open	7 Autologous Tissue Substitute J Synthetic Substitute K Nonautologous Tissue Substitute	Z No Qualifier
9 Hip Joint, Right B Hip Joint, Left	Ø Open	**1 Synthetic Substitute, Metal** **2 Synthetic Substitute, Metal on Polyethylene** **3 Synthetic Substitute, Ceramic** **4 Synthetic Substitute, Ceramic on Polyethylene** **J Synthetic Substitute**	9 Cemented **A Uncemented** Z No Qualifier
9 Hip Joint, Right B Hip Joint, Left	Ø Open	7 Autologous Tissue Substitute K Nonautologous Tissue Substitute	Z No Qualifier
A Hip Joint, Acetabular Surface, Right E Hip Joint, Acetabular Surface, Left	Ø Open	**Ø Synthetic Substitute, Polyethylene** **1 Synthetic Substitute, Metal** **3 Synthetic Substitute, Ceramic** **J Synthetic Substitute**	9 Cemented **A Uncemented** Z No Qualifier
A Hip Joint, Acetabular Surface, Right E Hip Joint, Acetabular Surface, Left	Ø Open	7 Autologous Tissue Substitute K Nonautologous Tissue Substitute	Z No Qualifier
C Knee Joint, Right D Knee Joint, Left F Ankle Joint, Right G Ankle Joint, Left T Knee Joint, Femoral Surface, Right U Knee Joint, Femoral Surface, Left V Knee Joint, Tibial Surface, Right W Knee Joint, Tibial Surface, Left	Ø Open	7 Autologous Tissue Substitute K Nonautologous Tissue Substitute	Z No Qualifier
C Knee Joint, Right D Knee Joint, Left F Ankle Joint, Right G Ankle Joint, Left T Knee Joint, Femoral Surface, Right U Knee Joint, Femoral Surface, Left V Knee Joint, Tibial Surface, Right W Knee Joint, Tibial Surface, Left	Ø Open	J Synthetic Substitute	9 Cemented **A Uncemented** Z No Qualifier
R Hip Joint, Femoral Surface, Right S Hip Joint, Femoral Surface, Left	Ø Open	**1 Synthetic Substitute, Metal** **3 Synthetic Substitute, Ceramic** **J Synthetic Substitute**	9 Cemented **A Uncemented** Z No Qualifier
R Hip Joint, Femoral Surface, Right S Hip Joint, Femoral Surface, Left	Ø Open	7 Autologous Tissue Substitute K Nonautologous Tissue Substitute	Z No Qualifier

Ø Medical and Surgical
S Lower Joints
S Reposition Moving to its normal location or other suitable location all or a portion of a body part

Body Part Character 4	Approach Character 5	Device Character 6	Qualifier Character 7
Ø Lumbar Vertebral Joint **3** Lumbosacral Joint **5** Sacrococcygeal Joint **6** Coccygeal Joint **7** Sacroiliac Joint, Right **8** Sacroiliac Joint, Left	**Ø** Open **3** Percutaneous **4** Percutaneous Endoscopic **X** External	**4** Internal Fixation Device **Z** No Device	**Z** No Qualifier
9 Hip Joint, Right **B** Hip Joint, Left **C** Knee Joint, Right **D** Knee Joint, Left **F** Ankle Joint, Right **G** Ankle Joint, Left **H** Tarsal Joint, Right **J** Tarsal Joint, Left **K** Metatarsal-Tarsal Joint, Right **L** Metatarsal-Tarsal Joint, Left **M** Metatarsal-Phalangeal Joint, Right **N** Metatarsal-Phalangeal Joint, Left **P** Toe Phalangeal Joint, Right **Q** Toe Phalangeal Joint, Left	**Ø** Open **3** Percutaneous **4** Percutaneous Endoscopic **X** External	**4** Internal Fixation Device **5** External Fixation Device **Z** No Device	**Z** No Qualifier

Ø Medical and Surgical
S Lower Joints
T Resection Cutting out or off, without replacement, all of a body part

Body Part Character 4	Approach Character 5	Device Character 6	Qualifier Character 7
2 Lumbar Vertebral Disc **4** Lumbosacral Disc **5** Sacrococcygeal Joint **6** Coccygeal Joint **7** Sacroiliac Joint, Right **8** Sacroiliac Joint, Left **9** Hip Joint, Right **B** Hip Joint, Left **C** Knee Joint, Right **D** Knee Joint, Left **F** Ankle Joint, Right **G** Ankle Joint, Left **H** Tarsal Joint, Right **J** Tarsal Joint, Left **K** Metatarsal-Tarsal Joint, Right **L** Metatarsal-Tarsal Joint, Left **M** Metatarsal-Phalangeal Joint, Right **N** Metatarsal-Phalangeal Joint, Left **P** Toe Phalangeal Joint, Right **Q** Toe Phalangeal Joint, Left	**Ø** Open	**Z** No Device	**Z** No Qualifier

0 Medical and Surgical
S Lower Joints
U Supplement Putting in or on biological or synthetic material that physically reinforces and/or augments the function of a portion of a body part

Body Part Character 4	Approach Character 5	Device Character 6	Qualifier Character 7
0 Lumbar Vertebral Joint **2** Lumbar Vertebral Disc **3** Lumbosacral Joint **4** Lumbosacral Disc **5** Sacrococcygeal Joint **6** Coccygeal Joint **7** Sacroiliac Joint, Right **8** Sacroiliac Joint, Left **F** Ankle Joint, Right **G** Ankle Joint, Left **H** Tarsal Joint, Right J Tarsal Joint, Left **K** Metatarsal-Tarsal Joint, Right **L** Metatarsal-Tarsal Joint, Left **M** Metatarsal-Phalangeal Joint, Right **N** Metatarsal-Phalangeal Joint, Left **P** Toe Phalangeal Joint, Right **Q** Toe Phalangeal Joint, Left	**0** Open **3** Percutaneous **4** Percutaneous Endoscopic	**7** Autologous Tissue Substitute **J** Synthetic Substitute **K** Nonautologous Tissue Substitute	**Z** No Qualifier
9 Hip Joint, Right **B** Hip Joint, Left	**0** Open	**7** Autologous Tissue Substitute **9** Liner **B** Resurfacing Device **J** Synthetic Substitute **K** Nonautologous Tissue Substitute	**Z** No Qualifier
9 Hip Joint, Right **B** Hip Joint, Left	**3** Percutaneous **4** Percutaneous Endoscopic	**7** Autologous Tissue Substitute **J** Synthetic Substitute **K** Nonautologous Tissue Substitute	**Z** No Qualifier
A Hip Joint, Acetabular Surface, Right **E** Hip Joint, Acetabular Surface, Left **R** Hip Joint, Femoral Surface, Right **S** Hip Joint, Femoral Surface, Left	**0** Open	**9** Liner **B** Resurfacing Device	**Z** No Qualifier
C Knee Joint, Right **D** Knee Joint, Left	**0** Open	**7** Autologous Tissue Substitute **J** Synthetic Substitute **K** Nonautologous Tissue Substitute	**Z** No Qualifier
C Knee Joint, Right **D** Knee Joint, Left	**0** Open	**9** Liner	**C** Patellar Surface **Z** No Qualifier
T Knee Joint, Femoral Surface, Right **U** Knee Joint, Femoral Surface, Left **V** Knee Joint, Tibial Surface, Right **W** Knee Joint, Tibial Surface, Left	**0** Open	**9** Liner	**Z** No Qualifier

Ø Medical and Surgical
S Lower Joints
W Revision Correcting, to the extent possible, a portion of a malfunctioning device or the position of a displaced device

Body Part Character 4	Approach Character 5	Device Character 6	Qualifier Character 7
Ø Lumbar Vertebral Joint **3** Lumbosacral Joint	**Ø** Open **3** Percutaneous **4** Percutaneous Endoscopic **X** External	**Ø** Drainage Device **3** Infusion Device **4** Internal Fixation Device **7** Autologous Tissue Substitute **8** Spacer **A** **Interbody Fusion Device** **J** Synthetic Substitute **K** Nonautologous Tissue Substitute	**Z** No Qualifier
2 Lumbar Vertebral Disc **4** Lumbosacral Disc	**Ø** Open **3** Percutaneous **4** Percutaneous Endoscopic **X** External	**Ø** Drainage Device **3** Infusion Device **7** Autologous Tissue Substitute **J** Synthetic Substitute **K** Nonautologous Tissue Substitute	**Z** No Qualifier
5 Sacrococcygeal Joint **6** Coccygeal Joint **7** Sacroiliac Joint, Right **8** Sacroiliac Joint, Left	**Ø** Open **3** Percutaneous **4** Percutaneous Endoscopic **X** External	**Ø** Drainage Device **3** Infusion Device **4** Internal Fixation Device **7** Autologous Tissue Substitute **8** Spacer **J** Synthetic Substitute **K** Nonautologous Tissue Substitute	**Z** No Qualifier
9 Hip Joint, Right **B** Hip Joint, Left	**Ø** Open	**Ø** Drainage Device **3** Infusion Device **4** Internal Fixation Device **5** External Fixation Device **7** Autologous Tissue Substitute **8** Spacer **9** Liner **B** Resurfacing Device **J** Synthetic Substitute **K** Nonautologous Tissue Substitute	**Z** No Qualifier
9 Hip Joint, Right **B** Hip Joint, Left **C** Knee Joint, Right **D** Knee Joint, Left	**3** Percutaneous **4** Percutaneous Endoscopic **X** External	**Ø** Drainage Device **3** Infusion Device **4** Internal Fixation Device **5** External Fixation Device **7** Autologous Tissue Substitute **8** Spacer **J** Synthetic Substitute **K** Nonautologous Tissue Substitute	**Z** No Qualifier
C Knee Joint, Right **D** Knee Joint, Left	**Ø** Open	**Ø** Drainage Device **3** Infusion Device **4** Internal Fixation Device **5** External Fixation Device **7** Autologous Tissue Substitute **8** Spacer **9** Liner **J** Synthetic Substitute **K** Nonautologous Tissue Substitute	**Z** No Qualifier
F Ankle Joint, Right **G** Ankle Joint, Left **H** Tarsal Joint, Right **J** Tarsal Joint, Left **K** Metatarsal-Tarsal Joint, Right **L** Metatarsal-Tarsal Joint, Left **M** Metatarsal-Phalangeal Joint, Right **N** Metatarsal-Phalangeal Joint, Left **P** Toe Phalangeal Joint, Right **Q** Toe Phalangeal Joint, Left	**Ø** Open **3** Percutaneous **4** Percutaneous Endoscopic **X** External	**Ø** Drainage Device **3** Infusion Device **4** Internal Fixation Device **5** External Fixation Device **7** Autologous Tissue Substitute **8** Spacer **J** Synthetic Substitute **K** Nonautologous Tissue Substitute	**Z** No Qualifier

Urinary System 0T1–0TY

0 Medical and Surgical
T Urinary System
1 Bypass Altering the route of passage of the contents of a tubular body part

Body Part Character 4	Approach Character 5	Device Character 6	Qualifier Character 7
3 Kidney Pelvis, Right 4 Kidney Pelvis, Left	0 Open 4 Percutaneous Endoscopic	7 Autologous Tissue Substitute J Synthetic Substitute K Nonautologous Tissue Substitute Z No Device	3 Kidney Pelvis, Right 4 Kidney Pelvis, Left 6 Ureter, Right 7 Ureter, Left 8 Colon 9 Colocutaneous A Ileum B Bladder C Ileocutaneous D Cutaneous
3 Kidney Pelvis, Right 4 Kidney Pelvis, Left 6 Ureter, Right 7 Ureter, Left 8 Ureters, Bilateral B Bladder	3 Percutaneous	J Synthetic Substitute	D Cutaneous
6 Ureter, Right 7 Ureter, Left 8 Ureters, Bilateral	0 Open 4 Percutaneous Endoscopic	7 Autologous Tissue Substitute J Synthetic Substitute K Nonautologous Tissue Substitute Z No Device	6 Ureter, Right 7 Ureter, Left 8 Colon 9 Colocutaneous A Ileum B Bladder C Ileocutaneous D Cutaneous
B Bladder	0 Open 4 Percutaneous Endoscopic	7 Autologous Tissue Substitute J Synthetic Substitute K Nonautologous Tissue Substitute Z No Device	9 Colocutaneous C Ileocutaneous D Cutaneous

0 Medical and Surgical
T Urinary System
2 Change Taking out or off a device from a body part and putting back an identical or similar device in or on the same body part without cutting or puncturing the skin or a mucous membrane

Body Part Character 4	Approach Character 5	Device Character 6	Qualifier Character 7
5 Kidney 9 Ureter B Bladder D Urethra	X External	0 Drainage Device Y Other Device	Z No Qualifier

0 Medical and Surgical
T Urinary System
5 Destruction Physical eradication of all or a portion of a body part by the direct use of energy, force, or a destructive agent

Body Part Character 4	Approach Character 5	Device Character 6	Qualifier Character 7
0 Kidney, Right 1 Kidney, Left 3 Kidney Pelvis, Right 4 Kidney Pelvis, Left 6 Ureter, Right 7 Ureter, Left B Bladder C Bladder Neck	0 Open 3 Percutaneous 4 Percutaneous Endoscopic 7 Via Natural or Artificial Opening 8 Via Natural or Artificial Opening Endoscopic	Z No Device	Z No Qualifier
D Urethra	0 Open 3 Percutaneous 4 Percutaneous Endoscopic 7 Via Natural or Artificial Opening 8 Via Natural or Artificial Opening Endoscopic X External	Z No Device	Z No Qualifier

Ø Medical and Surgical
T Urinary System
7 Dilation Expanding an orifice or the lumen of a tubular body part

Body Part Character 4	Approach Character 5	Device Character 6	Qualifier Character 7
3 Kidney Pelvis, Right **4** Kidney Pelvis, Left **6** Ureter, Right **7** Ureter, Left **8** Ureters, Bilateral **B** Bladder **C** Bladder Neck **D** Urethra	**Ø** Open **3** Percutaneous **4** Percutaneous Endoscopic **7** Via Natural or Artificial Opening **8** Via Natural or Artificial Opening Endoscopic	**D** Intraluminal Device **Z** No Device	**Z** No Qualifier

Ø Medical and Surgical
T Urinary System
8 Division Cutting into a body part without draining fluids and/or gases from the body part in order to separate or transect a body part

Body Part Character 4	Approach Character 5	Device Character 6	Qualifier Character 7
2 Kidneys, Bilateral **C** Bladder Neck	**Ø** Open **3** Percutaneous **4** Percutaneous Endoscopic	**Z** No Device	**Z** No Qualifier

Ø Medical and Surgical
T Urinary System
9 Drainage Taking or letting out fluids and/or gases from a body part

Body Part Character 4	Approach Character 5	Device Character 6	Qualifier Character 7
Ø Kidney, Right **1** Kidney, Left **3** Kidney Pelvis, Right **4** Kidney Pelvis, Left **6** Ureter, Right **7** Ureter, Left **8** Ureters, Bilateral **B** Bladder **C** Bladder Neck	**Ø** Open **3** Percutaneous **4** Percutaneous Endoscopic **7** Via Natural or Artificial Opening **8** Via Natural or Artificial Opening Endoscopic	**Ø** Drainage Device	**Z** No Qualifier
Ø Kidney, Right **1** Kidney, Left **3** Kidney Pelvis, Right **4** Kidney Pelvis, Left **6** Ureter, Right **7** Ureter, Left **8** Ureters, Bilateral **B** Bladder **C** Bladder Neck	**Ø** Open **3** Percutaneous **4** Percutaneous Endoscopic **7** Via Natural or Artificial Opening **8** Via Natural or Artificial Opening Endoscopic	**Z** No Device	**X** Diagnostic **Z** No Qualifier
D Urethra	**Ø** Open **3** Percutaneous **4** Percutaneous Endoscopic **7** Via Natural or Artificial Opening **8** Via Natural or Artificial Opening Endoscopic **X** External	**Ø** Drainage Device	**Z** No Qualifier
D Urethra	**Ø** Open **3** Percutaneous **4** Percutaneous Endoscopic **7** Via Natural or Artificial Opening **8** Via Natural or Artificial Opening Endoscopic **X** External	**Z** No Device	**X** Diagnostic **Z** No Qualifier

0 Medical and Surgical
T Urinary System
B Excision Cutting out or off, without replacement, a portion of a body part

Body Part Character 4	Approach Character 5	Device Character 6	Qualifier Character 7
0 Kidney, Right 1 Kidney, Left 3 Kidney Pelvis, Right 4 Kidney Pelvis, Left 6 Ureter, Right 7 Ureter, Left B Bladder C Bladder Neck	0 Open 3 Percutaneous 4 Percutaneous Endoscopic 7 Via Natural or Artificial Opening 8 Via Natural or Artificial Opening Endoscopic	Z No Device	X Diagnostic Z No Qualifier
D Urethra	0 Open 3 Percutaneous 4 Percutaneous Endoscopic 7 Via Natural or Artificial Opening 8 Via Natural or Artificial Opening Endoscopic X External	Z No Device	X Diagnostic Z No Qualifier

0 Medical and Surgical
T Urinary System
C Extirpation Taking or cutting out solid matter from a body part

Body Part Character 4	Approach Character 5	Device Character 6	Qualifier Character 7
0 Kidney, Right 1 Kidney, Left 3 Kidney Pelvis, Right 4 Kidney Pelvis, Left 6 Ureter, Right 7 Ureter, Left B Bladder C Bladder Neck	0 Open 3 Percutaneous 4 Percutaneous Endoscopic 7 Via Natural or Artificial Opening 8 Via Natural or Artificial Opening Endoscopic	Z No Device	Z No Qualifier
D Urethra	0 Open 3 Percutaneous 4 Percutaneous Endoscopic 7 Via Natural or Artificial Opening 8 Via Natural or Artificial Opening Endoscopic X External	Z No Device	Z No Qualifier

0 Medical and Surgical
T Urinary System
D Extraction Pulling or stripping out or off all or a portion of a body part by the use of force

Body Part Character 4	Approach Character 5	Device Character 6	Qualifier Character 7
0 Kidney, Right 1 Kidney, Left	0 Open 3 Percutaneous 4 Percutaneous Endoscopic	Z No Device	Z No Qualifier

0 Medical and Surgical
T Urinary System
F Fragmentation Breaking solid matter in a body part into pieces

Body Part Character 4	Approach Character 5	Device Character 6	Qualifier Character 7
3 Kidney Pelvis, Right 4 Kidney Pelvis, Left 6 Ureter, Right 7 Ureter, Left B Bladder C Bladder Neck D Urethra	0 Open 3 Percutaneous 4 Percutaneous Endoscopic 7 Via Natural or Artificial Opening 8 Via Natural or Artificial Opening Endoscopic X External	Z No Device	Z No Qualifier

Ø Medical and Surgical
T Urinary System
H Insertion Putting in a nonbiological appliance that monitors, assists, performs, or prevents a physiological function but does not physically take the place of a body part

Body Part Character 4	Approach Character 5	Device Character 6	Qualifier Character 7
5 Kidney	**Ø** Open **3** Percutaneous **4** Percutaneous Endoscopic **7** Via Natural or Artificial Opening **8** Via Natural or Artificial Opening Endoscopic	**2** Monitoring Device **3** Infusion Device	**Z** No Qualifier
9 Ureter	**Ø** Open **3** Percutaneous **4** Percutaneous Endoscopic **7** Via Natural or Artificial Opening **8** Via Natural or Artificial Opening Endoscopic	**2** Monitoring Device **3** Infusion Device **M** Stimulator Lead	**Z** No Qualifier
B Bladder	**Ø** Open **3** Percutaneous **4** Percutaneous Endoscopic **7** Via Natural or Artificial Opening **8** Via Natural or Artificial Opening Endoscopic	**2** Monitoring Device **3** Infusion Device **L** Artificial Sphincter **M** Stimulator Lead	**Z** No Qualifier
C Bladder Neck	**Ø** Open **3** Percutaneous **4** Percutaneous Endoscopic **7** Via Natural or Artificial Opening **8** Via Natural or Artificial Opening Endoscopic	**L** Artificial Sphincter	**Z** No Qualifier
D Urethra	**Ø** Open **3** Percutaneous **4** Percutaneous Endoscopic **7** Via Natural or Artificial Opening **8** Via Natural or Artificial Opening Endoscopic **X** External	**2** Monitoring Device **3** Infusion Device **L** Artificial Sphincter	**Z** No Qualifier

Ø Medical and Surgical
T Urinary System
J Inspection Visually and/or manually exploring a body part

Body Part Character 4	Approach Character 5	Device Character 6	Qualifier Character 7
5 Kidney **9** Ureter **B** Bladder **D** Urethra	**Ø** Open **3** Percutaneous **4** Percutaneous Endoscopic **7** Via Natural or Artificial Opening **8** Via Natural or Artificial Opening Endoscopic **X** External	**Z** No Device	**Z** No Qualifier

Ø Medical and Surgical
T Urinary System
L Occlusion Completely closing an orifice or the lumen of a tubular body part

Body Part Character 4	Approach Character 5	Device Character 6	Qualifier Character 7
3 Kidney Pelvis, Right **4** Kidney Pelvis, Left **6** Ureter, Right **7** Ureter, Left **B** Bladder **C** Bladder Neck	**Ø** Open **3** Percutaneous **4** Percutaneous Endoscopic	**C** Extraluminal Device **D** Intraluminal Device **Z** No Device	**Z** No Qualifier
3 Kidney Pelvis, Right **4** Kidney Pelvis, Left **6** Ureter, Right **7** Ureter, Left **B** Bladder **C** Bladder Neck **D** Urethra	**7** Via Natural or Artificial Opening **8** Via Natural or Artificial Opening Endoscopic	**D** Intraluminal Device **Z** No Device	**Z** No Qualifier
D Urethra	**Ø** Open **3** Percutaneous **4** Percutaneous Endoscopic **X** External	**C** Extraluminal Device **D** Intraluminal Device **Z** No Device	**Z** No Qualifier

0 Medical and Surgical
T Urinary System
M Reattachment Putting back in or on all or a portion of a separated body part to its normal location or other suitable location

Body Part Character 4	Approach Character 5	Device Character 6	Qualifier Character 7
0 Kidney, Right 1 Kidney, Left 2 Kidneys, Bilateral 3 Kidney Pelvis, Right 4 Kidney Pelvis, Left 6 Ureter, Right 7 Ureter, Left 8 Ureters, Bilateral B Bladder C Bladder Neck D Urethra	0 Open 4 Percutaneous Endoscopic	Z No Device	Z No Qualifier

0 Medical and Surgical
T Urinary System
N Release Freeing a body part from an abnormal physical constraint

Body Part Character 4	Approach Character 5	Device Character 6	Qualifier Character 7
0 Kidney, Right 1 Kidney, Left 3 Kidney Pelvis, Right 4 Kidney Pelvis, Left 6 Ureter, Right 7 Ureter, Left B Bladder C Bladder Neck	0 Open 3 Percutaneous 4 Percutaneous Endoscopic 7 Via Natural or Artificial Opening 8 Via Natural or Artificial Opening Endoscopic	Z No Device	Z No Qualifier
D Urethra	0 Open 3 Percutaneous 4 Percutaneous Endoscopic 7 Via Natural or Artificial Opening 8 Via Natural or Artificial Opening Endoscopic X External	Z No Device	Z No Qualifier

0 Medical and Surgical
T Urinary System
P Removal Taking out or off a device from a body part

Body Part Character 4	Approach Character 5	Device Character 6	Qualifier Character 7
5 Kidney	0 Open 3 Percutaneous 4 Percutaneous Endoscopic 7 Via Natural or Artificial Opening 8 Via Natural or Artificial Opening Endoscopic	0 Drainage Device 2 Monitoring Device 3 Infusion Device 7 Autologous Tissue Substitute C Extraluminal Device D Intraluminal Device J Synthetic Substitute K Nonautologous Tissue Substitute	Z No Qualifier
5 Kidney	X External	0 Drainage Device 2 Monitoring Device 3 Infusion Device D Intraluminal Device	Z No Qualifier
9 Ureter	0 Open 3 Percutaneous 4 Percutaneous Endoscopic 7 Via Natural or Artificial Opening 8 Via Natural or Artificial Opening Endoscopic	0 Drainage Device 2 Monitoring Device 3 Infusion Device 7 Autologous Tissue Substitute C Extraluminal Device D Intraluminal Device J Synthetic Substitute K Nonautologous Tissue Substitute M Stimulator Lead	Z No Qualifier
9 Ureter	X External	0 Drainage Device 2 Monitoring Device 3 Infusion Device D Intraluminal Device M Stimulator Lead	Z No Qualifier

0TP Continued on next page

ØTP Continued

Ø Medical and Surgical
T Urinary System
P Removal Taking out or off a device from a body part

Body Part Character 4	Approach Character 5	Device Character 6	Qualifier Character 7
B Bladder	**Ø** Open **3** Percutaneous **4** Percutaneous Endoscopic **7** Via Natural or Artificial Opening **8** Via Natural or Artificial Opening Endoscopic	**Ø** Drainage Device **2** Monitoring Device **3** Infusion Device **7** Autologous Tissue Substitute **C** Extraluminal Device **D** Intraluminal Device **J** Synthetic Substitute **K** Nonautologous Tissue Substitute **L** Artificial Sphincter **M** Stimulator Lead	**Z** No Qualifier
B Bladder	**X** External	**Ø** Drainage Device **2** Monitoring Device **3** Infusion Device **D** Intraluminal Device **L** Artificial Sphincter **M** Stimulator Lead	**Z** No Qualifier
D Urethra	**Ø** Open **3** Percutaneous **4** Percutaneous Endoscopic **7** Via Natural or Artificial Opening **8** Via Natural or Artificial Opening Endoscopic	**Ø** Drainage Device **2** Monitoring Device **3** Infusion Device **7** Autologous Tissue Substitute **C** Extraluminal Device **D** Intraluminal Device **J** Synthetic Substitute **K** Nonautologous Tissue Substitute **L** Artificial Sphincter	**Z** No Qualifier
D Urethra	**X** External	**Ø** Drainage Device **2** Monitoring Device **3** Infusion Device **D** Intraluminal Device **L** Artificial Sphincter	**Z** No Qualifier

Ø Medical and Surgical
T Urinary System
Q Repair Restoring, to the extent possible, a body part to its normal anatomic structure and function

Body Part Character 4	Approach Character 5	Device Character 6	Qualifier Character 7
Ø Kidney, Right **1** Kidney, Left **3** Kidney Pelvis, Right **4** Kidney Pelvis, Left **6** Ureter, Right **7** Ureter, Left **B** Bladder **C** Bladder Neck	**Ø** Open **3** Percutaneous **4** Percutaneous Endoscopic **7** Via Natural or Artificial Opening **8** Via Natural or Artificial Opening Endoscopic	**Z** No Device	**Z** No Qualifier
D Urethra	**Ø** Open **3** Percutaneous **4** Percutaneous Endoscopic **7** Via Natural or Artificial Opening **8** Via Natural or Artificial Opening Endoscopic **X** External	**Z** No Device	**Z** No Qualifier

Ø Medical and Surgical
T Urinary System
R Replacement Putting in or on biological or synthetic material that physically takes the place and/or function of all or a portion of a body part

Body Part Character 4	Approach Character 5	Device Character 6	Qualifier Character 7
3 Kidney Pelvis, Right **4** Kidney Pelvis, Left **6** Ureter, Right **7** Ureter, Left **B** Bladder **C** Bladder Neck	**Ø** Open **4** Percutaneous Endoscopic **7** Via Natural or Artificial Opening **8** Via Natural or Artificial Opening Endoscopic	**7** Autologous Tissue Substitute **J** Synthetic Substitute **K** Nonautologous Tissue Substitute	**Z** No Qualifier
D Urethra	**Ø** Open **4** Percutaneous Endoscopic **7** Via Natural or Artificial Opening **8** Via Natural or Artificial Opening Endoscopic **X** External	**7** Autologous Tissue Substitute **J** Synthetic Substitute **K** Nonautologous Tissue Substitute	**Z** No Qualifier

0 Medical and Surgical
T Urinary System
S Reposition Moving to its normal location or other suitable location all or a portion of a body part

Body Part Character 4	Approach Character 5	Device Character 6	Qualifier Character 7
0 Kidney, Right 1 Kidney, Left 2 Kidneys, Bilateral 3 Kidney Pelvis, Right 4 Kidney Pelvis, Left 6 Ureter, Right 7 Ureter, Left 8 Ureters, Bilateral B Bladder C Bladder Neck D Urethra	0 Open 4 Percutaneous Endoscopic	Z No Device	Z No Qualifier

0 Medical and Surgical
T Urinary System
T Resection Cutting out or off, without replacement, all of a body part

Body Part Character 4	Approach Character 5	Device Character 6	Qualifier Character 7
0 Kidney, Right 1 Kidney, Left 2 Kidneys, Bilateral	0 Open 4 Percutaneous Endoscopic	Z No Device	Z No Qualifier
3 Kidney Pelvis, Right 4 Kidney Pelvis, Left 6 Ureter, Right 7 Ureter, Left B Bladder C Bladder Neck D Urethra	0 Open 4 Percutaneous Endoscopic 7 Via Natural or Artificial Opening 8 Via Natural or Artificial Opening Endoscopic	Z No Device	Z No Qualifier

0 Medical and Surgical
T Urinary System
U Supplement Putting in or on biological or synthetic material that physically reinforces and/or augments the function of a portion of a body part

Body Part Character 4	Approach Character 5	Device Character 6	Qualifier Character 7
3 Kidney Pelvis, Right 4 Kidney Pelvis, Left 6 Ureter, Right 7 Ureter, Left B Bladder C Bladder Neck	0 Open 4 Percutaneous Endoscopic 7 Via Natural or Artificial Opening 8 Via Natural or Artificial Opening Endoscopic	7 Autologous Tissue Substitute J Synthetic Substitute K Nonautologous Tissue Substitute	Z No Qualifier
D Urethra	0 Open 4 Percutaneous Endoscopic 7 Via Natural or Artificial Opening 8 Via Natural or Artificial Opening Endoscopic X External	7 Autologous Tissue Substitute J Synthetic Substitute K Nonautologous Tissue Substitute	Z No Qualifier

0 Medical and Surgical
T Urinary System
V Restriction Partially closing an orifice or the lumen of a tubular body part

Body Part Character 4	Approach Character 5	Device Character 6	Qualifier Character 7
3 Kidney Pelvis, Right 4 Kidney Pelvis, Left 6 Ureter, Right 7 Ureter, Left B Bladder C Bladder Neck D Urethra	0 Open 3 Percutaneous 4 Percutaneous Endoscopic	C Extraluminal Device D Intraluminal Device Z No Device	Z No Qualifier
3 Kidney Pelvis, Right 4 Kidney Pelvis, Left 6 Ureter, Right 7 Ureter, Left B Bladder C Bladder Neck D Urethra	7 Via Natural or Artificial Opening 8 Via Natural or Artificial Opening Endoscopic	D Intraluminal Device Z No Device	Z No Qualifier
D Urethra	X External	Z No Device	Z No Qualifier

Ø Medical and Surgical
T Urinary System
W Revision Correcting, to the extent possible, a portion of a malfunctioning device or the position of a displaced device

Body Part Character 4	Approach Character 5	Device Character 6	Qualifier Character 7
5 Kidney	**Ø** Open **3** Percutaneous **4** Percutaneous Endoscopic **7** Via Natural or Artificial Opening **8** Via Natural or Artificial Opening Endoscopic **X** External	**Ø** Drainage Device **2** Monitoring Device **3** Infusion Device **7** Autologous Tissue Substitute **C** Extraluminal Device **D** Intraluminal Device **J** Synthetic Substitute **K** Nonautologous Tissue Substitute	**Z** No Qualifier
9 Ureter	**Ø** Open **3** Percutaneous **4** Percutaneous Endoscopic **7** Via Natural or Artificial Opening **8** Via Natural or Artificial Opening Endoscopic **X** External	**Ø** Drainage Device **2** Monitoring Device **3** Infusion Device **7** Autologous Tissue Substitute **C** Extraluminal Device **D** Intraluminal Device **J** Synthetic Substitute **K** Nonautologous Tissue Substitute **M** Stimulator Lead	**Z** No Qualifier
B Bladder	**Ø** Open **3** Percutaneous **4** Percutaneous Endoscopic **7** Via Natural or Artificial Opening **8** Via Natural or Artificial Opening Endoscopic **X** External	**Ø** Drainage Device **2** Monitoring Device **3** Infusion Device **7** Autologous Tissue Substitute **C** Extraluminal Device **D** Intraluminal Device **J** Synthetic Substitute **K** Nonautologous Tissue Substitute **L** Artificial Sphincter **M** Stimulator Lead	**Z** No Qualifier
D Urethra	**Ø** Open **3** Percutaneous **4** Percutaneous Endoscopic **7** Via Natural or Artificial Opening **8** Via Natural or Artificial Opening Endoscopic **X** External	**Ø** Drainage Device **2** Monitoring Device **3** Infusion Device **7** Autologous Tissue Substitute **C** Extraluminal Device **D** Intraluminal Device **J** Synthetic Substitute **K** Nonautologous Tissue Substitute **L** Artificial Sphincter	**Z** No Qualifier

Ø Medical and Surgical
T Urinary System
Y Transplantation Putting in or on all or a portion of a living body part taken from another individual or animal to physically take the place and/or function of all or a portion of a similar body part

Body Part Character 4	Approach Character 5	Device Character 6	Qualifier Character 7
Ø Kidney, Right **1** Kidney, Left	**Ø** Open	**Z** No Device	**Ø** Allogeneic **1** Syngeneic **2** Zooplastic

Female Reproductive System 0U1–0UY

0 Medical and Surgical
U Female Reproductive System
1 Bypass Altering the route of passage of the contents of a tubular body part

Body Part Character 4	Approach Character 5	Device Character 6	Qualifier Character 7
5 Fallopian Tube, Right 6 Fallopian Tube, Left	0 Open 4 Percutaneous Endoscopic	7 Autologous Tissue Substitute J Synthetic Substitute K Nonautologous Tissue Substitute Z No Device	5 Fallopian Tube, Right 6 Fallopian Tube, Left 9 Uterus

0 Medical and Surgical
U Female Reproductive System
2 Change Taking out or off a device from a body part and putting back an identical or similar device in or on the same body part without cutting or puncturing the skin or a mucous membrane

Body Part Character 4	Approach Character 5	Device Character 6	Qualifier Character 7
3 Ovary 8 Fallopian Tube M Vulva	X External	0 Drainage Device Y Other Device	Z No Qualifier
D Uterus and Cervix	X External	0 Drainage Device H Contraceptive Device Y Other Device	Z No Qualifier
H Vagina and Cul-de-sac	X External	0 Drainage Device G Pessary Y Other Device	Z No Qualifier

0 Medical and Surgical
U Female Reproductive System
5 Destruction Physical eradication of all or a portion of a body part by the direct use of energy, force, or a destructive agent

Body Part Character 4	Approach Character 5	Device Character 6	Qualifier Character 7
0 Ovary, Right 1 Ovary, Left 2 Ovaries, Bilateral 4 Uterine Supporting Structure	0 Open 3 Percutaneous 4 Percutaneous Endoscopic	Z No Device	Z No Qualifier
5 Fallopian Tube, Right 6 Fallopian Tube, Left 7 Fallopian Tubes, Bilateral 9 Uterus B Endometrium C Cervix F Cul-de-sac	0 Open 3 Percutaneous 4 Percutaneous Endoscopic 7 Via Natural or Artificial Opening 8 Via Natural or Artificial Opening Endoscopic	Z No Device	Z No Qualifier
G Vagina **K Hymen**	0 Open 3 Percutaneous 4 Percutaneous Endoscopic 7 Via Natural or Artificial Opening 8 Via Natural or Artificial Opening Endoscopic X External	Z No Device	Z No Qualifier
J Clitoris L Vestibular Gland M Vulva	0 Open X External	Z No Device	Z No Qualifier

Ø Medical and Surgical
U Female Reproductive System
7 Dilation Expanding an orifice or lumen of a tabular body part

Body Part Character 4	Approach Character 5	Device Character 6	Qualifier Character 7
5 Fallopian Tube, Right 6 Fallopian Tube, Left 7 Fallopian Tubes, Bilateral 9 Uterus C Cervix G Vagina	Ø Open 3 Percutaneous 4 Percutaneous Endoscopic 7 Via Natural or Artificial Opening 8 Via Natural or Artificial Opening Endoscopic	D Intraluminal Device Z No Device	Z No Qualifier
K Hymen	Ø Open 3 Percutaneous 4 Percutaneous Endoscopic 7 Via Natural or Artificial Opening 8 Via Natural or Artificial Opening Endoscopic X External	D Intraluminal Device Z No Device	Z No Qualifier

Ø Medical and Surgical
U Female Reproductive System
8 Division Cutting into a body part without draining fluids and/or gases from the body part in order to separate or transect a body part

Body Part Character 4	Approach Character 5	Device Character 6	Qualifier Character 7
Ø Ovary, Right 1 Ovary, Left 2 Ovaries, Bilateral 4 Uterine Supporting Structure	Ø Open 3 Percutaneous 4 Percutaneous Endoscopic	Z No Device	Z No Qualifier
K Hymen	7 Via Natural or Artificial Opening 8 Via Natural or Artificial Opening Endoscopic **X External**	Z No Device	Z No Qualifier

Ø Medical and Surgical
U Female Reproductive System
9 Drainage Taking or letting out fluids and/or gases from a body part

Body Part Character 4	Approach Character 5	Device Character 6	Qualifier Character 7
Ø Ovary, Right 1 Ovary, Left 2 Ovaries, Bilateral	X External	Z No Device	Z No Qualifier
Ø Ovary, Right 1 Ovary, Left 2 Ovaries, Bilateral 4 Uterine Supporting Structure	Ø Open 3 Percutaneous 4 Percutaneous Endoscopic	Ø Drainage Device	Z No Qualifier
Ø Ovary, Right 1 Ovary, Left 2 Ovaries, Bilateral 4 Uterine Supporting Structure	Ø Open 3 Percutaneous 4 Percutaneous Endoscopic	Z No Device	X Diagnostic Z No Qualifier
5 Fallopian Tube, Right 6 Fallopian Tube, Left 7 Fallopian Tubes, Bilateral 9 Uterus C Cervix F Cul-de-sac	Ø Open 3 Percutaneous 4 Percutaneous Endoscopic 7 Via Natural or Artificial Opening 8 Via Natural or Artificial Opening Endoscopic	Ø Drainage Device	Z No Qualifier
5 Fallopian Tube, Right 6 Fallopian Tube, Left 7 Fallopian Tubes, Bilateral 9 Uterus C Cervix F Cul-de-sac	Ø Open 3 Percutaneous 4 Percutaneous Endoscopic 7 Via Natural or Artificial Opening 8 Via Natural or Artificial Opening Endoscopic	Z No Device	X Diagnostic Z No Qualifier

ØU9 Continued on next page

0 Medical and Surgicall
U Female Reproductive System
9 Drainage Taking or letting out fluids and/or gases from a body part

0U9 Continued

Body Part Character 4	Approach Character 5	Device Character 6	Qualifier Character 7
G Vagina K **Hymen**	0 Open 3 Percutaneous 4 Percutaneous Endoscopic 7 Via Natural or Artificial Opening 8 Via Natural or Artificial Opening Endoscopic X External	0 Drainage Device	Z No Qualifier
G Vagina K **Hymen**	0 Open 3 Percutaneous 4 Percutaneous Endoscopic 7 Via Natural or Artificial Opening 8 Via Natural or Artificial Opening Endoscopic X External	Z No Device	X Diagnostic Z No Qualifier
J Clitoris L Vestibular Gland M Vulva	0 Open X External	0 Drainage Device	Z No Qualifier
J Clitoris L Vestibular Gland M Vulva	0 Open X External	Z No Device	X Diagnostic Z No Qualifier

0 Medical and Surgical
U Female Reproductive System
B Excision Cutting out or off, without replacement, a portion of a body part

Body Part Character 4	Approach Character 5	Device Character 6	Qualifier Character 7
0 Ovary, Right 1 Ovary, Left 2 Ovaries, Bilateral 4 Uterine Supporting Structure 5 Fallopian Tube, Right 6 Fallopian Tube, Left 7 Fallopian Tubes, Bilateral 9 Uterus C Cervix F Cul-de-sac	0 Open 3 Percutaneous 4 Percutaneous Endoscopic 7 Via Natural or Artificial Opening 8 Via Natural or Artificial Opening Endoscopic	Z No Device	X Diagnostic Z No Qualifier
G Vagina K **Hymen**	0 Open 3 Percutaneous 4 Percutaneous Endoscopic 7 Via Natural or Artificial Opening 8 Via Natural or Artificial Opening Endoscopic X External	Z No Device	X Diagnostic Z No Qualifier
J Clitoris L Vestibular Gland M Vulva	0 Open X External	Z No Device	X Diagnostic Z No Qualifier

Ø Medical and Surgical
U Female Reproductive System
C Extirpation Taking or cutting out solid matter from a body part

Body Part Character 4	Approach Character 5	Device Character 6	Qualifier Character 7
Ø Ovary, Right **1** Ovary, Left **2** Ovaries, Bilateral **4** Uterine Supporting Structure	**Ø** Open **3** Percutaneous **4** Percutaneous Endoscopic	**Z** No Device	**Z** No Qualifier
5 Fallopian Tube, Right **6** Fallopian Tube, Left **7** Fallopian Tubes, Bilateral **9** Uterus **B** Endometrium **C** Cervix **F** Cul-de-sac	**Ø** Open **3** Percutaneous **4** Percutaneous Endoscopic **7** Via Natural or Artificial Opening **8** Via Natural or Artificial Opening Endoscopic	**Z** No Device	**Z** No Qualifier
G Vagina **K** Hymen	**Ø** Open **3** Percutaneous **4** Percutaneous Endoscopic **7** Via Natural or Artificial Opening **8** Via Natural or Artificial Opening Endoscopic **X** External	**Z** No Device	**Z** No Qualifier
J Clitoris **L** Vestibular Gland **M** Vulva	**Ø** Open **X** External	**Z** No Device	**Z** No Qualifier

Ø Medical and Surgical
U Female Reproductive System
D Extraction Pulling or stripping out or off all or a portion of a body part by the use of force

Body Part Character 4	Approach Character 5	Device Character 6	Qualifier Character 7
B Endometrium	**7** Via Natural or Artificial Opening **8** Via Natural or Artificial Opening Endoscopic	**Z** No Device	**X** Diagnostic **Z** No Qualifier
N Ova	**Ø** Open **3** Percutaneous **4** Percutaneous Endoscopic	**Z** No Device	**Z** No Qualifier

Ø Medical and Surgical
U Female Reproductive System
F Fragmentation Breaking solid matter in a body part into pieces

Body Part Character 4	Approach Character 5	Device Character 6	Qualifier Character 7
5 Fallopian Tube, Right **6** Fallopian Tube, Left **7** Fallopian Tubes, Bilateral **9** Uterus	**Ø** Open **3** Percutaneous **4** Percutaneous Endoscopic **7** Via Natural or Artificial Opening **8** Via Natural or Artificial Opening Endoscopic **X** External	**Z** No Device	**Z** No Qualifier

0 Medical and Surgical
U Female Reproductive System
H Insertion Putting in a nonbiological appliance that monitors, assists, performs, or prevents a physiological function but does not physically take the place of a body part

Body Part Character 4	Approach Character 5	Device Character 6	Qualifier Character 7
3 Ovary	0 Open 3 Percutaneous 4 Percutaneous Endoscopic	3 Infusion Device	Z No Qualifier
8 Fallopian Tube D Uterus and Cervix H Vagina and Cul-de-sac	0 Open 3 Percutaneous 4 Percutaneous Endoscopic 7 Via Natural or Artificial Opening 8 Via Natural or Artificial Opening Endoscopic	3 Infusion Device	Z No Qualifier
9 Uterus C Cervix	7 Via Natural or Artificial Opening 8 Via Natural or Artificial Opening Endoscopic	H Contraceptive Device	Z No Qualifier
C Cervix	0 Open 3 Percutaneous 4 Percutaneous Endoscopic 7 Via Natural or Artificial Opening 8 Via Natural or Artificial Opening Endoscopic	**1 Radioactive Element**	Z No Qualifier
F Cul-de-sac	7 Via Natural or Artificial Opening 8 Via Natural or Artificial Opening Endoscopic	**G Intraluminal Device, Pessary**	Z No Qualifier
G Vagina	0 Open 3 Percutaneous 4 Percutaneous Endoscopic X External	1 Radioactive Element	Z No Qualifier
G Vagina	7 Via Natural or Artificial Opening 8 Via Natural or Artificial Opening Endoscopic	1 Radioactive Element **G Intraluminal Device, Pessary**	Z No Qualifier

0 Medical and Surgical
U Female Reproductive System
J Inspection Visually and/or manually exploring a body part

Body Part Character 4	Approach Character 5	Device Character 6	Qualifier Character 7
3 Ovary	0 Open 3 Percutaneous 4 Percutaneous Endoscopic X External	Z No Device	Z No Qualifier
8 Fallopian Tube D Uterus and Cervix H Vagina and Cul-de-sac	0 Open 3 Percutaneous 4 Percutaneous Endoscopic 7 Via Natural or Artificial Opening 8 Via Natural or Artificial Opening Endoscopic X External	Z No Device	Z No Qualifier
M Vulva	0 Open X External	Z No Device	Z No Qualifier

0 Medical and Surgical
U Female Reproductive System
L Occlusion Completely closing an orifice or the lumen of a tubular body part

Body Part Character 4	Approach Character 5	Device Character 6	Qualifier Character 7
5 Fallopian Tube, Right 6 Fallopian Tube, Left 7 Fallopian Tubes, Bilateral	0 Open 3 Percutaneous 4 Percutaneous Endoscopic	C Extraluminal Device D Intraluminal Device Z No Device	Z No Qualifier
5 Fallopian Tube, Right 6 Fallopian Tube, Left 7 Fallopian Tubes, Bilateral F Cul-de-sac G Vagina	7 Via Natural or Artificial Opening 8 Via Natural or Artificial Opening Endoscopic	D Intraluminal Device Z No Device	Z No Qualifier

Ø Medical and Surgical
U Female Reproductive System
M Reattachment Putting back in or on all or a portion of a separated body part to its normal location or other suitable location

Body Part Character 4	Approach Character 5	Device Character 6	Qualifier Character 7
Ø Ovary, Right **1** Ovary, Left **2** Ovaries, Bilateral **4** Uterine Supporting Structure **5** Fallopian Tube, Right **6** Fallopian Tube, Left **7** Fallopian Tubes, Bilateral **9** Uterus **C** Cervix **F** Cul-de-sac **G** Vagina **K** Hymen	**Ø** Open **4** Percutaneous Endoscopic	**Z** No Device	**Z** No Qualifier
J Clitoris **M** Vulva	**X** External	**Z** No Device	**Z** No Qualifier
K Hymen	**Ø** Open **4** Percutaneous **X** External	**Z** No Device	**Z** No Qualifier

Ø Medical and Surgical
U Female Reproductive System
N Release Freeing a body part from an abnormal physical constraint

Body Part Character 4	Approach Character 5	Device Character 6	Qualifier Character 7
Ø Ovary, Right **1** Ovary, Left **2** Ovaries, Bilateral **4** Uterine Supporting Structure	**Ø** Open **3** Percutaneous **4** Percutaneous Endoscopic	**Z** No Device	**Z** No Qualifier
5 Fallopian Tube, Right **6** Fallopian Tube, Left **7** Fallopian Tubes, Bilateral **9** Uterus **C** Cervix **F** Cul-de-sac	**Ø** Open **3** Percutaneous **4** Percutaneous Endoscopic **7** Via Natural or Artificial Opening **8** Via Natural or Artificial Opening Endoscopic	**Z** No Device	**Z** No Qualifier
G Vagina **K Hymen**	**Ø** Open **3** Percutaneous **4** Percutaneous Endoscopic **7** Via Natural or Artificial Opening **8** Via Natural or Artificial Opening Endoscopic **X** External	**Z** No Device	**Z** No Qualifier
J Clitoris **L** Vestibular Gland **M** Vulva	**Ø** Open **X** External	**Z** No Device	**Z** No Qualifier

0 Medical and Surgical
U Female Reproductive System
P Removal Taking out or off a device from a body part

Body Part Character 4	Approach Character 5	Device Character 6	Qualifier Character 7
3 Ovary	0 Open 3 Percutaneous 4 Percutaneous Endoscopic X External	0 Drainage Device 3 Infusion Device	Z No Qualifier
8 Fallopian Tube	0 Open 3 Percutaneous 4 Percutaneous Endoscopic 7 Via Natural or Artificial Opening 8 Via Natural or Artificial Opening Endoscopic	0 Drainage Device 3 Infusion Device 7 Autologous Tissue Substitute C Extraluminal Device D Intraluminal Device J Synthetic Substitute K Nonautologous Tissue Substitute	Z No Qualifier
8 Fallopian Tube	X External	0 Drainage Device 3 Infusion Device D Intraluminal Device	Z No Qualifier
D Uterus and Cervix	0 Open 3 Percutaneous 4 Percutaneous Endoscopic 7 Via Natural or Artificial Opening 8 Via Natural or Artificial Opening Endoscopic	0 Drainage Device **1 Radioactive Element** 3 Infusion Device 7 Autologous Tissue Substitute C Extraluminal Device D Intraluminal Device H Contraceptive Device J Synthetic Substitute K Nonautologous Tissue Substitute	Z No Qualifier
D Uterus and Cervix	X External	0 Drainage Device 3 Infusion Device D Intraluminal Device H Contraceptive Device	Z No Qualifier
H Vagina and Cul-de-sac	0 Open 3 Percutaneous 4 Percutaneous Endoscopic 7 Via Natural or Artificial Opening 8 Via Natural or Artificial Opening Endoscopic	0 Drainage Device **1 Radioactive Element** 3 Infusion Device 7 Autologous Tissue Substitute D Intraluminal Device J Synthetic Substitute K Nonautologous Tissue Substitute	Z No Qualifier
H Vagina and Cul-de-sac	X External	0 Drainage Device 1 Radioactive Element 3 Infusion Device D Intraluminal Device	Z No Qualifier
M Vulva	0 Open	0 Drainage Device 7 Autologous Tissue Substitute J Synthetic Substitute K Nonautologous Tissue Substitute	Z No Qualifier
M Vulva	X External	0 Drainage Device	Z No Qualifier

0 Medical and Surgical
U Female Reproductive System
Q Repair Restoring, to the extent possible, a body part to its normal anatomic structure and function

Body Part Character 4	Approach Character 5	Device Character 6	Qualifier Character 7
0 Ovary, Right 1 Ovary, Left 2 Ovaries, Bilateral 4 Uterine Supporting Structure	0 Open 3 Percutaneous 4 Percutaneous Endoscopic	Z No Device	Z No Qualifier
5 Fallopian Tube, Right 6 Fallopian Tube, Left 7 Fallopian Tubes, Bilateral 9 Uterus C Cervix F Cul-de-sac	0 Open 3 Percutaneous 4 Percutaneous Endoscopic 7 Via Natural or Artificial Opening 8 Via Natural or Artificial Opening Endoscopic	Z No Device	Z No Qualifier
G Vagina **K Hymen**	0 Open 3 Percutaneous 4 Percutaneous Endoscopic 7 Via Natural or Artificial Opening 8 Via Natural or Artificial Opening Endoscopic X External	Z No Device	Z No Qualifier
J Clitoris L Vestibular Gland M Vulva	0 Open X External	Z No Device	Z No Qualifier

Ø Medical and Surgical
U Female Reproductive System
S Reposition Moving to its normal location or other suitable location all or a portion of a body part

Body Part Character 4	Approach Character 5	Device Character 6	Qualifier Character 7
Ø Ovary, Right 1 Ovary, Left 2 Ovaries, Bilateral 4 Uterine Supporting Structure 5 Fallopian Tube, Right 6 Fallopian Tube, Left 7 Fallopian Tubes, Bilateral C Cervix F Cul-de-sac	Ø Open 4 Percutaneous Endoscopic	Z No Device	Z No Qualifier
9 Uterus G Vagina	Ø Open 4 Percutaneous Endoscopic X External	Z No Device	Z No Qualifier

Ø Medical and Surgical
U Female Reproductive System
T Resection Cutting out or off, without replacement, all of a body part

Body Part Character 4	Approach Character 5	Device Character 6	Qualifier Character 7
Ø Ovary, Right 1 Ovary, Left 2 Ovaries, Bilateral 5 Fallopian Tube, Right 6 Fallopian Tube, Left 7 Fallopian Tubes, Bilateral 9 Uterus	Ø Open 4 Percutaneous Endoscopic 7 Via Natural or Artificial Opening 8 Via Natural or Artificial Opening Endoscopic F Via Natural or Artificial Opening With Percutaneous Endoscopic Assistance	Z No Device	Z No Qualifier
4 Uterine Supporting Structure C Cervix F Cul-de-sac G Vagina K Hymen	Ø Open 4 Percutaneous Endoscopic 7 Via Natural or Artificial Opening 8 Via Natural or Artificial Opening Endoscopic	Z No Device	Z No Qualifier
J Clitoris L Vestibular Gland M Vulva	Ø Open X External	Z No Device	Z No Qualifier
K Hymen	Ø Open 4 Percutaneous Endoscopic 7 Via Natural or Artificial Opening 8 Via Natural or Artificial Opening Endoscopic X External	Z No Device	Z No Device

Ø Medical and Surgical
U Female Reproductive System
U Supplement Putting in or on biological or synthetic material that physically reinforces and/or augments the function of a portion of a body part

Body Part Character 4	Approach Character 5	Device Character 6	Qualifier Character 7
4 Uterine Supporting Structure	Ø Open 4 Percutaneous Endoscopic	7 Autologous Tissue Substitute J Synthetic Substitute K Nonautologous Tissue Substitute	Z No Qualifier
5 Fallopian Tube, Right 6 Fallopian Tube, Left 7 Fallopian Tubes, Bilateral F Cul-de-sac	Ø Open 4 Percutaneous Endoscopic 7 Via Natural or Artificial Opening 8 Via Natural or Artificial Opening Endoscopic	7 Autologous Tissue Substitute J Synthetic Substitute K Nonautologous Tissue Substitute	Z No Qualifier
G Vagina **K Hymen**	Ø Open 4 Percutaneous Endoscopic 7 Via Natural or Artificial Opening 8 Via Natural or Artificial Opening Endoscopic X External	7 Autologous Tissue Substitute J Synthetic Substitute K Nonautologous Tissue Substitute	Z No Qualifier
J Clitoris M Vulva	Ø Open X External	7 Autologous Tissue Substitute J Synthetic Substitute K Nonautologous Tissue Substitute	Z No Qualifier

0 Medical and Surgical
U Female Reproductive System
V Restriction Partially closing an orifice or the lumen of a tubular body part

Body Part Character 4	Approach Character 5	Device Character 6	Qualifier Character 7
C Cervix	0 Open 3 Percutaneous 4 Percutaneous Endoscopic	C Extraluminal Device D Intraluminal Device Z No Device	Z No Qualifier
C Cervix	7 Via Natural or Artificial Opening 8 Via Natural or Artificial Opening Endoscopic	D Intraluminal Device Z No Device	Z No Qualifier

0 Medical and Surgical
U Female Reproductive System
W Revision Correcting, to the extent possible, a portion of a malfunctioning device or the position of a displaced device

Body Part Character 4	Approach Character 5	Device Character 6	Qualifier Character 7
3 Ovary	0 Open 3 Percutaneous 4 Percutaneous Endoscopic X External	0 Drainage Device 3 Infusion Device	Z No Qualifier
8 Fallopian Tube	0 Open 3 Percutaneous 4 Percutaneous Endoscopic 7 Via Natural or Artificial Opening 8 Via Natural or Artificial Opening Endoscopic X External	0 Drainage Device 3 Infusion Device 7 Autologous Tissue Substitute C Extraluminal Device D Intraluminal Device J Synthetic Substitute K Nonautologous Tissue Substitute	Z No Qualifier
D Uterus and Cervix	0 Open 3 Percutaneous 4 Percutaneous Endoscopic 7 Via Natural or Artificial Opening 8 Via Natural or Artificial Opening Endoscopic X External	0 Drainage Device **1 Radioactive Element** 3 Infusion Device 7 Autologous Tissue Substitute C Extraluminal Device D Intraluminal Device H Contraceptive Device J Synthetic Substitute K Nonautologous Tissue Substitute	Z No Qualifier
H Vagina and Cul-de-sac	0 Open 3 Percutaneous 4 Percutaneous Endoscopic 7 Via Natural or Artificial Opening 8 Via Natural or Artificial Opening Endoscopic X External	0 Drainage Device **1 Radioactive Element** 3 Infusion Device 7 Autologous Tissue Substitute D Intraluminal Device J Synthetic Substitute K Nonautologous Tissue Substitute	Z No Qualifier
M Vulva	0 Open X External	0 Drainage Device 7 Autologous Tissue Substitute J Synthetic Substitute K Nonautologous Tissue Substitute	Z No Qualifier

0 Medical and Surgical
U Female Reproductive System
Y Transplantation Putting in or on all or a portion of a living body part taken from another individual or animal to physically take the place and/or function of all or a portion of a similar body part

Body Part Character 4	Approach Character 5	Device Character 6	Qualifier Character 7
0 Ovary, Right 1 Ovary, Left	0 Open	Z No Device	0 Allogeneic 1 Syngeneic 2 Zooplastic

Male Reproductive System ØV1–ØVW

Ø Medical and Surgical
V Male Reproductive System
1 Bypass Altering the route of passage of the contents of a tubular body part

Body Part Character 4	Approach Character 5	Device Character 6	Qualifier Character 7
N Vas Deferens, Right P Vas Deferens, Left Q Vas Deferens, Bilateral	Ø Open 4 Percutaneous Endoscopic	7 Autologous Tissue Substitute J Synthetic Substitute K Nonautologous Tissue Substitute Z No Device	J Epididymis, Right K Epididymis, Left N Vas Deferens, Right P Vas Deferens, Left

Ø Medical and Surgical
V Male Reproductive System
2 Change Taking out or off a device from a body part and putting back an identical or similar device in or on the same body part without cutting or puncturing the skin or a mucous membrane

Body Part Character 4	Approach Character 5	Device Character 6	Qualifier Character 7
4 Prostate and Seminal Vesicles 8 Scrotum and Tunica Vaginalis D Testis M Epididymis and Spermatic Cord R Vas Deferens S Penis	X External	Ø Drainage Device Y Other Device	Z No Qualifier

Ø Medical and Surgical
V Male Reproductive System
5 Destruction Physical eradication of all or a portion of a body part by the direct use of energy, force, or a destructive agent

Body Part Character 4	Approach Character 5	Device Character 6	Qualifier Character 7
Ø Prostate	Ø Open 3 Percutaneous 4 Percutaneous Endoscopic 7 Via Natural or Artificial Opening 8 Via Natural or Artificial Opening Endoscopic	Z No Device	Z No Qualifier
1 Seminal Vesicle, Right 2 Seminal Vesicle, Left 3 Seminal Vesicles, Bilateral 6 Tunica Vaginalis, Right 7 Tunica Vaginalis, Left 9 Testis, Right B Testis, Left C Testes, Bilateral F Spermatic Cord, Right G Spermatic Cord, Left H Spermatic Cords, Bilateral J Epididymis, Right K Epididymis, Left L Epididymis, Bilateral N Vas Deferens, Right P Vas Deferens, Left Q Vas Deferens, Bilateral	Ø Open 3 Percutaneous 4 Percutaneous Endoscopic	Z No Device	Z No Qualifier
5 Scrotum S Penis T Prepuce	Ø Open 3 Percutaneous 4 Percutaneous Endoscopic X External	Z No Device	Z No Qualifier

Ø Medical and Surgical
V Male Reproductive System
7 Dilation Expanding an orifice or the lumen of a tubular body part

Body Part Character 4	Approach Character 5	Device Character 6	Qualifier Character 7
N Vas Deferens, Right P Vas Deferens, Left Q Vas Deferens, Bilateral	Ø Open 3 Percutaneous 4 Percutaneous Endoscopic	D Intraluminal Device Z No Device	Z No Qualifier

0 Medical and Surgical
V Male Reproductive System
9 Drainage Taking or letting out fluids and/or gases from a body part

Body Part Character 4	Approach Character 5	Device Character 6	Qualifier Character 7
0 Prostate	0 Open 3 Percutaneous 4 Percutaneous Endoscopic 7 Via Natural or Artificial Opening 8 Via Natural or Artificial Opening Endoscopic	0 Drainage Device	Z No Qualifier
0 Prostate	0 Open 3 Percutaneous 4 Percutaneous Endoscopic 7 Via Natural or Artificial Opening 8 Via Natural or Artificial Opening Endoscopic	Z No Device	X Diagnostic Z No Qualifier
1 Seminal Vesicle, Right 2 Seminal Vesicle, Left 3 Seminal Vesicles, Bilateral 6 Tunica Vaginalis, Right 7 Tunica Vaginalis, Left 9 Testis, Right B Testis, Left C Testes, Bilateral F Spermatic Cord, Right G Spermatic Cord, Left H Spermatic Cords, Bilateral J Epididymis, Right K Epididymis, Left L Epididymis, Bilateral N Vas Deferens, Right P Vas Deferens, Left Q Vas Deferens, Bilateral	0 Open 3 Percutaneous 4 Percutaneous Endoscopic	0 Drainage Device	Z No Qualifier
1 Seminal Vesicle, Right 2 Seminal Vesicle, Left 3 Seminal Vesicles, Bilateral 6 Tunica Vaginalis, Right 7 Tunica Vaginalis, Left 9 Testis, Right B Testis, Left C Testes, Bilateral F Spermatic Cord, Right G Spermatic Cord, Left H Spermatic Cords, Bilateral J Epididymis, Right K Epididymis, Left L Epididymis, Bilateral N Vas Deferens, Right P Vas Deferens, Left Q Vas Deferens, Bilateral	0 Open 3 Percutaneous 4 Percutaneous Endoscopic	Z No Device	X Diagnostic Z No Qualifier
5 Scrotum S Penis T Prepuce	0 Open 3 Percutaneous 4 Percutaneous Endoscopic X External	0 Drainage Device	Z No Qualifier
5 Scrotum S Penis T Prepuce	0 Open 3 Percutaneous 4 Percutaneous Endoscopic X External	Z No Device	X Diagnostic Z No Qualifier

Ø Medical and Surgical
V Male Reproductive System
B Excision Cutting out or off, without replacement, a portion of a body part

Body Part Character 4	Approach Character 5	Device Character 6	Qualifier Character 7
Ø Prostate	**Ø** Open **3** Percutaneous **4** Percutaneous Endoscopic **7** Via Natural or Artificial Opening **8** Via Natural or Artificial Opening Endoscopic	**Z** No Device	**X** Diagnostic **Z** No Qualifier
1 Seminal Vesicle, Right **2** Seminal Vesicle, Left **3** Seminal Vesicles, Bilateral **6** Tunica Vaginalis, Right **7** Tunica Vaginalis, Left **9** Testis, Right **B** Testis, Left **C** Testes, Bilateral **F** Spermatic Cord, Right **G** Spermatic Cord, Left **H** Spermatic Cords, Bilateral **J** Epididymis, Right **K** Epididymis, Left **L** Epididymis, Bilateral **N** Vas Deferens, Right **P** Vas Deferens, Left **Q** Vas Deferens, Bilateral	**Ø** Open **3** Percutaneous **4** Percutaneous Endoscopic	**Z** No Device	**X** Diagnostic **Z** No Qualifier
5 Scrotum **S** Penis **T** Prepuce	**Ø** Open **3** Percutaneous **4** Percutaneous Endoscopic **X** External	**Z** No Device	**X** Diagnostic **Z** No Qualifier

Ø Medical and Surgical
V Male Reproductive System
C Extirpation Taking or cutting out solid matter from a body part

Body Part Character 4	Approach Character 5	Device Character 6	Qualifier Character 7
Ø Prostate	**Ø** Open **3** Percutaneous **4** Percutaneous Endoscopic **7** Via Natural or Artificial Opening **8** Via Natural or Artificial Opening Endoscopic	**Z** No Device	**Z** No Qualifier
1 Seminal Vesicle, Right **2** Seminal Vesicle, Left **3** Seminal Vesicles, Bilateral **6** Tunica Vaginalis, Right **7** Tunica Vaginalis, Left **9** Testis, Right **B** Testis, Left **C** Testes, Bilateral **F** Spermatic Cord, Right **G** Spermatic Cord, Left **H** Spermatic Cords, Bilateral **J** Epididymis, Right **K** Epididymis, Left **L** Epididymis, Bilateral **N** Vas Deferens, Right **P** Vas Deferens, Left **Q** Vas Deferens, Bilateral	**Ø** Open **3** Percutaneous **4** Percutaneous Endoscopic	**Z** No Device	**Z** No Qualifier
5 Scrotum **S** Penis **T** Prepuce	**Ø** Open **3** Percutaneous **4** Percutaneous Endoscopic **X** External	**Z** No Device	**Z** No Qualifier

0 Medical and Surgical
V Male Reproductive System
H Insertion Putting in a nonbiological appliance that monitors, assists, performs, or prevents a physiological function but does not physically take the place of a body part

Body Part Character 4	Approach Character 5	Device Character 6	Qualifier Character 7
0 Prostate	**0** Open **3** Percutaneous **4** Percutaneous Endoscopic **7** Via Natural or Artificial Opening **8** Via Natural or Artificial Opening Endoscopic	**1** Radioactive Element	**Z** No Qualifier
4 Prostate and Seminal Vesicles **8** Scrotum and Tunica Vaginalis **D** Testis **M** Epididymis and Spermatic Cord **R** Vas Deferens	**0** Open **3** Percutaneous **4** Percutaneous Endoscopic **7** Via Natural or Artificial Opening **8** Via Natural or Artificial Opening Endoscopic	**3** Infusion Device	**Z** No Qualifier
S Penis	**0** Open **3** Percutaneous **4** Percutaneous Endoscopic **X** External	**3** Infusion Device	**Z** No Qualifier

0 Medical and Surgical
V Male Reproductive System
J Inspection Visually and/or manually exploring a body part

Body Part Character 4	Approach Character 5	Device Character 6	Qualifier Character 7
4 Prostate and Seminal Vesicles **8** Scrotum and Tunica Vaginalis **D** Testis **M** Epididymis and Spermatic Cord **R** Vas Deferens **S** Penis	**0** Open **3** Percutaneous **4** Percutaneous Endoscopic **X** External	**Z** No Device	**Z** No Qualifier

0 Medical and Surgical
V Male Reproductive System
L Occlusion Completely closing an orifice or the lumen of a tubular body part

Body Part Character 4	Approach Character 5	Device Character 6	Qualifier Character 7
F Spermatic Cord, Right **G** Spermatic Cord, Left **H** Spermatic Cords, Bilateral **N** Vas Deferens, Right **P** Vas Deferens, Left **Q** Vas Deferens, Bilateral	**0** Open **3** Percutaneous **4** Percutaneous Endoscopic	**C** Extraluminal Device **D** Intraluminal Device **Z** No Device	**Z** No Qualifier

0 Medical and Surgical
V Male Reproductive System
M Reattachment Putting back in or on all or a portion of a separated body part to its normal location or other suitable location

Body Part Character 4	Approach Character 5	Device Character 6	Qualifier Character 7
5 Scrotum **S** Penis	**X** External	**Z** No Device	**Z** No Qualifier
6 Tunica Vaginalis, Right **7** Tunica Vaginalis, Left **9** Testis, Right **B** Testis, Left **C** Testes, Bilateral **F** Spermatic Cord, Right **G** Spermatic Cord, Left **H** Spermatic Cords, Bilateral	**0** Open **4** Percutaneous Endoscopic	**Z** No Device	**Z** No Qualifier

Ø Medical and Surgical
V Male Reproductive System
N Release Freeing a body part from an abnormal physical constraint

Body Part Character 4	Approach Character 5	Device Character 6	Qualifier Character 7
Ø Prostate	**Ø** Open **3** Percutaneous **4** Percutaneous Endoscopic **7** Via Natural or Artificial Opening **8** Via Natural or Artificial Opening Endoscopic	**Z** No Device	**Z** No Qualifier
1 Seminal Vesicle, Right **2** Seminal Vesicle, Left **3** Seminal Vesicles, Bilateral **6** Tunica Vaginalis, Right **7** Tunica Vaginalis, Left **9** Testis, Right **B** Testis, Left **C** Testes, Bilateral **F** Spermatic Cord, Right **G** Spermatic Cord, Left **H** Spermatic Cords, Bilateral **J** Epididymis, Right **K** Epididymis, Left **L** Epididymis, Bilateral **N** Vas Deferens, Right **P** Vas Deferens, Left **Q** Vas Deferens, Bilateral	**Ø** Open **3** Percutaneous **4** Percutaneous Endoscopic	**Z** No Device	**Z** No Qualifier
5 Scrotum **S** Penis **T** Prepuce	**Ø** Open **3** Percutaneous **4** Percutaneous Endoscopic **X** External	**Z** No Device	**Z** No Qualifier

Ø Medical and Surgical
V Male Reproductive System
P Removal Taking out or off a device from a body part

Body Part Character 4	Approach Character 5	Device Character 6	Qualifier Character 7
4 Prostate and Seminal Vesicles	**Ø** Open **3** Percutaneous **4** Percutaneous Endoscopic **7** Via Natural or Artificial Opening **8** Via Natural or Artificial Opening Endoscopic	**Ø** Drainage Device **1** Radioactive Element **3** Infusion Device **7** Autologous Tissue Substitute **J** Synthetic Substitute **K** Nonautologous Tissue Substitute	**Z** No Qualifier
4 Prostate and Seminal Vesicles	**X** External	**Ø** Drainage Device **1** Radioactive Element **3** Infusion Device	**Z** No Qualifier
8 Scrotum and Tunica Vaginalis **D** Testis **M** Epididymis and Spermatic Cord **S** Penis	**X** External	**Ø** Drainage Device **3** Infusion Device	**Z** No Qualifier
8 Scrotum and Tunica Vaginalis **D** Testis **S** Penis	**Ø** Open **3** Percutaneous **4** Percutaneous Endoscopic **7** Via Natural or Artificial Opening **8** Via Natural or Artificial Opening Endoscopic	**Ø** Drainage Device **3** Infusion Device **7** Autologous Tissue Substitute **J** Synthetic Substitute **K** Nonautologous Tissue Substitute	**Z** No Qualifier
M Epididymis and Spermatic Cord	**Ø** Open **3** Percutaneous **4** Percutaneous Endoscopic **7** Via Natural or Artificial Opening **8** Via Natural or Artificial Opening Endoscopic	**Ø** Drainage Device **3** Infusion Device **7** Autologous Tissue Substitute **C** Extraluminal Device **J** Synthetic Substitute **K** Nonautologous Tissue Substitute	**Z** No Qualifier
R Vas Deferens	**Ø** Open **3** Percutaneous **4** Percutaneous Endoscopic **7** Via Natural or Artificial Opening **8** Via Natural or Artificial Opening Endoscopic	**Ø** Drainage Device **3** Infusion Device **7** Autologous Tissue Substitute **C** Extraluminal Device **D** Intraluminal Device **J** Synthetic Substitute **K** Nonautologous Tissue Substitute	**Z** No Qualifier
R Vas Deferens	**X** External	**Ø** Drainage Device **3** Infusion Device **D** Intraluminal Device	**Z** No Qualifier

0 Medical and Surgical
V Male Reproductive System
Q Repair Restoring, to the extent possible, a body part to its normal anatomic structure and function

Body Part Character 4	Approach Character 5	Device Character 6	Qualifier Character 7
0 Prostate	0 Open 3 Percutaneous 4 Percutaneous Endoscopic 7 Via Natural or Artificial Opening 8 Via Natural or Artificial Opening Endoscopic	Z No Device	Z No Qualifier
1 Seminal Vesicle, Right 2 Seminal Vesicle, Left 3 Seminal Vesicles, Bilateral 6 Tunica Vaginalis, Right 7 Tunica Vaginalis, Left 9 Testis, Right B Testis, Left C Testes, Bilateral F Spermatic Cord, Right G Spermatic Cord, Left H Spermatic Cords, Bilateral J Epididymis, Right K Epididymis, Left L Epididymis, Bilateral N Vas Deferens, Right P Vas Deferens, Left Q Vas Deferens, Bilateral	0 Open 3 Percutaneous 4 Percutaneous Endoscopic	Z No Device	Z No Qualifier
5 Scrotum S Penis T Prepuce	0 Open 3 Percutaneous 4 Percutaneous Endoscopic X External	Z No Device	Z No Qualifier

0 Medical and Surgical
V Male Reproductive System
R Replacement Putting in or on biological or synthetic material that physically takes the place and/or function of all or a portion of a body part

Body Part Character 4	Approach Character 5	Device Character 6	Qualifier Character 7
9 Testis, Right B Testis, Left C Testes, Bilateral	0 Open	J Synthetic Substitute	Z No Qualifier

0 Medical and Surgical
V Male Reproductive System
S Reposition Moving to its normal location or other suitable location all or a portion of a body part

Body Part Character 4	Approach Character 5	Device Character 6	Qualifier Character 7
9 Testis, Right B Testis, Left C Testes, Bilateral F Spermatic Cord, Right G Spermatic Cord, Left H Spermatic Cords, Bilateral	0 Open 3 Percutaneous 4 Percutaneous Endoscopic	Z No Device	Z No Qualifier

Ø Medical and Surgical
V Male Reproductive System
T Resection Cutting out or off, without replacement, all of a body part

Body Part Character 4	Approach Character 5	Device Character 6	Qualifier Character 7
Ø Prostate	Ø Open 4 Percutaneous Endoscopic 7 Via Natural or Artificial Opening 8 Via Natural or Artificial Opening Endoscopic	Z No Device	Z No Qualifier
1 Seminal Vesicle, Right 2 Seminal Vesicle, Left 3 Seminal Vesicles, Bilateral 6 Tunica Vaginalis, Right 7 Tunica Vaginalis, Left 9 Testis, Right B Testis, Left C Testes, Bilateral F Spermatic Cord, Right G Spermatic Cord, Left H Spermatic Cords, Bilateral J Epididymis, Right K Epididymis, Left L Epididymis, Bilateral N Vas Deferens, Right P Vas Deferens, Left Q Vas Deferens, Bilateral	Ø Open 4 Percutaneous Endoscopic	Z No Device	Z No Qualifier
5 Scrotum S Penis T Prepuce	Ø Open 4 Percutaneous Endoscopic X External	Z No Device	Z No Qualifier

Ø Medical and Surgical
V Male Reproductive System
U Supplement Putting in or on biological or synthetic material that physically reinforces and/or augments the function of a portion of a body part

Body Part Character 4	Approach Character 5	Device Character 6	Qualifier Character 7
1 Seminal Vesicle, Right 2 Seminal Vesicle, Left 3 Seminal Vesicles, Bilateral 6 Tunica Vaginalis, Right 7 Tunica Vaginalis, Left F Spermatic Cord, Right G Spermatic Cord, Left H Spermatic Cords, Bilateral J Epididymis, Right K Epididymis, Left L Epididymis, Bilateral N Vas Deferens, Right P Vas Deferens, Left Q Vas Deferens, Bilateral	Ø Open 4 Percutaneous Endoscopic	7 Autologous Tissue Substitute J Synthetic Substitute K Nonautologous Tissue Substitute	Z No Qualifier
5 Scrotum S Penis T Prepuce	Ø Open 4 Percutaneous Endoscopic X External	7 Autologous Tissue Substitute J Synthetic Substitute K Nonautologous Tissue Substitute	Z No Qualifier
9 Testis, Right B Testis, Left C Testes, Bilateral	Ø Open	7 Autologous Tissue Substitute J Synthetic Substitute K Nonautologous Tissue Substitute	Z No Qualifier

0 Medical and Surgical
V Male Reproductive System
W Revision Correcting, to the extent possible, a portion of a malfunctioning device or the position of a displaced device

Body Part Character 4	Approach Character 5	Device Character 6	Qualifier Character 7
4 Prostate and Seminal Vesicles **8** Scrotum and Tunica Vaginalis **D** Testis **S** Penis	**0** Open **3** Percutaneous **4** Percutaneous Endoscopic **7** Via Natural or Artificial Opening **8** Via Natural or Artificial Opening Endoscopic **X** External	**0** Drainage Device **3** Infusion Device **7** Autologous Tissue Substitute **J** Synthetic Substitute **K** Nonautologous Tissue Substitute	**Z** No Qualifier
M Epididymis and Spermatic Cord	**0** Open **3** Percutaneous **4** Percutaneous Endoscopic **7** Via Natural or Artificial Opening **8** Via Natural or Artificial Opening Endoscopic **X** External	**0** Drainage Device **3** Infusion Device **7** Autologous Tissue Substitute **C** Extraluminal Device **J** Synthetic Substitute **K** Nonautologous Tissue Substitute	**Z** No Qualifier
R Vas Deferens	**0** Open **3** Percutaneous **4** Percutaneous Endoscopic **7** Via Natural or Artificial Opening **8** Via Natural or Artificial Opening Endoscopic **X** External	**0** Drainage Device **3** Infusion Device **7** Autologous Tissue Substitute **C** Extraluminal Device **D** Intraluminal Device **J** Synthetic Substitute **K** Nonautologous Tissue Substitute	**Z** No Qualifier

Anatomical Regions, General ØWØ–ØWW

Ø Medical and Surgical
W Anatomical Regions, General
Ø Alteration Modifying the anatomic structure of a body part without affecting the function of the body part

Body Part Character 4	Approach Character 5	Device Character 6	Qualifier Character 7
Ø Head **2** Face **4** Upper Jaw **5** Lower Jaw **6** Neck **8** Chest Wall **F** Abdominal Wall **K** Upper Back **L** Lower Back **M** Perineum, Male **N** Perineum, Female	**Ø** Open **3** Percutaneous **4** Percutaneous Endoscopic	**7** Autologous Tissue Substitute **J** Synthetic Substitute **K** Nonautologous Tissue Substitute **Z** No Device	**Z** No Qualifier

Ø Medical and Surgical
W Anatomical Regions, General
1 Bypass Altering the route of passage of the contents of a tubular body part

Body Part Character 4	Approach Character 5	Device Character 6	Qualifier Character 7
1 Cranial Cavity	**Ø** Open	**J** Synthetic Substitute	**9** Pleural Cavity, Right **B** Pleural Cavity, Left **G** Peritoneal Cavity **J** Pelvic Cavity
9 Pleural Cavity, Right **B** Pleural Cavity, Left **G** Peritoneal Cavity **J** Pelvic Cavity	**Ø** Open **4** Percutaneous Endoscopic	**J** Synthetic Substitute	**4** Cutaneous **9** Pleural Cavity, Right **B** Pleural Cavity, Left **G** Peritoneal Cavity **J** Pelvic Cavity **Y** Lower Vein
9 Pleural Cavity, Right **B** Pleural Cavity, Left **G** Peritoneal Cavity **J** Pelvic Cavity	**3** Percutaneous	**J** Synthetic Substitute	**4** Cutaneous

Ø Medical and Surgical
W Anatomical Regions, General
2 Change Taking out or off a device from a body part and putting back an identical or similar device in or on the same body part without cutting or puncturing the skin or a mucous membrane

Body Part Character 4	Approach Character 5	Device Character 6	Qualifier Character 7
Ø Head **1** Cranial Cavity **2** Face **4** Upper Jaw **5** Lower Jaw **6** Neck **8** Chest Wall **9** Pleural Cavity, Right **B** Pleural Cavity, Left **C** Mediastinum **D** Pericardial Cavity **F** Abdominal Wall **G** Peritoneal Cavity **H** Retroperitoneum **J** Pelvic Cavity **K** Upper Back **L** Lower Back **M** Perineum, Male **N** Perineum, Female	**X** External	**Ø** Drainage Device **Y** Other Device	**Z** No Qualifier

0 Medical and Surgical
W Anatomical Regions, General
3 Control Stopping, or attempting to stop, postprocedural bleeding

Body Part Character 4	Approach Character 5	Device Character 6	Qualifier Character 7
0 Head **1** Cranial Cavity **2** Face **4** Upper Jaw **5** Lower Jaw **6** Neck **8** Chest Wall **9** Pleural Cavity, Right **B** Pleural Cavity, Left **C** Mediastinum **D** Pericardial Cavity **F** Abdominal Wall **G** Peritoneal Cavity **H** Retroperitoneum **J** Pelvic Cavity **K** Upper Back **L** Lower Back **M** Perineum, Male **N** Perineum, Female	**0** Open **3** Percutaneous **4** Percutaneous Endoscopic	**Z** No Device	**Z** No Qualifier
3 Oral Cavity and Throat	**0** Open **3** Percutaneous **4** Percutaneous Endoscopic **7** Via Natural or Artificial Opening **8** Via Natural or Artificial Opening Endoscopic **X External**	**Z** No Device	**Z** No Qualifier
P Gastrointestinal Tract **Q** Respiratory Tract **R** Genitourinary Tract	**0** Open **3** Percutaneous **4** Percutaneous Endoscopic **7** Via Natural or Artificial Opening **8** Via Natural or Artificial Opening Endoscopic	**Z** No Device	**Z** No Qualifier

0 Medical and Surgical
W Anatomical Regions, General
4 Creation Making a new genital structure that does not take over the function of a body part

Body Part Character 4	Approach Character 5	Device Character 6	Qualifier Character 7
M Perineum, Male	**0** Open	**7** Autologous Tissue Substitute **J** Synthetic Substitute **K** Nonautologous Tissue Substitute **Z** No Device	**0** Vagina
N Perineum, Female	**0** Open	**7** Autologous Tissue Substitute **J** Synthetic Substitute **K** Nonautologous Tissue Substitute **Z** No Device	**1** Penis

0 Medical and Surgical
W Anatomical Regions, General
8 Division Cutting into a body part without draining fluids and/or gases from the body part in order to separate or transect a body part

Body Part Character 4	Approach Character 5	Device Character 6	Qualifier Character 7
N Perineum, Female	**X** External	**Z** No Device	**Z** No Qualifier

Ø Medical and Surgical
W Anatomical Regions, General
9 Drainage Taking or letting out fluids and/or gases from a body part

Body Part Character 4	Approach Character 5	Device Character 6	Qualifier Character 7
Ø Head **1** Cranial Cavity **2** Face **3** Oral Cavity and Throat **4** Upper Jaw **5** Lower Jaw **6** Neck **8** Chest Wall **9** Pleural Cavity, Right **B** Pleural Cavity, Left **C** Mediastinum **D** Pericardial Cavity **F** Abdominal Wall **G** Peritoneal Cavity **H** Retroperitoneum **J** Pelvic Cavity **K** Upper Back **L** Lower Back **M** Perineum, Male **N** Perineum, Female	**Ø** Open **3** Percutaneous **4** Percutaneous Endoscopic	**Ø** Drainage Device	**Z** No Qualifier
Ø Head **1** Cranial Cavity **2** Face **3** Oral Cavity and Throat **4** Upper Jaw **5** Lower Jaw **6** Neck **8** Chest Wall **9** Pleural Cavity, Right **B** Pleural Cavity, Left **C** Mediastinum **D** Pericardial Cavity **F** Abdominal Wall **G** Peritoneal Cavity **H** Retroperitoneum **J** Pelvic Cavity **K** Upper Back **L** Lower Back **M** Perineum, Male **N** Perineum, Female	**Ø** Open **3** Percutaneous **4** Percutaneous Endoscopic	**Z** No Device	**X** Diagnostic **Z** No Qualifier

Ø Medical and Surgical
W Anatomical Regions, General
B Excision Cutting out or off, without replacement, a portion of a body part

Body Part Character 4	Approach Character 5	Device Character 6	Qualifier Character 7
Ø Head **2** Face **4** Upper Jaw **5** Lower Jaw **8** Chest Wall **K** Upper Back **L** Lower Back **M** Perineum, Male **N** Perineum, Female	**Ø** Open **3** Percutaneous **4** Percutaneous Endoscopic **X** External	**Z** No Device	**X** Diagnostic **Z** No Qualifier
6 Neck **C** Mediastinum **F** Abdominal Wall **H** Retroperitoneum	**Ø** Open **3** Percutaneous **4** Percutaneous Endoscopic	**Z** No Device	**X** Diagnostic **Z** No Qualifier
6 Neck **F** Abdominal Wall	**X** External	**Z** No Device	**2** Stoma **X** Diagnostic **Z** No Qualifier

0 Medical and Surgical
W Anatomical Regions, General
C Extirpation Taking or cutting out solid matter from a body part

Body Part Character 4	Approach Character 5	Device Character 6	Qualifier Character 7
1 Cranial Cavity 3 Oral Cavity and Throat 9 Pleural Cavity, Right B Pleural Cavity, Left C Mediastinum D Pericardial Cavity G Peritoneal Cavity J Pelvic Cavity	0 Open 3 Percutaneous 4 Percutaneous Endoscopic X External	Z No Device	Z No Qualifier
P Gastrointestinal Tract Q Respiratory Tract R Genitourinary Tract	0 Open 3 Percutaneous 4 Percutaneous Endoscopic 7 Via Natural or Artificial Opening 8 Via Natural or Artificial Opening Endoscopic X External	Z No Device	Z No Qualifier

0 Medical and Surgical
W Anatomical Regions, General
F Fragmentation Breaking solid matter in a body part into pieces

Body Part Character 4	Approach Character 5	Device Character 6	Qualifier Character 7
1 Cranial Cavity 3 Oral Cavity and Throat 9 Pleural Cavity, Right B Pleural Cavity, Left C Mediastinum D Pericardial Cavity G Peritoneal Cavity J Pelvic Cavity	0 Open 3 Percutaneous 4 Percutaneous Endoscopic X External	Z No Device	Z No Qualifier
P Gastrointestinal Tract Q Respiratory Tract R Genitourinary Tract	0 Open 3 Percutaneous 4 Percutaneous Endoscopic 7 Via Natural or Artificial Opening 8 Via Natural or Artificial Opening Endoscopic X External	Z No Device	Z No Qualifier

0 Medical and Surgical
W Anatomical Regions, General
H Insertion Putting in a nonbiological appliance that monitors, assists, performs, or prevents a physiological function but does not physically take the place of a body part

Body Part Character 4	Approach Character 5	Device Character 6	Qualifier Character 7
0 Head 1 Cranial Cavity 2 Face 3 Oral Cavity and Throat 4 Upper Jaw 5 Lower Jaw 6 Neck 8 Chest Wall 9 Pleural Cavity, Right B Pleural Cavity, Left C Mediastinum D Pericardial Cavity F Abdominal Wall G Peritoneal Cavity H Retroperitoneum J Pelvic Cavity K Upper Back L Lower Back M Perineum, Male N Perineum, Female	0 Open 3 Percutaneous 4 Percutaneous Endoscopic	1 Radioactive Element 3 Infusion Device Y Other Device	Z No Qualifier
P Gastrointestinal Tract Q Respiratory Tract R Genitourinary Tract	0 Open 3 Percutaneous 4 Percutaneous Endoscopic 7 Via Natural or Artificial Opening 8 Via Natural or Artificial Opening Endoscopic	1 Radioactive Element 3 Infusion Device Y Other Device	Z No Qualifier

Ø Medical and Surgical
W Anatomical Regions, General
J Inspection Visually and/or manually exploring a body part

Body Part Character 4	Approach Character 5	Device Character 6	Qualifier Character 7
Ø Head **2** Face **3** Oral Cavity and Throat **4** Upper Jaw **5** Lower Jaw **6** Neck **8** Chest Wall **F** Abdominal Wall **K** Upper Back **L** Lower Back **M** Perineum, Male **N** Perineum, Female	**Ø** Open **3** Percutaneous **4** Percutaneous Endoscopic **X** External	**Z** No Device	**Z** No Qualifier
1 Cranial Cavity **9** Pleural Cavity, Right **B** Pleural Cavity, Left **C** Mediastinum **D** Pericardial Cavity **G** Peritoneal Cavity **H** Retroperitoneum **J** Pelvic Cavity	**Ø** Open **3** Percutaneous **4** Percutaneous Endoscopic	**Z** No Device	**Z** No Qualifier
P Gastrointestinal Tract **Q** Respiratory Tract **R** Genitourinary Tract	**Ø** Open **3** Percutaneous **4** Percutaneous Endoscopic **7** Via Natural or Artificial Opening **8** Via Natural or Artificial Opening Endoscopic	**Z** No Device	**Z** No Qualifier

Ø Medical and Surgical
W Anatomical Regions, General
M Reattachment Putting back in or on all or a portion of a separated body part to its normal location or other suitable location

Body Part Character 4	Approach Character 5	Device Character 6	Qualifier Character 7
2 Face **4** Upper Jaw **5** Lower Jaw **6** Neck **8** Chest Wall **F** Abdominal Wall **K** Upper Back **L** Lower Back **M** Perineum, Male **N** Perineum, Female	**Ø** Open	**Z** No Device	**Z** No Qualifier

0 Medical and Surgical
W Anatomical Regions, General
P Removal Taking out or off a device from a body part

Body Part Character 4	Approach Character 5	Device Character 6	Qualifier Character 7
0 Head 2 Face 4 Upper Jaw 5 Lower Jaw 6 Neck 8 Chest Wall C Mediastinum F Abdominal Wall K Upper Back L Lower Back M Perineum, Male N Perineum, Female	0 Open 3 Percutaneous 4 Percutaneous Endoscopic X External	0 Drainage Device 1 Radioactive Element 3 Infusion Device 7 Autologous Tissue Substitute J Synthetic Substitute K Nonautologous Tissue Substitute Y Other Device	Z No Qualifier
1 Cranial Cavity 9 Pleural Cavity, Right B Pleural Cavity, Left D Pericardial Cavity G Peritoneal Cavity H Retroperitoneum J Pelvic Cavity	X External	0 Drainage Device 1 Radioactive Element 3 Infusion Device	Z No Qualifier
1 Cranial Cavity 9 Pleural Cavity, Right B Pleural Cavity, Left G Peritoneal Cavity J Pelvic Cavity	0 Open 3 Percutaneous 4 Percutaneous Endoscopic	0 Drainage Device 1 Radioactive Element 3 Infusion Device J Synthetic Substitute Y Other Device	Z No Qualifier
D Pericardial Cavity H Retroperitoneum	0 Open 3 Percutaneous 4 Percutaneous Endoscopic	0 Drainage Device 1 Radioactive Element 3 Infusion Device Y Other Device	Z No Qualifier
P Gastrointestinal Tract Q Respiratory Tract R Genitourinary Tract	0 Open 3 Percutaneous 4 Percutaneous Endoscopic 7 Via Natural or Artificial Opening 8 Via Natural or Artificial Opening Endoscopic X External	1 Radioactive Element 3 Infusion Device Y Other Device	Z No Qualifier

0 Medical and Surgical
W Anatomical Regions, General
Q Repair Restoring, to the extent possible, a body part to its normal anatomic structure and function

Body Part Character 4	Approach Character 5	Device Character 6	Qualifier Character 7
0 Head 2 Face 4 Upper Jaw 5 Lower Jaw 8 Chest Wall K Upper Back L Lower Back M Perineum, Male N Perineum, Female	0 Open 3 Percutaneous 4 Percutaneous Endoscopic X External	Z No Device	Z No Qualifier
6 Neck C Mediastinum F Abdominal Wall	0 Open 3 Percutaneous 4 Percutaneous Endoscopic	Z No Device	Z No Qualifier
6 Neck F Abdominal Wall	X External	Z No Device	2 Stoma Z No Qualifier

Ø Medical and Surgical
W Anatomical Regions, General
U Supplement Putting in or on biological or synthetic material that physically reinforces and/or augments the function of a portion of a body part

Body Part Character 4	Approach Character 5	Device Character 6	Qualifier Character 7
Ø Head **2** Face **4** Upper Jaw **5** Lower Jaw **6** Neck **8** Chest Wall **C** Mediastinum **F** Abdominal Wall **K** Upper Back **L** Lower Back **M** Perineum, Male **N** Perineum, Female	**Ø** Open **4** Percutaneous Endoscopic	**7** Autologous Tissue Substitute **J** Synthetic Substitute **K** Nonautologous Tissue Substitute	**Z** No Qualifier

Ø Medical and Surgical
W Anatomical Regions, General
W Revision Correcting, to the extent possible, a portion of a malfunctioning device or the position of a displaced device

Body Part Character 4	Approach Character 5	Device Character 6	Qualifier Character 7
Ø Head **2** Face **4** Upper Jaw **5** Lower Jaw **6** Neck **8** Chest Wall **C** Mediastinum **F** Abdominal Wall **K** Upper Back **L** Lower Back **M** Perineum, Male **N** Perineum, Female	**Ø** Open **3** Percutaneous **4** Percutaneous Endoscopic **X** External	**Ø** Drainage Device **1** Radioactive Element **3** Infusion Device **7** Autologous Tissue Substitute **J** Synthetic Substitute **K** Nonautologous Tissue Substitute **Y** Other Device	**Z** No Qualifier
1 Cranial Cavity **9** Pleural Cavity, Right **B** Pleural Cavity, Left **G** Peritoneal Cavity **J** Pelvic Cavity	**Ø** Open **3** Percutaneous **4** Percutaneous Endoscopic **X** External	**Ø** Drainage Device **1** Radioactive Element **3** Infusion Device **J** Synthetic Substitute **Y** Other Device	**Z** No Qualifier
D Pericardial Cavity **H** Retroperitoneum	**Ø** Open **3** Percutaneous **4** Percutaneous Endoscopic **X** External	**Ø** Drainage Device **1** Radioactive Element **3** Infusion Device **Y** Other Device	**Z** No Qualifier
P Gastrointestinal Tract **Q** Respiratory Tract **R** Genitourinary Tract	**Ø** Open **3** Percutaneous **4** Percutaneous Endoscopic **7** Via Natural or Artificial Opening **8** Via Natural or Artificial Opening Endoscopic **X** External	**1** Radioactive Element **3** Infusion Device **Y** Other Device	**Z** No Qualifier

Anatomical Regions, Upper Extremities 0X0–0XX

0 Medical and Surgical
X Anatomical Regions, Upper Extremities
0 Alteration Modifying the anatomic structure of a body part without affecting the function of the body part

Body Part Character 4	Approach Character 5	Device Character 6	Qualifier Character 7
2 Shoulder Region, Right 3 Shoulder Region, Left 4 Axilla, Right 5 Axilla, Left 6 Upper Extremity, Right 7 Upper Extremity, Left 8 Upper Arm, Right 9 Upper Arm, Left B Elbow Region, Right C Elbow Region, Left D Lower Arm, Right F Lower Arm, Left G Wrist Region, Right H Wrist Region, Left	0 Open 3 Percutaneous 4 Percutaneous Endoscopic	7 Autologous Tissue Substitute J Synthetic Substitute K Nonautologous Tissue Substitute Z No Device	Z No Qualifier

0 Medical and Surgical
X Anatomical Regions, Upper Extremities
2 Change Taking out or off a device from a body part and putting back an identical or similar device in or on the same body part without cutting or puncturing the skin or a mucous membrane

Body Part Character 4	Approach Character 5	Device Character 6	Qualifier Character 7
6 Upper Extremity, Right 7 Upper Extremity, Left	X External	0 Drainage Device Y Other Device	Z No Qualifier

0 Medical and Surgical
X Anatomical Regions, Upper Extremities
3 Control Stopping, or attempting to stop, postprocedural bleeding

Body Part Character 4	Approach Character 5	Device Character 6	Qualifier Character 7
2 Shoulder Region, Right 3 Shoulder Region, Left 4 Axilla, Right 5 Axilla, Left 6 Upper Extremity, Right 7 Upper Extremity, Left 8 Upper Arm, Right 9 Upper Arm, Left B Elbow Region, Right C Elbow Region, Left D Lower Arm, Right F Lower Arm, Left G Wrist Region, Right H Wrist Region, Left J Hand, Right K Hand, Left	0 Open 3 Percutaneous 4 Percutaneous Endoscopic	Z No Device	Z No Qualifier

Ø Medical and Surgical
X Anatomical Regions, Upper Extremities
6 Detachment Cutting off all or a portion of the upper or lower extremities

Body Part Character 4	Approach Character 5	Device Character 6	Qualifier Character 7
Ø Forequarter, Right **1** Forequarter, Left **2** Shoulder Region, Right **3** Shoulder Region, Left **B** Elbow Region, Right **C** Elbow Region, Left	**Ø** Open	**Z** No Device	**Z** No Qualifier
8 Upper Arm, Right **9** Upper Arm, Left **D** Lower Arm, Right **F** Lower Arm, Left	**Ø** Open	**Z** No Device	**1** High **2** Mid **3** Low
J Hand, Right **K** Hand, Left	**Ø** Open	**Z** No Device	**Ø** Complete **4** Complete 1st Ray **5** Complete 2nd Ray **6** Complete 3rd Ray **7** Complete 4th Ray **8** Complete 5th Ray **9** Partial 1st Ray **B** Partial 2nd Ray **C** Partial 3rd Ray **D** Partial 4th Ray **F** Partial 5th Ray
L Thumb, Right **M** Thumb, Left **N** Index Finger, Right **P** Index Finger, Left **Q** Middle Finger, Right **R** Middle Finger, Left **S** Ring Finger, Right **T** Ring Finger, Left **V** Little Finger, Right **W** Little Finger, Left	**Ø** Open	**Z** No Device	**Ø** Complete **1** High **2** Mid **3** Low

Ø Medical and Surgical
X Anatomical Regions, Upper Extremities
9 Drainage Taking or letting out fluids and/or gases from a body part

Body Part Character 4	Approach Character 5	Device Character 6	Qualifier Character 7
2 Shoulder Region, Right **3** Shoulder Region, Left **4** Axilla, Right **5** Axilla, Left **6** Upper Extremity, Right **7** Upper Extremity, Left **8** Upper Arm, Right **9** Upper Arm, Left **B** Elbow Region, Right **C** Elbow Region, Left **D** Lower Arm, Right **F** Lower Arm, Left **G** Wrist Region, Right **H** Wrist Region, Left **J** Hand, Right **K** Hand, Left	**Ø** Open **3** Percutaneous **4** Percutaneous Endoscopic	**Ø** Drainage Device	**Z** No Qualifier
2 Shoulder Region, Right **3** Shoulder Region, Left **4** Axilla, Right **5** Axilla, Left **6** Upper Extremity, Right **7** Upper Extremity, Left **8** Upper Arm, Right **9** Upper Arm, Left **B** Elbow Region, Right **C** Elbow Region, Left **D** Lower Arm, Right **F** Lower Arm, Left **G** Wrist Region, Right **H** Wrist Region, Left **J** Hand, Right **K** Hand, Left	**Ø** Open **3** Percutaneous **4** Percutaneous Endoscopic	**Z** No Device	**X** Diagnostic **Z** No Qualifier

Ø Medical and Surgical
X Anatomical Regions, Upper Extremities
B Excision Cutting out or off, without replacement, a portion of a body part

Body Part Character 4	Approach Character 5	Device Character 6	Qualifier Character 7
2 Shoulder Region, Right 3 Shoulder Region, Left 4 Axilla, Right 5 Axilla, Left 6 Upper Extremity, Right 7 Upper Extremity, Left 8 Upper Arm, Right 9 Upper Arm, Left B Elbow Region, Right C Elbow Region, Left D Lower Arm, Right F Lower Arm, Left G Wrist Region, Right H Wrist Region, Left J Hand, Right K Hand, Left	Ø Open 3 Percutaneous 4 Percutaneous Endoscopic	Z No Device	X Diagnostic Z No Qualifier

Ø Medical and Surgical
X Anatomical Regions, Upper Extremities
H Insertion Putting in a nonbiological appliance that monitors, assists, performs, or prevents a physiological function but does not physically take the place of a body part

Body Part Character 4	Approach Character 5	Device Character 6	Qualifier Character 7
2 Shoulder Region, Right 3 Shoulder Region, Left 4 Axilla, Right 5 Axilla, Left 6 Upper Extremity, Right 7 Upper Extremity, Left 8 Upper Arm, Right 9 Upper Arm, Left B Elbow Region, Right C Elbow Region, Left D Lower Arm, Right F Lower Arm, Left G Wrist Region, Right H Wrist Region, Left J Hand, Right K Hand, Left	Ø Open 3 Percutaneous 4 Percutaneous Endoscopic	1 Radioactive Element 3 Infusion Device Y Other Device	Z No Qualifier

Ø Medical and Surgical
X Anatomical Regions, Upper Extremities
J Inspection Visually and/or manually exploring a body part

Body Part Character 4	Approach Character 5	Device Character 6	Qualifier Character 7
2 Shoulder Region, Right 3 Shoulder Region, Left 4 Axilla, Right 5 Axilla, Left 6 Upper Extremity, Right 7 Upper Extremity, Left 8 Upper Arm, Right 9 Upper Arm, Left B Elbow Region, Right C Elbow Region, Left D Lower Arm, Right F Lower Arm, Left G Wrist Region, Right H Wrist Region, Left J Hand, Right K Hand, Left	Ø Open 3 Percutaneous 4 Percutaneous Endoscopic X External	Z No Device	Z No Qualifier

Ø Medical and Surgical
X Anatomical Regions, Upper Extremities
M Reattachment Putting back in or on all or a portion of a separated body part to its normal location or other suitable location

Body Part Character 4	Approach Character 5	Device Character 6	Qualifier Character 7
Ø Forequarter, Right **1** Forequarter, Left **2** Shoulder Region, Right **3** Shoulder Region, Left **4** Axilla, Right **5** Axilla, Left **6** Upper Extremity, Right **7** Upper Extremity, Left **8** Upper Arm, Right **9** Upper Arm, Left **B** Elbow Region, Right **C** Elbow Region, Left **D** Lower Arm, Right **F** Lower Arm, Left **G** Wrist Region, Right **H** Wrist Region, Left **J** Hand, Right **K** Hand, Left **L** Thumb, Right **M** Thumb, Left **N** Index Finger, Right **P** Index Finger, Left **Q** Middle Finger, Right **R** Middle Finger, Left **S** Ring Finger, Right **T** Ring Finger, Left **V** Little Finger, Right **W** Little Finger, Left	**Ø** Open	**Z** No Device	**Z** No Qualifier

Ø Medical and Surgical
X Anatomical Regions, Upper Extremities
P Removal Taking out or off a device from a body part

Body Part Character 4	Approach Character 5	Device Character 6	Qualifier Character 7
6 Upper Extremity, Right **7** Upper Extremity, Left	**Ø** Open **3** Percutaneous **4** Percutaneous Endoscopic **X** External	**Ø** Drainage Device **1** Radioactive Element **3** Infusion Device **7** Autologous Tissue Substitute **J** Synthetic Substitute **K** Nonautologous Tissue Substitute **Y** Other Device	**Z** No Qualifier

0 Medical and Surgical
X Anatomical Regions, Upper Extremities
Q Repair Restoring, to the extent possible, a body part to its normal anatomic structure and function

Body Part Character 4	Approach Character 5	Device Character 6	Qualifier Character 7
2 Shoulder Region, Right **3** Shoulder Region, Left **4** Axilla, Right **5** Axilla, Left **6** Upper Extremity, Right **7** Upper Extremity, Left **8** Upper Arm, Right **9** Upper Arm, Left **B** Elbow Region, Right **C** Elbow Region, Left **D** Lower Arm, Right **F** Lower Arm, Left **G** Wrist Region, Right **H** Wrist Region, Left **J** Hand, Right **K** Hand, Left **L** Thumb, Right **M** Thumb, Left **N** Index Finger, Right **P** Index Finger, Left **Q** Middle Finger, Right **R** Middle Finger, Left **S** Ring Finger, Right **T** Ring Finger, Left **V** Little Finger, Right **W** Little Finger, Left	**0** Open **3** Percutaneous **4** Percutaneous Endoscopic **X** External	**Z** No Device	**Z** No Qualifier

0 Medical and Surgical
X Anatomical Regions, Upper Extremities
R Replacement Putting in or on biological or synthetic material that physically takes the place and/or function of all or a portion of a body part

Body Part Character 4	Approach Character 5	Device Character 6	Qualifier Character 7
L Thumb, Right **M** Thumb, Left	**0** Open **4** Percutaneous Endoscopic	**7** Autologous Tissue Substitute	**N** Toe, Right **P** Toe, Left

0 Medical and Surgical
X Anatomical Regions, Upper Extremities
U Supplement Putting in or on biological or synthetic material that physically reinforces and/or augments the function of a portion of a body part

Body Part Character 4	Approach Character 5	Device Character 6	Qualifier Character 7
2 Shoulder Region, Right **3** Shoulder Region, Left **4** Axilla, Right **5** Axilla, Left **6** Upper Extremity, Right **7** Upper Extremity, Left **8** Upper Arm, Right **9** Upper Arm, Left **B** Elbow Region, Right **C** Elbow Region, Left **D** Lower Arm, Right **F** Lower Arm, Left **G** Wrist Region, Right **H** Wrist Region, Left **J** Hand, Right **K** Hand, Left **L** Thumb, Right **M** Thumb, Left **N** Index Finger, Right **P** Index Finger, Left **Q** Middle Finger, Right **R** Middle Finger, Left **S** Ring Finger, Right **T** Ring Finger, Left **V** Little Finger, Right **W** Little Finger, Left	**0** Open **4** Percutaneous Endoscopic	**7** Autologous Tissue Substitute **J** Synthetic Substitute **K** Nonautologous Tissue Substitute	**Z** No Qualifier

Ø Medical and Surgical
X Anatomical Regions, Upper Extremities
W Revision Correcting, to the extent possible, a portion of a malfunctioning device or the position of a displaced device

Body Part Character 4	Approach Character 5	Device Character 6	Qualifier Character 7
6 Upper Extremity, Right **7** Upper Extremity, Left	**Ø** Open **3** Percutaneous **4** Percutaneous Endoscopic **X** External	**Ø** Drainage Device **3** Infusion Device **7** Autologous Tissue Substitute **J** Synthetic Substitute **K** Nonautologous Tissue Substitute **Y** Other Device	**Z** No Qualifier

Ø Medical and Surgical
X Anatomical Regions, Upper Extremities
X Transfer Moving, without taking out, all or a portion of a body part to another location to take over the function of all or a portion of a body part

Body Part Character 4	Approach Character 5	Device Character 6	Qualifier Character 7
N Index Finger, Right	**Ø** Open	**Z** No Device	**L** Thumb, Right
P Index Finger, Left	**Ø** Open	**Z** No Device	**M** Thumb, Left

Anatomical Regions, Lower Extremities ØYØ–ØYW

Ø Medical and Surgical
Y Anatomical Regions, Lower Extremities
Ø Alteration Modifying the anatomic structure of a body part without affecting the function of the body part

Body Part Character 4	Approach Character 5	Device Character 6	Qualifier Character 7
Ø Buttock, Right **1** Buttock, Left **9** Lower Extremity, Right **B** Lower Extremity, Left **C** Upper Leg, Right **D** Upper Leg, Left **F** Knee Region, Right **G** Knee Region, Left **H** Lower Leg, Right **J** Lower Leg, Left **K** Ankle Region, Right **L** Ankle Region, Left	**Ø** Open **3** Percutaneous **4** Percutaneous Endoscopic	**7** Autologous Tissue Substitute **J** Synthetic Substitute **K** Nonautologous Tissue Substitute **Z** No Device	**Z** No Qualifier

Ø Medical and Surgical
Y Anatomical Regions, Lower Extremities
2 Change Taking out or off a device from a body part and putting back an identical or similar device in or on the same body part without cutting or puncturing the skin or a mucous membrane

Body Part Character 4	Approach Character 5	Device Character 6	Qualifier Character 7
9 Lower Extremity, Right **B** Lower Extremity, Left	**X** External	**Ø** Drainage Device **Y** Other Device	**Z** No Qualifier

Ø Medical and Surgical
Y Anatomical Regions, Lower Extremities
3 Control Stopping, or attempting to stop, postprocedural bleeding

Body Part Character 4	Approach Character 5	Device Character 6	Qualifier Character 7
Ø Buttock, Right **1** Buttock, Left **5** Inguinal Region, Right **6** Inguinal Region, Left **7** Femoral Region, Right **8** Femoral Region, Left **9** Lower Extremity, Right **B** Lower Extremity, Left **C** Upper Leg, Right **D** Upper Leg, Left **F** Knee Region, Right **G** Knee Region, Left **H** Lower Leg, Right **J** Lower Leg, Left **K** Ankle Region, Right **L** Ankle Region, Left **M** Foot, Right **N** Foot, Left	**Ø** Open **3** Percutaneous **4** Percutaneous Endoscopic	**Z** No Device	**Z** No Qualifier

Ø Medical and Surgical
Y Anatomical Regions, Lower Extremities
6 Detachment Cutting off all or a portion of the upper or lower extremities

Body Part Character 4	Approach Character 5	Device Character 6	Qualifier Character 7
2 Hindquarter, Right **3** Hindquarter, Left **4** Hindquarter, Bilateral **7** Femoral Region, Right **8** Femoral Region, Left **F** Knee Region, Right **G** Knee Region, Left	**Ø** Open	**Z** No Device	**Z** No Qualifier
C Upper Leg, Right **D** Upper Leg, Left **H** Lower Leg, Right **J** Lower Leg, Left	**Ø** Open	**Z** No Device	**1** High **2** Mid **3** Low

ØY6 Continued on next page

ØY6 Continued

Ø Medical and Surgical
Y Anatomical Regions, Lower Extremities
6 Detachment Cutting off all or a portion of the upper or lower extremities

Body Part Character 4	Approach Character 5	Device Character 6	Qualifier Character 7
M Foot, Right **N** Foot, Left	**Ø** Open	**Z** No Device	**Ø** Complete **4** Complete 1st Ray **5** Complete 2nd Ray **6** Complete 3rd Ray **7** Complete 4th Ray **8** Complete 5th Ray **9** Partial 1st Ray **B** Partial 2nd Ray **C** Partial 3rd Ray **D** Partial 4th Ray **F** Partial 5th Ray
P 1st Toe, Right **Q** 1st Toe, Left **R** 2nd Toe, Right **S** 2nd Toe, Left **T** 3rd Toe, Right **U** 3rd Toe, Left **V** 4th Toe, Right **W** 4th Toe, Left **X** 5th Toe, Right **Y** 5th Toe, Left	**Ø** Open	**Z** No Device	**Ø** Complete **1** High **2** Mid **3** Low

Ø Medical and Surgical
Y Anatomical Regions, Lower Extremities
9 Drainage Taking or letting out fluids and/or gases from a body part

Body Part Character 4	Approach Character 5	Device Character 6	Qualifier Character 7
Ø Buttock, Right **1** Buttock, Left **5** Inguinal Region, Right **6** Inguinal Region, Left **7** Femoral Region, Right **8** Femoral Region, Left **9** Lower Extremity, Right **B** Lower Extremity, Left **C** Upper Leg, Right **D** Upper Leg, Left **F** Knee Region, Right **G** Knee Region, Left **H** Lower Leg, Right **J** Lower Leg, Left **K** Ankle Region, Right **L** Ankle Region, Left **M** Foot, Right **N** Foot, Left	**Ø** Open **3** Percutaneous **4** Percutaneous Endoscopic	**Ø** Drainage Device	**Z** No Qualifier
Ø Buttock, Right **1** Buttock, Left **5** Inguinal Region, Right **6** Inguinal Region, Left **7** Femoral Region, Right **8** Femoral Region, Left **9** Lower Extremity, Right **B** Lower Extremity, Left **C** Upper Leg, Right **D** Upper Leg, Left **F** Knee Region, Right **G** Knee Region, Left **H** Lower Leg, Right **J** Lower Leg, Left **K** Ankle Region, Right **L** Ankle Region, Left **M** Foot, Right **N** Foot, Left	**Ø** Open **3** Percutaneous **4** Percutaneous Endoscopic	**Z** No Device	**X** Diagnostic **Z** No Qualifier

Ø Medical and Surgical
Y Anatomical Regions, Lower Extremities
B Excision Cutting out or off, without replacement, a portion of a body part

Body Part Character 4	Approach Character 5	Device Character 6	Qualifier Character 7
Ø Buttock, Right 1 Buttock, Left 5 Inguinal Region, Right 6 Inguinal Region, Left 7 Femoral Region, Right 8 Femoral Region, Left 9 Lower Extremity, Right B Lower Extremity, Left C Upper Leg, Right D Upper Leg, Left F Knee Region, Right G Knee Region, Left H Lower Leg, Right J Lower Leg, Left K Ankle Region, Right L Ankle Region, Left M Foot, Right N Foot, Left	Ø Open 3 Percutaneous 4 Percutaneous Endoscopic	Z No Device	X Diagnostic Z No Qualifier

Ø Medical and Surgical
Y Anatomical Regions, Lower Extremities
H Insertion Putting in a nonbiological appliance that monitors, assists, performs, or prevents a physiological function but does not physically take the place of a body part

Body Part Character 4	Approach Character 5	Device Character 6	Qualifier Character 7
Ø Buttock, Right 1 Buttock, Left 5 Inguinal Region, Right 6 Inguinal Region, Left 7 Femoral Region, Right 8 Femoral Region, Left 9 Lower Extremity, Right B Lower Extremity, Left C Upper Leg, Right D Upper Leg, Left F Knee Region, Right G Knee Region, Left H Lower Leg, Right J Lower Leg, Left K Ankle Region, Right L Ankle Region, Left M Foot, Right N Foot, Left	Ø Open 3 Percutaneous 4 Percutaneous Endoscopic	1 Radioactive Element 3 Infusion Device Y Other Device	Z No Qualifier

Ø Medical and Surgical
Y Anatomical Regions, Lower Extremities
J Inspection Visually and/or manually exploring a body part

Body Part Character 4	Approach Character 5	Device Character 6	Qualifier Character 7
Ø Buttock, Right 1 Buttock, Left 5 Inguinal Region, Right 6 Inguinal Region, Left 7 Femoral Region, Right 8 Femoral Region, Left 9 Lower Extremity, Right A Inguinal Region, Bilateral B Lower Extremity, Left C Upper Leg, Right D Upper Leg, Left E Femoral Region, Bilateral F Knee Region, Right G Knee Region, Left H Lower Leg, Right J Lower Leg, Left K Ankle Region, Right L Ankle Region, Left M Foot, Right N Foot, Left	Ø Open 3 Percutaneous 4 Percutaneous Endoscopic X External	Z No Device	Z No Qualifier

Ø Medical and Surgical
Y Anatomical Regions, Lower Extremities
M Reattachment Putting back in or on all or a portion of a separated body part to its normal location or other suitable location

Body Part Character 4	Approach Character 5	Device Character 6	Qualifier Character 7
Ø Buttock, Right **1** Buttock, Left **2** Hindquarter, Right **3** Hindquarter, Left **4** Hindquarter, Bilateral **5** Inguinal Region, Right **6** Inguinal Region, Left **7** Femoral Region, Right **8** Femoral Region, Left **9** Lower Extremity, Right **B** Lower Extremity, Left **C** Upper Leg, Right **D** Upper Leg, Left **F** Knee Region, Right **G** Knee Region, Left **H** Lower Leg, Right **J** Lower Leg, Left **K** Ankle Region, Right **L** Ankle Region, Left **M** Foot, Right **N** Foot, Left **P** 1st Toe, Right **Q** 1st Toe, Left **R** 2nd Toe, Right **S** 2nd Toe, Left **T** 3rd Toe, Right **U** 3rd Toe, Left **V** 4th Toe, Right **W** 4th Toe, Left **X** 5th Toe, Right **Y** 5th Toe, Left	**Ø** Open	**Z** No Device	**Z** No Qualifier

Ø Medical and Surgical
Y Anatomical Regions, Lower Extremities
P Removal Taking out or off a device from a body part

Body Part Character 4	Approach Character 5	Device Character 6	Qualifier Character 7
9 Lower Extremity, Right **B** Lower Extremity, Left	**Ø** Open **3** Percutaneous **4** Percutaneous Endoscopic **X** External	**Ø** Drainage Device **1** Radioactive Element **3** Infusion Device **7** Autologous Tissue Substitute **J** Synthetic Substitute **K** Nonautologous Tissue Substitute **Y** Other Device	**Z** No Qualifier

Ø Medical and Surgical
Y Anatomical Regions, Lower Extremities
Q Repair Restoring, to the extent possible, a body part to its normal anatomic structure and function

Body Part Character 4	Approach Character 5	Device Character 6	Qualifier Character 7
Ø Buttock, Right **1** Buttock, Left **5** Inguinal Region, Right **6** Inguinal Region, Left **7** Femoral Region, Right **8** Femoral Region, Left **9** Lower Extremity, Right **A** Inguinal Region, Bilateral **B** Lower Extremity, Left **C** Upper Leg, Right **D** Upper Leg, Left **E** Femoral Region, Bilateral **F** Knee Region, Right **G** Knee Region, Left **H** Lower Leg, Right **J** Lower Leg, Left **K** Ankle Region, Right **L** Ankle Region, Left **M** Foot, Right **N** Foot, Left **P** 1st Toe, Right **Q** 1st Toe, Left **R** 2nd Toe, Right **S** 2nd Toe, Left **T** 3rd Toe, Right **U** 3rd Toe, Left **V** 4th Toe, Right **W** 4th Toe, Left **X** 5th Toe, Right **Y** 5th Toe, Left	**Ø** Open **3** Percutaneous **4** Percutaneous Endoscopic **X** External	**Z** No Device	**Z** No Qualifier

Ø Medical and Surgical
Y Anatomical Regions, Lower Extremities
U Supplement Putting in or on biological or synthetic material that physically reinforces and/or augments the function of a portion of a body part

Body Part Character 4	Approach Character 5	Device Character 6	Qualifier Character 7
Ø Buttock, Right **1** Buttock, Left **5** Inguinal Region, Right **6** Inguinal Region, Left **7** Femoral Region, Right **8** Femoral Region, Left **9** Lower Extremity, Right **A** Inguinal Region, Bilateral **B** Lower Extremity, Left **C** Upper Leg, Right **D** Upper Leg, Left **E** Femoral Region, Bilateral **F** Knee Region, Right **G** Knee Region, Left **H** Lower Leg, Right **J** Lower Leg, Left **K** Ankle Region, Right **L** Ankle Region, Left **M** Foot, Right **N** Foot, Left **P** 1st Toe, Right **Q** 1st Toe, Left **R** 2nd Toe, Right **S** 2nd Toe, Left **T** 3rd Toe, Right **U** 3rd Toe, Left **V** 4th Toe, Right **W** 4th Toe, Left **X** 5th Toe, Right **Y** 5th Toe, Left	**Ø** Open **4** Percutaneous Endoscopic	**7** Autologous Tissue Substitute **J** Synthetic Substitute **K** Nonautologous Tissue Substitute	**Z** No Qualifier

Ø Medical and Surgical
Y Anatomical Regions, Lower Extremities
W Revision Correcting, to the extent possible, a portion of a malfunctioning device or the position of a displaced device

Body Part Character 4	Approach Character 5	Device Character 6	Qualifier Character 7
9 Lower Extremity, Right **B** Lower Extremity, Left	**Ø** Open **3** Percutaneous **4** Percutaneous Endoscopic **X** External	**Ø** Drainage Device **3** Infusion Device **7** Autologous Tissue Substitute **J** Synthetic Substitute **K** Nonautologous Tissue Substitute **Y** Other Device	**Z** No Qualifier

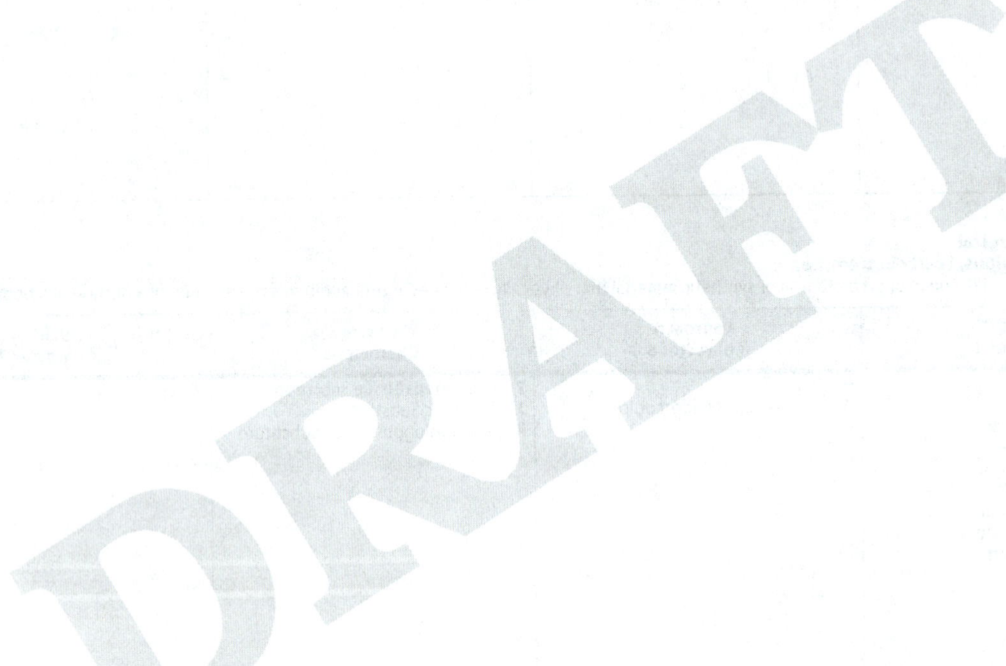

Obstetrics 102–10Y

1 **Obstetrics**
0 **Pregnancy**
2 **Change** Taking out or off a device from a body part and putting back an identical or similar device in or on the same body part without cutting or puncturing the skin or a mucous membrane

Body Part Character 4	Approach Character 5	Device Character 6	Qualifier Character 7
0 Products of Conception	7 Via Natural or Artificial Opening	3 Monitoring Electrode Y Other Device	Z No Qualifier

1 **Obstetrics**
0 **Pregnancy**
9 **Drainage** Taking or letting out fluids and/or gases from a body part

Body Part Character 4	Approach Character 5	Device Character 6	Qualifier Character 7
0 Products of Conception	0 Open 3 Percutaneous 4 Percutaneous Endoscopic 7 Via Natural or Artificial Opening 8 Via Natural or Artificial Opening Endoscopic	Z No Device	9 Fetal Blood A Fetal Cerebrospinal Fluid B Fetal Fluid, Other C Amniotic Fluid, Therapeutic D Fluid, Other U Amniotic Fluid, Diagnostic

1 **Obstetrics**
0 **Pregnancy**
A **Abortion** Artificially terminating a pregnancy

Body Part Character 4	Approach Character 5	Device Character 6	Qualifier Character 7
0 Products of Conception	0 Open 3 Percutaneous 4 Percutaneous Endoscopic 8 Via Natural or Artificial Opening Endoscopic	Z No Device	Z No Qualifier
0 Products of Conception	7 Via Natural or Artificial Opening	Z No Device	6 Vacuum W Laminaria X Abortifacient Z No Qualifier

1 **Obstetrics**
0 **Pregnancy**
D **Extraction** Pulling or stripping out or off all or a portion of a body part

Body Part Character 4	Approach Character 5	Device Character 6	Qualifier Character 7
0 Products of Conception	0 Open	Z No Device	0 Classical 1 Low Cervical 2 Extraperitoneal
0 Products of Conception	7 Via Natural or Artificial Opening	Z No Device	3 Low Forceps 4 Mid Forceps 5 High Forceps 6 Vacuum 7 Internal Version 8 Other
1 Products of Conception, Retained 2 Products of Conception, Ectopic	7 Via Natural or Artificial Opening 8 Via Natural or Artificial Opening Endoscopic	Z No Device	Z No Qualifier

1 **Obstetrics**
0 **Pregnancy**
E **Delivery** Assisting the passage of the products of conception from the genital canal

Body Part Character 4	Approach Character 5	Device Character 6	Qualifier Character 7
0 Products of Conception	X External	Z No Device	Z No Qualifier

1 Obstetrics
Ø Pregnancy
H Insertion Putting in a nonbiological appliance that monitors, assists, performs, or prevents a physiological function but does not physically take the place of a body part

Body Part Character 4	Approach Character 5	Device Character 6	Qualifier Character 7
Ø Products of Conception	**Ø** Open **7** Via Natural or Artificial Opening	**3** Monitoring Electrode **Y** Other Device	**Z** No Qualifier

1 Obstetrics
Ø Pregnancy
J Inspection Visually and/or manually exploring a body part

Body Part Character 4	Approach Character 5	Device Character 6	Qualifier Character 7
Ø Products of Conception **1** Products of Conception, Retained **2** Products of Conception, Ectopic	**Ø** Open **3** Percutaneous **4** Percutaneous Endoscopic **7** Via Natural or Artificial Opening **8** Via Natural or Artificial Opening Endoscopic **X** External	**Z** No Device	**Z** No Qualifier

1 Obstetrics
Ø Pregnancy
P Removal Taking out or off a device from a body part, region or orifice

Body Part Character 4	Approach Character 5	Device Character 6	Qualifier Character 7
Ø Products of Conception	**Ø** Open **7** Via Natural or Artificial Opening	**3** Monitoring Electrode **Y** Other Device	**Z** No Qualifier

1 Obstetrics
Ø Pregnancy
Q Repair Restoring, to the extent possible, a body part to its normal anatomic structure and function

Body Part Character 4	Approach Character 5	Device Character 6	Qualifier Character 7
Ø Products of Conception	**Ø** Open **3** Percutaneous **4** Percutaneous Endoscopic **7** Via Natural or Artificial Opening **8** Via Natural or Artificial Opening Endoscopic	**Y** Other Device **Z** No Device	**E** Nervous System **F** Cardiovascular System **G** Lymphatics and Hemic **H** Eye **J** Ear, Nose and Sinus **K** Respiratory System **L** Mouth and Throat **M** Gastrointestinal System **N** Hepatobiliary and Pancreas **P** Endocrine System **Q** Skin **R** Musculoskeletal System **S** Urinary System **T** Female Reproductive System **V** Male Reproductive System **Y** Other Body System

1 Obstetrics
Ø Pregnancy
S Reposition Moving to its normal location or other suitable location all or a portion of a body part

Body Part Character 4	Approach Character 5	Device Character 6	Qualifier Character 7
Ø Products of Conception	**7** Via Natural or Artificial Opening **X** External	**Z** No Device	**Z** No Qualifier
2 Products of Conception, Ectopic	**Ø** Open **3** Percutaneous **4** Percutaneous Endoscopic **7** Via Natural or Artificial Opening **8** Via Natural or Artificial Opening Endoscopic	**Z** No Device	**Z** No Qualifier

1 Obstetrics
0 Pregnancy
T Resection Cutting out or off, without replacement, all of a body part

Body Part Character 4	Approach Character 5	Device Character 6	Qualifier Character 7
2 Products of Conception, Ectopic	**0** Open **3** Percutaneous **4** Percutaneous Endoscopic **7** Via Natural or Artificial Opening **8** Via Natural or Artificial Opening Endoscopic	**Z** No Device	**Z** No Qualifier

1 Obstetrics
0 Pregnancy
Y Transplantation Putting in or on all or a portion of a living body part taken from another individual or animal to physically take the place and/or function of all or a portion of a similar body part

Body Part Character 4	Approach Character 5	Device Character 6	Qualifier Character 7
0 Products of Conception	**3** Percutaneous **4** Percutaneous Endoscopic **7** Via Natural or Artificial Opening	**Z** No Device	**E** Nervous System **F** Cardiovascular System **G** Lymphatics and Hemic **H** Eye **J** Ear, Nose and Sinus **K** Respiratory System **L** Mouth and Throat **M** Gastrointestinal System **N** Hepatobiliary and Pancreas **P** Endocrine System **Q** Skin **R** Musculoskeletal System **S** Urinary System **T** Female Reproductive System **V** Male Reproductive System **Y** Other Body System

Placement—Anatomical Regions 2WØ–2W6

2 Placement
W Anatomical Regions Body S
Ø Change Taking out or off a device from a body part and putting back an identical or similar device in or on the same body part without cutting or puncturing the skin or a mucous membrane

Body Region Character 4	Approach Character 5	Device Character 6	Qualifier Character 7
Ø Head **1** Face **2** Neck **3** Abdominal Wall **4** Chest Wall **5** Back **6** Inguinal Region, Right **7** Inguinal Region, Left **8** Upper Extremity, Right **9** Upper Extremity, Left **A** Upper Arm, Right **B** Upper Arm, Left **C** Lower Arm, Right **D** Lower Arm, Left **E** Hand, Right **F** Hand, Left **G** Thumb, Right **H** Thumb, Left **J** Finger, Right **K** Finger, Left **L** Lower Extremity, Right **M** Lower Extremity, Left **N** Upper Leg, Right **P** Upper Leg, Left **Q** Lower Leg, Right **R** Lower Leg, Left **S** Foot, Right **T** Foot, Left **U** Toe, Right **V** Toe, Left	**X** External	**Ø** Traction Apparatus **1** Splint **2** Cast **3** Brace **4** Bandage **5** Packing Material **6** Pressure Dressing **7** Intermittent Pressure Device **Y** Other Device	**Z** No Qualifier
1 Face	**X** External	**Ø** Traction Apparatus **1** Splint **2** Cast **3** Brace **4** Bandage **5** Packing Material **6** Pressure Dressing **7** Intermittent Pressure Device **9** Wire **Y** Other Device	**Z** No Qualifier

2 Placement
W Anatomical Regions
1 Compression Putting pressure on a body region

Body Region Character 4	Approach Character 5	Device Character 6	Qualifier Character 7
0 Head **1** Face **2** Neck **3** Abdominal Wall **4** Chest Wall **5** Back **6** Inguinal Region, Right **7** Inguinal Region, Left **8** Upper Extremity, Right **9** Upper Extremity, Left **A** Upper Arm, Right **B** Upper Arm, Left **C** Lower Arm, Right **D** Lower Arm, Left **E** Hand, Right **F** Hand, Left **G** Thumb, Right **H** Thumb, Left **J** Finger, Right **K** Finger, Left **L** Lower Extremity, Right **M** Lower Extremity, Left **N** Upper Leg, Right **P** Upper Leg, Left **Q** Lower Leg, Right **R** Lower Leg, Left **S** Foot, Right **T** Foot, Left **U** Toe, Right **V** Toe, Left	**X** External	**6** Pressure Dressing **7** Intermittent Pressure Device	**Z** No Qualifier

2 Placement
W Anatomical Regions
2 Dressing Putting material on a body region for protection

Body Region Character 4	Approach Character 5	Device Character 6	Qualifier Character 7
0 Head **1** Face **2** Neck **3** Abdominal Wall **4** Chest Wall **5** Back **6** Inguinal Region, Right **7** Inguinal Region, Left **8** Upper Extremity, Right **9** Upper Extremity, Left **A** Upper Arm, Right **B** Upper Arm, Left **C** Lower Arm, Right **D** Lower Arm, Left **E** Hand, Right **F** Hand, Left **G** Thumb, Right **H** Thumb, Left **J** Finger, Right **K** Finger, Left **L** Lower Extremity, Right **M** Lower Extremity, Left **N** Upper Leg, Right **P** Upper Leg, Left **Q** Lower Leg, Right **R** Lower Leg, Left **S** Foot, Right **T** Foot, Left **U** Toe, Right **V** Toe, Left	**X** External	**4** Bandage	**Z** No Qualifier

2 Placement
W Anatomical Regions
3 Immobilization Limiting or preventing motion of a body region

Body Region Character 4	Approach Character 5	Device Character 6	Qualifier Character 7
Ø Head **2** Neck **3** Abdominal Wall **4** Chest Wall **5** Back **6** Inguinal Region, Right **7** Inguinal Region, Left **8** Upper Extremity, Right **9** Upper Extremity, Left **A** Upper Arm, Right **B** Upper Arm, Left **C** Lower Arm, Right **D** Lower Arm, Left **E** Hand, Right **F** Hand, Left **G** Thumb, Right **H** Thumb, Left **J** Finger, Right **K** Finger, Left **L** Lower Extremity, Right **M** Lower Extremity, Left **N** Upper Leg, Right **P** Upper Leg, Left **Q** Lower Leg, Right **R** Lower Leg, Left **S** Foot, Right **T** Foot, Left **U** Toe, Right **V** Toe, Left	**X** External	**1** Splint **2** Cast **3** Brace **Y** Other Device	**Z** No Qualifier
1 Face	**X** External	**1** Splint **2** Cast **3** Brace **9** Wire **Y** Other Device	**Z** No Qualifier

2 Placement
W Anatomical Regions
4 Packing Putting material in a body region or orifice

Body Region Character 4	Approach Character 5	Device Character 6	Qualifier Character 7
Ø Head **1** Face **2** Neck **3** Abdominal Wall **4** Chest Wall **5** Back **6** Inguinal Region, Right **7** Inguinal Region, Left **8** Upper Extremity, Right **9** Upper Extremity, Left **A** Upper Arm, Right **B** Upper Arm, Left **C** Lower Arm, Right **D** Lower Arm, Left **E** Hand, Right **F** Hand, Left **G** Thumb, Right **H** Thumb, Left **J** Finger, Right **K** Finger, Left **L** Lower Extremity, Right **M** Lower Extremity, Left **N** Upper Leg, Right **P** Upper Leg, Left **Q** Lower Leg, Right **R** Lower Leg, Left **S** Foot, Right **T** Foot, Left **U** Toe, Right **V** Toe, Left	**X** External	**5** Packing Material	**Z** No Qualifier

2 Placement
W Anatomical Regions
5 Removal Taking out or off a device from a body part

Body Region Character 4	Approach Character 5	Device Character 6	Qualifier Character 7
Ø Head **2** Neck **3** Abdominal Wall **4** Chest Wall **5** Back **6** Inguinal Region, Right **7** Inguinal Region, Left **8** Upper Extremity, Right **9** Upper Extremity, Left **A** Upper Arm, Right **B** Upper Arm, Left **C** Lower Arm, Right **D** Lower Arm, Left **E** Hand, Right **F** Hand, Left **G** Thumb, Right **H** Thumb, Left **J** Finger, Right **K** Finger, Left **L** Lower Extremity, Right **M** Lower Extremity, Left **N** Upper Leg, Right **P** Upper Leg, Left **Q** Lower Leg, Right **R** Lower Leg, Left **S** Foot, Right **T** Foot, Left **U** Toe, Right **V** Toe, Left	**X** External	**Ø** Traction Apparatus **1** Splint **2** Cast **3** Brace **4** Bandage **5** Packing Material **6** Pressure Dressing **7** Intermittent Pressure Device **Y** Other Device	**Z** No Qualifier
1 Face	**X** External	**Ø** Traction Apparatus **1** Splint **2** Cast **3** Brace **4** Bandage **5** Packing Material **6** Pressure Dressing **7** Intermittent Pressure Device **9** Wire **Y** Other Device	**Z** No Qualifier

2 Placement
W Anatomical Regions
6 Traction Exerting a pulling force on a body region in a distal direction

Body Region Character 4	Approach Character 5	Device Character 6	Qualifier Character 7
Ø Head **1** Face **2** Neck **3** Abdominal Wall **4** Chest Wall **5** Back **6** Inguinal Region, Right **7** Inguinal Region, Left **8** Upper Extremity, Right **9** Upper Extremity, Left **A** Upper Arm, Right **B** Upper Arm, Left **C** Lower Arm, Right **D** Lower Arm, Left **E** Hand, Right **F** Hand, Left **G** Thumb, Right **H** Thumb, Left **J** Finger, Right **K** Finger, Left **L** Lower Extremity, Right **M** Lower Extremity, Left **N** Upper Leg, Right **P** Upper Leg, Left **Q** Lower Leg, Right **R** Lower Leg, Left **S** Foot, Right **T** Foot, Left **U** Toe, Right **V** Toe, Left	**X** External	**Ø** Traction Apparatus **Z** No Device	**Z** No Qualifier

Placement—Anatomical Orifices 2YØ–2Y5

2 Placement
Y Anatomical Orifices
Ø Change Taking out or off a device from a body part and putting back an identical or similar device in or on the same body part without cutting or puncturing the skin or a mucous membrane

Body Region Character 4	Approach Character 5	Device Character 6	Qualifier Character 7
Ø Mouth and Pharynx **1** Nasal **2** Ear **3** Anorectal **4** Female Genital Tract **5** Urethra	**X** External	**5** Packing Material	**Z** No Qualifier

2 Placement
Y Anatomical Orifices
4 Packing Putting material in a body region or orifice

Body Region Character 4	Approach Character 5	Device Character 6	Qualifier Character 7
Ø Mouth and Pharynx **1** Nasal **2** Ear **3** Anorectal **4** Female Genital Tract **5** Urethra	**X** External	**5** Packing Material	**Z** No Qualifier

2 Placement
Y Anatomical Orifices
5 Removal Taking out or off a device from a body part

Body Region Character 4	Approach Character 5	Device Character 6	Qualifier Character 7
Ø Mouth and Pharynx **1** Nasal **2** Ear **3** Anorectal **4** Female Genital Tract **5** Urethra	**X** External	**5** Packing Material	**Z** No Qualifier

Administration 3Ø2–3E1

3 Administration
Ø Circulatory
2 Transfusion Putting in blood or blood products

Body System/Region Character 4	Approach Character 5	Substance Character 6	Qualifier Character 7
3 Peripheral Vein **4** Central Vein	**Ø** Open **3** Percutaneous	**A** Stem Cells, Embryonic	**Z** No Qualifier
3 Peripheral Vein **4** Central Vein **5** Peripheral Artery **6** Central Artery	**Ø** Open **3** Percutaneous	**G** Bone Marrow **H** Whole Blood **J** Serum Albumin **K** Frozen Plasma **L** Fresh Plasma **M** Plasma Cryoprecipitate **N** Red Blood Cells **P** Frozen Red Cells **Q** White Cells **R** Platelets **S** Globulin **T** Fibrinogen **V** Antihemophilic Factors **W** Factor IX **X** Stem Cells, Cord Blood **Y** Stem Cells, Hematopoietic	**Ø** Autologous **1** Nonautologous
7 Products of Conception, Circulatory	**3** Percutaneous **7** Via Natural or Artificial Opening	**H** Whole Blood **J** Serum Albumin **K** Frozen Plasma **L** Fresh Plasma **M** Plasma Cryoprecipitate **N** Red Blood Cells **P** Frozen Red Cells **Q** White Cells **R** Platelets **S** Globulin **T** Fibrinogen **V** Antihemophilic Factors **W** Factor IX	**1** Nonautologous

3 Administration
C Indwelling Device
1 Irrigation Putting in or on a cleansing substance

Body System/Region Character 4	Approach Character 5	Substance Character 6	Qualifier Character 7
Z None	**X** External	**8** Irrigating Substance	**Z** No Qualifier

3 Administration
E Physiological Systems and Anatomical Regions
Ø Introduction Putting in or on a therapeutic, diagnostic, nutritional, physiological, or prophylactic substance except blood or blood products

Body System/Region Character 4	Approach Character 5	Substance Character 6	Qualifier Character 7
Ø Skin and Mucous Membranes	**X** External	**Ø** Antineoplastic	**5** Other Antineoplastic **M** Monoclonal Antibody
Ø Skin and Mucous Membranes	**X** External	**2** Anti-infective	**8** Oxazolidinones **9** Other Anti-infective
Ø Skin and Mucous Membranes	**X** External	**3** Anti-inflammatory **4** Serum, Toxoid and Vaccine **B** Local Anesthetic **K** Other Diagnostic Substance **M** Pigment **N** Analgesics, Hypnotics, Sedatives **T** Destructive Agent	**Z** No Qualifier
Ø Skin and Mucous Membranes	**X** External	**G** Other Therapeutic Substance	**C** Other Substance
1 Subcutaneous Tissue	**Ø** Open	**2** Infective	**A** Infective Envelope
1 Subcutaneous Tissue	**3** Percutaneous	**V** Hormone	**G** Insulin **J** Other Hormone
1 Subcutaneous Tissue	**3** Percutaneous	**2** Anti-infective	**8** Oxazolidinones **9** Other Anti-infective **A** **Anti-Infective Envelope**

3EØ Continued on next page

3EØ Continued

3 Administration
E Physiological Systems and Anatomical Regions
Ø Introduction Putting in or on a therapeutic, diagnostic, nutritional, physiological, or prophylactic substance except blood or blood products

Body System/Region Character 4	Approach Character 5	Substance Character 6	Qualifier Character 7
1 Subcutaneous Tissue **2** Muscle	**3** Percutaneous	**3** Anti-inflammatory **4** Serum, Toxoid and Vaccine **6** Nutritional Substance **7** Electrolytic and Water Balance Substance **B** Local Anesthetic **H** Radioactive Substance **K** Other Diagnostic Substance **N** Analgesics, Hypnotics, Sedatives **T** Destructive Agent	**Z** No Qualifier
1 Subcutaneous Tissue **2** Muscle **A** Bone Marrow **F** Respiratory Tract **L** Pleural Cavity **M** Peritoneal Cavity **Q** Cranial Cavity and Brain **R** Spinal Canal **S** Epidural Space **T** Peripheral Nerves and Plexi **W** Lymphatics **X** Cranial Nerves **Y** Pericardial Cavity	**3** Percutaneous	**G** Other Therapeutic Substance	**C** Other Substance
1 Subcutaneous Tissue **2** Muscle **A** Bone Marrow **V** Bones **W** Lymphatics	**3** Percutaneous	**Ø** Antineoplastic	**5** Other Antineoplastic **M** Monoclonal Antibody
1 Subcutaneous Tissue **2** Muscle **F** Respiratory Tract **L** Pleural Cavity **M** Peritoneal Cavity **Q** Cranial Cavity and Brain **R** Spinal Canal **S** Epidural Space **U** Joints **V** Bones **W** Lymphatics **Y** Pericardial Cavity	**3** Percutaneous	**2** Anti-infective	**8** Oxazolidinones **9** Other Anti-infective
3 Peripheral Vein	**Ø** Open **3** Percutaneous	**U** Pancreatic Islet Cells	**Ø** Autologous **1** Nonautologous
3 Peripheral Vein **4** Central Vein **5** Peripheral Artery **6** Central Artery	**Ø** Open **3** Percutaneous	**Ø** Antineoplastic	**2** High-dose Interleukin-2 **3** Low-dose Interleukin-2 **5** Other Antineoplastic **M** Monoclonal Antibody **P** Clofarabine
3 Peripheral Vein **4** Central Vein **5** Peripheral Artery **6** Central Artery	**Ø** Open **3** Percutaneous	**2** Anti-infective	**8** Oxazolidinones **9** Other Anti-infective
3 Peripheral Vein **4** Central Vein **5** Peripheral Artery **6** Central Artery	**Ø** Open **3** Percutaneous	**3** Anti-inflammatory **4** Serum, Toxoid and Vaccine **6** Nutritional Substance **7** Electrolytic and Water Balance Substance **F** Intracirculatory Anesthetic **H** Radioactive Substance **K** Other Diagnostic Substance **N** Analgesics, Hypnotics, Sedatives **P** Platelet Inhibitor **R** Antiarrhythmic **T** Destructive Agent **X** Vasopressor	**Z** No Qualifier
3 Peripheral Vein **4** Central Vein **5** Peripheral Artery **6** Central Artery	**Ø** Open **3** Percutaneous	**G** Other Therapeutic Substance	**C** Other Substance **N** Blood Brain Barrier Disruption
3 Peripheral Vein **4** Central Vein **5** Peripheral Artery **6** Central Artery	**Ø** Open **3** Percutaneous	**V** Hormone	**G** Insulin **H** Human B-type Natriuretic Peptide **J** Other Hormone

3EØ Continued on next page

3 Administration
E Physiological Systems and Anatomical Regions
0 Introduction Putting in or on a therapeutic, diagnostic, nutritional, physiological, or prophylactic substance except blood or blood products

3E0 Continued

Body System/Region Character 4	Approach Character 5	Substance Character 6	Qualifier Character 7
3 Peripheral Vein **4** Central Vein **5** Peripheral Artery **6** Central Artery	**0** Open **3** Percutaneous	**W** Immunotherapeutic	**K** Immunostimulator **L** Immunosuppressive
3 Peripheral Vein **4** Central Vein **5** Peripheral Artery **6** Central Artery **7** Coronary Artery **8** Heart	**0** Open **3** Percutaneous	**1** Thrombolytic	**6** Recombinant Human-activated Protein C **7** Other Thrombolytic
7 Coronary Artery **8** Heart	**0** Open **3** Percutaneous	**G** Other Therapeutic Substance	**C** Other Substance
7 Coronary Artery **8** Heart	**0** Open **3** Percutaneous	**K** Other Diagnostic Substance **P** Platelet Inhibitor	**Z** No Qualifier
9 Nose	**3** Percutaneous **7** Via Natural or Artificial Opening **X** External	**0** Antineoplastic	**5** Other Antineoplastic **M** Monoclonal Antibody
9 Nose	**3** Percutaneous **7** Via Natural or Artificial Opening **X** External	**3** Anti-inflammatory **4** Serum, Toxoid and Vaccine **B** Local Anesthetic **H** Radioactive Substance **K** Other Diagnostic Substance **N** Analgesics, Hypnotics, Sedatives **T** Destructive Agent	**Z** No Qualifier
9 Nose **B** Ear **C** Eye **D** Mouth and Pharynx	**3** Percutaneous **7** Via Natural or Artificial Opening **X** External	**2** Anti-infective	**8** Oxazolidinones **9** Other Anti-infective
9 Nose **B** Ear **C** Eye **D** Mouth and Pharynx	**3** Percutaneous **7** Via Natural or Artificial Opening **X** External	**G** Other Therapeutic Substance	**C** Other Substance
B Ear	**3** Percutaneous **7** Via Natural or Artificial Opening **X** External	**3** Anti-inflammatory **B** Local Anesthetic **H** Radioactive Substance **K** Other Diagnostic Substance **N** Analgesics, Hypnotics, Sedatives **T** Destructive Agent	**Z** No Qualifier
B Ear **C** Eye **D** Mouth and Pharynx	**3** Percutaneous **7** Via Natural or Artificial Opening **X** External	**0** Antineoplastic	**4** Liquid Brachytherapy Radioisotope **5** Other Antineoplastic **M** Monoclonal Antibody
C Eye	**3** Percutaneous **7** Via Natural or Artificial Opening **X** External	**3** Anti-inflammatory **B** Local Anesthetic **H** Radioactive Substance **K** Other Diagnostic Substance **M** Pigment **N** Analgesics, Hypnotics, Sedatives **T** Destructive Agent	**Z** No Qualifier
C Eye	**3** Percutaneous **7** Via Natural or Artificial Opening **X** External	**S** Gas	**F** Other Gas
D Mouth and Pharynx	**3** Percutaneous **7** Via Natural or Artificial Opening **X** External	**3** Anti-inflammatory **4** Serum, Toxoid and Vaccine **6** Nutritional Substance **7** Electrolytic and Water Balance Substance **B** Local Anesthetic **H** Radioactive Substance **K** Other Diagnostic Substance **N** Analgesics, Hypnotics, Sedatives **R** Antiarrhythmic **T** Destructive Agent	**Z** No Qualifier
E Products of Conception **F** Respiratory Tract **G** Upper GI **H** Lower GI **J** Biliary and Pancreatic Tract **K** Genitourinary Tract **N** Male Reproductive **P** Female Reproductive	**3** Percutaneous **7** Via Natural or Artificial Opening **8** Via Natural or Artificial Opening Endoscopic	**0** Antineoplastic	**4** Liquid Brachytherapy Radioisotope **5** Other Antineoplastic **M** Monoclonal Antibody

3E0 Continued on next page

 Revised Text in **BLUE**

3EØ Continued

3 Administration
E Physiological Systems and Anatomical Regions
Ø Introduction Putting in or on a therapeutic, diagnostic, nutritional, physiological, or prophylactic substance except blood or blood products

Body System/Region Character 4	Approach Character 5	Substance Character 6	Qualifier Character 7
E Products of Conception **F** Respiratory Tract **G** Upper GI **H** Lower GI **J** Biliary and Pancreatic Tract **K** Genitourinary Tract **N** Male Reproductive **P** Female Reproductive	**3** Percutaneous **7** Via Natural or Artificial Opening **8** Via Natural or Artificial Opening Endoscopic	**2** Anti-infective	**8** Oxazolidinones **9** Other Anti-infective
E Products of Conception **F** Respiratory Tract **G** Upper GI **H** Lower GI **J** Biliary and Pancreatic Tract **K** Genitourinary Tract **N** Male Reproductive **P** Female Reproductive	**3** Percutaneous **7** Via Natural or Artificial Opening **8** Via Natural or Artificial Opening Endoscopic	**G** Other Therapeutic Substance	**C** Other Substance
E Products of Conception **G** Upper GI **H** Lower GI **J** Biliary and Pancreatic Tract **K** Genitourinary Tract **N** Male Reproductive	**3** Percutaneous **7** Via Natural or Artificial Opening **8** Via Natural or Artificial Opening Endoscopic	**3** Anti-inflammatory **6** Nutritional Substance **7** Electrolytic and Water Balance Substance **B** Local Anesthetic **H** Radioactive Substance **K** Other Diagnostic Substance **N** Analgesics, Hypnotics, Sedatives **T** Destructive Agent	**Z** No Qualifier
E Products of Conception **G** Upper GI **H** Lower GI **J** Biliary and Pancreatic Tract **K** Genitourinary Tract **N** Male Reproductive **P** Female Reproductive	**3** Percutaneous **7** Via Natural or Artificial Opening **8** Via Natural or Artificial Opening Endoscopic	**S** Gas	**F** Other Gas
F Respiratory Tract	**3** Percutaneous **7** Via Natural or Artificial Opening **8** Via Natural or Artificial Opening Endoscopic	**S** Gas	**D** Nitric Oxide **F** Other Gas
F Respiratory Tract	**7** Via Natural or Artificial Opening **8** Via Natural or Artificial Opening Endoscopic	**3** Anti-inflammatory **6** Nutritional Substance **7** Electrolytic and Water Balance Substance **B** Local Anesthetic **D** Inhalation Anesthetic **H** Radioactive Substance **K** Other Diagnostic Substance **N** Analgesics, Hypnotics, Sedatives **T** Destructive Agent	**Z** No Qualifier
F Respiratory Tract **L** Pleural Cavity **M** Peritoneal Cavity **W** Lymphatics **Y** Pericardial Cavity	**3** Percutaneous	**3** Anti-inflammatory **6** Nutritional Substance **7** Electrolytic and Water Balance Substance **B** Local Anesthetic **H** Radioactive Substance **K** Other Diagnostic Substance **N** Analgesics, Hypnotics, Sedatives **T** Destructive Agent	**Z** No Qualifier
J Biliary and Pancreatic Tract	**3** Percutaneous **7** Via Natural or Artificial Opening **8** Via Natural or Artificial Opening Endoscopic	**U** Pancreatic Islet Cells	**Ø** Autologous **1** Nonautologous
L Pleural Cavity **M** Peritoneal Cavity **P** Female Reproductive	**Ø** Open	**5** Adhesion Barrier	**Z** No Qualifier
L Pleural Cavity **M** Peritoneal Cavity **Q** Cranial Cavity and Brain **R** Spinal Canal **S** Epidural Space **Y** Pericardial Cavity	**3** Percutaneous **7** Via Natural or Artificial Opening	**S** Gas	**F** Other Gas
L Pleural Cavity **M** Peritoneal Cavity **Q** Cranial Cavity and Brain **Y** Pericardial Cavity	**3** Percutaneous **7** Via Natural or Artificial Opening	**Ø** Antineoplastic	**4** Liquid Brachytherapy Radioisotope **5** Other Antineoplastic **M** Monoclonal Antibody

3EØ Continued on next page

3 Administration
E Physiological Systems and Anatomical Regions
0 Introduction Putting in or on a therapeutic, diagnostic, nutritional, physiological, or prophylactic substance except blood or blood products

3E0 Continued

Body System/Region Character 4	Approach Character 5	Substance Character 6	Qualifier Character 7
P Female Reproductive	**3** Percutaneous **7** Via Natural or Artificial Opening	**3** Anti-inflammatory **6** Nutritional Substance **7** Electrolytic and Water Balance Substance **B** Local Anesthetic **H** Radioactive Substance **K** Other Diagnostic Substance **L** Sperm **N** Analgesics, Hypnotics, Sedatives **T** Destructive Agent	**Z** No Qualifier
P Female Reproductive	**3** Percutaneous **7** Via Natural or Artificial Opening	**Q** Fertilized Ovum	**0** Autologous **1** Nonautologous
P Female Reproductive	**8** Via Natural or Artificial Opening Endoscopic	**3** Anti-inflammatory **6** Nutritional Substance **7** Electrolytic and Water Balance Substance **B** Local Anesthetic **H** Radioactive Substance **K** Other Diagnostic Substance **N** Analgesics, Hypnotics, Sedatives **T** Destructive Agent	**Z** No Qualifier
Q Cranial Cavity and Brain	**3** Percutaneous	**3** Anti-inflammatory **6** Nutritional Substance **7** Electrolytic and Water Balance Substance **A** Stem Cells, Embryonic **B** Local Anesthetic **H** Radioactive Substance **K** Other Diagnostic Substance **N** Analgesics, Hypnotics, Sedatives **T** Destructive Agent	**Z** No Qualifier
Q Cranial Cavity and Brain **R** Spinal Canal	**0** Open	**A** Stem Cells, Embryonic	**Z** No Qualifier
Q Cranial Cavity and Brain **R** Spinal Canal	**0** Open **3** Percutaneous	**E** Stem Cells, Somatic	**0** Autologous **1** Nonautologous
R Spinal Canal	**3** Percutaneous	**3** Anti-inflammatory **6** Nutritional Substance **7** Electrolytic and Water Balance Substance **A** Stem Cells, Embryonic **B** Local Anesthetic **C** Regional Anesthetic **H** Radioactive Substance **K** Other Diagnostic Substance **N** Analgesics, Hypnotics, Sedatives **T** Destructive Agent	**Z** No Qualifier
R Spinal Canal **S** Epidural Space	**3** Percutaneous	**0** Antineoplastic	**2** High-dose Interleukin-2 **3** Low-dose Interleukin-2 **4** Liquid Brachytherapy Radioisotope **5** Other Antineoplastic **M** Monoclonal Antibody
S Epidural Space	**3** Percutaneous	**3** Anti-inflammatory **6** Nutritional Substance **7** Electrolytic and Water Balance Substance **B** Local Anesthetic **C** Regional Anesthetic **H** Radioactive Substance **K** Other Diagnostic Substance **N** Analgesics, Hypnotics, Sedatives **T** Destructive Agent	**Z** No Qualifier
T Peripheral Nerves and Plexi **X** Cranial Nerves	**3** Percutaneous	**3** Anti-inflammatory **C** Regional Anesthetic **T** Destructive Agent	**Z** No Qualifier
U Joints **V** Bones	**0** Open	**G** Other Therapeutic Substance	**B** Recombinant Bone Morphogenetic Protein
U Joints	**0** Open	**2** Anti-infective	**8** Oxazolidinones **9** Other Anti-infective
U Joints	**3** Percutaneous	**0** Antineoplastic	**4** Liquid Brachytherapy Radioisotope **5** Other Antineoplastic **M** Monoclonal Antibody
U Joints	**3** Percutaneous	**2** Anti-infective	**8** Oxazolidinones 9 Other Anti-infective
U Joints	**3** Percutaneous	**S** Gas	**F** **Other Gas**

3E0 Continued on next page

3EØ Continued

3 Administration
E Physiological Systems and Anatomical Regions
Ø Introduction Putting in or on a therapeutic, diagnostic, nutritional, physiological, or prophylactic substance except blood or blood products

Body System/Region Character 4	Approach Character 5	Substance Character 6	Qualifier Character 7
U Joints **V** Bones	**3** Percutaneous	**3** Anti-inflammatory **6** Nutritional Substance **7** Electrolytic and Water Balance Substance **B** Local Anesthetic **H** Radioactive Substance **K** Other Diagnostic Substance **N** Analgesics, Hypnotics, Sedatives **T** Destructive Agent	**Z** No Qualifier
V Bones	**3** Percutaneous	**Ø** Antineoplastic	**5** Other Antineoplastic **M** Monoclonal Antibody
V Bones	**3** Percutaneous	**2** Anti-infective	**8** Oxazolidinones **9** Other Anti-infective
U Joints **V** Bones	**3** Percutaneous	**G** Other Therapeutic Substance	**B** Recombinant Bone Morphogenetic Protein **C** Other Substance

3 Administration
E Physiological Systems and Anatomical Regions
1 Irrigation Putting in or on a cleansing substance

Body System/Region Character 4	Approach Character 5	Substance Character 6	Qualifier Character 7
Ø Skin and Mucous Membranes **C** Eye	**3** Percutaneous **X** External	**8** Irrigating Substance	**X** Diagnostic **Z** No Qualifier
9 Nose **B** Ear **F** Respiratory Tract **G** Upper GI **H** Lower GI **J** Biliary and Pancreatic Tract **K** Genitourinary Tract **N** Male Reproductive **P** Female Reproductive	**3** Percutaneous **7** Via Natural or Artificial Opening **8** Via Natural or Artificial Opening Endoscopic	**8** Irrigating Substance	**X** Diagnostic **Z** No Qualifier
L Pleural Cavity **M** Peritoneal Cavity **Q** Cranial Cavity and Brain **R** Spinal Canal **S** Epidural Space **U** Joints **Y** Pericardial Cavity	**3** Percutaneous	**8** Irrigating Substance	**X** Diagnostic **Z** No Qualifier
M Peritoneal Cavity	**3** Percutaneous	**9** Dialysate	**Z** No Qualifier

Measurement and Monitoring 4A0–4B0

4 Measurement and Monitoring
A Physiological Systems
0 Measurement Determining the level of a physiological or physical function at a point in time

Body System Character 4	Approach Character 5	Function/Device Character 6	Qualifier Character 7
0 Central Nervous	0 Open	2 Conductivity 4 Electrical Activity B Pressure	Z No Qualifier
0 Central Nervous	**3 Percutaneous**	**4 Electrical Activity**	**Z No Qualifier**
0 Central Nervous	3 Percutaneous 7 Via Natural or Artificial Opening	B Pressure K Temperature R Saturation	D Intracranial
0 Central Nervous	X External	2 Conductivity 4 Electrical Activity	Z No Qualifier
1 Peripheral Nervous	0 Open 3 Percutaneous X External	2 Conductivity	9 Sensory B Motor
1 Peripheral Nervous	0 Open 3 Percutaneous X External	**4 Electrical Activity**	Z No Qualifier
2 Cardiac	0 Open 3 Percutaneous	N Sampling and Pressure	6 Right Heart 7 Left Heart 8 Bilateral
2 Cardiac	0 Open 3 Percutaneous	4 Electrical Activity 9 Output C Rate F Rhythm H Sound P Action Currents	Z No Qualifier
2 Cardiac	X External	9 Output C Rate F Rhythm H Sound P Action Currents	Z No Qualifier
2 Cardiac	X External	M Total Activity	4 Stress
2 Cardiac	X External	4 Electrical Activity	A Guidance Z No Qualifier
3 Arterial	0 Open 3 Percutaneous	5 Flow J Pulse	1 Peripheral 3 Pulmonary C Coronary
3 Arterial	0 Open 3 Percutaneous	B Pressure	1 Peripheral 3 Pulmonary C Coronary F Other Thoracic
3 Arterial	0 Open 3 Percutaneous	H Sound R Saturation	1 Peripheral
3 Arterial	X External	5 Flow B Pressure H Sound J Pulse R Saturation	1 Peripheral
4 Venous	0 Open 3 Percutaneous	5 Flow B Pressure J Pulse	0 Central 1 Peripheral 2 Portal 3 Pulmonary
4 Venous	0 Open 3 Percutaneous	R Saturation	1 Peripheral
4 Venous	X External	5 Flow B Pressure J Pulse R Saturation	1 Peripheral
5 Circulatory	X External	L Volume	Z No Qualifier
6 Lymphatic	0 Open 3 Percutaneous	5 Flow B Pressure	Z No Qualifier
7 Visual	X External	0 Acuity 7 Mobility B Pressure	Z No Qualifier

4A0 Continued on next page

4AØ Continued

4 Measurement and Monitoring
A Physiological Systems
Ø Measurement Determining the level of a physiological or physical function at a point in time

Body System Character 4	Approach Character 5	Function/Device Character 6	Qualifier Character 7
8 Olfactory	X External	Ø Acuity	Z No Qualifier
9 Respiratory	7 Via Natural or Artificial Opening 8 Via Natural or Artificial Opening Endoscopic X External	1 Capacity 5 Flow C Rate D Resistance L Volume M Total Activity	Z No Qualifier
B Gastrointestinal	7 Via Natural or Artificial Opening 8 Via Natural or Artificial Opening Endoscopic	8 Motility B Pressure G Secretion	Z No Qualifier
C Biliary	3 Percutaneous 4 Percutaneous Endoscopic 7 Via Natural or Artificial Opening 8 Via Natural or Artificial Opening Endoscopic	5 Flow B Pressure	Z No Qualifier
D Urinary	7 Via Natural or Artificial Opening	3 Contractility 5 Flow B Pressure D Resistance L Volume	Z No Qualifier
F Musculoskeletal	3 Percutaneous X External	3 Contractility	Z No Qualifier
H Products of Conception, Cardiac	7 Via Natural or Artificial Opening 8 Via Natural or Artificial Opening Endoscopic X External	4 Electrical Activity C Rate F Rhythm H Sound	Z No Qualifier
J Products of Conception, Nervous	7 Via Natural or Artificial Opening 8 Via Natural or Artificial Opening Endoscopic X External	2 Conductivity 4 Electrical Activity B Pressure	Z No Qualifier
Z None	7 Via Natural or Artificial Opening	6 Metabolism K Temperature	Z No Qualifier
Z None	X External	6 Metabolism K Temperature Q Sleep	Z No Qualifier

4 Measurement and Monitoring
A Physiological Systems
1 Monitoring Determining the level of a physiological or physical function repetitively over a period of time

Body System Character 4	Approach Character 5	Function/Device Character 6	Qualifier Character 7
Ø Central Nervous	Ø Open	2 Conductivity B Pressure	Z No Qualifier
Ø Central Nervous	Ø Open X External	4 Electrical Activity	G Intraoperative Z No Qualifier
Ø Central Nervous	3 Percutaneous 7 Via Natural or Artificial Opening	B Pressure K Temperature R Saturation	D Intracranial
Ø Central Nervous	**3 Percutaneous**	4 Electrical Activity	G Intraoperative Z No Qualifier
Ø Central Nervous	X External	2 Conductivity	Z No Qualifier
1 Peripheral Nervous	Ø Open 3 Percutaneous X External	2 Conductivity	9 Sensory B Motor
1 Peripheral Nervous	Ø Open 3 Percutaneous X External	**4 Electrical Activity**	G Intraoperative Z No Qualifier
2 Cardiac	Ø Open 3 Percutaneous	4 Electrical Activity 9 Output C Rate F Rhythm H Sound	Z No Qualifier
2 Cardiac	X External	4 Electrical Activity	5 Ambulatory Z No Qualifier

4A1 Continued on next page

4 Measurement and Monitoring
A Physiological Systems
1 Monitoring Determining the level of a physiological or physical function repetitively over a period of time

4A1 Continued

Body System Character 4	Approach Character 5	Function/Device Character 6	Qualifier Character 7
2 Cardiac	**X** External	**9** Output **C** Rate **F** Rhythm **H** Sound	**Z** No Qualifier
2 Cardiac	**X** External	**M** Total Activity	**4** Stress
3 Arterial	**0** Open **3** Percutaneous	**5** Flow **B** Pressure **J** Pulse	**1** Peripheral **3** Pulmonary **C** Coronary
3 Arterial	**0** Open **3** Percutaneous	**H** Sound **R** Saturation	**1** Peripheral
3 Arterial	**X** External	**5** Flow **B** Pressure **H** Sound **J** Pulse **R** Saturation	**1** Peripheral
4 Venous	**0** Open **3** Percutaneous	**5** Flow **B** Pressure **J** Pulse	**0** Central **1** Peripheral **2** Portal **3** Pulmonary
4 Venous	**0** Open **3** Percutaneous	**R** Saturation	**0** Central **2** Portal **3** Pulmonary
4 Venous	**X** External	**5** Flow **B** Pressure **J** Pulse	**1** Peripheral
6 Lymphatic	**0** Open **3** Percutaneous	**5** Flow **B** Pressure	**Z** No Qualifier
9 Respiratory	**7** Via Natural or Artificial Opening **X** External	**1** Capacity **5** Flow **C** Rate **D** Resistance **L** Volume	**Z** No Qualifier
B Gastrointestinal	**7** Via Natural or Artificial Opening **8** Via Natural or Artificial Opening Endoscopic	**8** Motility **B** Pressure **G** Secretion	**Z** No Qualifier
D Urinary	**7** Via Natural or Artificial Opening	**3** Contractility **5** Flow **B** Pressure **D** Resistance **L** Volume	**Z** No Qualifier
H Products of Conception, Cardiac	**7** Via Natural or Artificial Opening **8** Via Natural or Artificial Opening Endoscopic **X** External	**4** Electrical Activity **C** Rate **F** Rhythm **H** Sound	**Z** No Qualifier
J Products of Conception, Nervous	**7** Via Natural or Artificial Opening **8** Via Natural or Artificial Opening Endoscopic **X** External	**2** Conductivity **4** Electrical Activity **B** Pressure	**Z** No Qualifier
Z None	**7** Via Natural or Artificial Opening	**K** Temperature	**Z** No Qualifier
Z None	**X** External	**K** Temperature **Q** Sleep	**Z** No Qualifier

4 Measurement and Monitoring
B Physiological Devices
0 Measurement Determining the level of a physiological or physical function repetitively over a period of time

Body System Character 4	Approach Character 5	Function/Device Character 6	Qualifier Character 7
0 Central Nervous **1** Peripheral Nervous **F** Musculoskeletal	**X** External	**V** Stimulator	**Z** No Qualifier
2 Cardiac	**X** External	**S** Pacemaker **T** Defibrillator	**Z** No Qualifier
9 Respiratory	**X** External	**S** Pacemaker	**Z** No Qualifier

Extracorporeal Assistance and Performance 5AØ–5A2

5 Extracorporeal Assistance and Performance
A Physiological Systems
Ø Assistance Taking over a portion of a physiological function by extracorporeal means

Body System Character 4	Duration Character 5	Function Character 6	Qualifier Character 7
2 Cardiac	1 Intermittent 2 Continuous	1 Output	Ø Balloon Pump 5 Pulsatile Compression 6 Other Pump D Impeller Pump
5 Circulatory	1 Intermittent 2 Continuous	2 Oxygenation	1 Hyperbaric C Supersaturated
9 Respiratory	3 Less than 24 Consecutive Hours 4 24-96 Consecutive Hours 5 Greater than 96 Consecutive Hours	5 Ventilation	7 Continuous Positive Airway Pressure 8 Intermittent Positive Airway Pressure 9 Continuous Negative Airway Pressure B Intermittent Negative Airway Pressure Z No Qualifier

5 Extracorporeal Assistance and Performance
A Physiological Systems
1 Performance Completely taking over a physiological function by extracorporeal means

Body System Character 4	Duration Character 5	Function Character 6	Qualifier Character 7
2 Cardiac	Ø Single	1 Output	2 Manual
2 Cardiac	1 Intermittent	3 Pacing	Z No Qualifier
2 Cardiac	2 Continuous	1 Output 3 Pacing	Z No Qualifier
5 Circulatory	2 Continuous	2 Oxygenation	3 Membrane
9 Respiratory	Ø Single	5 Ventilation	4 Nonmechanical
9 Respiratory	3 Less than 24 Consecutive Hours 4 24-96 Consecutive Hours 5 Greater than 96 Consecutive Hours	5 Ventilation	Z No Qualifier
C Biliary D Urinary	Ø Single 6 Multiple	Ø Filtration	Z No Qualifier

5 Extracorporeal Assistance and Performance
A Physiological Systems
2 Restoration Returning, or attempting to return, a physiological function to its original state by extracorporeal means.

Body System Character 4	Duration Character 5	Function Character 6	Qualifier Character 7
2 Cardiac	Ø Single	4 Rhythm	Z No Qualifier

Extracorporeal Therapies 6A0–6A9

6 Extracorporeal Therapies
A Physiological Systems
0 Atmospheric Control Extracorporeal control of atmospheric pressure and composition

Body System Character 4	Duration Character 5	Qualifier Character 6	Qualifier Character 7
Z None	0 Single 1 Multiple	Z No Qualifier	Z No Qualifier

6 Extracorporeal Therapies
A Physiological Systems
1 Decompression Extracorporeal elimination of undissolved gas from body fluids

Body System Character 4	Duration Character 5	Qualifier Character 6	Qualifier Character 7
5 Circulatory	0 Single 1 Multiple	Z No Qualifier	Z No Qualifier

6 Extracorporeal Therapies
A Physiological Systems
2 Electromagnetic Therapy Extracorporeal treatment by electromagnetic rays

Body System Character 4	Duration Character 5	Qualifier Character 6	Qualifier Character 7
1 Urinary 2 Central Nervous	0 Single 1 Multiple	Z No Qualifier	Z No Qualifier

6 Extracorporeal Therapies
A Physiological Systems
3 Hyperthermia Extracorporeal raising of body temperature

Body System Character 4	Duration Character 5	Qualifier Character 6	Qualifier Character 7
Z None	0 Single 1 Multiple	Z No Qualifier	Z No Qualifier

6 Extracorporeal Therapies
A Physiological Systems
4 Hypothermia Extracorporeal lowering of body temperature

Body System Character 4	Duration Character 5	Qualifier Character 6	Qualifier Character 7
Z None	0 Single 1 Multiple	Z No Qualifier	Z No Qualifier

6 Extracorporeal Therapies
A Physiological Systems
5 Pheresis Extracorporeal separation of blood products

Body System Character 4	Duration Character 5	Qualifier Character 6	Qualifier Character 7
5 Circulatory	0 Single 1 Multiple	Z No Qualifier	0 Erythrocytes 1 Leukocytes 2 Platelets 3 Plasma T Stem Cells, Cord Blood V Stem Cells, Hematopoietic

6 Extracorporeal Therapies
A Physiological Systems
6 Phototherapy Extracorporeal treatment by light rays

Body System Character 4	Duration Character 5	Qualifier Character 6	Qualifier Character 7
0 Skin 5 Circulatory	0 Single 1 Multiple	Z No Qualifier	Z No Qualifier

6 Extracorporeal Therapies
A Physiological Systems
7 Ultrasound Therapy Extracorporeal treatment by ultrasound

Body System Character 4	Duration Character 5	Qualifier Character 6	Qualifier Character 7
5 Circulatory	**Ø** Single **1** Multiple	**Z** No Qualifier	**4** Head and Neck Vessels **5** Heart **6** Peripheral Vessels **7** Other Vessels **Z** No Qualifier

6 Extracorporeal Therapies
A Physiological Systems
8 Ultraviolet Light Therapy Extracorporeal treatment by ultraviolet light

Body System Character 4	Duration Character 5	Qualifier Character 6	Qualifier Character 7
Ø Skin	**Ø** Single **1** Multiple	**Z** No Qualifier	**Z** No Qualifier

6 Extracorporeal Therapies
A Physiological Systems
9 Shock Wave Therapy Extracorporeal treatment by shock waves

Body System Character 4	Duration Character 5	Qualifier Character 6	Qualifier Character 7
3 Musculoskeletal	**Ø** Single **1** Multiple	**Z** No Qualifier	**Z** No Qualifier

Osteopathic 7WØ

7 Osteopathic
W Anatomical Regions
Ø Treatment Manual treatment to eliminate or alleviate somatic dysfunction and related disorders

Body Region Character 4	Approach Character 5	Method Character 6	Qualifier Character 7
Ø Head	**X** External	**Ø** Articulatory-Raising	**Z** None
1 Cervical		**1** Fascial Release	
2 Thoracic		**2** General Mobilization	
3 Lumbar		**3** High Velocity-Low Amplitude	
4 Sacrum		**4** Indirect	
5 Pelvis		**5** Low Velocity-High Amplitude	
6 Lower Extremities		**6** Lymphatic Pump	
7 Upper Extremities		**7** Muscle Energy-Isometric	
8 Rib Cage		**8** Muscle Energy-Isotonic	
9 Abdomen		**9** Other Method	

Other Procedures 8CØ–8EØ

8 Other Procedures
C Indwelling Device
Ø Other Procedures Methodologies which attempt to remediate or cure a disorder or disease

Body Region Character 4	Approach Character 5	Method Character 6	Qualifier Character 7
1 Nervous System	**X** External	**6** Collection	**J** Cerebrospinal Fluid **L** Other Fluid
2 Circulatory System	**X** External	**6** Collection	**K** Blood **L** Other Fluid

8 Other Procedures
E Physiological Systems and Anatomical Regions
Ø Other Procedures Methodologies which attempt to remediate or cure a disorder or disease

Body Region Character 4	Approach Character 5	Method Character 6	Qualifier Character 7
1 Nervous System **K** Musculoskeletal System **U** Female Reproductive System	**X** External	**Y** Other Method	**7** Examination
2 Circulatory System	**3** Percutaneous	**D** Near Infrared Spectroscopy	**Z** No Qualifier
9 Head and Neck Region **W** Trunk Region	**Ø** Open **3** Percutaneous **4** Percutaneous Endoscopic **7** Via Natural or Artificial Opening **8** Via Natural or Artificial Opening Endoscopic **X** External	**C** Robotic Assisted Procedure	**Z** No Qualifier
9 Head and Neck Region **W** Trunk Region **X** Upper Extremity **Y** Lower Extremity	**X** External	**B** Computer Assisted Procedure	**F** With Fluoroscopy **G** With Computerized Tomography **H** With Magnetic Resonance Imaging **Z** No Qualifier
9 Head and Neck Region **W** Trunk Region **X** Upper Extremity **Y** Lower Extremity	**X** External	**Y** Other Method	**8** Suture Removal
H Integumentary System and Breast	**3** Percutaneous	**Ø** Acupuncture	**Ø** Anesthesia **Z** No Qualifier
H Integumentary System and Breast	**X** External	**6** Collection	**2** Breast Milk
H Integumentary System and Breast	**X** External	**Y** Other Method	**9** Piercing
K Musculoskeletal System	**X** External	**1** Therapeutic Massage	**Z** No Qualifier
V Male Reproductive System	**X** External	**1** Therapeutic Massage	**C** Prostate **D** Rectum
V Male Reproductive System	**X** External	**6** Collection	**3** Sperm
X Upper Extremity **Y** Lower Extremity	**Ø** Open **3** Percutaneous **4** Percutaneous Endoscopic **X** External	**C** Robotic Assisted Procedure	**Z** No Qualifier
Z None	**X** External	**Y** Other Method	**1** In Vitro Fertilization **4** Yoga Therapy **5** Meditation **6** Isolation

Chiropractic 9WB

9 Chiropractic
W Anatomical Regions
B Manipulation Manual procedure that involves a directed thrust to move a joint past the physiological range of motion, without exceeding the anatomical limit

Body Region Character 4	Approach Character 5	Method Character 6	Qualifier Character 7
Ø Head **1** Cervical **2** Thoracic **3** Lumbar **4** Sacrum **5** Pelvis **6** Lower Extremities **7** Upper Extremities **8** Rib Cage **9** Abdomen	**X** External	**B** Non-Manual **C** Indirect Visceral **D** Extra-Articular **F** Direct Visceral **G** Long Lever Specific Contact **H** Short Lever Specific Contact **J** Long and Short Lever Specific Contact **K** Mechanically Assisted **L** Other Method	**Z** None

Imaging B00–BY4

B Imaging
0 Central Nervous System
0 Plain Radiography Planar display of an image developed from the capture of external ionizing radiation on photographic or photoconductive plate

Body Part Character 4	Contrast Character 5	Qualifier Character 6	Qualifier Character 7
B Spinal Cord	**0** High Osmolar **1** Low Osmolar **Y** Other Contrast **Z** None	**Z** None	**Z** None

B Imaging
0 Central Nervous System
1 Fluoroscopy Single plane or bi-plane real time display of an image developed from the capture of external ionizing radioation on a fluorescent screen. The image may also be stored by either digital or analog means

Body Part Character 4	Contrast Character 5	Qualifier Character 6	Qualifier Character 7
B Spinal Cord	**0** High Osmolar **1** Low Osmolar **Y** Other Contrast **Z** None	**Z** None	**Z** None

B Imaging
0 Central Nervous System
2 Computerized Tomography (CT Scan) Computer reformatted digital display of multiplanar images developed from the capture of multiple exposures of external ionizing radiation

Body Part Character 4	Contrast Character 5	Qualifier Character 6	Qualifier Character 7
0 Brain **7** Cisterna **8** Cerebral Ventricle(s) **9** Sella Turcica/Pituitary Gland **B** Spinal Cord	**0** High Osmolar **1** Low Osmolar **Y** Other Contrast	**0** Unenhanced and Enhanced **Z** None	**Z** None
0 Brain **7** Cisterna **8** Cerebral Ventricle(s) **9** Sella Turcica/Pituitary Gland **B** Spinal Cord	**Z** None	**Z** None	**Z** None

B Imaging
0 Central Nervous System
3 Magnetic Resonance Imaging (MRI) Computer reformatted digital display of multiplanar images developed from the capture of radio-frequency signals emitted by nuclei in a body site excited within a magnetic field

Body Part Character 4	Contrast Character 5	Qualifier Character 6	Qualifier Character 7
0 Brain **9** Sella Turcica/Pituitary Gland **B** Spinal Cord **C** Acoustic Nerves	**Y** Other Contrast	**0** Unenhanced and Enhanced **Z** None	**Z** None
0 Brain **9** Sella Turcica/Pituitary Gland **B** Spinal Cord **C** Acoustic Nerves	**Z** None	**Z** None	**Z** None

B Imaging
0 Central Nervous System
4 Ultrasonography Real time display of images of anatomy or flow information developed from the capture of relected and attenuated high frequency sound waves

Body Part Character 4	Contrast Character 5	Qualifier Character 6	Qualifier Character 7
0 Brain **B** Spinal Cord	**Z** None	**Z** None	**Z** None

B Imaging
2 Heart
0 Plain Radiography Planar display of an image developed from the capture of external ionizing radiation on photographic or photoconductive plate

Body Part Character 4	Contrast Character 5	Qualifier Character 6	Qualifier Character 7
0 Coronary Artery, Single 1 Coronary Arteries, Multiple 2 Coronary Artery Bypass Graft, Single 3 Coronary Artery Bypass Grafts, Multiple 4 Heart, Right 5 Heart, Left 6 Heart, Right and Left 7 Internal Mammary Bypass Graft, Right 8 Internal Mammary Bypass Graft, Left F Bypass Graft, Other	0 High Osmolar 1 Low Osmolar Y Other Contrast	Z None	Z None

B Imaging
2 Heart
1 Fluoroscopy Single plane or bi-plane real time display of an image developed from the capture of external ionizing radioation on a fluorescent screen. The image may also be stored by either digital or analog means

Body Part Character 4	Contrast Character 5	Qualifier Character 6	Qualifier Character 7
0 Coronary Artery, Single 1 Coronary Arteries, Multiple 2 Coronary Artery Bypass Graft, Single 3 Coronary Artery Bypass Grafts, Multiple	0 High Osmolar 1 Low Osmolar Y Other Contrast	1 Laser	0 Intraoperative
0 Coronary Artery, Single 1 Coronary Arteries, Multiple 2 Coronary Artery Bypass Graft, Single 3 Coronary Artery Bypass Grafts, Multiple 4 Heart, Right 5 Heart, Left 6 Heart, Right and Left 7 Internal Mammary Bypass Graft, Right 8 Internal Mammary Bypass Graft, Left F Bypass Graft, Other	0 High Osmolar 1 Low Osmolar Y Other Contrast	Z None	Z None

B Imaging
2 Heart
2 Computerized Tomography (CT Scan) Computer reformatted digital display of multiplanar images developed from the capture of multiple exposures of external ionizing radiation

Body Part Character 4	Contrast Character 5	Qualifier Character 6	Qualifier Character 7
1 Coronary Arteries, Multiple 3 Coronary Artery Bypass Grafts, Multiple 6 Heart, Right and Left	0 High Osmolar 1 Low Osmolar Y Other Contrast	0 Unenhanced and Enhanced Z None	Z None
1 Coronary Arteries, Multiple 3 Coronary Artery Bypass Grafts, Multiple 6 Heart, Right and Left	Z None	2 Intravascular Optical Coherence Z None	Z None

B Imaging
2 Heart
3 Magnetic Resonance Imaging (MRI) Computer reformatted digital display of multiplanar images developed from the capture of radio-frequency signals emitted by nuclei in a body site excited within a magnetic field

Body Part Character 4	Contrast Character 5	Qualifier Character 6	Qualifier Character 7
1 Coronary Arteries, Multiple 3 Coronary Artery Bypass Grafts, Multiple 6 Heart, Right and Left	Y Other Contrast	0 Unenhanced and Enhanced Z None	Z None
1 Coronary Arteries, Multiple 3 Coronary Artery Bypass Grafts, Multiple 6 Heart, Right and Left	Z None	Z None	Z None

B Imaging
2 Heart
4 Ultrasonography Real time display of images of anatomy or flow information developed from the capture of relected and attenuated high frequency sound waves

Body Part Character 4	Contrast Character 5	Qualifier Character 6	Qualifier Character 7
Ø Coronary Artery, Single **1** Coronary Arteries, Multiple **4** Heart, Right **5** Heart, Left **6** Heart, Right and Left **B** Heart with Aorta **C** Pericardium **D** Pediatric Heart	**Y** Other Contrast	**Z** None	**Z** None
Ø Coronary Artery, Single **1** Coronary Arteries, Multiple **4** Heart, Right **5** Heart, Left **6** Heart, Right and Left **B** Heart with Aorta **C** Pericardium **D** Pediatric Heart	**Z** None	**Z** None	**3** Intravascular **4** Transesophageal **Z** None

B Imaging
3 Upper Arteries
Ø Plain Radiography Planar display of an image developed from the capture of external ionizing radiation on photographic or photoconductive plate

Body Part Character 4	Contrast Character 5	Qualifier Character 6	Qualifier Character 7
Ø Thoracic Aorta **1** Brachiocephalic-Subclavian Artery, Right **2** Subclavian Artery, Left **3** Common Carotid Artery, Right **4** Common Carotid Artery, Left **5** Common Carotid Arteries, Bilateral **6** Internal Carotid Artery, Right **7** Internal Carotid Artery, Left **8** Internal Carotid Arteries, Bilateral **9** External Carotid Artery, Right **B** External Carotid Artery, Left **C** External Carotid Arteries, Bilateral **D** Vertebral Artery, Right **F** Vertebral Artery, Left **G** Vertebral Arteries, Bilateral **H** Upper Extremity Arteries, Right **J** Upper Extremity Arteries, Left **K** Upper Extremity Arteries, Bilateral **L** Intercostal and Bronchial Arteries **M** Spinal Arteries **N** Upper Arteries, Other **P** Thoraco-Abdominal Aorta **Q** Cervico-Cerebral Arch **R** Intracranial Arteries **S** Pulmonary Artery, Right **T** Pulmonary Artery, Left	**Ø** High Osmolar **1** Low Osmolar **Y** Other Contrast **Z** None	**Z** None	**Z** None

B Imaging
3 Upper Arteries
1 Fluoroscopy Fluoroscopy: Single plane or bi-plane real time display of an image developed from the capture of external ionizing radiation on a fluorescent screen. The image may also be stored by either digital or analog means

Body Part Character 4	Contrast Character 5	Qualifier Character 6	Qualifier Character 7
Ø Thoracic Aorta **1** Brachiocephalic-Subclavian Artery, Right **2** Subclavian Artery, Left **3** Common Carotid Artery, Right **4** Common Carotid Artery, Left **5** Common Carotid Arteries, Bilateral **6** Internal Carotid Artery, Right **7** Internal Carotid Artery, Left **8** Internal Carotid Arteries, Bilateral **9** External Carotid Artery, Right **B** External Carotid Artery, Left **C** External Carotid Arteries, Bilateral **D** Vertebral Artery, Right **F** Vertebral Artery, Left **G** Vertebral Arteries, Bilateral **H** Upper Extremity Arteries, Right **J** Upper Extremity Arteries, Left **K** Upper Extremity Arteries, Bilateral **L** Intercostal and Bronchial Arteries **M** Spinal Arteries **N** Upper Arteries, Other **P** Thoraco-Abdominal Aorta **Q** Cervico-Cerebral Arch **R** Intracranial Arteries **S** Pulmonary Artery, Right **T** Pulmonary Artery, Left	**Ø** High Osmolar **1** Low Osmolar **Y** Other Contrast	**1** Laser	**Ø** Intraoperative
Ø Thoracic Aorta **1** Brachiocephalic-Subclavian Artery, Right **2** Subclavian Artery, Left **3** Common Carotid Artery, Right **4** Common Carotid Artery, Left **5** Common Carotid Arteries, Bilateral **6** Internal Carotid Artery, Right **7** Internal Carotid Artery, Left **8** Internal Carotid Arteries, Bilateral **9** External Carotid Artery, Right **B** External Carotid Artery, Left **C** External Carotid Arteries, Bilateral **D** Vertebral Artery, Right **F** Vertebral Artery, Left **G** Vertebral Arteries, Bilateral **H** Upper Extremity Arteries, Right **J** Upper Extremity Arteries, Left **K** Upper Extremity Arteries, Bilateral **L** Intercostal and Bronchial Arteries **M** Spinal Arteries **N** Upper Arteries, Other **P** Thoraco-Abdominal Aorta **Q** Cervico-Cerebral Arch **R** Intracranial Arteries **S** Pulmonary Artery, Right **T** Pulmonary Artery, Left	**Ø** High Osmolar **1** Low Osmolar **Y** Other Contrast	**Z** None	**Z** None

B31 Continued on next page

B31 Continued

B Imaging
3 Upper Arteries
1 Fluoroscopy Fluoroscopy: Single plane or bi-plane real time display of an image developed from the capture of external ionizing radiation on a fluorescent screen. The image may also be stored by either digital or analog means

Body Part Character 4	Contrast Character 5	Qualifier Character 6	Qualifier Character 7
0 Thoracic Aorta **1** Brachiocephalic-Subclavian Artery, Right **2** Subclavian Artery, Left **3** Common Carotid Artery, Right **4** Common Carotid Artery, Left **5** Common Carotid Arteries, Bilateral **6** Internal Carotid Artery, Right **7** Internal Carotid Artery, Left **8** Internal Carotid Arteries, Bilateral **9** External Carotid Artery, Right **B** External Carotid Artery, Left **C** External Carotid Arteries, Bilateral **D** Vertebral Artery, Right **F** Vertebral Artery, Left **G** Vertebral Arteries, Bilateral **H** Upper Extremity Arteries, Right **J** Upper Extremity Arteries, Left **K** Upper Extremity Arteries, Bilateral **L** Intercostal and Bronchial Arteries **M** Spinal Arteries **N** Upper Arteries, Other **P** Thoraco-Abdominal Aorta **Q** Cervico-Cerebral Arch **R** Intracranial Arteries **S** Pulmonary Artery, Right **T** Pulmonary Artery, Left	**Z** None	**Z** None	**Z** None

B Imaging
3 Upper Arteries
2 Computerized Tomography (CT Scan) Computer reformatted digital display of multiplanar images developed from the capture of multiple exposures of external ionizing radiation

Body Part Character 4	Contrast Character 5	Qualifier Character 6	Qualifier Character 7
0 Thoracic Aorta **5** Common Carotid Arteries, Bilateral **8** Internal Carotid Arteries, Bilateral **G** Vertebral Arteries, Bilateral **R** Intracranial Arteries **S** Pulmonary Artery, Right **T** Pulmonary Artery, Left	**0** High Osmolar **1** Low Osmolar **Y** Other Contrast	**Z** None	**Z** None
0 Thoracic Aorta **5** Common Carotid Arteries, Bilateral **8** Internal Carotid Arteries, Bilateral **G** Vertebral Arteries, Bilateral **R** Intracranial Arteries **S** Pulmonary Artery, Right **T** Pulmonary Artery, Left	**Z** None	**2** Intravascular Optical Coherence **Z** None	**Z** None

B Imaging
3 Upper Arteries
3 Magnetic Resonance Imaging (MRI) Computer reformatted digital display of multiplanar images developed from the capture of radio-frequency signals emitted by nuclei in a body site excited within a magnetic field

Body Part Character 4	Contrast Character 5	Qualifier Character 6	Qualifier Character 7
0 Thoracic Aorta **5** Common Carotid Arteries, Bilateral **8** Internal Carotid Arteries, Bilateral **G** Vertebral Arteries, Bilateral **H** Upper Extremity Arteries, Right **J** Upper Extremity Arteries, Left **K** Upper Extremity Arteries, Bilateral **M** Spinal Arteries **Q** Cervico-Cerebral Arch **R** Intracranial Arteries	**Y** Other Contrast	**0** Unenhanced and Enhanced **Z** None	**Z** None
0 Thoracic Aorta **5** Common Carotid Arteries, Bilateral **8** Internal Carotid Arteries, Bilateral **G** Vertebral Arteries, Bilateral **H** Upper Extremity Arteries, Right **J** Upper Extremity Arteries, Left **K** Upper Extremity Arteries, Bilateral **M** Spinal Arteries **Q** Cervico-Cerebral Arch **R** Intracranial Arteries	**Z** None	**Z** None	**Z** None

B Imaging
3 Upper Arteries
4 Ultrasonography Real time display of images of anatomy or flow information developed from the capture of relected and attenuated high frequency sound waves

Body Part Character 4	Contrast Character 5	Qualifier Character 6	Qualifier Character 7
0 Thoracic Aorta **1** Brachiocephalic-Subclavian Artery, Right **2** Subclavian Artery, Left **3** Common Carotid Artery, Right **4** Common Carotid Artery, Left **5** Common Carotid Arteries, Bilateral **6** Internal Carotid Artery, Right **7** Internal Carotid Artery, Left **8** Internal Carotid Arteries, Bilateral **H** Upper Extremity Arteries, Right **J** Upper Extremity Arteries, Left **K** Upper Extremity Arteries, Bilateral **R** Intracranial Arteries **S** Pulmonary Artery, Right **T** Pulmonary Artery, Left **V** Ophthalmic Arteries	**Z** None	**Z** None	**3** Intravascular **Z** None

B Imaging
4 Lower Arteries
0 Plain Radiography Planar display of an image developed from the capture of external ionizing radiation on photographic or photoconductive plate

Body Part Character 4	Contrast Character 5	Qualifier Character 6	Qualifier Character 7
0 Abdominal Aorta **2** Hepatic Artery **3** Splenic Arteries **4** Superior Mesenteric Artery **5** Inferior Mesenteric Artery **6** Renal Artery, Right **7** Renal Artery, Left **8** Renal Arteries, Bilateral **9** Lumbar Arteries **B** Intra-Abdominal Arteries, Other **C** Pelvic Arteries **D** Aorta and Bilateral Lower Extremity Arteries **F** Lower Extremity Arteries, Right **G** Lower Extremity Arteries, Left **J** Lower Arteries, Other **M** Renal Artery Transplant	**0** High Osmolar **1** Low Osmolar **Y** Other Contrast	**Z** None	**Z** None

B Imaging
4 Lower Arteries
1 Fluoroscopy Single plane or bi-plane real time display of an image developed from the capture of external ionizing radiation on a fluorescent screen. The image may also be stored by either digital or analog means

Body Part Character 4	Contrast Character 5	Qualifier Character 6	Qualifier Character 7
Ø Abdominal Aorta **2** Hepatic Artery **3** Splenic Arteries **4** Superior Mesenteric Artery **5** Inferior Mesenteric Artery **6** Renal Artery, Right **7** Renal Artery, Left **8** Renal Arteries, Bilateral **9** Lumbar Arteries **B** Intra-Abdominal Arteries, Other **C** Pelvic Arteries **D** Aorta and Bilateral Lower Extremity Arteries **F** Lower Extremity Arteries, Right **G** Lower Extremity Arteries, Left **J** Lower Arteries, Other	**Ø** High Osmolar **1** Low Osmolar **Y** Other Contrast	**1** Laser	**Ø** Intraoperative
Ø Abdominal Aorta **2** Hepatic Artery **3** Splenic Arteries **4** Superior Mesenteric Artery **5** Inferior Mesenteric Artery **6** Renal Artery, Right **7** Renal Artery, Left **8** Renal Arteries, Bilateral **9** Lumbar Arteries **B** Intra-Abdominal Arteries, Other **C** Pelvic Arteries **D** Aorta and Bilateral Lower Extremity Arteries **F** Lower Extremity Arteries, Right **G** Lower Extremity Arteries, Left **J** Lower Arteries, Other	**Ø** High Osmolar **1** Low Osmolar **Y** Other Contrast	**Z** None	**Z** None
Ø Abdominal Aorta **2** Hepatic Artery **3** Splenic Arteries **4** Superior Mesenteric Artery **5** Inferior Mesenteric Artery **6** Renal Artery, Right **7** Renal Artery, Left **8** Renal Arteries, Bilateral **9** Lumbar Arteries **B** Intra-Abdominal Arteries, Other **C** Pelvic Arteries **D** Aorta and Bilateral Lower Extremity Arteries **F** Lower Extremity Arteries, Right **G** Lower Extremity Arteries, Left **J** Lower Arteries, Other	**Z** None	**Z** None	**Z** None

B Imaging
4 Lower Arteries
2 Computerized Tomography (CT Scan) Computer reformatted digital display of multiplanar images developed from the capture of multiple exposures of external ionizing radiation

Body Part Character 4	Contrast Character 5	Qualifier Character 6	Qualifier Character 7
Ø Abdominal Aorta **1** Celiac Artery **4** Superior Mesenteric Artery **8** Renal Arteries, Bilateral **C** Pelvic Arteries **F** Lower Extremity Arteries, Right **G** Lower Extremity Arteries, Left **H** Lower Extremity Arteries, Bilateral **M** Renal Artery Transplant	**Ø** High Osmolar **1** Low Osmolar **Y** Other Contrast	**Z** None	**Z** None
Ø Abdominal Aorta **1** Celiac Artery **4** Superior Mesenteric Artery **8** Renal Arteries, Bilateral **C** Pelvic Arteries **F** Lower Extremity Arteries, Right **G** Lower Extremity Arteries, Left **H** Lower Extremity Arteries, Bilateral **M** Renal Artery Transplant	**Z** None	**2** Intravascular Optical Coherence **Z** None	**Z** None

B Imaging
4 Lower Arteries
3 Magnetic Resonance Imaging (MRI) Computer reformatted digital display of multiplanar images developed from the capture of radio-frequency signals emitted by nuclei in a body site excited within a magnetic field

Body Part Character 4	Contrast Character 5	Qualifier Character 6	Qualifier Character 7
0 Abdominal Aorta **1** Celiac Artery **4** Superior Mesenteric Artery **8** Renal Arteries, Bilateral **C** Pelvic Arteries **F** Lower Extremity Arteries, Right **G** Lower Extremity Arteries, Left **H** Lower Extremity Arteries, Bilateral	**Y** Other Contrast	**0** Unenhanced and Enhanced **Z** None	**Z** None
0 Abdominal Aorta **1** Celiac Artery **4** Superior Mesenteric Artery **8** Renal Arteries, Bilateral **C** Pelvic Arteries **F** Lower Extremity Arteries, Right **G** Lower Extremity Arteries, Left **H** Lower Extremity Arteries, Bilateral	**Z** None	**Z** None	**Z** None

B Imaging
4 Lower Arteries
4 Ultrasonography Real time display of images of anatomy or flow information developed from the capture of relected and attenuated high frequency sound waves

Body Part Character 4	Contrast Character 5	Qualifier Character 6	Qualifier Character 7
0 Abdominal Aorta **4** Superior Mesenteric Artery **5** Inferior Mesenteric Artery **6** Renal Artery, Right **7** Renal Artery, Left **8** Renal Arteries, Bilateral **B** Intra-Abdominal Arteries, Other **F** Lower Extremity Arteries, Right **G** Lower Extremity Arteries, Left **H** Lower Extremity Arteries, Bilateral **K** Celiac and Mesenteric Arteries **L** Femoral Artery **N** Penile Arteries	**Z** None	**Z** None	**3** Intravascular **Z** None

B Imaging
5 Veins
0 Plain Radiography Planar display of an image developed from the capture of external ionizing radiation on photographic or photoconductive plate

Body Part Character 4	Contrast Character 5	Qualifier Character 6	Qualifier Character 7
0 Epidural Veins **1** Cerebral and Cerebellar Veins **2** Intracranial Sinuses **3** Jugular Veins, Right **4** Jugular Veins, Left **5** Jugular Veins, Bilateral **6** Subclavian Vein, Right **7** Subclavian Vein, Left **8** Superior Vena Cava **9** Inferior Vena Cava **B** Lower Extremity Veins, Right **C** Lower Extremity Veins, Left **D** Lower Extremity Veins, Bilateral **F** Pelvic (Iliac) Veins, Right **G** Pelvic (Iliac) Veins, Left **H** Pelvic (Iliac) Veins, Bilateral **J** Renal Vein, Right **K** Renal Vein, Left **L** Renal Veins, Bilateral **M** Upper Extremity Veins, Right **N** Upper Extremity Veins, Left **P** Upper Extremity Veins, Bilateral **Q** Pulmonary Vein, Right **R** Pulmonary Vein, Left **S** Pulmonary Veins, Bilateral **T** Portal and Splanchnic Veins **V** Veins, Other **W** Dialysis Shunt/Fistula	**0** High Osmolar **1** Low Osmolar **Y** Other Contrast	**Z** None	**Z** None

B Imaging
5 Veins
1 Fluoroscopy Single plane or bi-plane real time display of an image developed from the capture of external ionizing radioation on a fluorescent screen. The image may also be stored by either digital or analog means

Body Part Character 4	Contrast Character 5	Qualifier Character 6	Qualifier Character 7
Ø Epidural Veins **1** Cerebral and Cerebellar Veins **2** Intracranial Sinuses **3** Jugular Veins, Right **4** Jugular Veins, Left **5** Jugular Veins, Bilateral **6** Subclavian Vein, Right **7** Subclavian Vein, Left **8** Superior Vena Cava **9** Inferior Vena Cava **B** Lower Extremity Veins, Right **C** Lower Extremity Veins, Left **D** Lower Extremity Veins, Bilateral **F** Pelvic (Iliac) Veins, Right **G** Pelvic (Iliac) Veins, Left **H** Pelvic (Iliac) Veins, Bilateral **J** Renal Vein, Right **K** Renal Vein, Left **L** Renal Veins, Bilateral **M** Upper Extremity Veins, Right **N** Upper Extremity Veins, Left **P** Upper Extremity Veins, Bilateral **Q** Pulmonary Vein, Right **R** Pulmonary Vein, Left **S** Pulmonary Veins, Bilateral **T** Portal and Splanchnic Veins **V** Veins, Other **W** Dialysis Shunt/Fistula	**Ø** High Osmolar **1** Low Osmolar **Y** Other Contrast **Z** None	**Z** None	**A** Guidance **Z** None

B Imaging
5 Veins
2 Computerized Tomography (CT Scan) Computer reformatted digital display of multiplanar images developed from the capture of multiple exposures of external ionizing radiation

Body Part Character 4	Contrast Character 5	Qualifier Character 6	Qualifier Character 7
2 Intracranial Sinuses **8** Superior Vena Cava **9** Inferior Vena Cava **F** Pelvic (Iliac) Veins, Right **G** Pelvic (Iliac) Veins, Left **H** Pelvic (Iliac) Veins, Bilateral **J** Renal Vein, Right **K** Renal Vein, Left **L** Renal Veins, Bilateral **Q** Pulmonary Vein, Right **R** Pulmonary Vein, Left **S** Pulmonary Veins, Bilateral **T** Portal and Splanchnic Veins	**Ø** High Osmolar **1** Low Osmolar **Y** Other Contrast	**Ø** Unenhanced and Enhanced **Z** None	**Z** None
2 Intracranial Sinuses **8** Superior Vena Cava **9** Inferior Vena Cava **F** Pelvic (Iliac) Veins, Right **G** Pelvic (Iliac) Veins, Left **H** Pelvic (Iliac) Veins, Bilateral **J** Renal Vein, Right **K** Renal Vein, Left **L** Renal Veins, Bilateral **Q** Pulmonary Vein, Right **R** Pulmonary Vein, Left **S** Pulmonary Veins, Bilateral **T** Portal and Splanchnic Veins	**Z** None	**2** Intravascular Optical Coherence **Z** None	**Z** None

B Imaging
5 Veins
3 Magnetic Resonance Imaging (MRI) Computer reformatted digital display of multiplanar images developed from the capture of radio-frequency signals emitted by nuclei in a body site excited within a magnetic field

Body Part Character 4	Contrast Character 5	Qualifier Character 6	Qualifier Character 7
1 Cerebral and Cerebellar Veins **2** Intracranial Sinuses **5** Jugular Veins, Bilateral **8** Superior Vena Cava **9** Inferior Vena Cava **B** Lower Extremity Veins, Right **C** Lower Extremity Veins, Left **D** Lower Extremity Veins, Bilateral **H** Pelvic (Iliac) Veins, Bilateral **L** Renal Veins, Bilateral **M** Upper Extremity Veins, Right **N** Upper Extremity Veins, Left **P** Upper Extremity Veins, Bilateral **S** Pulmonary Veins, Bilateral **T** Portal and Splanchnic Veins **V** Veins, Other	**Y** Other Contrast	**Ø** Unenhanced and Enhanced **Z** None	**Z** None
1 Cerebral and Cerebellar Veins **2** Intracranial Sinuses **5** Jugular Veins, Bilateral **8** Superior Vena Cava **9** Inferior Vena Cava **B** Lower Extremity Veins, Right **C** Lower Extremity Veins, Left **D** Lower Extremity Veins, Bilateral **H** Pelvic (Iliac) Veins, Bilateral **L** Renal Veins, Bilateral **M** Upper Extremity Veins, Right **N** Upper Extremity Veins, Left **P** Upper Extremity Veins, Bilateral **S** Pulmonary Veins, Bilateral **T** Portal and Splanchnic Veins **V** Veins, Other	**Z** None	**Z** None	**Z** None

B Imaging
5 Veins
4 Ultrasonography Real time display of images of anatomy or flow information developed from the capture of relected and attenuated high frequency sound waves

Body Part Character 4	Contrast Character 5	Qualifier Character 6	Qualifier Character 7
3 Jugular Veins, Right **4** Jugular Veins, Left **6** Subclavian Vein, Right **7** Subclavian Vein, Left **9** Inferior Vena Cava **B** Lower Extremity Veins, Right **C** Lower Extremity Veins, Left **D** Lower Extremity Veins, Bilateral **J** Renal Vein, Right **K** Renal Vein, Left **L** Renal Veins, Bilateral **M** Upper Extremity Veins, Right **N** Upper Extremity Veins, Left **P** Upper Extremity Veins, Bilateral **T** Portal and Splanchnic Veins	**Z** None	**Z** None	**3** Intravascular **A** Guidance **Z** None

B Imaging
7 Lymphatic System
0 Plain Radiography Planar display of an image developed from the capture of external ionizing radiation on photographic or photoconductive plate

Body Part Character 4	Contrast Character 5	Qualifier Character 6	Qualifier Character 7
0 Abdominal/Retroperitoneal Lymphatics, Unilateral 1 Abdominal/Retroperitoneal Lymphatics, Bilateral 4 Lymphatics, Head and Neck 5 Upper Extremity Lymphatics, Right 6 Upper Extremity Lymphatics, Left 7 Upper Extremity Lymphatics, Bilateral 8 Lower Extremity Lymphatics, Right 9 Lower Extremity Lymphatics, Left B Lower Extremity Lymphatics, Bilateral C Lymphatics, Pelvic	0 High Osmolar 1 Low Osmolar Y Other Contrast	Z None	Z None

B Imaging
8 Eye
0 Plain Radiography Planar display of an image developed from the capture of external ionizing radiation on photographic or photoconductive plate

Body Part Character 4	Contrast Character 5	Qualifier Character 6	Qualifier Character 7
0 Lacrimal Duct, Right 1 Lacrimal Duct, Left 2 Lacrimal Ducts, Bilateral	0 High Osmolar 1 Low Osmolar Y Other Contrast	Z None	Z None
3 Optic Foramina, Right 4 Optic Foramina, Left 5 Eye, Right 6 Eye, Left 7 Eyes, Bilateral	Z None	Z None	Z None

B Imaging
8 Eye
2 Computerized Tomography (CT Scan) Computer reformatted digital display of multiplanar images developed from the capture of multiple exposures of external ionizing radiation

Body Part Character 4	Contrast Character 5	Qualifier Character 6	Qualifier Character 7
5 Eye, Right 6 Eye, Left 7 Eyes, Bilateral	0 High Osmolar 1 Low Osmolar Y Other Contrast	0 Unenhanced and Enhanced Z None	Z None
5 Eye, Right 6 Eye, Left 7 Eyes, Bilateral	Z None	Z None	Z None

B Imaging
8 Eye
3 Magnetic Resonance Imaging (MRI) Computer reformatted digital display of multiplanar images developed from the capture of radio-frequency signals emitted by nuclei in a body site excited within a magnetic field

Body Part Character 4	Contrast Character 5	Qualifier Character 6	Qualifier Character 7
5 Eye, Right 6 Eye, Left 7 Eyes, Bilateral	Y Other Contrast	0 Unenhanced and Enhanced Z None	Z None
5 Eye, Right 6 Eye, Left 7 Eyes, Bilateral	Z None	Z None	Z None

B Imaging
8 Eye
4 Ultrasonography Real time display of images of anatomy or flow information developed from the capture of relected and attenuated high frequency sound waves

Body Part Character 4	Contrast Character 5	Qualifier Character 6	Qualifier Character 7
5 Eye, Right 6 Eye, Left 7 Eyes, Bilateral	Z None	Z None	Z None

B Imaging
9 Ear, Nose, Mouth and Throat
0 Plain Radiography Planar display of an image developed from the capture of external ionizing radiation on photographic or photoconductive plate

Body Part Character 4	Contrast Character 5	Qualifier Character 6	Qualifier Character 7
2 Paranasal Sinuses **F** Nasopharynx/Oropharynx **H** Mastoids	**Z** None	**Z** None	**Z** None
4 Parotid Gland, Right **5** Parotid Gland, Left **6** Parotid Glands, Bilateral **7** Submandibular Gland, Right **8** Submandibular Gland, Left **9** Submandibular Glands, Bilateral **B** Salivary Gland, Right **C** Salivary Gland, Left **D** Salivary Glands, Bilateral	**0** High Osmolar **1** Low Osmolar **Y** Other Contrast	**Z** None	**Z** None

B Imaging
9 Ear, Nose, Mouth and Throat
1 Fluoroscopy Single plane or bi-plane real time display of an image developed from the capture of external ionizing radioation on a fluorescent screen. The image may also be stored by either digital or analog means

Body Part Character 4	Contrast Character 5	Qualifier Character 6	Qualifier Character 7
G Pharynx and Epiglottis **J** Larynx	**Y** Other Contrast **Z** None	**Z** None	**Z** None

B Imaging
9 Ear, Nose, Mouth and Throat
2 Computerized Tomography (CT Scan) Computer reformatted digital display of multiplanar images developed from the capture of multiple exposures of external ionizing radiation

Body Part Character 4	Contrast Character 5	Qualifier Character 6	Qualifier Character 7
0 Ear **2** Paranasal Sinuses **6** Parotid Glands, Bilateral **9** Submandibular Glands, Bilateral **D** Salivary Glands, Bilateral **F** Nasopharynx/Oropharynx **J** Larynx	**0** High Osmolar **1** Low Osmolar **Y** Other Contrast	**0** Unenhanced and Enhanced **Z** None	**Z** None
0 Ear **2** Paranasal Sinuses **6** Parotid Glands, Bilateral **9** Submandibular Glands, Bilateral **D** Salivary Glands, Bilateral **F** Nasopharynx/Oropharynx **J** Larynx	**Z** None	**Z** None	**Z** None

B Imaging
9 Ear, Nose, Mouth and Throat
3 Magnetic Resonance Imaging (MRI) Computer reformatted digital display of multiplanar images developed from the capture of radio-frequency signals emitted by nuclei in a body site excited within a magnetic field

Body Part Character 4	Contrast Character 5	Qualifier Character 6	Qualifier Character 7
0 Ear **2** Paranasal Sinuses **6** Parotid Glands, Bilateral **9** Submandibular Glands, Bilateral **D** Salivary Glands, Bilateral **F** Nasopharynx/Oropharynx **J** Larynx	**Y** Other Contrast	**0** Unenhanced and Enhanced **Z** None	**Z** None
0 Ear **2** Paranasal Sinuses **6** Parotid Glands, Bilateral **9** Submandibular Glands, Bilateral **D** Salivary Glands, Bilateral **F** Nasopharynx/Oropharynx **J** Larynx	**Z** None	**Z** None	**Z** None

B Imaging
B Respiratory System
Ø Plain Radiography Planar display of an image developed from the capture of external ionizing radiation on photographic or photoconductive plate

Body Part Character 4	Contrast Character 5	Qualifier Character 6	Qualifier Character 7
7 Tracheobronchial Tree, Right **8** Tracheobronchial Tree, Left **9** Tracheobronchial Trees, Bilateral	**Y** Other Contrast	**Z** None	**Z** None
D Upper Airways	**Z** None	**Z** None	**Z** None

B Imaging
B Respiratory System
1 Fluoroscopy Single plane or bi-plane real time display of an image developed from the capture of external ionizing radioation on a fluorescent screen. The image may also be stored by either digital or analog means

Body Part Character 4	Contrast Character 5	Qualifier Character 6	Qualifier Character 7
2 Lung, Right **3** Lung, Left **4** Lungs, Bilateral **6** Diaphragm **C** Mediastinum **D** Upper Airways	**Z** None	**Z** None	**Z** None
7 Tracheobronchial Tree, Right **8** Tracheobronchial Tree, Left **9** Tracheobronchial Trees, Bilateral	**Y** Other Contrast	**Z** None	**Z** None

B Imaging
B Respiratory System
2 Computerized Tomography (CT Scan) Computer reformatted digital display of multiplanar images developed from the capture of multiple exposures of external ionizing radiation

Body Part Character 4	Contrast Character 5	Qualifier Character 6	Qualifier Character 7
4 Lungs, Bilateral **7** Tracheobronchial Tree, Right **8** Tracheobronchial Tree, Left **9** Tracheobronchial Trees, Bilateral **F** Trachea/Airways	**Ø** High Osmolar **1** Low Osmolar **Y** Other Contrast	**Ø** Unenhanced and Enhanced **Z** None	**Z** None
4 Lungs, Bilateral **7** Tracheobronchial Tree, Right **8** Tracheobronchial Tree, Left **9** Tracheobronchial Trees, Bilateral **F** Trachea/Airways	**Z** None	**Z** None	**Z** None

B Imaging
B Respiratory System
3 Magnetic Resonance Imaging (MRI) Computer reformatted digital display of multiplanar images developed from the capture of radio-frequency signals emitted by nuclei in a body site excited within a magnetic field

Body Part Character 4	Contrast Character 5	Qualifier Character 6	Qualifier Character 7
G Lung Apices	**Y** Other Contrast	**Ø** Unenhanced and Enhanced **Z** None	**Z** None
G Lung Apices	**Z** None	**Z** None	**Z** None

B Imaging
B Respiratory System
4 Ultrasonography Real time display of images of anatomy or flow information developed from the capture of relected and attenuated high frequency sound waves

Body Part Character 4	Contrast Character 5	Qualifier Character 6	Qualifier Character 7
B Pleura **C** Mediastinum	**Z** None	**Z** None	**Z** None

B Imaging
D Gastrointestinal System
1 Fluoroscopy Single plane or bi-plane real time display of an image developed from the capture of external ionizing radioation on a fluorescent screen. The image may also be stored by either digital or analog means

Body Part Character 4	Contrast Character 5	Qualifier Character 6	Qualifier Character 7
1 Esophagus **2** Stomach **3** Small Bowel **4** Colon **5** Upper GI **6** Upper GI and Small Bowel **9** Duodenum **B** Mouth/Oropharynx	**Y** Other Contrast **Z** None	**Z** None	**Z** None

B Imaging
D Gastrointestinal System
2 Computerized Tomography (CT Scan) Computer reformatted digital display of multiplanar images developed from the capture of multiple exposures of external ionizing radiation

Body Part Character 4	Contrast Character 5	Qualifier Character 6	Qualifier Character 7
4 Colon	**0** High Osmolar **1** Low Osmolar **Y** Other Contrast	**0** Unenhanced and Enhanced **Z** None	**Z** None
4 Colon	**Z** None	**Z** None	**Z** None

B Imaging
D Gastrointestinal System
4 Ultrasonography Real time display of images of anatomy or flow information developed from the capture of relected and attenuated high frequency sound waves

Body Part Character 4	Contrast Character 5	Qualifier Character 6	Qualifier Character 7
1 Esophagus **2** Stomach **7** Gastrointestinal Tract **8** Appendix **9** Duodenum **C** Rectum	**Z** None	**Z** None	**Z** None

B Imaging
F Hepatobiliary System and Pancreas
0 Plain Radiography Planar display of an image developed from the capture of external ionizing radiation on photographic or photoconductive plate

Body Part Character 4	Contrast Character 5	Qualifier Character 6	Qualifier Character 7
0 Bile Ducts **3** Gallbladder and Bile Ducts **C** Hepatobiliary System, All	**0** High Osmolar **1** Low Osmolar **Y** Other Contrast	**Z** None	**Z** None

B Imaging
F Hepatobiliary System and Pancreas
1 Fluoroscopy Single plane or bi-plane real time display of an image developed from the capture of external ionizing radioation on a fluorescent screen. The image may also be stored by either digital or analog means

Body Part Character 4	Contrast Character 5	Qualifier Character 6	Qualifier Character 7
0 Bile Ducts **1** Biliary and Pancreatic Ducts **2** Gallbladder **3** Gallbladder and Bile Ducts **4** Gallbladder, Bile Ducts and Pancreatic Ducts **8** Pancreatic Ducts	**0** High Osmolar **1** Low Osmolar **Y** Other Contrast	**Z** None	**Z** None

B Imaging
F Hepatobiliary System and Pancreas
2 Computerized Tomography (CT Scan) Computer reformatted digital display of multiplanar images developed from the capture of multiple exposures of external ionizing radiation

Body Part Character 4	Contrast Character 5	Qualifier Character 6	Qualifier Character 7
5 Liver **6** Liver and Spleen **7** Pancreas **C** Hepatobiliary System, All	**Ø** High Osmolar **1** Low Osmolar **Y** Other Contrast	**Ø** Unenhanced and Enhanced **Z** None	**Z** None
5 Liver **6** Liver and Spleen **7** Pancreas **C** Hepatobiliary System, All	**Z** None	**Z** None	**Z** None

B Imaging
F Hepatobiliary System and Pancreas
3 Magnetic Resonance Imaging (MRI) Computer reformatted digital display of multiplanar images developed from the capture of radio-frequency signals emitted by nuclei in a body site excited within a magnetic field

Body Part Character 4	Contrast Character 5	Qualifier Character 6	Qualifier Character 7
5 Liver **6** Liver and Spleen **7** Pancreas	**Y** Other Contrast	**Ø** Unenhanced and Enhanced **Z** None	**Z** None
5 Liver **6** Liver and Spleen **7** Pancreas	**Z** None	**Z** None	**Z** None

B Imaging
F Hepatobiliary System and Pancreas
4 Ultrasonography Real time display of images of anatomy or flow information developed from the capture of relected and attenuated high frequency sound waves

Body Part Character 4	Contrast Character 5	Qualifier Character 6	Qualifier Character 7
Ø Bile Ducts **2** Gallbladder **3** Gallbladder and Bile Ducts **5** Liver **6** Liver and Spleen **7** Pancreas **C** Hepatobiliary System, All	**Z** None	**Z** None	**Z** None

B Imaging
G Endocrine System
2 Computerized Tomography (CT Scan) Computer reformatted digital display of multiplanar images developed from the capture of multiple exposures of external ionizing radiation

Body Part Character 4	Contrast Character 5	Qualifier Character 6	Qualifier Character 7
2 Adrenal Glands, Bilateral **3** Parathyroid Glands **4** Thyroid Gland	**Ø** High Osmolar **1** Low Osmolar **Y** Other Contrast	**Ø** Unenhanced and Enhanced **Z** None	**Z** None
2 Adrenal Glands, Bilateral **3** Parathyroid Glands **4** Thyroid Gland	**Z** None	**Z** None	**Z** None

B Imaging
G Endocrine System
3 Magnetic Resonance Imaging (MRI) Computer reformatted digital display of multiplanar images developed from the capture of radio-frequency signals emitted by nuclei in a body site excited within a magnetic field

Body Part Character 4	Contrast Character 5	Qualifier Character 6	Qualifier Character 7
2 Adrenal Glands, Bilateral **3** Parathyroid Glands **4** Thyroid Gland	**Y** Other Contrast	**Ø** Unenhanced and Enhanced **Z** None	**Z** None
2 Adrenal Glands, Bilateral **3** Parathyroid Glands **4** Thyroid Gland	**Z** None	**Z** None	**Z** None

B Imaging
G Endocrine System
4 Ultrasonography Real time display of images of anatomy or flow information developed from the capture of relected and attenuated high frequency sound waves

Body Part Character 4	Contrast Character 5	Qualifier Character 6	Qualifier Character 7
0 Adrenal Gland, Right **1** Adrenal Gland, Left **2** Adrenal Glands, Bilateral **3** Parathyroid Glands **4** Thyroid Gland	**Z** None	**Z** None	**Z** None

B Imaging
H Skin, Subcutaneous Tissue and Breast
0 Plain Radiography Planar display of an image developed from the capture of external ionizing radiation on photographic or photoconductive plate

Body Part Character 4	Contrast Character 5	Qualifier Character 6	Qualifier Character 7
0 Breast, Right **1** Breast, Left **2** Breasts, Bilateral	**Z** None	**Z** None	**Z** None
3 Single Mammary Duct, Right **4** Single Mammary Duct, Left **5** Multiple Mammary Ducts, Right **6** Multiple Mammary Ducts, Left	**0** High Osmolar **1** Low Osmolar **Y** Other Contrast **Z** None	**Z** None	**Z** None

B Imaging
H Skin, Subcutaneous Tissue and Breast
3 Magnetic Resonance Imaging (MRI) Computer reformatted digital display of multiplanar images developed from the capture of radio-frequency signals emitted by nuclei in a body site excited within a magnetic field

Body Part Character 4	Contrast Character 5	Qualifier Character 6	Qualifier Character 7
0 Breast, Right **1** Breast, Left **2** Breasts, Bilateral **D** Subcutaneous Tissue, Head/Neck **F** Subcutaneous Tissue, Upper Extremity **G** Subcutaneous Tissue, Thorax **H** Subcutaneous Tissue, Abdomen and Pelvis **J** Subcutaneous Tissue, Lower Extremity	**Y** Other Contrast	**0** Unenhanced and Enhanced **Z** None	**Z** None
0 Breast, Right **1** Breast, Left **2** Breasts, Bilateral **D** Subcutaneous Tissue, Head/Neck **F** Subcutaneous Tissue, Upper Extremity **G** Subcutaneous Tissue, Thorax **H** Subcutaneous Tissue, Abdomen and Pelvis **J** Subcutaneous Tissue, Lower Extremity	**Z** None	**Z** None	**Z** None

B Imaging
H Skin, Subcutaneous Tissue and Breast
4 Ultrasonography Real time display of images of anatomy or flow information developed from the capture of relected and attenuated high frequency sound waves

Body Part Character 4	Contrast Character 5	Qualifier Character 6	Qualifier Character 7
0 Breast, Right **1** Breast, Left **2** Breasts, Bilateral **7** Extremity, Upper **8** Extremity, Lower **9** Abdominal Wall **B** Chest Wall **C** Head and Neck	**Z** None	**Z** None	**Z** None

B Imaging
L Connective Tissue
3 Magnetic Resonance Imaging (MRI) Computer reformatted digital display of multiplanar images developed from the capture of radio-frequency signals emitted by nuclei in a body site excited within a magnetic field

Body Part Character 4	Contrast Character 5	Qualifier Character 6	Qualifier Character 7
Ø Connective Tissue, Upper Extremity **1** Connective Tissue, Lower Extremity **2** Tendons, Upper Extremity **3** Tendons, Lower Extremity	**Y** Other Contrast	**Ø** Unenhanced and Enhanced **Z** None	**Z** None
Ø Connective Tissue, Upper Extremity **1** Connective Tissue, Lower Extremity **2** Tendons, Upper Extremity **3** Tendons, Lower Extremity	**Z** None	**Z** None	**Z** None

B Imaging
L Connective Tissue
4 Ultrasonography Real time display of images of anatomy or flow information developed from the capture of relected and attenuated high frequency sound waves

Body Part Character 4	Contrast Character 5	Qualifier Character 6	Qualifier Character 7
Ø Connective Tissue, Upper Extremity **1** Connective Tissue, Lower Extremity **2** Tendons, Upper Extremity **3** Tendons, Lower Extremity	**Z** None	**Z** None	**Z** None

B Imaging
N Skull and Facial Bones
Ø Plain Radiography Planar display of an image developed from the capture of external ionizing radiation on photographic or photoconductive plate

Body Part Character 4	Contrast Character 5	Qualifier Character 6	Qualifier Character 7
Ø Skull **1** Orbit, Right **2** Orbit, Left **3** Orbits, Bilateral **4** Nasal Bones **5** Facial Bones **6** Mandible **B** Zygomatic Arch, Right **C** Zygomatic Arch, Left **D** Zygomatic Arches, Bilateral **G** Tooth, Single **H** Teeth, Multiple **J** Teeth, All	**Z** None	**Z** None	**Z** None
7 Temporomandibular Joint, Right **8** Temporomandibular Joint, Left **9** Temporomandibular Joints, Bilateral	**Ø** High Osmolar **1** Low Osmolar **Y** Other Contrast **Z** None	**Z** None	**Z** None

B Imaging
N Skull and Facial Bones
1 Fluoroscopy Single plane or bi-plane real time display of an image developed from the capture of external ionizing radioation on a fluorescent screen. The image may also be stored by either digital or analog means

Body Part Character 4	Contrast Character 5	Qualifier Character 6	Qualifier Character 7
7 Temporomandibular Joint, Right **8** Temporomandibular Joint, Left **9** Temporomandibular Joints, Bilateral	**Ø** High Osmolar **1** Low Osmolar **Y** Other Contrast **Z** None	**Z** None	**Z** None

B Imaging
N Skull and Facial Bones
2 Computerized Tomography (CT Scan) Computer reformatted digital display of multiplanar images developed from the capture of multiple exposures of external ionizing radiation

Body Part Character 4	Contrast Character 5	Qualifier Character 6	Qualifier Character 7
0 Skull 3 Orbits, Bilateral 5 Facial Bones 6 Mandible 9 Temporomandibular Joints, Bilateral F Temporal Bones	0 High Osmolar 1 Low Osmolar Y Other Contrast Z None	Z None	Z None

B Imaging
N Skull and Facial Bones
3 Magnetic Resonance Imaging (MRI) Computer reformatted digital display of multiplanar images developed from the capture of radio-frequency signals emitted by nuclei in a body site excited within a magnetic field

Body Part Character 4	Contrast Character 5	Qualifier Character 6	Qualifier Character 7
9 Temporomandibular Joints, Bilateral	Y Other Contrast Z None	Z None	Z None

B Imaging
P Non-Axial Upper Bones
0 Plain Radiography Planar display of an image developed from the capture of external ionizing radiation on photographic or photoconductive plate

Body Part Character 4	Contrast Character 5	Qualifier Character 6	Qualifier Character 7
0 Sternoclavicular Joint, Right 1 Sternoclavicular Joint, Left 2 Sternoclavicular Joints, Bilateral 3 Acromioclavicular Joints, Bilateral 4 Clavicle, Right 5 Clavicle, Left 6 Scapula, Right 7 Scapula, Left A Humerus, Right B Humerus, Left E Upper Arm, Right F Upper Arm, Left J Forearm, Right K Forearm, Left N Hand, Right P Hand, Left R Finger(s), Right S Finger(s), Left X Ribs, Right Y Ribs, Left	Z None	Z None	Z None
8 Shoulder, Right 9 Shoulder, Left C Hand/Finger Joint, Right D Hand/Finger Joint, Left G Elbow, Right H Elbow, Left L Wrist, Right M Wrist, Left	0 High Osmolar 1 Low Osmolar Y Other Contrast Z None	Z None	Z None

B Imaging
P Non-Axial Upper Bones
1 Fluoroscopy Single plane or bi-plane real time display of an image developed from the capture of external ionizing radioation on a fluorescent screen. The image may also be stored by either digital or analog means

Body Part Character 4	Contrast Character 5	Qualifier Character 6	Qualifier Character 7
Ø Sternoclavicular Joint, Right **1** Sternoclavicular Joint, Left **2** Sternoclavicular Joints, Bilateral **3** Acromioclavicular Joints, Bilateral **4** Clavicle, Right **5** Clavicle, Left **6** Scapula, Right **7** Scapula, Left **A** Humerus, Right **B** Humerus, Left **E** Upper Arm, Right **F** Upper Arm, Left **J** Forearm, Right **K** Forearm, Left **N** Hand, Right **P** Hand, Left **R** Finger(s), Right **S** Finger(s), Left **X** Ribs, Right **Y** Ribs, Left	**Z** None	**Z** None	**Z** None
8 Shoulder, Right **9** Shoulder, Left **L** Wrist, Right **M** Wrist, Left	**Ø** High Osmolar **1** Low Osmolar **Y** Other Contrast **Z** None	**Z** None	**Z** None
C Hand/Finger Joint, Right **D** Hand/Finger Joint, Left **G** Elbow, Right **H** Elbow, Left	**Ø** High Osmolar **1** Low Osmolar **Y** Other Contrast	**Z** None	**Z** None

B Imaging
P Non-Axial Upper Bones
2 Computerized Tomography (CT Scan) Computer reformatted digital display of multiplanar images developed from the capture of multiple exposures of external ionizing radiation

Body Part Character 4	Contrast Character 5	Qualifier Character 6	Qualifier Character 7
Ø Sternoclavicular Joint, Right **1** Sternoclavicular Joint, Left **W** Thorax	**Ø** High Osmolar **1** Low Osmolar **Y** Other Contrast	**Z** None	**Z** None
2 Sternoclavicular Joints, Bilateral **3** Acromioclavicular Joints, Bilateral **4** Clavicle, Right **5** Clavicle, Left **6** Scapula, Right **7** Scapula, Left **8** Shoulder, Right **9** Shoulder, Left **A** Humerus, Right **B** Humerus, Left **E** Upper Arm, Right **F** Upper Arm, Left **G** Elbow, Right **H** Elbow, Left **J** Forearm, Right **K** Forearm, Left **L** Wrist, Right **M** Wrist, Left **N** Hand, Right **P** Hand, Left **Q** Hands and Wrists, Bilateral **R** Finger(s), Right **S** Finger(s), Left **T** Upper Extremity, Right **U** Upper Extremity, Left **V** Upper Extremities, Bilateral **X** Ribs, Right **Y** Ribs, Left	**Ø** High Osmolar **1** Low Osmolar **Y** Other Contrast **Z** None	**Z** None	**Z** None
C Hand/Finger Joint, Right **D** Hand/Finger Joint, Left	**Z** None	**Z** None	**Z** None

B Imaging
P Non-Axial Upper Bones
3 Magnetic Resonance Imaging (MRI) Computer reformatted digital display of multiplanar images developed from the capture of radio-frequency signals emitted by nuclei in a body site excited within a magnetic field

Body Part Character 4	Contrast Character 5	Qualifier Character 6	Qualifier Character 7
8 Shoulder, Right **9** Shoulder, Left **C** Hand/Finger Joint, Right **D** Hand/Finger Joint, Left **E** Upper Arm, Right **F** Upper Arm, Left **G** Elbow, Right **H** Elbow, Left **J** Forearm, Right **K** Forearm, Left **L** Wrist, Right **M** Wrist, Left	**Y** Other Contrast	**0** Unenhanced and Enhanced **Z** None	**Z** None
8 Shoulder, Right **9** Shoulder, Left **C** Hand/Finger Joint, Right **D** Hand/Finger Joint, Left **E** Upper Arm, Right **F** Upper Arm, Left **G** Elbow, Right **H** Elbow, Left **J** Forearm, Right **K** Forearm, Left **L** Wrist, Right **M** Wrist, Left	**Z** None	**Z** None	**Z** None

B Imaging
P Non-Axial Upper Bones
4 Ultrasonography Real time display of images of anatomy or flow information developed from the capture of relected and attenuated high frequency sound waves

Body Part Character 4	Contrast Character 5	Qualifier Character 6	Qualifier Character 7
8 Shoulder, Right **9** Shoulder, Left **G** Elbow, Right **H** Elbow, Left **L** Wrist, Right **M** Wrist, Left **N** Hand, Right **P** Hand, Left	**Z** None	**Z** None	**1** Densitometry **Z** None

B Imaging
Q Non-Axial Lower Bones
0 Plain Radiography Planar display of an image developed from the capture of external ionizing radiation on photographic or photoconductive plate

Body Part Character 4	Contrast Character 5	Qualifier Character 6	Qualifier Character 7
0 Hip, Right **1** Hip, Left **3** Femur, Right **4** Femur, Left	**Z** None	**Z** None	**1** Densitometry **Z** None
0 Hip, Right **1** Hip, Left **X** Foot/Toe Joint, Right **Y** Foot/Toe Joint, Left	**0** High Osmolar **1** Low Osmolar **Y** Other Contrast	**Z** None	**Z** None
7 Knee, Right **8** Knee, Left **G** Ankle, Right **H** Ankle, Left	**0** High Osmolar **1** Low Osmolar **Y** Other Contrast **Z** None	**Z** None	**Z** None
D Lower Leg, Right **F** Lower Leg, Left **J** Calcaneus, Right **K** Calcaneus, Left **L** Foot, Right **M** Foot, Left **P** Toe(s), Right **Q** Toe(s), Left **V** Patella, Right **W** Patella, Left	**Z** None	**Z** None	**Z** None

B Imaging
Q Non-Axial Lower Bones
1 Fluoroscopy Single plane or bi-plane real time display of an image developed from the capture of external ionizing radioation on a fluorescent screen. The image may also be stored by either digital or analog means

Body Part Character 4	Contrast Character 5	Qualifier Character 6	Qualifier Character 7
Ø Hip, Right **1** Hip, Left **7** Knee, Right **8** Knee, Left **G** Ankle, Right **H** Ankle, Left **X** Foot/Toe Joint, Right **Y** Foot/Toe Joint, Left	**Ø** High Osmolar **1** Low Osmolar **Y** Other Contrast **Z** None	**Z** None	**Z** None
3 Femur, Right **4** Femur, Left **D** Lower Leg, Right **F** Lower Leg, Left **J** Calcaneus, Right **K** Calcaneus, Left **L** Foot, Right **M** Foot, Left **P** Toe(s), Right **Q** Toe(s), Left **V** Patella, Right **W** Patella, Left	**Z** None	**Z** None	**Z** None

B Imaging
Q Non-Axial Lower Bones
2 Computerized Tomography (CT Scan) Computer reformatted digital display of multiplanar images developed from the capture of multiple exposures of external ionizing radiation

Body Part Character 4	Contrast Character 5	Qualifier Character 6	Qualifier Character 7
Ø Hip, Right **1** Hip, Left **3** Femur, Right **4** Femur, Left **7** Knee, Right **8** Knee, Left **D** Lower Leg, Right **F** Lower Leg, Left **G** Ankle, Right **H** Ankle, Left **J** Calcaneus, Right **K** Calcaneus, Left **L** Foot, Right **M** Foot, Left **P** Toe(s), Right **Q** Toe(s), Left **R** Lower Extremity, Right **S** Lower Extremity, Left **V** Patella, Right **W** Patella, Left **X** Foot/Toe Joint, Right **Y** Foot/Toe Joint, Left	**Ø** High Osmolar **1** Low Osmolar **Y** Other Contrast **Z** None	**Z** None	**Z** None
B Tibia/Fibula, Right **C** Tibia/Fibula, Left	**Ø** High Osmolar **1** Low Osmolar **Y** Other Contrast	**Z** None	**Z** None

B Imaging
Q Non-Axial Lower Bones
3 Magnetic Resonance Imaging (MRI) Computer reformatted digital display of multiplanar images developed from the capture of radio-frequency signals emitted by nuclei in a body site excited within a magnetic field

Body Part Character 4	Contrast Character 5	Qualifier Character 6	Qualifier Character 7
Ø Hip, Right 1 Hip, Left 3 Femur, Right 4 Femur, Left 7 Knee, Right 8 Knee, Left D Lower Leg, Right F Lower Leg, Left G Ankle, Right H Ankle, Left J Calcaneus, Right K Calcaneus, Left L Foot, Right M Foot, Left P Toe(s), Right Q Toe(s), Left V Patella, Right W Patella, Left	Y Other Contrast	Ø Unenhanced and Enhanced Z None	Z None
Ø Hip, Right 1 Hip, Left 3 Femur, Right 4 Femur, Left 7 Knee, Right 8 Knee, Left D Lower Leg, Right F Lower Leg, Left G Ankle, Right H Ankle, Left J Calcaneus, Right K Calcaneus, Left L Foot, Right M Foot, Left P Toe(s), Right Q Toe(s), Left V Patella, Right W Patella, Left	Z None	Z None	Z None

B Imaging
Q Non-Axial Lower Bones
4 Ultrasonography Real time display of images of anatomy or flow information developed from the capture of relected and attenuated high frequency sound waves

Body Part Character 4	Contrast Character 5	Qualifier Character 6	Qualifier Character 7
Ø Hip, Right 1 Hip, Left 2 Hips, Bilateral 7 Knee, Right 8 Knee, Left 9 Knees, Bilateral	Z None	Z None	Z None

B Imaging
R Axial Skeleton, Except Skull and Facial Bones
Ø Plain Radiography Planar display of an image developed from the capture of external ionizing radiation on photographic or photoconductive plate

Body Part Character 4	Contrast Character 5	Qualifier Character 6	Qualifier Character 7
Ø Cervical Spine **7** Thoracic Spine **9** Lumbar Spine **G** Whole Spine	**Z** None	**Z** None	**1** Densitometry **Z** None
1 Cervical Disc(s) **2** Thoracic Disc(s) **3** Lumbar Disc(s) **4** Cervical Facet Joint(s) **5** Thoracic Facet Joint(s) **6** Lumbar Facet Joint(s) **D** Sacroiliac Joints	**Ø** High Osmolar **1** Low Osmolar **Y** Other Contrast **Z** None	**Z** None	**Z** None
8 Thoracolumbar Joint **B** Lumbosacral Joint **C** Pelvis **F** Sacrum and Coccyx **H** Sternum	**Z** None	**Z** None	**Z** None

B Imaging
R Axial Skeleton, Except Skull and Facial Bones
1 Fluoroscopy Single plane or bi-plane real time display of an image developed from the capture of external ionizing radioation on a fluorescent screen. The image may also be stored by either digital or analog means

Body Part Character 4	Contrast Character 5	Qualifier Character 6	Qualifier Character 7
Ø Cervical Spine **1** Cervical Disc(s) **2** Thoracic Disc(s) **3** Lumbar Disc(s) **4** Cervical Facet Joint(s) **5** Thoracic Facet Joint(s) **6** Lumbar Facet Joint(s) **7** Thoracic Spine **8** Thoracolumbar Joint **9** Lumbar Spine **B** Lumbosacral Joint **C** Pelvis **D** Sacroiliac Joints **F** Sacrum and Coccyx **G** Whole Spine **H** Sternum	**Ø** High Osmolar **1** Low Osmolar **Y** Other Contrast **Z** None	**Z** None	**Z** None

B Imaging
R Axial Skeleton, Except Skull and Facial Bones
2 Computerized Tomography (CT Scan) Computer reformatted digital display of multiplanar images developed from the capture of multiple exposures of external ionizing radiation

Body Part Character 4	Contrast Character 5	Qualifier Character 6	Qualifier Character 7
Ø Cervical Spine **7** Thoracic Spine **9** Lumbar Spine **C** Pelvis **D** Sacroiliac Joints **F** Sacrum and Coccyx	**Ø** High Osmolar **1** Low Osmolar **Y** Other Contrast **Z** None	**Z** None	**Z** None

B Imaging
R Axial Skeleton, Except Skull and Facial Bones
3 Magnetic Resonance Imaging (MRI) Computer reformatted digital display of multiplanar images developed from the capture of radio-frequency signals emitted by nuclei in a body site excited within a magnetic field

Body Part Character 4	Contrast Character 5	Qualifier Character 6	Qualifier Character 7
Ø Cervical Spine **1** Cervical Disc(s) **2** Thoracic Disc(s) **3** Lumbar Disc(s) **7** Thoracic Spine **9** Lumbar Spine **C** Pelvis **F** Sacrum and Coccyx	**Y** Other Contrast	**Ø** Unenhanced and Enhanced **Z** None	**Z** None
Ø Cervical Spine **1** Cervical Disc(s) **2** Thoracic Disc(s) **3** Lumbar Disc(s) **7** Thoracic Spine **9** Lumbar Spine **C** Pelvis **F** Sacrum and Coccyx	**Z** None	**Z** None	**Z** None

B Imaging
R Axial Skeleton, Except Skull and Facial Bones
4 Ultrasonography Real time display of images of anatomy or flow information developed from the capture of relected and attenuated high frequency sound waves

Body Part Character 4	Contrast Character 5	Qualifier Character 6	Qualifier Character 7
Ø Cervical Spine **7** Thoracic Spine **9** Lumbar Spine **F** Sacrum and Coccyx	**Z** None	**Z** None	**Z** None

B Imaging
T Urinary System
Ø Plain Radiography Planar display of an image developed from the capture of external ionizing radiation on photographic or photoconductive plate

Body Part Character 4	Contrast Character 5	Qualifier Character 6	Qualifier Character 7
Ø Bladder **1** Kidney, Right **2** Kidney, Left **3** Kidneys, Bilateral **4** Kidneys, Ureters and Bladder **5** Urethra **6** Ureter, Right **7** Ureter, Left **8** Ureters, Bilateral **B** Bladder and Urethra **C** Ileal Diversion Loop	**Ø** High Osmolar **1** Low Osmolar **Y** Other Contrast **Z** None	**Z** None	**Z** None

B Imaging
T Urinary System
1 Fluoroscopy Single plane or bi-plane real time display of an image developed from the capture of external ionizing radioation on a fluorescent screen. The image may also be stored by either digital or analog means

Body Part Character 4	Contrast Character 5	Qualifier Character 6	Qualifier Character 7
Ø Bladder **1** Kidney, Right **2** Kidney, Left **3** Kidneys, Bilateral **4** Kidneys, Ureters and Bladder **5** Urethra **6** Ureter, Right **7** Ureter, Left **B** Bladder and Urethra **C** Ileal Diversion Loop **D** Kidney, Ureter and Bladder, Right **F** Kidney, Ureter and Bladder, Left **G** Ileal Loop, Ureters and Kidneys	**Ø** High Osmolar **1** Low Osmolar **Y** Other Contrast **Z** None	**Z** None	**Z** None

B Imaging
T Urinary System
2 Computerized Tomography (CT Scan) Computer reformatted digital display of multiplanar images developed from the capture of multiple exposures of external ionizing radiation

Body Part Character 4	Contrast Character 5	Qualifier Character 6	Qualifier Character 7
Ø Bladder **1** Kidney, Right **2** Kidney, Left **3** Kidneys, Bilateral **9** Kidney Transplant	**Ø** High Osmolar **1** Low Osmolar **Y** Other Contrast	**Ø** Unenhanced and Enhanced **Z** None	**Z** None
Ø Bladder **1** Kidney, Right **2** Kidney, Left **3** Kidneys, Bilateral **9** Kidney Transplant	**Z** None	**Z** None	**Z** None

B Imaging
T Urinary System
3 Magnetic Resonance Imaging (MRI) Computer reformatted digital display of multiplanar images developed from the capture of radio-frequency signals emitted by nuclei in a body site excited within a magnetic field

Body Part Character 4	Contrast Character 5	Qualifier Character 6	Qualifier Character 7
Ø Bladder **1** Kidney, Right **2** Kidney, Left **3** Kidneys, Bilateral **9** Kidney Transplant	**Y** Other Contrast	**Ø** Unenhanced and Enhanced **Z** None	**Z** None
Ø Bladder **1** Kidney, Right **2** Kidney, Left **3** Kidneys, Bilateral **9** Kidney Transplant	**Z** None	**Z** None	**Z** None

B Imaging
T Urinary System
4 Ultrasonography Real time display of images of anatomy or flow information developed from the capture of relected and attenuated high frequency sound waves

Body Part Character 4	Contrast Character 5	Qualifier Character 6	Qualifier Character 7
Ø Bladder **1** Kidney, Right **2** Kidney, Left **3** Kidneys, Bilateral **5** Urethra **6** Ureter, Right **7** Ureter, Left **8** Ureters, Bilateral **9** Kidney Transplant **J** Kidneys and Bladder	**Z** None	**Z** None	**Z** None

B Imaging
U Female Reproductive System
Ø Plain Radiography Planar display of an image developed from the capture of external ionizing radiation on photographic or photoconductive plate

Body Part Character 4	Contrast Character 5	Qualifier Character 6	Qualifier Character 7
Ø Fallopian Tube, Right **1** Fallopian Tube, Left **2** Fallopian Tubes, Bilateral **6** Uterus **8** Uterus and Fallopian Tubes **9** Vagina	**Ø** High Osmolar **1** Low Osmolar **Y** Other Contrast	**Z** None	**Z** None

B Imaging
U Female Reproductive System
1 Fluoroscopy Single plane or bi-plane real time display of an image developed from the capture of external ionizing radioation on a fluorescent screen. The image may also be stored by either digital or analog means

Body Part Character 4	Contrast Character 5	Qualifier Character 6	Qualifier Character 7
Ø Fallopian Tube, Right **1** Fallopian Tube, Left **2** Fallopian Tubes, Bilateral **6** Uterus **8** Uterus and Fallopian Tubes **9** Vagina	**Ø** High Osmolar **1** Low Osmolar **Y** Other Contrast **Z** None	**Z** None	**Z** None

B Imaging
U Female Reproductive System
3 Magnetic Resonance Imaging (MRI) Computer reformatted digital display of multiplanar images developed from the capture of radio-frequency signals emitted by nuclei in a body site excited within a magnetic field

Body Part Character 4	Contrast Character 5	Qualifier Character 6	Qualifier Character 7
3 Ovary, Right **4** Ovary, Left **5** Ovaries, Bilateral **6** Uterus **9** Vagina **B** Pregnant Uterus **C** Uterus and Ovaries	**Y** Other Contrast	**Ø** Unenhanced and Enhanced **Z** None	**Z** None
3 Ovary, Right **4** Ovary, Left **5** Ovaries, Bilateral **6** Uterus **9** Vagina **B** Pregnant Uterus **C** Uterus and Ovaries	**Z** None	**Z** None	**Z** None

B Imaging
U Female Reproductive System
4 Ultrasonography Real time display of images of anatomy or flow information developed from the capture of relected and attenuated high frequency sound waves

Body Part Character 4	Contrast Character 5	Qualifier Character 6	Qualifier Character 7
Ø Fallopian Tube, Right **1** Fallopian Tube, Left **2** Fallopian Tubes, Bilateral **3** Ovary, Right **4** Ovary, Left **5** Ovaries, Bilateral **6** Uterus **C** Uterus and Ovaries	**Y** Other Contrast **Z** None	**Z** None	**Z** None

B Imaging
V Male Reproductive System
Ø Plain Radiography Planar display of an image developed from the capture of external ionizing radiation on photographic or photoconductive plate

Body Part Character 4	Contrast Character 5	Qualifier Character 6	Qualifier Character 7
Ø Corpora Cavernosa **1** Epididymis, Right **2** Epididymis, Left **3** Prostate **5** Testicle, Right **6** Testicle, Left **8** Vasa Vasorum	**Ø** High Osmolar **1** Low Osmolar **Y** Other Contrast	**Z** None	**Z** None

B Imaging
V Male Reproductive System
1 Fluoroscopy Single plane or bi-plane real time display of an image developed from the capture of external ionizing radioation on a fluorescent screen. The image may also be stored by either digital or analog means

Body Part Character 4	Contrast Character 5	Qualifier Character 6	Qualifier Character 7
Ø Corpora Cavernosa **8** Vasa Vasorum	**Ø** High Osmolar **1** Low Osmolar **Y** Other Contrast **Z** None	**Z** None	**Z** None

B Imaging
V Male Reproductive System
2 Computerized Tomography (CT Scan) Computer reformatted digital display of multiplanar images developed from the capture of multiple exposures of external ionizing radiation

Body Part Character 4	Contrast Character 5	Qualifier Character 6	Qualifier Character 7
3 Prostate	**Ø** High Osmolar **1** Low Osmolar **Y** Other Contrast	**Ø** Unenhanced and Enhanced **Z** None	**Z** None
3 Prostate	**Z** None	**Z** None	**Z** None

B Imaging
V Male Reproductive System
3 Magnetic Resonance Imaging (MRI) Computer reformatted digital display of multiplanar images developed from the capture of radio-frequency signals emitted by nuclei in a body site excited within a magnetic field

Body Part Character 4	Contrast Character 5	Qualifier Character 6	Qualifier Character 7
Ø Corpora Cavernosa **3** Prostate **4** Scrotum **5** Testicle, Right **6** Testicle, Left **7** Testicles, Bilateral	**Y** Other Contrast	**Ø** Unenhanced and Enhanced **Z** None	**Z** None
Ø Corpora Cavernosa **3** Prostate **4** Scrotum **5** Testicle, Right **6** Testicle, Left **7** Testicles, Bilateral	**Z** None	**Z** None	**Z** None

B Imaging
V Male Reproductive System
4 Ultrasonography Real time display of images of anatomy or flow information developed from the capture of relected and attenuated high frequency sound waves

Body Part Character 4	Contrast Character 5	Qualifier Character 6	Qualifier Character 7
4 Scrotum **9** Prostate and Seminal Vesicles **B** Penis	**Z** None	**Z** None	**Z** None

B Imaging
W Anatomical Regions
Ø Plain Radiography Planar display of an image developed from the capture of external ionizing radiation on photographic or photoconductive plate

Body Part Character 4	Contrast Character 5	Qualifier Character 6	Qualifier Character 7
Ø Abdomen **1** Abdomen and Pelvis **3** Chest **B** Long Bones, All **C** Lower Extremity **J** Upper Extremity **K** Whole Body **L** Whole Skeleton **M** Whole Body, Infant	**Z** None	**Z** None	**Z** None

B Imaging
W Anatomical Regions
1 Fluoroscopy Single plane or bi-plane real time display of an image developed from the capture of external ionizing radioation on a fluorescent screen. The image may also be stored by either digital or analog means

Body Part Character 4	Contrast Character 5	Qualifier Character 6	Qualifier Character 7
1 Abdomen and Pelvis **9** Head and Neck **C** Lower Extremity **J** Upper Extremity	**Ø** High Osmolar **1** Low Osmolar **Y** Other Contrast **Z** None	**Z** None	**Z** None

B Imaging
W Anatomical Regions
2 Computerized Tomography (CT Scan) Computer reformatted digital display of multiplanar images developed from the capture of multiple exposures of external ionizing radiation

Body Part Character 4	Contrast Character 5	Qualifier Character 6	Qualifier Character 7
Ø Abdomen **1** Abdomen and Pelvis **4** Chest and Abdomen **5** Chest, Abdomen and Pelvis **8** Head **9** Head and Neck **F** Neck **G** Pelvic Region	**Ø** High Osmolar **1** Low Osmolar **Y** Other Contrast	**Ø** Unenhanced and Enhanced **Z** None	**Z** None
Ø Abdomen **1** Abdomen and Pelvis **4** Chest and Abdomen **5** Chest, Abdomen and Pelvis **8** Head **9** Head and Neck **F** Neck **G** Pelvic Region	**Z** None	**Z** None	**Z** None

B Imaging
W Anatomical Regions
3 Magnetic Resonance Imaging (MRI) Computer reformatted digital display of multiplanar images developed from the capture of radio-frequency signals emitted by nuclei in a body site excited within a magnetic field

Body Part Character 4	Contrast Character 5	Qualifier Character 6	Qualifier Character 7
Ø Abdomen **3** Chest **8** Head **F** Neck **G** Pelvic Region **H** Retroperitoneum **P** Brachial Plexus	**Y** Other Contrast	**Ø** Unenhanced and Enhanced **Z** None	**Z** None
Ø Abdomen **8** Head **F** Neck **G** Pelvic Region **H** Retroperitoneum **P** Brachial Plexus	**Z** None	**Z** None	**Z** None

B Imaging
W Anatomical Regions
4 Ultrasonography Real time display of images of anatomy or flow information developed from the capture of relected and attenuated high frequency sound waves

Body Part Character 4	Contrast Character 5	Qualifier Character 6	Qualifier Character 7
Ø Abdomen **1** Abdomen and Pelvis **F** Neck **G** Pelvic Region	**Z** None	**Z** None	**Z** None

B Imaging
Y Fetus and Obstetrical
3 Magnetic Resonance Imaging (MRI) Computer reformatted digital display of multiplanar images developed from the capture of radio-frequency signals emitted by nuclei in a body site excited within a magnetic field

Body Part Character 4	Contrast Character 5	Qualifier Character 6	Qualifier Character 7
Ø Fetal Head **1** Fetal Heart **2** Fetal Thorax **3** Fetal Abdomen **4** Fetal Spine **5** Fetal Extremities **6** Whole Fetus	**Y** Other Contrast	**Ø** Unenhanced and Enhanced **Z** None	**Z** None
Ø Fetal Head **1** Fetal Heart **2** Fetal Thorax **3** Fetal Abdomen **4** Fetal Spine **5** Fetal Extremities **6** Whole Fetus	**Z** None	**Z** None	**Z** None

B Imaging
Y Fetus and Obstetrical
4 Ultrasonography Real time display of images of anatomy or flow information developed from the capture of relected and attenuated high frequency sound waves

Body Part Character 4	Contrast Character 5	Qualifier Character 6	Qualifier Character 7
7 Fetal Umbilical Cord **8** Placenta **9** First Trimester, Single Fetus **B** First Trimester, Multiple Gestation **C** Second Trimester, Single Fetus **D** Second Trimester, Multiple Gestation **F** Third Trimester, Single Fetus **G** Third Trimester, Multiple Gestation	**Z** None	**Z** None	**Z** None

Nuclear Medicine C01–CW7

C Nuclear Medicine
0 Central Nervous System
1 Planar Nuclear Medicine Imaging Introduction of radioactive materials into the body for single plane display of images developed from the capture of radioactive emissions

Body Part Character 4	Radionuclide Character 5	Qualifier Character 6	Qualifier Character 7
0 Brain	1 Technetium 99m (Tc-99m) Y Other Radionuclide	Z None	Z None
5 Cerebrospinal Fluid	D Indium 111 (In-111) Y Other Radionuclide	Z None	Z None
Y Central Nervous System	Y Other Radionuclide	Z None	Z None

C Nuclear Medicine
0 Central Nervous System
2 Tomographic (Tomo) Nuclear Medicine Imaging Introduction of radioactive materials into the body for three dimensional display of images developed from the capture of radioactive emissions

Body Part Character 4	Radionuclide Character 5	Qualifier Character 6	Qualifier Character 7
0 Brain	1 Technetium 99m (Tc-99m) F Iodine 123 (I-123) S Thallium 201 (Tl-201) Y Other Radionuclide	Z None	Z None
5 Cerebrospinal Fluid	D Indium 111 (In-111) Y Other Radionuclide	Z None	Z None
Y Central Nervous System	Y Other Radionuclide	Z None	Z None

C Nuclear Medicine
0 Central Nervous System
3 Positron Emission Tomographic (PET) Imaging Introduction of radioactive materials into the body for three dimensional display of images developed from the simultaneous capture, 180 degrees apart, of radioactive emissions

Body Part Character 4	Radionuclide Character 5	Qualifier Character 6	Qualifier Character 7
0 Brain	B Carbon 11 (C-11) K Fluorine 18 (F-18) M Oxygen 15 (O-15) Y Other Radionuclide	Z None	Z None
Y Central Nervous System	Y Other Radionuclide	Z None	Z None

C Nuclear Medicine
0 Central Nervous System
5 Nonimaging Nuclear Medicine Probe Introduction of radioactive materials into the body for the study of distribution and fate of certain substances by the detection of radioactive emissions; or, alternatively, measurement of absorption of radioactive emissions from an external source

Body Part Character 4	Radionuclide Character 5	Qualifier Character 6	Qualifier Character 7
0 Brain	V Xenon 133 (Xe-133) Y Other Radionuclide	Z None	Z None
Y Central Nervous System	Y Other Radionuclide	Z None	Z None

C Nuclear Medicine
2 Heart
1 Planar Nuclear Medicine Imaging Introduction of radioactive materials into the body for single plane display of images developed from the capture of radioactive emissions

Body Part Character 4	Radionuclide Character 5	Qualifier Character 6	Qualifier Character 7
6 Heart, Right and Left	1 Technetium 99m (Tc-99m) Y Other Radionuclide	Z None	Z None
G Myocardium	1 Technetium 99m (Tc-99m) D Indium 111 (In-111) S Thallium 201 (Tl-201) Y Other Radionuclide Z None	Z None	Z None
Y Heart	Y Other Radionuclide	Z None	Z None

C Nuclear Medicine
2 Heart
2 Tomographic (Tomo) Nuclear Medicine Imaging Introduction of radioactive materials into the body for three dimensional display of images developed from the capture of radioactive emissions

Body Part Character 4	Radionuclide Character 5	Qualifier Character 6	Qualifier Character 7
6 Heart, Right and Left	**1** Technetium 99m (Tc-99m) **Y** Other Radionuclide	**Z** None	**Z** None
G Myocardium	**1** Technetium 99m (Tc-99m) **D** Indium 111 (In-111) **K** Fluorine 18 (F-18) **S** Thallium 201 (Tl-201) **Y** Other Radionuclide **Z** None	**Z** None	**Z** None
Y Heart	**Y** Other Radionuclide	**Z** None	**Z** None

C Nuclear Medicine
2 Heart
3 Positron Emission Tomographic (PET) Imaging Introduction of radioactive materials into the body for three dimensional display of images developed from the simultaneous capture, 180 degrees apart, of radioactive emissions

Body Part Character 4	Radionuclide Character 5	Qualifier Character 6	Qualifier Character 7
G Myocardium	**K** Fluorine 18 (F-18) **M** Oxygen 15 (O-15) **Q** Rubidium 82 (Rb-82) **R** Nitrogen 13 (N-13) **Y** Other Radionuclide	**Z** None	**Z** None
Y Heart	**Y** Other Radionuclide	**Z** None	**Z** None

C Nuclear Medicine
2 Heart
5 Nonimaging Nuclear Medicine Probe Introduction of radioactive materials into the body for the study of distribution and fate of certain substances by the detection of radioactive emissions; or, alternatively, measurement of absorption of radioactive emissions from an external source

Body Part Character 4	Radionuclide Character 5	Qualifier Character 6	Qualifier Character 7
6 Heart, Right and Left	**1** Technetium 99m (Tc-99m) **Y** Other Radionuclide	**Z** None	**Z** None
Y Heart	**Y** Other Radionuclide	**Z** None	**Z** None

C Nuclear Medicine
5 Veins
1 Planar Nuclear Medicine Imaging Introduction of radioactive materials into the body for single plane display of images developed from the capture of radioactive emissions

Body Part Character 4	Radionuclide Character 5	Qualifier Character 6	Qualifier Character 7
B Lower Extremity Veins, Right **C** Lower Extremity Veins, Left **D** Lower Extremity Veins, Bilateral **N** Upper Extremity Veins, Right **P** Upper Extremity Veins, Left **Q** Upper Extremity Veins, Bilateral **R** Central Veins	**1** Technetium 99m (Tc-99m) **Y** Other Radionuclide	**Z** None	**Z** None
Y Veins	**Y** Other Radionuclide	**Z** None	**Z** None

C Nuclear Medicine
7 Lymphatic and Hematologic System
1 Planar Nuclear Medicine Imaging Introduction of radioactive materials into the body for single plane display of images developed from the capture of radioactive emissions

Body Part Character 4	Radionuclide Character 5	Qualifier Character 6	Qualifier Character 7
Ø Bone Marrow	**1** Technetium 99m (Tc-99m) **D** Indium 111 (In-111) **Y** Other Radionuclide	**Z** None	**Z** None
2 Spleen **5** Lymphatics, Head and Neck **D** Lymphatics, Pelvic **J** Lymphatics, Head **K** Lymphatics, Neck **L** Lymphatics, Upper Chest **M** Lymphatics, Trunk **N** Lymphatics, Upper Extremity **P** Lymphatics, Lower Extremity	**1** Technetium 99m (Tc-99m) **Y** Other Radionuclide	**Z** None	**Z** None
3 Blood	**D** Indium 111 (In-111) **Y** Other Radionuclide	**Z** None	**Z** None
Y Lymphatic and Hematologic System	**Y** Other Radionuclide	**Z** None	**Z** None

C Nuclear Medicine
7 Lymphatic and Hematologic System
2 Tomographic (Tomo) Nuclear Medicine Imaging Introduction of radioactive materials into the body for three dimensional display of images developed from the capture of radioactive emissions

Body Part Character 4	Radionuclide Character 5	Qualifier Character 6	Qualifier Character 7
2 Spleen	**1** Technetium 99m (Tc-99m) **Y** Other Radionuclide	**Z** None	**Z** None
Y Lymphatic and Hematologic System	**Y** Other Radionuclide	**Z** None	**Z** None

C Nuclear Medicine
7 Lymphatic and Hematologic System
5 Nonimaging Nuclear Medicine Probe Introduction of radioactive materials into the body for the study of distribution and fate of certain substances by the detection of radioactive emissions; or, alternatively, measurement of absorption of radioactive emissions from an external source

Body Part Character 4	Radionuclide Character 5	Qualifier Character 6	Qualifier Character 7
5 Lymphatics, Head and Neck **D** Lymphatics, Pelvic **J** Lymphatics, Head **K** Lymphatics, Neck **L** Lymphatics, Upper Chest **M** Lymphatics, Trunk **N** Lymphatics, Upper Extremity **P** Lymphatics, Lower Extremity	**1** Technetium 99m (Tc-99m) **Y** Other Radionuclide	**Z** None	**Z** None
Y Lymphatic and Hematologic System	**Y** Other Radionuclide	**Z** None	**Z** None

C Nuclear Medicine
7 Lymphatic and Hematologic System
6 Nonimaging Nuclear Medicine Assay Introduction of radioactive materials into the body for the study of body fluids and blood elements, by the detection of radioactive emissions

Body Part Character 4	Radionuclide Character 5	Qualifier Character 6	Qualifier Character 7
3 Blood	**1** Technetium 99m (Tc-99m) **7** Cobalt 58 (Co-58) **C** Cobalt 57 (Co-57) **D** Indium 111 (In-111) **H** Iodine 125 (I-125) **W** Chromium (Cr-51) **Y** Other Radionuclide	**Z** None	**Z** None
Y Lymphatic and Hematologic System	**Y** Other Radionuclide	**Z** None	**Z** None

C Nuclear Medicine
8 Eye
1 Planar Nuclear Medicine Imaging Introduction of radioactive materials into the body for single plane display of images developed from the capture of radioactive emissions

Body Part Character 4	Radionuclide Character 5	Qualifier Character 6	Qualifier Character 7
9 Lacrimal Ducts, Bilateral	**1** Technetium 99m (Tc-99m) **Y** Other Radionuclide	**Z** None	**Z** None
Y Eye	**Y** Other Radionuclide	**Z** None	**Z** None

C Nuclear Medicine
9 Ear, Nose, Mouth and Throat
1 Planar Nuclear Medicine Imaging Introduction of radioactive materials into the body for single plane display of images developed from the capture of radioactive emissions

Body Part Character 4	Radionuclide Character 5	Qualifier Character 6	Qualifier Character 7
B Salivary Glands, Bilateral	**1** Technetium 99m (Tc-99m) **Y** Other Radionuclide	**Z** None	**Z** None
Y Ear, Nose, Mouth and Throat	**Y** Other Radionuclide	**Z** None	**Z** None

C Nuclear Medicine
B Respiratory System
1 Planar Nuclear Medicine Imaging Introduction of radioactive materials into the body for single plane display of images developed from the capture of radioactive emissions

Body Part Character 4	Radionuclide Character 5	Qualifier Character 6	Qualifier Character 7
2 Lungs and Bronchi	**1** Technetium 99m (Tc-99m) **9** Krypton (Kr-81m) **T** Xenon 127 (Xe-127) **V** Xenon 133 (Xe-133) **Y** Other Radionuclide	**Z** None	**Z** None
Y Respiratory System	**Y** Other Radionuclide	**Z** None	**Z** None

C Nuclear Medicine
B Respiratory System
2 Tomographic (Tomo) Nuclear Medicine Imaging Introduction of radioactive materials into the body for three dimensional display of images developed from the capture of radioactive emissions

Body Part Character 4	Radionuclide Character 5	Qualifier Character 6	Qualifier Character 7
2 Lungs and Bronchi	**1** Technetium 99m (Tc-99m) **9** Krypton (Kr-81m) **Y** Other Radionuclide	**Z** None	**Z** None
Y Respiratory System	**Y** Other Radionuclide	**Z** None	**Z** None

C Nuclear Medicine
B Respiratory System
3 Positron Emission Tomographic (PET) Imaging Introduction of radioactive materials into the body for three dimensional display of images developed from the simultaneous capture, 180 degrees apart, of radioactive emissions

Body Part Character 4	Radionuclide Character 5	Qualifier Character 6	Qualifier Character 7
2 Lungs and Bronchi	**K** Fluorine 18 (F-18) **Y** Other Radionuclide	**Z** None	**Z** None
Y Respiratory System	**Y** Other Radionuclide	**Z** None	**Z** None

C Nuclear Medicine
D Gastrointestinal System
1 Planar Nuclear Medicine Imaging Introduction of radioactive materials into the body for single plane display of images developed from the capture of radioactive emissions

Body Part Character 4	Radionuclide Character 5	Qualifier Character 6	Qualifier Character 7
5 Upper Gastrointestinal Tract **7** Gastrointestinal Tract	**1** Technetium 99m (Tc-99m) **D** Indium 111 (In-111) **Y** Other Radionuclide	**Z** None	**Z** None
Y Digestive System	**Y** Other Radionuclide	**Z** None	**Z** None

C Nuclear Medicine
D Gastrointestinal System
2 Tomographic (Tomo) Nuclear Medicine Imaging Introduction of radioactive materials into the body for three dimensional display of images developed from the capture of radioactive emissions

Body Part Character 4	Radionuclide Character 5	Qualifier Character 6	Qualifier Character 7
7 Gastrointestinal Tract	**1** Technetium 99m (Tc-99m) **D** Indium 111 (In-111) **Y** Other Radionuclide	**Z** None	**Z** None
Y Digestive System	**Y** Other Radionuclide	**Z** None	**Z** None

C Nuclear Medicine
F Hepatobiliary System and Pancreas
1 Planar Nuclear Medicine Imaging Introduction of radioactive materials into the body for single plane display of images developed from the capture of radioactive emissions

Body Part Character 4	Radionuclide Character 5	Qualifier Character 6	Qualifier Character 7
4 Gallbladder **5** Liver **6** Liver and Spleen **C** Hepatobiliary System, All	**1** Technetium 99m (Tc-99m) **Y** Other Radionuclide	**Z** None	**Z** None
Y Hepatobiliary System and Pancreas	**Y** Other Radionuclide	**Z** None	**Z** None

C Nuclear Medicine
F Hepatobiliary System and Pancreas
2 Tomographic (Tomo) Nuclear Medicine Imaging Introduction of radioactive materials into the body for three dimensional display of images developed from the capture of radioactive emissions

Body Part Character 4	Radionuclide Character 5	Qualifier Character 6	Qualifier Character 7
4 Gallbladder **5** Liver **6** Liver and Spleen	**1** Technetium 99m (Tc-99m) **Y** Other Radionuclide	**Z** None	**Z** None
Y Hepatobiliary System and Pancreas	**Y** Other Radionuclide	**Z** None	**Z** None

C Nuclear Medicine
G Endocrine System
1 Planar Nuclear Medicine Imaging Introduction of radioactive materials into the body for single plane display of images developed from the capture of radioactive emissions

Body Part Character 4	Radionuclide Character 5	Qualifier Character 6	Qualifier Character 7
1 Parathyroid Glands	**1** Technetium 99m (Tc-99m) **S** Thallium 201 (Tl-201) **Y** Other Radionuclide	**Z** None	**Z** None
2 Thyroid Gland	**1** Technetium 99m (Tc-99m) **F** Iodine 123 (I-123) **G** Iodine 131 (I-131) **Y** Other Radionuclide	**Z** None	**Z** None
4 Adrenal Glands, Bilateral	**G** Iodine 131 (I-131) **Y** Other Radionuclide	**Z** None	**Z** None
Y Endocrine System	**Y** Other Radionuclide	**Z** None	**Z** None

C Nuclear Medicine
G Endocrine System
2 Tomographic (Tomo) Nuclear Medicine Imaging Introduction of radioactive materials into the body for three dimensional display of images developed from the capture of radioactive emissions

Body Part Character 4	Radionuclide Character 5	Qualifier Character 6	Qualifier Character 7
1 Parathyroid Glands	**1** Technetium 99m (Tc-99m) **S** Thallium 201 (Tl-201) **Y** Other Radionuclide	**Z** None	**Z** None
Y Endocrine System	**Y** Other Radionuclide	**Z** None	**Z** None

C Nuclear Medicine
G Endocrine System
4 Nonimaging Nuclear Medicine Uptake Introduction of radioactive materials into the body for measurements of organ function, from the detection of radioactive emmissions

Body Part Character 4	Radionuclide Character 5	Qualifier Character 6	Qualifier Character 7
2 Thyroid Gland	1 Technetium 99m (Tc-99m) F Iodine 123 (I-123) G Iodine 131 (I-131) Y Other Radionuclide	Z None	Z None
Y Endocrine System	Y Other Radionuclide	Z None	Z None

C Nuclear Medicine
H Skin, Subcutaneous Tissue and Breast
1 Planar Nuclear Medicine Imaging Introduction of radioactive materials into the body for single plane display of images developed from the capture of radioactive emissions

Body Part Character 4	Radionuclide Character 5	Qualifier Character 6	Qualifier Character 7
0 Breast, Right 1 Breast, Left 2 Breasts, Bilateral	1 Technetium 99m (Tc-99m) S Thallium 201 (Tl-201) Y Other Radionuclide	Z None	Z None
Y Skin, Subcutaneous Tissue and Breast	Y Other Radionuclide	Z None	Z None

C Nuclear Medicine
H Skin, Subcutaneous Tissue and Breast
2 Tomographic (Tomo) Nuclear Medicine Imaging Introduction of radioactive materials into the body for three dimensional display of images developed from the capture of radioactive emissions

Body Part Character 4	Radionuclide Character 5	Qualifier Character 6	Qualifier Character 7
0 Breast, Right 1 Breast, Left 2 Breasts, Bilateral	1 Technetium 99m (Tc-99m) S Thallium 201 (Tl-201) Y Other Radionuclide	Z None	Z None
Y Skin, Subcutaneous Tissue and Breast	Y Other Radionuclide	Z None	Z None

C Nuclear Medicine
P Musculoskeletal System
1 Planar Nuclear Medicine Imaging Introduction of radioactive materials into the body for single plane display of images developed from the capture of radioactive emissions

Body Part Character 4	Radionuclide Character 5	Qualifier Character 6	Qualifier Character 7
1 Skull 4 Thorax 5 Spine 6 Pelvis 7 Spine and Pelvis 8 Upper Extremity, Right 9 Upper Extremity, Left B Upper Extremities, Bilateral C Lower Extremity, Right D Lower Extremity, Left F Lower Extremities, Bilateral Z Musculoskeletal System, All	1 Technetium 99m (Tc-99m) Y Other Radionuclide	Z None	Z None
Y Musculoskeletal System, Other	Y Other Radionuclide	Z None	Z None

C Nuclear Medicine
P Musculoskeletal System
2 Tomographic (Tomo) Nuclear Medicine Imaging Introduction of radioactive materials into the body for three dimensional display of images developed from the capture of radioactive emissions

Body Part Character 4	Radionuclide Character 5	Qualifier Character 6	Qualifier Character 7
1 Skull **2** Cervical Spine **3** Skull and Cervical Spine **4** Thorax **6** Pelvis **7** Spine and Pelvis **8** Upper Extremity, Right **9** Upper Extremity, Left **B** Upper Extremities, Bilateral **C** Lower Extremity, Right **D** Lower Extremity, Left **F** Lower Extremities, Bilateral **G** Thoracic Spine **H** Lumbar Spine **J** Thoracolumbar Spine	**1** Technetium 99m (Tc-99m) **Y** Other Radionuclide	**Z** None	**Z** None
Y Musculoskeletal System, Other	**Y** Other Radionuclide	**Z** None	**Z** None

C Nuclear Medicine
P Musculoskeletal System
5 Nonimaging Nuclear Medicine Probe Introduction of radioactive materials into the body for the study of distribution and fate of certain substances by the detection of radioactive emissions; or, alternatively, measurement of absorption of radioactive emissions from an external source

Body Part Character 4	Radionuclide Character 5	Qualifier Character 6	Qualifier Character 7
5 Spine **N** Upper Extremities **P** Lower Extremities	**Z** None	**Z** None	**Z** None
Y Musculoskeletal System, Other	**Y** Other Radionuclide	**Z** None	**Z** None

C Nuclear Medicine
T Urinary System
1 Planar Nuclear Medicine Imaging Introduction of radioactive materials into the body for single plane display of images developed from the capture of radioactive emissions

Body Part Character 4	Radionuclide Character 5	Qualifier Character 6	Qualifier Character 7
3 Kidneys, Ureters and Bladder	**1** Technetium 99m (Tc-99m) **F** Iodine 123 (I-123) **G** Iodine 131 (I-131) **Y** Other Radionuclide	**Z** None	**Z** None
H Bladder and Ureters	**1** Technetium 99m (Tc-99m) **Y** Other Radionuclide	**Z** None	**Z** None
Y Urinary System	**Y** Other Radionuclide	**Z** None	**Z** None

C Nuclear Medicine
T Urinary System
2 Tomographic (Tomo) Nuclear Medicine Imaging Introduction of radioactive materials into the body for three dimensional display of images developed from the capture of radioactive emissions

Body Part Character 4	Radionuclide Character 5	Qualifier Character 6	Qualifier Character 7
3 Kidneys, Ureters and Bladder	**1** Technetium 99m (Tc-99m) **Y** Other Radionuclide	**Z** None	**Z** None
Y Urinary System	**Y** Other Radionuclide	**Z** None	**Z** None

C Nuclear Medicine
T Urinary System
6 Nonimaging Nuclear Medicine Assay Introduction of radioactive materials into the body for the study of body fluids and blood elements, by the detection of radioactive emissions

Body Part Character 4	Radionuclide Character 5	Qualifier Character 6	Qualifier Character 7
3 Kidneys, Ureters and Bladder	**1** Technetium 99m (Tc-99m) **F** Iodine 123 (I-123) **G** Iodine 131 (I-131) **H** Iodine 125 (I-125) **Y** Other Radionuclide	**Z** None	**Z** None
Y Urinary System	**Y** Other Radionuclide	**Z** None	**Z** None

C Nuclear Medicine
V Male Reproductive System
1 Planar Nuclear Medicine Imaging Introduction of radioactive materials into the body for single plane display of images developed from the capture of radioactive emissions

Body Part Character 4	Radionuclide Character 5	Qualifier Character 6	Qualifier Character 7
9 Testicles, Bilateral	**1** Technetium 99m (Tc-99m) **Y** Other Radionuclide	**Z** None	**Z** None
Y Male Reproductive System	**Y** Other Radionuclide	**Z** None	**Z** None

C Nuclear Medicine
W Anatomical Regions
1 Planar Nuclear Medicine Imaging Introduction of radioactive materials into the body for single plane display of images developed from the capture of radioactive emissions

Body Part Character 4	Radionuclide Character 5	Qualifier Character 6	Qualifier Character 7
Ø Abdomen **1** Abdomen and Pelvis **4** Chest and Abdomen **6** Chest and Neck **B** Head and Neck **D** Lower Extremity **J** Pelvic Region **M** Upper Extremity **N** Whole Body	**1** Technetium 99m (Tc-99m) **D** Indium 111 (In-111) **F** Iodine 123 (I-123) **G** Iodine 131 (I-131) **L** Gallium 67 (Ga-67) **S** Thallium 2Ø1 (Tl-2Ø1) **Y** Other Radionuclide	**Z** None	**Z** None
3 Chest	**1** Technetium 99m (Tc-99m) **D** Indium 111 (In-111) **F** Iodine 123 (I-123) **G** Iodine 131 (I-131) **K** Fluorine 18 (F-18) **L** Gallium 67 (Ga-67) **S** Thallium 2Ø1 (Tl-2Ø1) **Y** Other Radionuclide	**Z** None	**Z** None
Y Anatomical Regions, Multiple	**Y** Other Radionuclide	**Z** None	**Z** None
Z Anatomical Region, Other	**Z** None	**Z** None	**Z** None

C Nuclear Medicine
W Anatomical Regions
2 Tomographic (Tomo) Nuclear Medicine Imaging Introduction of radioactive materials into the body for three dimensional display of images developed from the capture of radioactive emissions

Body Part Character 4	Radionuclide Character 5	Qualifier Character 6	Qualifier Character 7
Ø Abdomen **1** Abdomen and Pelvis **3** Chest **4** Chest and Abdomen **6** Chest and Neck **B** Head and Neck **D** Lower Extremity **J** Pelvic Region **M** Upper Extremity	**1** Technetium 99m (Tc-99m) **D** Indium 111 (In-111) **F** Iodine 123 (I-123) **G** Iodine 131 (I-131) **K** Fluorine 18 (F-18) **L** Gallium 67 (Ga-67) **S** Thallium 2Ø1 (Tl-2Ø1) **Y** Other Radionuclide	**Z** None	**Z** None
Y Anatomical Regions, Multiple	**Y** Other Radionuclide	**Z** None	**Z** None

C Nuclear Medicine
W Anatomical Regions
3 Positron Emission Tomographic (PET) Imaging Introduction of radioactive materials into the body for three dimensional display of images developed from the simultaneous capture, 180 degrees apart, of radioactive emissions

Body Part Character 4	Radionuclide Character 5	Qualifier Character 6	Qualifier Character 7
N Whole Body	**Y** Other Radionuclide	**Z** None	**Z** None

C Nuclear Medicine
W Anatomical Regions
5 Nonimaging Nuclear Medicine Probe Introduction of radioactive materials into the body for the study of distribution and fate of certain substances by the detection of radioactive emissions; or, alternatively, measurement of absorption of radioactive emissions from an external source

Body Part Character 4	Radionuclide Character 5	Qualifier Character 6	Qualifier Character 7
0 Abdomen **1** Abdomen and Pelvis **3** Chest **4** Chest and Abdomen **6** Chest and Neck **B** Head and Neck **D** Lower Extremity **J** Pelvic Region **M** Upper Extremity	**1** Technetium 99m (Tc-99m) **D** Indium 111 (In-111) **Y** Other Radionuclide	**Z** None	**Z** None

C Nuclear Medicine
W Anatomical Regions
7 Systemic Nuclear Medicine Therapy Introduction of radioactive materials into the body for treatment

Body Part Character 4	Radionuclide Character 5	Qualifier Character 6	Qualifier Character 7
0 Abdomen **3** Chest	**N** Phosphorus 32 (P-32) **Y** Other Radionuclide	**Z** None	**Z** None
G Thyroid	**G** Iodine 131 (I-131) **Y** Other Radionuclide	**Z** None	**Z** None
N Whole Body	**8** Samarium 153 (Sm-153) **G** Iodine 131 (I-131) **N** Phosphorus 32 (P-32) **P** Strontium 89 (Sr-89) **Y** Other Radionuclide	**Z** None	**Z** None
Y Anatomical Regions, Multiple	**Y** Other Radionuclide	**Z** None	**Z** None

Radiation Oncology DØØ–DWY

D Radiation Oncology
Ø Central and Peripheral Nervous System
Ø Beam Radiation

Treatment Site Character 4	Modal. Qualifier Character 5	Isotope Character 6	Qualifier Character 7
Ø Brain **1** Brain Stem **6** Spinal Cord **7** Peripheral Nerve	**Ø** Photons <1 MeV **1** Photons 1- 1Ø MeV **2** Photons >1Ø MeV **4** Heavy Particles (Protons, Ions) **5** Neutrons **6** Neutron Capture	**Z** None	**Z** None
Ø Brain **1** Brain Stem **6** Spinal Cord **7** Peripheral Nerve	**3** Electrons	**Z** None	**Ø** Intraoperative **Z** None

D Radiation Oncology
Ø Central and Peripheral Nervous System
1 Brachytherapy

Treatment Site Character 4	Modal. Qualifier Character 5	Isotope Character 6	Qualifier Character 7
Ø Brain **1** Brain Stem **6** Spinal Cord **7** Peripheral Nerve	**9** High Dose Rate (HDR) **B** Low Dose Rate (LDR)	**7** Cesium 137 (Cs-137) **8** Iridium 192 (Ir-192) **9** Iodine 125 (I-125) **B** Palladium 1Ø3 (Pd-1Ø3) **C** Californium 252 (Cf-252) **Y** Other Isotope	**Z** None

D Radiation Oncology
Ø Central and Peripheral Nervous System
2 Stereotactic Radiosurgery

Treatment Site Character 4	Modal. Qualifier Character 5	Isotope Character 6	Qualifier Character 7
Ø Brain **1** Brain Stem **6** Spinal Cord **7** Peripheral Nerve	**D** Stereotactic Other Photon Radiosurgery **H** Stereotactic Particulate Radiosurgery **J** Stereotactic Gamma Beam Radiosurgery	**Z** None	**Z** None

D Radiation Oncology
Ø Central and Peripheral Nervous System
Y Other Radiation

Treatment Site Character 4	Modal. Qualifier Character 5	Isotope Character 6	Qualifier Character 7
Ø Brain **1** Brain Stem **6** Spinal Cord **7** Peripheral Nerve	**7** Contact Radiation **8** Hyperthermia **F** Plaque Radiation **K** Laser Interstitial Thermal Therapy	**Z** None	**Z** None

D Radiation Oncology
7 Lymphatic and Hematologic System
Ø Beam Radiation

Treatment Site Character 4	Modal. Qualifier Character 5	Isotope Character 6	Qualifier Character 7
Ø Bone Marrow **1** Thymus **2** Spleen **3** Lymphatics, Neck **4** Lymphatics, Axillary **5** Lymphatics, Thorax **6** Lymphatics, Abdomen **7** Lymphatics, Pelvis **8** Lymphatics, Inguinal	**Ø** Photons <1 MeV **1** Photons 1- 1Ø MeV **2** Photons >1Ø MeV **4** Heavy Particles (Protons, Ions) **5** Neutrons **6** Neutron Capture	**Z** None	**Z** None
Ø Bone Marrow **1** Thymus **2** Spleen **3** Lymphatics, Neck **4** Lymphatics, Axillary **5** Lymphatics, Thorax **6** Lymphatics, Abdomen **7** Lymphatics, Pelvis **8** Lymphatics, Inguinal	**3** Electrons	**Z** None	**Ø** Intraoperative **Z** None

D Radiation Oncology
7 Lymphatic and Hematologic System
1 Brachytherapy

Treatment Site Character 4	Modal. Qualifier Character 5	Isotope Character 6	Qualifier Character 7
Ø Bone Marrow **1** Thymus **2** Spleen **3** Lymphatics, Neck **4** Lymphatics, Axillary **5** Lymphatics, Thorax **6** Lymphatics, Abdomen **7** Lymphatics, Pelvis **8** Lymphatics, Inguinal	**9** High Dose Rate (HDR) **B** Low Dose Rate (LDR)	**7** Cesium 137 (Cs-137) **8** Iridium 192 (Ir-192) **9** Iodine 125 (I-125) **B** Palladium 1Ø3 (Pd-1Ø3) **C** Californium 252 (Cf-252) **Y** Other Isotope	**Z** None

D Radiation Oncology
7 Lymphatic and Hematologic System
2 Stereotactic Radiosurgery

Treatment Site Character 4	Modal. Qualifier Character 5	Isotope Character 6	Qualifier Character 7
Ø Bone Marrow **1** Thymus **2** Spleen **3** Lymphatics, Neck **4** Lymphatics, Axillary **5** Lymphatics, Thorax **6** Lymphatics, Abdomen **7** Lymphatics, Pelvis **8** Lymphatics, Inguinal	**D** Stereotactic Other Photon Radiosurgery **H** Stereotactic Particulate Radiosurgery **J** Stereotactic Gamma Beam Radiosurgery	**Z** None	**Z** None

D Radiation Oncology
7 Lymphatic and Hematologic System
Y Other Radiation

Treatment Site Character 4	Modal. Qualifier Character 5	Isotope Character 6	Qualifier Character 7
Ø Bone Marrow **1** Thymus **2** Spleen **3** Lymphatics, Neck **4** Lymphatics, Axillary **5** Lymphatics, Thorax **6** Lymphatics, Abdomen **7** Lymphatics, Pelvis **8** Lymphatics, Inguinal	**8** Hyperthermia **F** Plaque Radiation	**Z** None	**Z** None

D Radiation Oncology
8 Eye
Ø Beam Radiation

Treatment Site Character 4	Modal. Qualifier Character 5	Isotope Character 6	Qualifier Character 7
Ø Eye	**Ø** Photons <1 MeV **1** Photons 1- 1Ø MeV **2** Photons >1Ø MeV **4** Heavy Particles (Protons, Ions) **5** Neutrons **6** Neutron Capture	**Z** None	**Z** None
Ø Eye	**3** Electrons	**Z** None	**Ø** Intraoperative **Z** None

D Radiation Oncology
8 Eye
1 Brachytherapy

Treatment Site Character 4	Modal. Qualifier Character 5	Isotope Character 6	Qualifier Character 7
Ø Eye	**9** High Dose Rate (HDR) **B** Low Dose Rate (LDR)	**7** Cesium 137 (Cs-137) **8** Iridium 192 (Ir-192) **9** Iodine 125 (I-125) **B** Palladium 1Ø3 (Pd-1Ø3) **C** Californium 252 (Cf-252) **Y** Other Isotope	**Z** None

D Radiation Oncology
8 Eye
2 Stereotactic Radiosurgery

Treatment Site Character 4	Modal. Qualifier Character 5	Isotope Character 6	Qualifier Character 7
Ø Eye	**D** Stereotactic Other Photon Radiosurgery **H** Stereotactic Particulate Radiosurgery **J** Stereotactic Gamma Beam Radiosurgery	**Z** None	**Z** None

D Radiation Oncology
8 Eye
Y Other Radiation

Treatment Site Character 4	Modal. Qualifier Character 5	Isotope Character 6	Qualifier Character 7
Ø Eye	**7** Contact Radiation **8** Hyperthermia **F** Plaque Radiation	**Z** None	**Z** None

D Radiation Oncology
9 Ear, Nose, Mouth and Throat
0 Beam Radiation

Treatment Site Character 4	Modal. Qualifier Character 5	Isotope Character 6	Qualifier Character 7
0 Ear **1** Nose **3** Hypopharynx **4** Mouth **5** Tongue **6** Salivary Glands **7** Sinuses **8** Hard Palate **9** Soft Palate **B** Larynx **D** Nasopharynx **F** Oropharynx	**0** Photons <1 MeV **1** Photons 1- 10 MeV **2** Photons >10 MeV **4** Heavy Particles (Protons, Ions) **5** Neutrons **6** Neutron Capture	**Z** None	**Z** None
0 Ear **1** Nose **3** Hypopharynx **4** Mouth **5** Tongue **6** Salivary Glands **7** Sinuses **8** Hard Palate **9** Soft Palate **B** Larynx **D** Nasopharynx **F** Oropharynx	**3** Electrons	**Z** None	**0** Intraoperative **Z** None

D Radiation Oncology
9 Ear, Nose, Mouth and Throat
1 Brachytherapy

Treatment Site Character 4	Modal. Qualifier Character 5	Isotope Character 6	Qualifier Character 7
0 Ear **1** Nose **3** Hypopharynx **4** Mouth **5** Tongue **6** Salivary Glands **7** Sinuses **8** Hard Palate **9** Soft Palate **B** Larynx **D** Nasopharynx **F** Oropharynx	**9** High Dose Rate (HDR) **B** Low Dose Rate (LDR)	**7** Cesium 137 (Cs-137) **8** Iridium 192 (Ir-192) **9** Iodine 125 (I-125) **B** Palladium 103 (Pd-103) **C** Californium 252 (Cf-252) **Y** Other Isotope	**Z** None

D Radiation Oncology
9 Ear, Nose, Mouth and Throat
2 Stereotactic Radiosurgery

Treatment Site Character 4	Modal. Qualifier Character 5	Isotope Character 6	Qualifier Character 7
0 Ear **1** Nose **4** Mouth **5** Tongue **6** Salivary Glands **7** Sinuses **8** Hard Palate **9** Soft Palate **B** Larynx **C** Pharynx **D** Nasopharynx	**D** Stereotactic Other Photon Radiosurgery **H** Stereotactic Particulate Radiosurgery **J** Stereotactic Gamma Beam Radiosurgery	**Z** None	**Z** None

D Radiation Oncology
9 Ear, Nose, Mouth and Throat
Y Other Radiation

Treatment Site Character 4	Modal. Qualifier Character 5	Isotope Character 6	Qualifier Character 7
0 Ear **1** Nose **5** Tongue **6** Salivary Glands **7** Sinuses **8** Hard Palate **9** Soft Palate	**7** Contact Radiation **8** Hyperthermia **F** Plaque Radiation	**Z** None	**Z** None
3 Hypopharynx **F** Oropharynx	**7** Contact Radiation **8** Hyperthermia	**Z** None	**Z** None
4 Mouth **B** Larynx **D** Nasopharynx	**7** Contact Radiation **8** Hyperthermia **C** Intraoperative Radiation Therapy (IORT) **F** Plaque Radiation	**Z** None	**Z** None
C Pharynx	**C** Intraoperative Radiation Therapy (IORT) **F** Plaque Radiation	**Z** None	**Z** None

D Radiation Oncology
B Respiratory System
0 Beam Radiation

Treatment Site Character 4	Modal. Qualifier Character 5	Isotope Character 6	Qualifier Character 7
0 Trachea **1** Bronchus **2** Lung **5** Pleura **6** Mediastinum **7** Chest Wall **8** Diaphragm	**0** Photons <1 MeV **1** Photons 1- 10 MeV **2** Photons >10 MeV **4** Heavy Particles (Protons, Ions) **5** Neutrons **6** Neutron Capture	**Z** None	**Z** None
0 Trachea **1** Bronchus **2** Lung **5** Pleura **6** Mediastinum **7** Chest Wall **8** Diaphragm	**3** Electrons	**Z** None	**0** Intraoperative **Z** None

D Radiation Oncology
B Respiratory System
1 Brachytherapy

Treatment Site Character 4	Modal. Qualifier Character 5	Isotope Character 6	Qualifier Character 7
0 Trachea **1** Bronchus **2** Lung **5** Pleura **6** Mediastinum **7** Chest Wall **8** Diaphragm	**9** High Dose Rate (HDR) **B** Low Dose Rate (LDR)	**7** Cesium 137 (Cs-137) **8** Iridium 192 (Ir-192) **9** Iodine 125 (I-125) **B** Palladium 103 (Pd-103) **C** Californium 252 (Cf-252) **Y** Other Isotope	**Z** None

D Radiation Oncology
B Respiratory System
2 Stereotactic Radiosurgery

Treatment Site Character 4	Modal. Qualifier Character 5	Isotope Character 6	Qualifier Character 7
0 Trachea **1** Bronchus **2** Lung **5** Pleura **6** Mediastinum **7** Chest Wall **8** Diaphragm	**D** Stereotactic Other Photon Radiosurgery **H** Stereotactic Particulate Radiosurgery **J** Stereotactic Gamma Beam Radiosurgery	**Z** None	**Z** None

D Radiation Oncology
B Respiratory System
Y Other Radiation

Treatment Site Character 4	Modal. Qualifier Character 5	Isotope Character 6	Qualifier Character 7
0 Trachea 1 Bronchus 2 Lung 5 Pleura 6 Mediastinum 7 Chest Wall 8 Diaphragm	7 Contact Radiation 8 Hyperthermia F Plaque Radiation **K Laser Interstitial Thermal Therapy**	Z None	Z None

D Radiation Oncology
D Gastrointestinal System
0 Beam Radiation

Treatment Site Character 4	Modal. Qualifier Character 5	Isotope Character 6	Qualifier Character 7
0 Esophagus 1 Stomach 2 Duodenum 3 Jejunum 4 Ileum 5 Colon 7 Rectum	0 Photons <1 MeV 1 Photons 1- 10 MeV 2 Photons >10 MeV 4 Heavy Particles (Protons, Ions) 5 Neutrons 6 Neutron Capture	Z None	Z None
0 Esophagus 1 Stomach 2 Duodenum 3 Jejunum 4 Ileum 5 Colon 7 Rectum	3 Electrons	Z None	0 Intraoperative Z None

D Radiation Oncology
D Gastrointestinal System
1 Brachytherapy

Treatment Site Character 4	Modal. Qualifier Character 5	Isotope Character 6	Qualifier Character 7
0 Esophagus 1 Stomach 2 Duodenum 3 Jejunum 4 Ileum 5 Colon 7 Rectum	9 High Dose Rate (HDR) B Low Dose Rate (LDR)	7 Cesium 137 (Cs-137) 8 Iridium 192 (Ir-192) 9 Iodine 125 (I-125) B Palladium 103 (Pd-103) C Californium 252 (Cf-252) Y Other Isotope	Z None

D Radiation Oncology
D Gastrointestinal System
2 Stereotactic Radiosurgery

Treatment Site Character 4	Modal. Qualifier Character 5	Isotope Character 6	Qualifier Character 7
0 Esophagus 1 Stomach 2 Duodenum 3 Jejunum 4 Ileum 5 Colon 7 Rectum	D Stereotactic Other Photon Radiosurgery H Stereotactic Particulate Radiosurgery J Stereotactic Gamma Beam Radiosurgery	Z None	Z None

D Radiation Oncology
D Gastrointestinal System
Y Other Radiation

Treatment Site Character 4	Modal. Qualifier Character 5	Isotope Character 6	Qualifier Character 7
0 Esophagus	**7** Contact Radiation **8** Hyperthermia **F** Plaque Radiation **K** Laser Interstitial Thermal Therapy	**Z** None	**Z** None
1 Stomach **2** Duodenum **3** Jejunum **4** Ileum **5** Colon **7** Rectum	**7** Contact Radiation **8** Hyperthermia **C** Intraoperative Radiation Therapy (IORT) **F** Plaque Radiation **K** Laser Interstitial Thermal Therapy	**Z** None	**Z** None
8 Anus	**C** Intraoperative Radiation Therapy (IORT) **F** Plaque Radiation **K** Laser Interstitial Thermal Therapy	**Z** None	**Z** None

D Radiation Oncology
F Hepatobiliary System and Pancreas
0 Beam Radiation

Treatment Site Character 4	Modal. Qualifier Character 5	Isotope Character 6	Qualifier Character 7
0 Liver **1** Gallbladder **2** Bile Ducts **3** Pancreas	**0** Photons <1 MeV **1** Photons 1- 10 MeV **2** Photons >10 MeV **4** Heavy Particles (Protons, Ions) **5** Neutrons **6** Neutron Capture	**Z** None	**Z** None
0 Liver **1** Gallbladder **2** Bile Ducts **3** Pancreas	**3** Electrons	**Z** None	**0** Intraoperative **Z** None

D Radiation Oncology
F Hepatobiliary System and Pancreas
1 Brachytherapy

Treatment Site Character 4	Modal. Qualifier Character 5	Isotope Character 6	Qualifier Character 7
0 Liver **1** Gallbladder **2** Bile Ducts **3** Pancreas	**9** High Dose Rate (HDR) **B** Low Dose Rate (LDR)	**7** Cesium 137 (Cs-137) **8** Iridium 192 (Ir-192) **9** Iodine 125 (I-125) **B** Palladium 103 (Pd-103) **C** Californium 252 (Cf-252) **Y** Other Isotope	**Z** None

D Radiation Oncology
F Hepatobiliary System and Pancreas
2 Stereotactic Radiosurgery

Treatment Site Character 4	Modal. Qualifier Character 5	Isotope Character 6	Qualifier Character 7
0 Liver **1** Gallbladder **2** Bile Ducts **3** Pancreas	**D** Stereotactic Other Photon Radiosurgery **H** Stereotactic Particulate Radiosurgery **J** Stereotactic Gamma Beam Radiosurgery	**Z** None	**Z** None

D Radiation Oncology
F Hepatobiliary System and Pancreas
Y Other Radiation

Treatment Site Character 4	Modal. Qualifier Character 5	Isotope Character 6	Qualifier Character 7
0 Liver **1** Gallbladder **2** Bile Ducts **3** Pancreas	**7** Contact Radiation **8** Hyperthermia **C** Intraoperative Radiation Therapy (IORT) **F** Plaque Radiation **K** Laser Interstitial Thermal Therapy	**Z** None	**Z** None

D Radiation Oncology
G Endocrine System
0 Beam Radiation

Treatment Site Character 4	Modal. Qualifier Character 5	Isotope Character 6	Qualifier Character 7
0 Pituitary Gland **1** Pineal Body **2** Adrenal Glands **4** Parathyroid Glands **5** Thyroid	**0** Photons <1 MeV **1** Photons 1- 10 MeV **2** Photons >10 MeV **5** Neutrons **6** Neutron Capture	**Z** None	**Z** None
0 Pituitary Gland **1** Pineal Body **2** Adrenal Glands **4** Parathyroid Glands **5** Thyroid	**3** Electrons	**Z** None	**0** Intraoperative **Z** None

D Radiation Oncology
G Endocrine System
1 Brachytherapy

Treatment Site Character 4	Modal. Qualifier Character 5	Isotope Character 6	Qualifier Character 7
0 Pituitary Gland **1** Pineal Body **2** Adrenal Glands **4** Parathyroid Glands **5** Thyroid	**9** High Dose Rate (HDR) **B** Low Dose Rate (LDR)	**7** Cesium 137 (Cs-137) **8** Iridium 192 (Ir-192) **9** Iodine 125 (I-125) **B** Palladium 103 (Pd-103) **C** Californium 252 (Cf-252) **Y** Other Isotope	**Z** None

D Radiation Oncology
G Endocrine System
2 Stereotactic Radiosurgery

Treatment Site Character 4	Modal. Qualifier Character 5	Isotope Character 6	Qualifier Character 7
0 Pituitary Gland **1** Pineal Body **2** Adrenal Glands **4** Parathyroid Glands **5** Thyroid	**D** Stereotactic Other Photon Radiosurgery **H** Stereotactic Particulate Radiosurgery **J** Stereotactic Gamma Beam Radiosurgery	**Z** None	**Z** None

D Radiation Oncology
G Endocrine System
Y Other Radiation

Treatment Site Character 4	Modal. Qualifier Character 5	Isotope Character 6	Qualifier Character 7
0 Pituitary Gland **1** Pineal Body **2** Adrenal Glands **4** Parathyroid Glands **5** Thyroid	**7** Contact Radiation **8** Hyperthermia **F** Plaque Radiation **K** Laser Interstitial Thermal Therapy	**Z** None	**Z** None

D Radiation Oncology
H Skin
Ø Beam Radiation

Treatment Site Character 4	Modal. Qualifier Character 5	Isotope Character 6	Qualifier Character 7
2 Skin, Face 3 Skin, Neck 4 Skin, Arm 6 Skin, Chest 7 Skin, Back 8 Skin, Abdomen 9 Skin, Buttock B Skin, Leg	Ø Photons <1 MeV 1 Photons 1- 1Ø MeV 2 Photons >1Ø MeV 4 Heavy Particles (Protons, Ions) 5 Neutrons 6 Neutron Capture	Z None	Z None
2 Skin, Face 3 Skin, Neck 4 Skin, Arm 6 Skin, Chest 7 Skin, Back 8 Skin, Abdomen 9 Skin, Buttock B Skin, Leg	3 Electrons	Z None	Ø Intraoperative Z None

D Radiation Oncology
H Skin
Y Other Radiation

Treatment Site Character 4	Modal. Qualifier Character 5	Isotope Character 6	Qualifier Character 7
2 Skin, Face 3 Skin, Neck 4 Skin, Arm 6 Skin, Chest 7 Skin, Back 8 Skin, Abdomen 9 Skin, Buttock B Skin, Leg	7 Contact Radiation 8 Hyperthermia F Plaque Radiation	Z None	Z None
5 Skin, Hand C Skin, Foot	F Plaque Radiation	Z None	Z None

D Radiation Oncology
M Breast
Ø Beam Radiation

Treatment Site Character 4	Modal. Qualifier Character 5	Isotope Character 6	Qualifier Character 7
Ø Breast, Left 1 Breast, Right	Ø Photons <1 MeV 1 Photons 1- 1Ø MeV 2 Photons >1Ø MeV 4 Heavy Particles (Protons, Ions) 5 Neutrons 6 Neutron Capture	Z None	Z None
Ø Breast, Left 1 Breast, Right	3 Electrons	Z None	Ø Intraoperative Z None

D Radiation Oncology
M Breast
1 Brachytherapy

Treatment Site Character 4	Modal. Qualifier Character 5	Isotope Character 6	Qualifier Character 7
Ø Breast, Left 1 Breast, Right	9 High Dose Rate (HDR) B Low Dose Rate (LDR)	7 Cesium 137 (Cs-137) 8 Iridium 192 (Ir-192) 9 Iodine 125 (I-125) B Palladium 1Ø3 (Pd-1Ø3) C Californium 252 (Cf-252) Y Other Isotope	Z None

D Radiation Oncology
M Breast
2 Stereotactic Radiosurgery

Treatment Site Character 4	Modal. Qualifier Character 5	Isotope Character 6	Qualifier Character 7
0 Breast, Left 1 Breast, Right	D Stereotactic Other Photon Radiosurgery H Stereotactic Particulate Radiosurgery J Stereotactic Gamma Beam Radiosurgery	Z None	Z None

D Radiation Oncology
M Breast
Y Other Radiation

Treatment Site Character 4	Modal. Qualifier Character 5	Isotope Character 6	Qualifier Character 7
0 Breast, Left 1 Breast, Right	7 Contact Radiation 8 Hyperthermia F Plaque Radiation **K Laser Interstitial Thermal Therapy**	Z None	Z None

D Radiation Oncology
P Musculoskeletal System
0 Beam Radiation

Treatment Site Character 4	Modal. Qualifier Character 5	Isotope Character 6	Qualifier Character 7
0 Skull 2 Maxilla 3 Mandible 4 Sternum 5 Rib(s) 6 Humerus 7 Radius/Ulna 8 Pelvic Bones 9 Femur B Tibia/Fibula C Other Bone	0 Photons <1 MeV 1 Photons 1- 10 MeV 2 Photons >10 MeV 4 Heavy Particles (Protons, Ions) 5 Neutrons 6 Neutron Capture	Z None	Z None
0 Skull 2 Maxilla 3 Mandible 4 Sternum 5 Rib(s) 6 Humerus 7 Radius/Ulna 8 Pelvic Bones 9 Femur B Tibia/Fibula C Other Bone	3 Electrons	Z None	0 Intraoperative Z None

D Radiation Oncology
P Musculoskeletal System
Y Other Radiation

Treatment Site Character 4	Modal. Qualifier Character 5	Isotope Character 6	Qualifier Character 7
0 Skull 2 Maxilla 3 Mandible 4 Sternum 5 Rib(s) 6 Humerus 7 Radius/Ulna 8 Pelvic Bones 9 Femur B Tibia/Fibula C Other Bone	7 Contact Radiation 8 Hyperthermia F Plaque Radiation	Z None	Z None

D Radiation Oncology
T Urinary System
Ø Beam Radiation

Treatment Site Character 4	Modal. Qualifier Character 5	Isotope Character 6	Qualifier Character 7
Ø Kidney **1** Ureter **2** Bladder **3** Urethra	**Ø** Photons <1 MeV **1** Photons 1- 1Ø MeV **2** Photons >1Ø MeV **4** Heavy Particles (Protons, Ions) **5** Neutrons **6** Neutron Capture	**Z** None	**Z** None
Ø Kidney **1** Ureter **2** Bladder **3** Urethra	**3** Electrons	**Z** None	**Ø** Intraoperative **Z** None

D Radiation Oncology
T Urinary System
1 Brachytherapy

Treatment Site Character 4	Modal. Qualifier Character 5	Isotope Character 6	Qualifier Character 7
Ø Kidney **1** Ureter **2** Bladder **3** Urethra	**9** High Dose Rate (HDR) **B** Low Dose Rate (LDR)	**7** Cesium 137 (Cs-137) **8** Iridium 192 (Ir-192) **9** Iodine 125 (I-125) **B** Palladium 1Ø3 (Pd-1Ø3) **C** Californium 252 (Cf-252) **Y** Other Isotope	**Z** None

D Radiation Oncology
T Urinary System
2 Stereotactic Radiosurgery

Treatment Site Character 4	Modal. Qualifier Character 5	Isotope Character 6	Qualifier Character 7
Ø Kidney **1** Ureter **2** Bladder **3** Urethra	**D** Stereotactic Other Photon Radiosurgery **H** Stereotactic Particulate Radiosurgery **J** Stereotactic Gamma Beam Radiosurgery	**Z** None	**Z** None

D Radiation Oncology
T Urinary System
Y Other Radiation

Treatment Site Character 4	Modal. Qualifier Character 5	Isotope Character 6	Qualifier Character 7
Ø Kidney **1** Ureter **2** Bladder **3** Urethra	**7** Contact Radiation **8** Hyperthermia **C** Intraoperative Radiation Therapy (IORT) **F** Plaque Radiation	**Z** None	**Z** None

D Radiation Oncology
U Female Reproductive System
Ø Beam Radiation

Treatment Site Character 4	Modal. Qualifier Character 5	Isotope Character 6	Qualifier Character 7
Ø Ovary **1** Cervix **2** Uterus	**Ø** Photons <1 MeV **1** Photons 1- 1Ø MeV **2** Photons >1Ø MeV **4** Heavy Particles (Protons, Ions) **5** Neutrons **6** Neutron Capture	**Z** None	**Z** None
Ø Ovary **1** Cervix **2** Uterus	**3** Electrons	**Z** None	**Ø** Intraoperative **Z** None

D Radiation Oncology
U Female Reproductive System
1 Brachytherapy

Treatment Site Character 4	Modal. Qualifier Character 5	Isotope Character 6	Qualifier Character 7
0 Ovary **1** Cervix **2** Uterus	**9** High Dose Rate (HDR) **B** Low Dose Rate (LDR)	**7** Cesium 137 (Cs-137) **8** Iridium 192 (Ir-192) **9** Iodine 125 (I-125) **B** Palladium 103 (Pd-103) **C** Californium 252 (Cf-252) **Y** Other Isotope	**Z** None

D Radiation Oncology
U Female Reproductive System
2 Stereotactic Radiosurgery

Treatment Site Character 4	Modal. Qualifier Character 5	Isotope Character 6	Qualifier Character 7
0 Ovary **1** Cervix **2** Uterus	**D** Stereotactic Other Photon Radiosurgery **H** Stereotactic Particulate Radiosurgery **J** Stereotactic Gamma Beam Radiosurgery	**Z** None	**Z** None

D Radiation Oncology
U Female Reproductive System
Y Other Radiation

Treatment Site Character 4	Modal. Qualifier Character 5	Isotope Character 6	Qualifier Character 7
0 Ovary **1** Cervix **2** Uterus	**7** Contact Radiation **8** Hyperthermia **C** Intraoperative Radiation Therapy (IORT) **F** Plaque Radiation	**Z** None	**Z** None

D Radiation Oncology
V Male Reproductive System
0 Beam Radiation

Treatment Site Character 4	Modal. Qualifier Character 5	Isotope Character 6	Qualifier Character 7
0 Prostate **1** Testis	**0** Photons <1 MeV **1** Photons 1- 10 MeV **2** Photons >10 MeV **4** Heavy Particles (Protons, Ions) **5** Neutrons **6** Neutron Capture	**Z** None	**Z** None
0 Prostate **1** Testis	**3** Electrons	**Z** None	**0** Intraoperative **Z** None

D Radiation Oncology
V Male Reproductive System
1 Brachytherapy

Treatment Site Character 4	Modal. Qualifier Character 5	Isotope Character 6	Qualifier Character 7
0 Prostate **1** Testis	**9** High Dose Rate (HDR) **B** Low Dose Rate (LDR)	**7** Cesium 137 (Cs-137) **8** Iridium 192 (Ir-192) **9** Iodine 125 (I-125) **B** Palladium 103 (Pd-103) **C** Californium 252 (Cf-252) **Y** Other Isotope	**Z** None

D Radiation Oncology
V Male Reproductive System
2 Stereotactic Radiosurgery

Treatment Site Character 4	Modal. Qualifier Character 5	Isotope Character 6	Qualifier Character 7
0 Prostate **1** Testis	**D** Stereotactic Other Photon Radiosurgery **H** Stereotactic Particulate Radiosurgery **J** Stereotactic Gamma Beam Radiosurgery	**Z** None	**Z** None

D Radiation Oncology
V Male Reproductive System
Y Other Radiation

Treatment Site Character 4	Modal. Qualifier Character 5	Isotope Character 6	Qualifier Character 7
0 Prostate	**7** Contact Radiation **8** Hyperthermia **C** Intraoperative Radiation Therapy (IORT) **F** Plaque Radiation **K Laser Interstitial Thermal Therapy**	**Z** None	**Z** None
1 Testis	**7** Contact Radiation **8** Hyperthermia **F** Plaque Radiation	**Z** None	**Z** None

D Radiation Oncology
W Anatomical Regions
0 Beam Radiation

Treatment Site Character 4	Modal. Qualifier Character 5	Isotope Character 6	Qualifier Character 7
1 Head and Neck **2** Chest **3** Abdomen **4** Hemibody **5** Whole Body **6** Pelvic Region	**0** Photons <1 MeV **1** Photons 1- 10 MeV **2** Photons >10 MeV **4** Heavy Particles (Protons, Ions) **5** Neutrons **6** Neutron Capture	**Z** None	**Z** None
1 Head and Neck **2** Chest **3** Abdomen **4** Hemibody **5** Whole Body **6** Pelvic Region	**3** Electrons	**Z** None	**0** Intraoperative **Z** None

D Radiation Oncology
W Anatomical Regions
1 Brachytherapy

Treatment Site Character 4	Modal. Qualifier Character 5	Isotope Character 6	Qualifier Character 7
1 Head and Neck **2** Chest **3** Abdomen **6** Pelvic Region	**9** High Dose Rate (HDR) **B** Low Dose Rate (LDR)	**7** Cesium 137 (Cs-137) **8** Iridium 192 (Ir-192) **9** Iodine 125 (I-125) **B** Palladium 103 (Pd-103) **C** Californium 252 (Cf-252) **Y** Other Isotope	**Z** None

D Radiation Oncology
W Anatomical Regions
2 Stereotactic Radiosurgery

Treatment Site Character 4	Modal. Qualifier Character 5	Isotope Character 6	Qualifier Character 7
1 Head and Neck **2** Chest **3** Abdomen **6** Pelvic Region	**D** Stereotactic Other Photon Radiosurgery **H** Stereotactic Particulate Radiosurgery **J** Stereotactic Gamma Beam Radiosurgery	**Z** None	**Z** None

D Radiation Oncology
W Anatomical Regions
Y Other Radiation

Treatment Site Character 4	Modal. Qualifier Character 5	Isotope Character 6	Qualifier Character 7
1 Head and Neck **2** Chest **3** Abdomen **4** Hemibody **5** Whole Body **6** Pelvic Region	**7** Contact Radiation **8** Hyperthermia **F** Plaque Radiation	**Z** None	**Z** None
5 Whole Body	**G** Isotope Administration	**D** Iodine 131 (I-131) **F** Phosphorus 32 (P-32) **G** Strontium 89 (Sr-89) **H** Strontium 90 (Sr-90) **Y** Other Isotope	**Z** None

Physical Rehabilitation and Diagnostic Audiology FØØ–F15

F Physical Rehabilitation and Diagnostic Audiology
Ø Rehabilitation
Ø Speech Assessment Measurement of speech and related functions

Body System/Region Character 4	Type Qualifier Character 5	Equipment Character 6	Qualifier Character 7
3 Neurological System - Whole Body	**G** Communicative/Cognitive Integration Skills	**K** Audiovisual **M** Augmentative / Alternative Communication **P** Computer **Y** Other Equipment **Z** None	**Z** None
Z None	**Ø** Filtered Speech **3** Staggered Spondaic Word **Q** Performance Intensity Phonetically Balanced Speech Discrimination **R** Brief Tone Stimuli **S** Distorted Speech **T** Dichotic Stimuli **V** Temporal Ordering of Stimuli **W** Masking Patterns	**1** Audiometer **2** Sound Field / Booth **K** Audiovisual **Z** None	**Z** None
Z None	**1** Speech Threshold **2** Speech/Word Recognition	**1** Audiometer **2** Sound Field / Booth **9** Cochlear Implant **K** Audiovisual **Z** None	**Z** None
Z None	**4** Sensorineural Acuity Level	**1** Audiometer **2** Sound Field / Booth **Z** None	**Z** None
Z None	**5** Synthetic Sentence Identification	**1** Audiometer **2** Sound Field / Booth **9** Cochlear Implant **K** Audiovisual	**Z** None
Z None	**6** Speech and/or Language Screening **7** Nonspoken Language **8** Receptive/Expressive Language **C** Aphasia **G** Communicative/Cognitive Integration Skills **L** Augmentative/Alternative Communication System	**K** Audiovisual **M** Augmentative / Alternative Communication **P** Computer **Y** Other Equipment **Z** None	**Z** None
Z None	**9** Articulation/Phonology	**K** Audiovisual **P** Computer **Q** Speech Analysis **Y** Other Equipment **Z** None	**Z** None
Z None	**B** Motor Speech	**K** Audiovisual **N** Biosensory Feedback **P** Computer **Q** Speech Analysis **T** Aerodynamic Function **Y** Other Equipment **Z** None	**Z** None
Z None	**D** Fluency	**K** Audiovisual **N** Biosensory Feedback **P** Computer **Q** Speech Analysis **S** Voice Analysis **T** Aerodynamic Function **Y** Other Equipment **Z** None	**Z** None
Z None	**F** Voice	**K** Audiovisual **N** Biosensory Feedback **P** Computer **S** Voice Analysis **T** Aerodynamic Function **Y** Other Equipment **Z** None	**Z** None
Z None	**H** Bedside Swallowing and Oral Function **P** Oral Peripheral Mechanism	**Y** Other Equipment **Z** None	**Z** None
Z None	**J** Instrumental Swallowing and Oral Function	**T** Aerodynamic Function **W** Swallowing **Y** Other Equipment	**Z** None

FØØ Continued on next page

F Physical Rehabilitation and Diagnostic Audiology
0 Rehabilitation
0 Speech Assessment Measurement of speech and related functions

F00 Continued

Body System/Region Character 4	Type Qualifier Character 5	Equipment Character 6	Qualifier Character 7
Z None	K Orofacial Myofunctional	K Audiovisual P Computer Y Other Equipment Z None	Z None
Z None	M Voice Prosthetic	K Audiovisual P Computer S Voice Analysis V Speech Prosthesis Y Other Equipment Z None	Z None
Z None	N Non-invasive Instrumental Status	N Biosensory Feedback P Computer Q Speech Analysis S Voice Analysis T Aerodynamic Function Y Other Equipment	Z None
Z None	X Other Specified Central Auditory Processing	Z None	Z None

F Physical Rehabilitation and Diagnostic Audiology
0 Rehabilitation
1 Motor and/or Nerve Function Assessment Measurement of motor, nerve, and related functions

Body System/Region Character 4	Type Qualifier Character 5	Equipment Character 6	Qualifier Character 7
0 Neurological System - Head and Neck 1 Neurological System - Upper Back / Upper Extremity 2 Neurological System - Lower Back / Lower Extremity 3 Neurological System - Whole Body	1 Integumentary Integrity 3 Coordination/Dexterity 4 Motor Function G Reflex Integrity	Z None	Z None
0 Neurological System - Head and Neck 1 Neurological System - Upper Back / Upper Extremity 2 Neurological System - Lower Back / Lower Extremity 3 Neurological System - Whole Body D Integumentary System - Head and Neck F Integumentary System - Upper Back / Upper Extremity G Integumentary System - Lower Back / Lower Extremity H Integumentary System - Whole Body J Musculoskeletal System - Head and Neck K Musculoskeletal System - Upper Back / Upper Extremity L Musculoskeletal System - Lower Back / Lower Extremity M Musculoskeletal System - Whole Body	5 Range of Motion and Joint Integrity 6 Sensory Awareness/Processing/ Integrity	Y Other Equipment Z None	Z None
0 Neurological System - Head and Neck 1 Neurological System - Upper Back / Upper Extremity 2 Neurological System - Lower Back / Lower Extremity 3 Neurological System - Whole Body D Integumentary System - Head and Neck F Integumentary System - Upper Back / Upper Extremity G Integumentary System - Lower Back / Lower Extremity H Integumentary System - Whole Body J Musculoskeletal System - Head and Neck K Musculoskeletal System - Upper Back / Upper Extremity L Musculoskeletal System - Lower Back / Lower Extremity M Musculoskeletal System - Whole Body N Genitourinary System	0 Muscle Performance	E Orthosis F Assistive, Adaptive, Supportive or Protective U Prosthesis Y Other Equipment Z None	Z None

F01 Continued on next page

F01 Continued

F Physical Rehabilitation and Diagnostic Audiology
0 Rehabilitation
1 Motor and/or Nerve Function Assessment Measurement of motor, nerve, and related functions

Body System/Region Character 4	Type Qualifier Character 5	Equipment Character 6	Qualifier Character 7
D Integumentary System - Head and Neck **F** Integumentary System - Upper Back / Upper Extremity **G** Integumentary System - Lower Back / Lower Extremity **H** Integumentary System - Whole Body **J** Musculoskeletal System - Head and Neck **K** Musculoskeletal System - Upper Back / Upper Extremity **L** Musculoskeletal System - Lower Back / Lower Extremity **M** Musculoskeletal System - Whole Body	**1** Integumentary Integrity	**Z** None	**Z** None
Z None	**2** Visual Motor Integration	**K** Audiovisual **M** Augmentative / Alternative Communication **N** Biosensory Feedback **P** Computer **Q** Speech Analysis **S** Voice Analysis **Y** Other Equipment **Z** None	**Z** None
Z None	**7** Facial Nerve Function	**7** Electrophysiologic	**Z** None
Z None	**9** Somatosensory Evoked Potentials	**J** Somatosensory	**Z** None
Z None	**B** Bed Mobility **C** Transfer **F** Wheelchair Mobility	**E** Orthosis **F** Assistive, Adaptive, Supportive or Protective **U** Prosthesis **Z** None	**Z** None
Z None	**D** Gait and/or Balance	**E** Orthosis **F** Assistive, Adaptive, Supportive or Protective **U** Prosthesis **Y** Other Equipment **Z** None	**Z** None

F Physical Rehabilitation and Diagnostic Audiology
0 Rehabilitation
2 Activities of Daily Living Assessment Measurement of functional level for activities of daily living

Body System/Region Character 4	Type Qualifier Character 5	Equipment Character 6	Qualifier Character 7
0 Neurological System - Head and Neck	**9** Cranial Nerve Integrity **D** Neuromotor Development	**Y** Other Equipment **Z** None	**Z** None
1 Neurological System - Upper Back / Upper Extremity **2** Neurological System - Lower Back / Lower Extremity **3** Neurological System - Whole Body	**D** Neuromotor Development	**Y** Other Equipment **Z** None	**Z** None
4 Circulatory System - Head and Neck **5** Circulatory System - Upper Back / Upper Extremity **6** Circulatory System - Lower Back / Lower Extremity **7** Circulatory System - Whole Body **8** Respiratory System - Head and Neck **9** Respiratory System - Upper Back / Upper Extremity **B** Respiratory System - Lower Back / Lower Extremity **C** Respiratory System - Whole Body	**G** Ventilation, Respiration and Circulation	**C** Mechanical **G** Aerobic Endurance and Conditioning **Y** Other Equipment **Z** None	**Z** None
7 Circulatory System - Whole Body **C** Respiratory System - Whole Body	**7** Aerobic Capacity and Endurance	**E** Orthosis **G** Aerobic Endurance and Conditioning **U** Prosthesis **Y** Other Equipment **Z** None	**Z** None

F02 Continued on next page

F02 Continued

F Physical Rehabilitation and Diagnostic Audiology
0 Rehabilitation
2 Activities of Daily Living Assessment Measurement of functional level for activities of daily living

Body System/Region Character 4	Type Qualifier Character 5	Equipment Character 6	Qualifier Character 7
Z None	0 Bathing/Showering 1 Dressing 3 Grooming/Personal Hygiene 4 Home Management	E Orthosis F Assistive, Adaptive, Supportive or Protective U Prosthesis Z None	Z None
Z None	2 Feeding/Eating 8 Anthropometric Characteristics F Pain	Y Other Equipment Z None	Z None
Z None	5 Perceptual Processing	K Audiovisual M Augmentative / Alternative Communication N Biosensory Feedback P Computer Q Speech Analysis S Voice Analysis Y Other Equipment Z None	Z None
Z None	6 Psychosocial Skills	Z None	Z None
Z None	B Environmental, Home and Work Barriers C Ergonomics and Body Mechanics	E Orthosis F Assistive, Adaptive, Supportive or Protective U Prosthesis Y Other Equipment Z None	Z None
Z None	H Vocational Activities and Functional Community or Work Reintegration Skills	E Orthosis F Assistive, Adaptive, Supportive or Protective G Aerobic Endurance and Conditioning U Prosthesis Y Other Equipment Z None	Z None

F Physical Rehabilitation and Diagnostic Audiology
0 Rehabilitation
6 Speech Treatment Application of techniques to improve, augment, or compensate for speech and related functional impairment

Body System/Region Character 4	Type Qualifier Character 5	Equipment Character 6	Qualifier Character 7
3 Neurological System - Whole Body	6 Communicative/Cognitive Integration Skills	K Audiovisual M Augmentative / Alternative Communication P Computer Y Other Equipment Z None	Z None
Z None	0 Nonspoken Language 3 Aphasia 6 Communicative/Cognitive Integration Skills	K Audiovisual M Augmentative / Alternative Communication P Computer Y Other Equipment Z None	Z None
Z None	1 Speech-Language Pathology and Related Disorders Counseling 2 Speech-Language Pathology and Related Disorders Prevention	K Audiovisual Z None	Z None
Z None	4 Articulation/Phonology	K Audiovisual P Computer Q Speech Analysis T Aerodynamic Function Y Other Equipment Z None	Z None
Z None	5 Aural Rehabilitation	K Audiovisual L Assistive Listening M Augmentative / Alternative Communication N Biosensory Feedback P Computer Q Speech Analysis S Voice Analysis Y Other Equipment Z None	Z None

F06 Continued on next page

FØ6 Continued

F Physical Rehabilitation and Diagnostic Audiology
Ø Rehabilitation
6 Speech Treatment Application of techniques to improve, augment, or compensate for speech and related functional impairment

Body System/Region Character 4	Type Qualifier Character 5	Equipment Character 6	Qualifier Character 7
Z None	**7** Fluency	**4** Electroacoustic Immitance / Acoustic Reflex **K** Audiovisual **N** Biosensory Feedback **Q** Speech Analysis **S** Voice Analysis **T** Aerodynamic Function **Y** Other Equipment **Z** None	**Z** None
Z None	**8** Motor Speech	**K** Audiovisual **N** Biosensory Feedback **P** Computer **Q** Speech Analysis **S** Voice Analysis **T** Aerodynamic Function **Y** Other Equipment **Z** None	**Z** None
Z None	**9** Orofacial Myofunctional	**K** Audiovisual **P** Computer **Y** Other Equipment **Z** None	**Z** None
Z None	**B** Receptive/Expressive Language	**K** Audiovisual **L** Assistive Listening **M** Augmentative / Alternative Communication **P** Computer **Y** Other Equipment **Z** None	**Z** None
Z None	**C** Voice	**K** Audiovisual **N** Biosensory Feedback **P** Computer **S** Voice Analysis **T** Aerodynamic Function **V** Speech Prosthesis **Y** Other Equipment **Z** None	**Z** None
Z None	**D** Swallowing Dysfunction	**M** Augmentative / Alternative Communication **T** Aerodynamic Function **V** Speech Prosthesis **Y** Other Equipment **Z** None	**Z** None

F Physical Rehabilitation and Diagnostic Audiology
0 Rehabilitation
7 Motor Treatment Exercise or activities to increase or facilitate motor function

Body System/Region Character 4	Type Qualifier Character 5	Equipment Character 6	Qualifier Character 7
0 Neurological System - Head and Neck **1** Neurological System - Upper Back / Upper Extremity **2** Neurological System - Lower Back / Lower Extremity **3** Neurological System - Whole Body **4** Circulatory System - Head and Neck **5** Circulatory System - Upper Back / Upper Extremity **6** Circulatory System - Lower Back / Lower Extremity **7** Circulatory System - Whole Body **8** Respiratory System - Head and Neck **9** Respiratory System - Upper Back / Upper Extremity **B** Respiratory System - Lower Back / Lower Extremity **C** Respiratory System - Whole Body **D** Integumentary System - Head and Neck **F** Integumentary System - Upper Back / Upper Extremity **G** Integumentary System - Lower Back / Lower Extremity **H** Integumentary System - Whole Body **J** Musculoskeletal System - Head and Neck **K** Musculoskeletal System - Upper Back / Upper Extremity **L** Musculoskeletal System - Lower Back / Lower Extremity **M** Musculoskeletal System - Whole Body **N** Genitourinary System	**6** Therapeutic Exercise	**B** Physical Agents **C** Mechanical **D** Electrotherapeutic **E** Orthosis **F** Assistive, Adaptive, Supportive or Protective **G** Aerobic Endurance and Conditioning **H** Mechanical or Electromechanical **U** Prosthesis **Y** Other Equipment **Z** None	**Z** None
0 Neurological System - Head and Neck **1** Neurological System - Upper Back / Upper Extremity **2** Neurological System - Lower Back / Lower Extremity **3** Neurological System - Whole Body **D** Integumentary System - Head and Neck **F** Integumentary System - Upper Back / Upper Extremity **G** Integumentary System - Lower Back / Lower Extremity **H** Integumentary System - Whole Body **J** Musculoskeletal System - Head and Neck **K** Musculoskeletal System - Upper Back / Upper Extremity **L** Musculoskeletal System - Lower Back / Lower Extremity **M** Musculoskeletal System - Whole Body	**0** Range of Motion and Joint Mobility **1** Muscle Performance **2** Coordination/Dexterity **3** Motor Function	**E** Orthosis **F** Assistive, Adaptive, Supportive or Protective **U** Prosthesis **Y** Other Equipment **Z** None	**Z** None
0 Neurological System - Head and Neck **1** Neurological System - Upper Back / Upper Extremity **2** Neurological System - Lower Back / Lower Extremity **3** Neurological System - Whole Body **D** Integumentary System - Head and Neck **F** Integumentary System - Upper Back / Upper Extremity **G** Integumentary System - Lower Back / Lower Extremity **H** Integumentary System - Whole Body **J** Musculoskeletal System - Head and Neck **K** Musculoskeletal System - Upper Back / Upper Extremity **L** Musculoskeletal System - Lower Back / Lower Extremity **M** Musculoskeletal System - Whole Body	**7** Manual Therapy Techniques	**Z** None	**Z** None

F07 Continued on next page

F07 Continued

F Physical Rehabilitation and Diagnostic Audiology
0 Rehabilitation
7 Motor Treatment Exercise or activities to increase or facilitate motor function

Body System/Region Character 4	Type Qualifier Character 5	Equipment Character 6	Qualifier Character 7
N Genitourinary System	1 Muscle Performance	E Orthosis F Assistive, Adaptive, Supportive or Protective U Prosthesis Y Other Equipment Z None	Z None
Z None	4 Wheelchair Mobility	D Electrotherapeutic E Orthosis F Assistive, Adaptive, Supportive or Protective U Prosthesis Y Other Equipment Z None	Z None
Z None	5 Bed Mobility	C Mechanical E Orthosis F Assistive, Adaptive, Supportive or Protective U Prosthesis Y Other Equipment Z None	Z None
Z None	8 Transfer Training	C Mechanical D Electrotherapeutic E Orthosis F Assistive, Adaptive, Supportive or Protective U Prosthesis Y Other Equipment Z None	Z None
Z None	9 Gait Training/Functional Ambulation	C Mechanical D Electrotherapeutic E Orthosis F Assistive, Adaptive, Supportive or Protective G Aerobic Endurance and Conditioning U Prosthesis Y Other Equipment Z None	Z None

F Physical Rehabilitation and Diagnostic Audiology
0 Rehabilitation
8 Activities of Daily Living Treatment Exercise or activities to facilitate functional competence for activities of daily living

Body System/Region Character 4	Type Qualifier Character 5	Equipment Character 6	Qualifier Character 7
D Integumentary System - Head and Neck F Integumentary System - Upper Back / Upper Extremity G Integumentary System - Lower Back / Lower Extremity H Integumentary System - Whole Body J Musculoskeletal System - Head and Neck K Musculoskeletal System - Upper Back / Upper Extremity L Musculoskeletal System - Lower Back / Lower Extremity M Musculoskeletal System - Whole Body	5 Wound Management	B Physical Agents C Mechanical D Electrotherapeutic E Orthosis F Assistive, Adaptive, Supportive or Protective U Prosthesis Y Other Equipment Z None	Z None
Z None	0 Bathing/Showering Techniques 1 Dressing Techniques 2 Grooming/Personal Hygiene	E Orthosis F Assistive, Adaptive, Supportive or Protective U Prosthesis Y Other Equipment Z None	Z None
Z None	3 Feeding/Eating	C Mechanical D Electrotherapeutic E Orthosis F Assistive, Adaptive, Supportive or Protective U Prosthesis Y Other Equipment Z None	Z None

F08 Continued on next page

F Physical Rehabilitation and Diagnostic Audiology
0 Rehabilitation
8 Activities of Daily Living Treatment Exercise or activities to facilitate functional competence for activities of daily living

F08 Continued

Body System/Region Character 4	Type Qualifier Character 5	Equipment Character 6	Qualifier Character 7
Z None	**4** Home Management	**D** Electrotherapeutic **E** Orthosis **F** Assistive, Adaptive, Supportive or Protective **U** Prosthesis **Y** Other Equipment **Z** None	**Z** None
Z None	**6** Psychosocial Skills	**Z** None	**Z** None
Z None	**7** Vocational Activities and Functional Community or Work Reintegration Skills	**B** Physical Agents **C** Mechanical **D** Electrotherapeutic **E** Orthosis **F** Assistive, Adaptive, Supportive or Protective **G** Aerobic Endurance and Conditioning **U** Prosthesis **Y** Other Equipment **Z** None	**Z** None

F Physical Rehabilitation and Diagnostic Audiology
0 Rehabilitation
9 Hearing Treatment Application of techniques to improve, augment, or compensate for hearing and related functional impairment

Body System/Region Character 4	Type Qualifier Character 5	Equipment Character 6	Qualifier Character 7
Z None	**0** Hearing and Related Disorders Counseling **1** Hearing and Related Disorders Prevention	**K** Audiovisual **Z** None	**Z** None
Z None	**2** Auditory Processing	**K** Audiovisual **L** Assistive Listening **P** Computer **Y** Other Equipment **Z** None	**Z** None
Z None	**3** Cerumen Management	**X** Cerumen Management **Z** None	**Z** None

F Physical Rehabilitation and Diagnostic Audiology
0 Rehabilitation
B Cochlear Implant Treatment Application of techniques to improve the communication abilities of individuals with cochlear implant

Body System/Region Character 4	Type Qualifier Character 5	Equipment Character 6	Qualifier Character 7
Z None	**0** Cochlear Implant Rehabilitation	**1** Audiometer **2** Sound Field / Booth **9** Cochlear Implant **K** Audiovisual **P** Computer **Y** Other Equipment	**Z** None

F Physical Rehabilitation and Diagnostic Audiology
Ø Rehabilitation
C Vestibular Treatment Application of techniques to improve, augment, or compensate for vestibular and related functional impairment

Body System/Region Character 4	Type Qualifier Character 5	Equipment Character 6	Qualifier Character 7
3 Neurological System - Whole Body **H** Integumentary System - Whole Body **M** Musculoskeletal System - Whole Body	**3** Postural Control	**E** Orthosis **F** Assistive, Adaptive, Supportive or Protective **U** Prosthesis **Y** Other Equipment **Z** None	**Z** None
Z None	**Ø** Vestibular	**8** Vestibular / Balance **Z** None	**Z** None
Z None	**1** Perceptual Processing **2** Visual Motor Integration	**K** Audiovisual **L** Assistive Listening **N** Biosensory Feedback **P** Computer **Q** Speech Analysis **S** Voice Analysis **T** Aerodynamic Function **Y** Other Equipment **Z** None	**Z** None

F Physical Rehabilitation and Diagnostic Audiology
Ø Rehabilitation
D Device Fitting Fitting of a device designed to facilitate or support achievement of a higher level of function

Body System/Region Character 4	Type Qualifier Character 5	Equipment Character 6	Qualifier Character 7
Z None	**Ø** Tinnitus Masker	**5** Hearing Aid Selection / Fitting / Test **Z** None	**Z** None
Z None	**1** Monaural Hearing Aid **2** Binaural Hearing Aid **5** Assistive Listening Device	**1** Audiometer **2** Sound Field / Booth **5** Hearing Aid Selection / Fitting / Test **K** Audiovisual **L** Assistive Listening **Z** None	**Z** None
Z None	**3** Augmentative/Alternative Communication System	**M** Augmentative / Alternative Communication	**Z** None
Z None	**4** Voice Prosthetic	**S** Voice Analysis **V** Speech Prosthesis	**Z** None
Z None	**6** Dynamic Orthosis **7** Static Orthosis **8** Prosthesis **9** Assistive, Adaptive,Supportive or Protective Devices	**E** Orthosis **F** Assistive, Adaptive, Supportive or Protective **U** Prosthesis **Z** None	**Z** None

F Physical Rehabilitation and Diagnostic Audiology
0 Rehabilitation
F Caregiver Training Training in activities to support patient's optimal level of function

Body System/Region Character 4	Type Qualifier Character 5	Equipment Character 6	Qualifier Character 7
Z None	0 Bathing/Showering Technique 1 Dressing 2 Feeding and Eating 3 Grooming/Personal Hygiene 4 Bed Mobility 5 Transfer 6 Wheelchair Mobility 7 Therapeutic Exercise 8 Airway Clearance Techniques 9 Wound Management B Vocational Activities and Functional Community or Work Reintegration Skills C Gait Training/Functional Ambulation D Application, Proper Use and Care of Assistive, Adaptive, Supportive or Protective Devices F Application, Proper Use and Care of Orthoses G Application, Proper Use and Care of Prosthesis H Home Management	E Orthosis F Assistive, Adaptive, Supportive or Protective U Prosthesis Z None	Z None
Z None	J Communication Skills	K Audiovisual L Assistive Listening M Augmentative / Alternative Communication P Computer Z None	Z None

F Physical Rehabilitation and Diagnostic Audiology
1 Diagnostic Audiology
3 Hearing Assessment Measurement of hearing and related functions

Body System/Region Character 4	Type Qualifier Character 5	Equipment Character 6	Qualifier Character 7
Z None	0 Hearing Screening	0 Occupational Hearing 1 Audiometer 2 Sound Field / Booth 3 Tympanometer 8 Vestibular / Balance 9 Cochlear Implant Z None	Z None
Z None	1 Pure Tone Audiometry, Air 2 Pure Tone Audiometry, Air and Bone	0 Occupational Hearing 1 Audiometer 2 Sound Field / Booth Z None	Z None
Z None	3 Bekesy Audiometry 6 Visual Reinforcement Audiometry 9 Short Increment Sensitivity Index B Stenger C Pure Tone Stenger	1 Audiometer 2 Sound Field / Booth Z None	Z None
Z None	4 Conditioned Play Audiometry 5 Select Picture Audiometry	1 Audiometer 2 Sound Field / Booth K Audiovisual Z None	Z None
Z None	7 Alternate Binaural or Monaural Loudness Balance	1 Audiometer K Audiovisual Z None	Z None
Z None	8 Tone Decay D Tympanometry F Eustachian Tube Function G Acoustic Reflex Patterns H Acoustic Reflex Threshold J Acoustic Reflex Decay	3 Tympanometer 4 Electroacoustic Immitance / Acoustic Reflex Z None	Z None
Z None	K Electrocochleography L Auditory Evoked Potentials	7 Electrophysiologic Z None	Z None
Z None	M Evoked Otoacoustic Emissions, Screening N Evoked Otoacoustic Emissions, Diagnostic	6 Otoacoustic Emission (OAE) Z None	Z None

F13 Continued on next page

 Revised Text in **BLUE**

F13 Continued

F Physical Rehabilitation and Diagnostic Audiology
1 Diagnostic Audiology
3 Hearing Assessment Measurement of hearing and related functions

Body System/Region Character 4	Type Qualifier Character 5	Equipment Character 6	Qualifier Character 7
Z None	**P** Aural Rehabilitation Status	**1** Audiometer **2** Sound Field / Booth **4** Electroacoustic Immitance / Acoustic Reflex **9** Cochlear Implant **K** Audiovisual **L** Assistive Listening **P** Computer **Z** None	**Z** None
Z None	**Q** Auditory Processing	**K** Audiovisual **P** Computer **Y** Other Equipment **Z** None	**Z** None

F Physical Rehabilitation and Diagnostic Audiology
1 Diagnostic Audiology
4 Hearing Aid Assessment Measurement of the appropriateness and/or effectiveness of a hearing device

Body System/Region Character 4	Type Qualifier Character 5	Equipment Character 6	Qualifier Character 7
Z None	**Ø** Cochlear Implant	**1** Audiometer **2** Sound Field / Booth **3** Tympanometer **4** Electroacoustic Immitance / Acoustic Reflex **5** Hearing Aid Selection / Fitting / Test **7** Electrophysiologic **9** Cochlear Implant **K** Audiovisual **L** Assistive Listening **P** Computer **Y** Other Equipment **Z** None	**Z** None
Z None	**1** Ear Canal Probe Microphone **6** Binaural Electroacoustic Hearing Aid Check **8** Monaural Electroacoustic Hearing Aid Check	**5** Hearing Aid Selection / Fitting / Test **Z** None	**Z** None
Z None	**2** Monaural Hearing Aid **3** Binaural Hearing Aid	**1** Audiometer **2** Sound Field / Booth **3** Tympanometer **4** Electroacoustic Immitance / Acoustic Reflex **5** Hearing Aid Selection / Fitting / Test **K** Audiovisual **L** Assistive Listening **P** Computer **Z** None	**Z** None
Z None	**4** Assistive Listening System/Device Selection	**1** Audiometer **2** Sound Field / Booth **3** Tympanometer **4** Electroacoustic Immitance / Acoustic Reflex **K** Audiovisual **L** Assistive Listening **Z** None	**Z** None
Z None	**5** Sensory Aids	**1** Audiometer **2** Sound Field / Booth **3** Tympanometer **4** Electroacoustic Immitance / Acoustic Reflex **5** Hearing Aid Selection / Fitting / Test **K** Audiovisual **L** Assistive Listening **Z** None	**Z** None
Z None	**7** Ear Protector Attentuation	**Ø** Occupational Hearing **Z** None	**Z** None

F Physical Rehabilitation and Diagnostic Audiology
1 Diagnostic Audiology
5 Vestibular Assessment Measurement of the vestibular system and related functions

Body System/Region Character 4	Type Qualifier Character 5	Equipment Character 6	Qualifier Character 7
Z None	**0** Bithermal, Binaural Caloric Irrigation **1** Bithermal, Monaural Caloric Irrigation **2** Unithermal Binaural Screen **3** Oscillating Tracking **4** Sinusoidal Vertical Axis Rotational **5** Dix-Hallpike Dynamic **6** Computerized Dynamic Posturography	**8** Vestibular / Balance **Z** None	**Z** None
Z None	**7** Tinnitus Masker	**5** Hearing Aid Selection / Fitting / Test **Z** None	**Z** None

Mental Health GZ1–GZJ

G Mental Health
Z None
1 Psychological Tests The administration and interpretation of standardized psychological tests and measurement instruments for the assessment of psychological function

Type Qualifier Character 4	Qualifier Character 5	Qualifier Character 6	Qualifier Character 7
0 Developmental 1 Personality and Behavioral 2 Intellectual and Psychoeducational 3 Neuropsychological 4 Neurobehavioral and Cognitive Status	Z None	Z None	Z None

G Mental Health
Z None
2 Crisis Intervention Treatment of a traumatized, acutely disturbed or distressed individual for the purpose of short-term stabilization

Type Qualifier Character 4	Qualifier Character 5	Qualifier Character 6	Qualifier Character 7
Z None	Z None	Z None	Z None

G Mental Health
Z None
3 Medication Management Monitoring and adjusting the use of medications for the treatment of a mental health disorder

Type Qualifier Character 4	Qualifier Character 5	Qualifier Character 6	Qualifier Character 7
Z None	Z None	Z None	Z None

G Mental Health
Z None
5 Individual Psychotherapy Treatment of an individual with a mental health disorder by behavioral, cognitive, psychoanalytic, psychodynamic or psychophysiological means to improve functioning or well-being

Type Qualifier Character 4	Qualifier Character 5	Qualifier Character 6	Qualifier Character 7
0 Interactive 1 Behavioral 2 Cognitive 3 Interpersonal 4 Psychoanalysis 5 Psychodynamic 6 Supportive 8 Cognitive-Behavioral 9 Psychophysiological	Z None	Z None	Z None

G Mental Health
Z None
6 Counseling The application of psychological methods to treat an individual with normal developmental issues and psychological problems in order to increase function, improve well-being, alleviate distress, maladjustment or resolve crises

Type Qualifier Character 4	Qualifier Character 5	Qualifier Character 6	Qualifier Character 7
0 Educational 1 Vocational 3 Other Counseling	Z None	Z None	Z None

G Mental Health
Z None
7 Family Psychotherapy Treatment that includes one or more family members of an individual with a mental health disorder by behavioral, cognitive, psychoanalytic, psychodynamic or psychophysiological means to improve functioning or well-being

Type Qualifier Character 4	Qualifier Character 5	Qualifier Character 6	Qualifier Character 7
2 Other Family Psychotherapy	Z None	Z None	Z None

G Mental Health
Z None
B Electroconvulsive Therapy The application of controlled electrical voltages to treat a mental health disorder

Type Qualifier Character 4	Qualifier Character 5	Qualifier Character 6	Qualifier Character 7
Ø Unilateral-Single Seizure **1** Unilateral-Multiple Seizure **2** Bilateral-Single Seizure **3** Bilateral-Multiple Seizure **4** Other Electroconvulsive Therapy	**Z** None	**Z** None	**Z** None

G Mental Health
Z None
C Biofeedback Provision of information from the monitoring and regulating of physiological processes in conjunction with cognitive-behavioral techniques to improve patient functioning or well-being

Type Qualifier Character 4	Qualifier Character 5	Qualifier Character 6	Qualifier Character 7
9 Other Biofeedback	**Z** None	**Z** None	**Z** None

G Mental Health
Z None
F Hypnosis Induction of a state of heightened suggestibility by auditory, visual and tactile techniques to elicit an emotional or behavioral response

Type Qualifier Character 4	Qualifier Character 5	Qualifier Character 6	Qualifier Character 7
Z None	**Z** None	**Z** None	**Z** None

G Mental Health
Z None
G Narcosynthesis Administration of intravenous barbiturates in order to release suppressed or repressed thoughts

Type Qualifier Character 4	Qualifier Character 5	Qualifier Character 6	Qualifier Character 7
Z None	**Z** None	**Z** None	**Z** None

G Mental Health
Z None
H Group Psychotherapy Treatment of two or more individuals with a mental health disorder by behavioral, cognitive, psychoanalytic, psychodynamic or psychophysiological means to improve functioning or well-being

Type Qualifier Character 4	Qualifier Character 5	Qualifier Character 6	Qualifier Character 7
Z None	**Z** None	**Z** None	**Z** None

G Mental Health
Z None
J Light Therapy Application of specialized light treatments to improve functioning or well-being

Type Qualifier Character 4	Qualifier Character 5	Qualifier Character 6	Qualifier Character 7
Z None	**Z** None	**Z** None	**Z** None

Substance Abuse HZ2–HZ9

H Substance Abuse Treatment
Z None
2 Detoxification Services Detoxification from alcohol and/or drugs

Type Qualifier Character 4	Qualifier Character 5	Qualifier Character 6	Qualifier Character 7
Z None	Z None	Z None	Z None

H Substance Abuse Treatment
Z None
3 Individual Counseling The application of psychological methods to treat an individual with addictive behavior

Type Qualifier Character 4	Qualifier Character 5	Qualifier Character 6	Qualifier Character 7
Ø Cognitive 1 Behavioral 2 Cognitive-Behavioral 3 12-Step 4 Interpersonal 5 Vocational 6 Psychoeducation 7 Motivational Enhancement 8 Confrontational 9 Continuing Care B Spiritual C Pre/Post-Test Infectious Disease	Z None	Z None	Z None

H Substance Abuse Treatment
Z None
4 Group Counseling The application of psychological methods to treat two or more individuals with addictive behavior

Type Qualifier Character 4	Qualifier Character 5	Qualifier Character 6	Qualifier Character 7
Ø Cognitive 1 Behavioral 2 Cognitive-Behavioral 3 12-Step 4 Interpersonal 5 Vocational 6 Psychoeducation 7 Motivational Enhancement 8 Confrontational 9 Continuing Care B Spiritual C Pre/Post-Test Infectious Disease	Z None	Z None	Z None

H Substance Abuse Treatment
Z None
5 Individual Psychotherapy Treatment of an individual with addictive behavior by behavioral, cognitive, psychoanalytic, psychodynamic or psychophysiological means

Type Qualifier Character 4	Qualifier Character 5	Qualifier Character 6	Qualifier Character 7
Ø Cognitive 1 Behavioral 2 Cognitive-Behavioral 3 12-Step 4 Interpersonal 5 Interactive 6 Psychoeducation 7 Motivational Enhancement 8 Confrontational 9 Supportive B Psychoanalysis C Psychodynamic D Psychophysiological	Z None	Z None	Z None

H Substance Abuse Treatment
Z None
6 Family Counseling The application of psychological methods that includes one or more family members to treat an individual with addictive behavior

Type Qualifier Character 4	Qualifier Character 5	Qualifier Character 6	Qualifier Character 7
3 Other Family Counseling	Z None	Z None	Z None

H Substance Abuse Treatment
Z None
8 Medication Management Monitoring or adjusting the use of replacment medications for the treatment of addiction

Type Qualifier Character 4	Qualifier Character 5	Qualifier Character 6	Qualifier Character 7
Ø Nicotine Replacement 1 Methadone Maintenance 2 Levo-alpha-acetyl-methadol (LAAM) 3 Antabuse 4 Naltrexone 5 Naloxone 6 Clonidine 7 Bupropion 8 Psychiatric Medication 9 Other Replacement Medication	Z None	Z None	Z None

H Substance Abuse Treatment
Z None
9 Pharmacotherapy The use of replacement medications for the treatment of addiction

Type Qualifier Character 4	Qualifier Character 5	Qualifier Character 6	Qualifier Character 7
Ø Nicotine Replacement 1 Methadone Maintenance 2 Levo-alpha-acetyl-methadol (LAAM) 3 Antabuse 4 Naltrexone 5 Naloxone 6 Clonidine 7 Bupropion 8 Psychiatric Medication 9 Other Replacement Medication	Z None	Z None	Z None

Appendix A: Root Operations Definitions

Ø	Medical and Surgical		
Ø	Alteration	Definition:	Modifying the natural anatomic structure of a body part without affecting the function of the body part
		Explanation:	Principal purpose is to improve appearance
		Examples:	Face lift, breast augmentation
1	Bypass	Definition:	Altering the route of passage of the contents of a tubular body part
		Explanation:	Rerouting contents of a body part to a downstream area of the normal route, to a similar route and body part, or to an abnormal route and dissimilar body part. Includes one or more anastomoses, with or without the use of a device
		Examples:	Coronary artery bypass, colostomy formation
2	Change	Definition:	Taking out or off a device from a body part and putting back an identical or similar device in or on the same body part without cutting or puncturing the skin or a mucous membrane
		Explanation:	All CHANGE procedures are coded using the approach EXTERNAL
		Example:	Urinary catheter change, gastrostomy tube change
3	Control	Definition:	Stopping, or attempting to stop, postprocedural bleeding
		Explanation:	The site of the bleeding is coded as an anatomical region and not to a specific body part.
		Examples:	Control of post-prostatectomy hemorrhage, control of post-tonsillectomy hemorrhage
4	Creation	Definition:	Making a new genital structure that does not take over the function of a body part
		Explanation:	Used only for sex change operations
		Examples:	Creation of vagina in a male, creation of penis in a female
5	Destruction	Definition:	Physical eradication of all or a portion of a body part by the direct use of energy, force, or a destructive agent
		Explanation:	None of the body part is physically taken out.
		Examples:	Fulguration of rectal polyp, cautery of skin lesion
6	Detachment	Definition:	Cutting off all or part of the upper or lower extremities
		Explanation:	The body part value is the site of the detachment, with a qualifier if applicable to further specify the level where the extremity was detached
		Examples:	Below knee amputation, disarticulation of shoulder
7	Dilation	Definition:	Expanding an orifice or the lumen of a tubular body part
		Explanation:	The orifice can be a natural orifice or an artificially created orifice. Accomplished by stretching a tubular body part using intraluminal pressure or by cutting part of the orifice or wall of the tubular body part.
		Examples:	Percutaneous transluminal angioplasty, pyloromyotomy
8	Division	Definition:	Cutting into a body part without draining fluids and/or gases from the body part in order to separate or transect a body part
		Explanation:	All or a portion of the body part is separated into two or more portions.
		Examples:	Spinal cordotomy, osteotomy
9	Drainage	Definition:	Taking or letting out fluids and/or gases from a body part
		Explanation:	The qualifier *diagnostic* is used to identify drainage procedures that are biopsies.
		Examples:	Thoracentesis, incision and drainage
B	Excision	Definition:	Cutting out or off, without replacement, a portion of a body part
		Explanation:	The qualifier *diagnostic* is used to identify excision procedures that are biopsies.
		Examples:	Partial nephrectomy, liver biopsy
C	Extirpation	Definition:	Taking or cutting out solid matter from a body part
		Explanation:	The solid matter may be an abnormal byproduct of a biological function or a foreign body; it may be imbedded in a body part or in the lumen of a tubular body part. The solid matter may or may not have been previously broken into pieces.
		Examples:	Thrombectomy, choledocholithotomy, endarterectomy

Continued on next page

Ø Medical and Surgical

Continued from previous page

D	Extraction	Definition:	Pulling or stripping out or off all or a portion of a body part by the use of force
		Explanation:	The qualifier DIAGNOSTIC is used to identify extractions that are biopsies.
		Examples:	Dilation and curettage, vein stripping
F	Fragmentation	Definition:	Breaking solid matter in a body part into pieces
		Explanation:	Physical force (e.g., manual, ultrasonic) applied directly or indirectly through intervening body parts are used to break the solid matter into pieces. The solid matter may be an abnormal byproduct of a biological function or a foreign body. The pieces of solid matter are not taken out, but are eliminated or absorbed through normal biological functions.
		Examples:	Extracorporeal shockwave lithotripsy, transurethral lithotripsy
G	Fusion	Definition:	Joining together portions of an articular body part, rendering the articular body part immobile
		Explanation:	The body part is joined together by fixation device, bone graft, or other means.
		Examples:	Spinal fusion, ankle arthrodesis
H	Insertion	Definition:	Putting in a nonbiological appliance that monitors, assists, performs, or prevents a physiological function but does not physically take the place of a body part
		Explanation:	None
		Examples:	Insertion of radioactive implant, insertion of central venous catheter
J	Inspection	Definition:	Visually and/or manually exploring a body part
		Explanation:	Visual exploration may be performed with or without optical instrumentation. Manual exploration may be performed directly or through intervening body layers.
		Examples:	Diagnostic arthroscopy, exploratory laparotomy
K	Map	Definition:	Locating the route of passage of electrical impulses and/or locating functional areas in a body part
		Explanation:	Applicable only to the cardiac conduction mechanism and the central nervous system
		Examples:	Cardiac mapping, cortical mapping
L	Occlusion	Definition:	Completely closing an orifice or lumen of a tubular body part
		Explanation:	The orifice can be a natural orifice or an artificially created orifice.
		Examples:	Fallopian tube ligation, ligation of inferior vena cava
M	Reattachment	Definition:	Putting back in or on all or a portion of a separated body part to its normal location or other suitable location
		Explanation:	Vascular circulation and nervous pathways may or may not be reestablished.
		Examples:	Reattachment of hand, reattachment of avulsed kidney
N	Release	Definition:	Freeing a body part from an abnormal physical constraint by cutting or by use of force
		Explanation:	Some of the restraining tissue may be taken out but none of the body part is taken out.
		Examples:	Adhesiolysis, carpal tunnel release
P	Removal	Definition:	Taking out or off a device from a body part
		Explanation:	If a device is taken out and a similar device put in without cutting or puncturing the skin or mucous membrane, the procedure is coded to the root operation CHANGE. Otherwise, the procedure for taking out the device is coded to the root operation REMOVAL, and the procedure for putting in the new device is coded to the root operation performed.
		Examples:	Drainage tube removal, cardiac pacemaker removal
Q	Repair	Definition:	Restoring, to the extent possible, a body part to its normal anatomic structure and function
		Explanation:	Used only when the method to accomplish the repair is not one of the other root operations
		Examples:	Colostomy takedown, herniorrhaphy, suture of laceration
R	Replacement	Definition:	Putting in or on a biological or synthetic material that physically takes the place and/or function of all or a portion of a body part
		Explanation:	The body part may have been taken out or replaced, or may be taken out, physically eradicated, or rendered nonfunctional during the REPLACEMENT procedure. A REMOVAL procedure is coded for taking out the device used in a previous replacement procedure
		Examples:	Total hip replacement, free skin graft
S	Reposition	Definition:	Moving to its normal location or other suitable location all or a portion of a body part
		Explanation:	The body part is moved to a new location from an abnormal location, or from a normal location where it is not functioning correctly. The body part may or may not be cut out or off to be moved to the new location.
		Examples:	Reposition of undescended testicle, fracture reduction

Continued on next page

Ø	Medical and Surgical		Continued from previous page
T	Resection	Definition:	Cutting out or off, without replacement, all of a body part
		Explanation:	None
		Examples:	Total nephrectomy, total lobectomy of lung
V	Restriction	Definition:	Partially closing an orifice or the lumen of a tubular body part
		Explanation:	The orifice can be a natural orifice or an artificially created orifice.
		Examples:	Esophagogastric fundoplication, cervical cerclage
W	Revision	Definition:	Correcting, to the extent possible, a portion of a malfunctioning device or the position of a displaced device
		Explanation:	Revision can include correcting a malfunctioning or displaced device by taking out or putting in components of the device such as a screw or pin.
		Examples:	Adjustment of position of pacemaker lead, recementing of hip prosthesis
U	Supplement	Definition:	Putting in or on biological or synthetic material that physically reinforces and/or augments the function of a portion of a body part
		Explanation:	The biological material is non-living, or is living and from the same individual. The body part may have been previously replaced, and the SUPPLEMENT procedure is performed to physically reinforce and/or augment the function of the replaced body part
		Examples:	Herniorrhaphy using mesh, free nerve graft, mitral valve ring annuloplasty, put a new acetabular liner in a previous hip replacement
X	Transfer	Definition:	Moving, without taking out, all or a portion of a body part to another location to take over the function of all or a portion of a body part
		Explanation:	The body part transferred remains connected to its vascular and nervous supply.
		Examples:	Tendon transfer, skin pedicle flap transfer
Y	Transplantation	Definition:	Putting in or on all or a portion of a living body part taken from another individual or animal to physically take the place and/or function of all or a portion of a similar body part
		Explanation:	The native body part may or may not be taken out, and the transplanted body part may take over all or a portion of its function.
		Examples:	Kidney transplant, heart transplant

Root Operation Definitions for Other Sections

1	Obstetrics		
A	Abortion	Definition:	Artificially terminating a pregnancy
		Explanation:	Subdivided according to whether an additional device such as a laminaria or abortifacient is used, or whether the abortion was performed by mechanical means
		Examples:	Transvaginal abortion using vacuum aspiration technique
E	Delivery	Definition:	Assisting the passage of the products of conception from the genital canal
		Explanation:	Applies only to manually-assisted, vaginal delivery
		Examples:	Manually-assisted delivery

2	Placement		
Ø	Change	Definition:	Taking out or off a device from a body region and putting back an identical or similar device in or on the same body region without cutting or puncturing the skin or a mucous membrane
		Explanation:	Procedures performed without making an incision or a puncture.
		Examples:	Change of vaginal packing
1	Compression	Definition:	Putting pressure on a body region
		Explanation:	Procedures performed without making an incision or a puncture
		Examples:	Placement of pressure dressing on abdominal wall
2	Dressing	Definition:	Putting material on a body region for protection
		Explanation:	Procedures performed without making an incision or a puncture
		Examples:	Application of sterile dressing to head wound

Continued on next page

Continued from previous page

2	Placement		
3	Immobilization	Definition:	Limiting or preventing motion of a body region
		Explanation:	Procedures to fit a device, such as splints and braces, as described in FØDZ6EZ and FØDZ7EZ, apply only to the rehabilitation setting.
		Examples:	Placement of splint on left finger
4	Packing	Definition:	Putting material in a body region or orifice
		Explanation:	Procedures performed without making an incision or a puncture
		Examples:	Placement of nasal packing
5	Removal	Definition:	Taking out or off a device from a body region
		Explanation:	Procedures performed without making an incision or a puncture
		Examples:	Removal of stereotactic head frame
6	Traction	Definition:	Exerting a pulling force on a body region in a distal direction
		Explanation:	Traction in this section includes only the task performed using a mechanical traction apparatus.
		Examples:	Lumbar traction using motorized split-traction table

3	Administration		
Ø	Introduction	Definition:	Putting in or on a therapeutic, diagnostic, nutritional, physiological, or prophylactic substance except blood or blood products
		Explanation:	All other substances administered, such as antineoplastic substance
		Examples:	Nerve block injection to median nerve
1	Irrigation	Definition:	Putting in or on a cleansing substance
		Explanation:	Substance given is a cleansing substance or dialysate
		Examples:	Flushing of eye
2	Transfusion	Definition:	Putting in blood or blood products
		Explanation:	Substance given is a blood product or a stem cell substance
		Examples:	Transfusion of cell saver red cells into central venous line

4	Measurement and Monitoring		
Ø	Measurement	Definition:	Determining the level of a physiological or physical function at a point in time
		Explanation:	A single temperature reading is considered measurement.
		Examples:	External electrocardiogram(EKG), single reading
1	Monitoring	Definition:	Determining the level of a physiological or physical function repetitively over a period of time
		Explanation:	Temperature taken every half hour for 8 hours is considered monitoring
		Examples:	Urinary pressure monitoring

5	Extracorporeal Assistance and Performance		
Ø	Assistance	Definition:	Taking over a portion of a physiological function by extracorporeal means
		Explanation:	Procedures that support a physiological function but do not take complete control of it, such as intra-aortic balloon pump to support cardiac output and hyperbaric oxygen treatment
		Examples:	Hyperbaric oxygenation of wound
1	Performance	Definition:	Completely taking over a physiological function by extracorporeal means
		Explanation:	Procedures in which complete control is exercised over a physiological function, such as total mechanical ventilation, cardiac pacing, and cardiopulmonary bypass
		Examples:	Cardiopulmonary bypass in conjunction with CABG
2	Restoration	Definition:	Returning, or attempting to return, a physiological function to its original state by extracorporeal means
		Explanation:	Only external cardioversion and defibrillation procedures. Failed cardioversion procedures are also included in the definition of restoration, and are coded the same as successful procedures
		Examples:	Attempted cardiac defibrillation, unsuccessful

6 Extracorporeal Therapies

Ø	Atmospheric Control	Definition:	Extracorporeal control of atmospheric pressure and composition
		Explanation:	None
		Examples:	Antigen-free air conditioning, series treatment
1	Decompression	Definition:	Extracorporeal elimination of undissolved gas from body fluids
		Explanation:	A single type of procedure—treatment for decompression sickness (the bends) in a hyperbaric chamber
		Examples:	Hyperbaric decompression treatment, single
2	Electromagnetic Therapy	Definition:	Extracorporeal treatment by electromagnetic rays
		Explanation:	None
		Examples:	TMS (transcranial magnetic stimulation), series treatment
3	Hyperthermia	Definition:	Extracorporeal raising of body temperature
		Explanation:	To treat temperature imbalance, and as an adjunct radiation treatment for cancer. When performed to treat temperature imbalance, the procedure is coded to this section. When performed for cancer treatment, whole-body hyperthermia is classified as a modality qualifier in section D, "Radiation Oncology."
		Examples:	None
4	Hypothermia	Definition:	Extracorporeal lowering of body temperature
		Explanation:	None
		Examples:	Whole body hypothermia treatment for temperature imbalances, series
5	Pheresis	Definition:	Extracorporeal separation of blood products
		Explanation:	Used in medical practice for two main purposes: to treat diseases where too much of a blood component is produced, such as leukemia, or to remove a blood product such as platelets from a donor, for transfusion into a patient who needs them
		Examples:	Therapeutic leukopheresis, single treatment
6	Phototherapy	Definition:	Extracorporeal treatment by light rays
		Explanation:	Phototherapy to the circulatory system means exposing the blood to light rays outside the body, using a machine that recirculates the blood and returns it to the body after phototherapy.
		Examples:	Phototherapy of circulatory system, series treatment
7	Ultrasound Therapy	Definition:	Extracorporeal treatment by ultrasound
		Explanation:	None
		Examples:	Therapeutic ultrasound of peripheral vessels, single treatment
8	Ultraviolet Light Therapy	Definition:	Extracorporeal treatment by ultraviolet light
		Explanation:	None
		Examples:	Ultraviolet light phototherapy, series treatment
9	Shock Wave Therapy	Definition:	Extracorporeal treatment by shockwaves
		Explanation:	None
		Examples:	Shockwave therapy of plantar fascia, single treatment

7 Osteopathic

Ø	Treatment	Definition:	Manual treatment to eliminate or alleviate somatic dysfunction and related disorders
		Explanation:	None
		Examples:	Fascial release of abdomen, osteopathic treatment

8 Other Procedures

Ø	Other Procedures	Definition:	Methodologies that attempt to remediate or cure a disorder or disease
		Explanation:	For nontraditional, whole-body therapies including acupuncture and meditation
		Examples:	Acupuncture

9	Chiropractic		
B	Manipulation	Definition:	Manual procedure that involves a directed thrust to move a joint past the physiological range of motion, without exceeding the anatomical limit
		Explanation:	None
		Examples:	Chiropractic treatment of cervical spine, short lever specific contact

Note: Sections B-H (Imaging through Substance Abuse Treatment) do not include root operations. Character 3 position represents type of procedure, therefore those definitions are not included in this appendix. See appendix D for definitions of the type (character 3) or type qualifiers (character 5) that provide details of the procedures performed.

Appendix B: Comparison of Medical and Surgical Root Operations

Note: the character associated with each operation appears in parentheses after its title.

Procedures That Take Out Some or All of a Body Part

Operation	Action	Target	Clarification	Example
Excision (B)	Cutting out or off	Some of a body part	Without replacing body part	Breast lumpectomy
Resection (T)	Cutting out or off	All of a body part	Without replacing body part	Total nephrectomy
Extraction (D)	Pulling out or off	All or a portion of a body part	Without replacing body part	Suction D&C
Destruction (5)	Eradicating	All or a portion of a body part	Without taking out or replacing body part	Rectal polyp fulguration
Detachment (6)	Cutting out/off	Extremity only, any level	Without replacing extremity	Below knee amputation

Procedures That Put in/Put Back or Move Some/All of a Body Part

Operation	Action	Target	Clarification	Example
Transplantation (Y)	Putting in	All or a portion of a living body part from other individual or animal	Physically takes the place and/or function of all or a portion of a body part	Heart transplant, kidney transplant
Reattachment (M)	Putting back in or on	All or a portion of a separated body part	Put in its normal or other suitable location. The vascular circulation and nervous pathways may or may not be reestablished.	Finger reattachment
Reposition (S)	Moving	All or a portion of a body part	Moving to its normal or other suitable location. Body part may or may not be cut out or off	Reposition undescended testicle
Transfer (X)	Moving to function for a similar body part	All or a portion of a body part	Without taking out body part; assumes function of similar body part and remains connected to its vascular and nervous supply	Tendon transfer, skin transfer flap

Procedures That Take Out or Eliminate Solid Matter, Fluids, or Gases From a Body Part

Operation	Action	Target	Clarification	Example
Drainage (9)	Taking or letting out	Fluids and/or gases from a body part	Without taking out any of the body part. The qualifier DIAGNOSTIC is used to identify drainage procedures that are biopsies.	Incision and drainage
Extirpation (C)	Taking or cutting out	Solid matter in a body part	Without taking out any of the body part. The solid matter may be an abnormal byproduct of a biological function or a foreign body; it may be imbedded in a body part or in the lumen of a tubular body part. The solid matter may or may not have been previously broken into pieces.	Thrombectomy
Fragmentation (F)	Breaking down	Solid matter into pieces within a body part	The physical force (e.g., manual, ultrasonic) is applied directly or indirectly, without taking out any of the body part or any solid matter. The solid matter may be an abnormal byproduct of a biological function or a foreign body. The pieces of solid matter are not taken out.	Lithotripsy

Procedures That Involve Only Examination of Body Parts and Regions

Operation	Action	Target	Clarification	Example
Inspection (J)	Visual and/or manual exploration	Some or all of a body part	Performed with or without optical instrumentation, directly or through body layers	Diagnostic arthroscopy, diagnostic cystoscopy
Map (K)	Locating	Route of passage of electrical impulses or functional areas in a body part	Applicable only to cardiac conduction mechanism and central nervous system	Cardiac mapping

Procedures That Alter the Diameter/Route of a Tubular Body Part

Operation	Action	Target	Clarification	Example
Bypass (1)	Altering the route of passage	Contents of tubular body part	May include use of living tissue, nonliving biological material or synthetic material which does not take the place of the body part. Includes one or more anastomoses, with or without the use of a device.	Gastrojejunal bypass, coronary artery bypass (CABG)
Dilation (7)	Expanding	Orifice or lumen of tubular body part	By application of intraluminal pressure or by cutting the wall of the orifice	Percutaneous transluminal angioplasty
Occlusion (L)	Completely closing	Orifice or lumen of tubular body part	Orifice may be natural or artificially created	Fallopian tube ligation
Restriction (V)	Partially closing	Orifice or lumen of tubular body part	Orifice may be natural or artificially created	Cervical cerclage, gastroesophageal fundoplication

Procedures That Always Involve Devices

Operation	Action	Target	Clarification	Example
Insertion (H) DVC	Putting in non-biological device	Device in or on a body part	Putting in a non-biological device that monitors, performs, assists, or prevents a physical function, does not physically take the place of a body part	Pacemaker insertion, central line insertion
Replacement (R) DVC	Putting in or on	Biological or synthetic material; living tissue taken from same individual	Physically takes the place of all or a portion of a body part. A REMOVAL procedure is assigned for taking out the device used in a previous replacement procedure.	Total hip replacement
Supplement (U) DVC	Putting in or on	Device that reinforces or augments a body part	Biological material is nonliving or living and from the same individual	Herniorrhaphy using mesh
Removal (P) DVC	Taking a device out or off	Device from a body part	If a new device is inserted via an incision or puncture, that procedure is coded separately	Cardiac pacemaker removal, central line removal
Change (2) DVC	Taking a device out or off and putting back an indentical or similar device	Identical or similar device in or on a body part	Without cutting or puncturing skin or mucous membrane; all *change* procedures are coded using the *External* approach	Drainage tube change
Revision (W) DVC	Correcting	Malfunctioning or displaced device in or on a body part	To the extent possible	Hip prosthesis adjustment, revision of pacemaker lead

Procedures Involving Cutting or Separation Only

Operation	Action	Target	Clarification	Example
Division (8)	Cutting into/Separating	A body part	Without taking out any of the body part or draining fluids and/or gases. All or a portion of the body part is separated into two or more portions.	Osteotomy, neurotomy
Release (N)	Freeing, by cutting or by the use of force	A body part	Eliminating abnormal constraint without taking out any of the body part. Some of the restraining tissue may be taken out, but none of the body part is taken out.	Peritoneal adhesiolysis

Procedures That Define Other Repairs

Operation	Action	Target	Clarification	Example
Control (3)	Stopping or attempting to stop	Postprocedural bleeding	Limited to anatomic regions not specific body parts	Control of postprostatectomy bleeding
Repair (Q)	Restoring	A body part to its natural anatomic structure and function	To the extent possible	Hernia repair, suture laceration

Procedures That Define Objectives

Operation	Action	Target	Clarification	Example
Alteration (Ø)	Modifying	Natural anatomical structure of a body part	Without affecting function of body part, performed for cosmetic purposes	Face lift
Creation (4)	Making	New genital structure	Does not physically take the place of a body part, used only for sex change operations	Artificial vagina creation
Fusion (G)	Unification and immobilization	Joint or articular body part	Stabilization of damaged joints by graft and/or fixation	Spinal fusion

Appendix C: Body Part Key

Anatomical Term	PCS Description
Abdominal aortic plexus	Abdominal Sympathetic Nerve
Abdominal esophagus	Esophagus, Lower
Abductor hallucis muscle	Foot Muscle, Right
	Foot Muscle, Left
Accessory cephalic vein	Cephalic Vein, Right
	Cephalic Vein, Left
Accessory obturator nerve	Lumbar Plexus
Accessory phrenic nerve	Phrenic nerve
Accessory spleen	Spleen
Acetabulofemoral joint	Hip Joint, Left
	Hip Joint, Right
Achilles tendon	Lower Leg Tendon, Right
	Lower Leg Tendon, Left
Acromioclavicular ligament	Shoulder Bursa and Ligament, Right
	Shoulder Bursa and Ligament, Left
Acromion (process)	Scapula, Left
	Scapula, Right
Adductor brevis muscle	Upper Leg Muscle, Right
	Upper Leg Muscle, Left
Adductor hallucis muscle	Foot Muscle, Right
	Foot Muscle, Left
Adductor longus muscle	Upper Leg Muscle, Right
	Upper Leg Muscle, Left
Adductor magnus muscle	Upper Leg Muscle, Right
	Upper Leg Muscle, Left
Adenohypophysis	Pituitary Gland
Alar ligament of axis	Head and Neck Bursa and Ligament
Alveolar process of mandible	Mandible, Left
	Mandible, Right
Alveolar process of maxilla	Maxilla, Left
	Maxilla, Right
Anal orifice	Anus
Anatomical snuffbox	Lower Arm and Wrist Tendon, Right
	Lower Arm and Wrist Tendon, Left
Angular artery	Face Artery
Angular vein	Face Vein, Left
	Face Vein, Right
Annular ligament	Elbow Bursa and Ligament, Right
	Elbow Bursa and Ligament, Left
Anorectal junction	Rectum
Ansa cervicalis	Cervical Plexus
Antebrachial fascia	Subcutaneous Tissue and Fascia, Right Lower Arm
	Subcutaneous Tissue and Fascia, Left Lower Arm
Anterior (pectoral) lymph node	Lymphatic, Left Axillary
	Lymphatic, Right Axillary

Anatomical Term	PCS Description
Anterior cerebral artery	Intracranial Artery
Anterior cerebral vein	Intracranial Vein
Anterior choroidal artery	Intracranial Artery
Anterior circumflex humeral artery	Axillary Artery, Right
	Axillary Artery, Left
Anterior communicating artery	Intracranial Artery
Anterior cruciate ligament (ACL)	Knee Bursa and Ligament, Right
	Knee Bursa and Ligament, Left
Anterior crural nerve	Femoral Nerve
Anterior facial vein	Face Vein, Left
	Face Vein, Right
Anterior intercostal artery	Internal Mammary Artery, Right
	Internal Mammary Artery, Left
Anterior interosseous nerve	Median Nerve
Anterior lateral malleolar artery	Anterior Tibial Artery, Right
	Anterior Tibial Artery, Left
Anterior lingual gland	Minor Salivary Gland
Anterior medial malleolar artery	Anterior Tibial Artery, Right
	Anterior Tibial Artery, Left
Anterior spinal artery	Vertebral Artery, Right
	Vertebral Artery, Left
Anterior tibial recurrent artery	Anterior Tibial Artery, Right
	Anterior Tibial Artery, Left
Anterior ulnar recurrent artery	Ulnar Artery, Right
	Ulnar Artery, Left
Anterior vagal trunk	Vagus Nerve
Anterior vertebral muscle	Neck Muscle, Right
	Neck Muscle, Left
Antihelix	External Ear, Right
	External Ear, Left
	External Ear, Bilateral
Antitragus	External Ear, Right
	External Ear, Left
	External Ear, Bilateral
Antrum of Highmore	Maxillary Sinus, Right
	Maxillary Sinus, Left
Aortic annulus	Aortic Valve
Aortic arch	Thoracic Aorta
Aortic intercostal artery	Thoracic Aorta
Apical (subclavicular) lymph node	Lymphatic, Left Axillary
	Lymphatic, Right Axillary
Apneustic center	Pons
Aqueduct of Sylvius	Cerebral Ventricle
Aqueous humour	Anterior Chamber, Right
	Anterior Chamber, Left

Anatomical Term	PCS Description
Arachnoid mater	Cerebral Meninges
	Spinal Meninges
Arcuate artery	Foot Artery, Right
	Foot Artery, Right
Areola	Nipple, Left
	Nipple, Right
Arterial canal (duct)	Pulmonary Artery, Left
Aryepiglottic fold	Larynx
Arytenoid cartilage	Larynx
Arytenoid muscle	Neck Muscle, Right
	Neck Muscle, Left
Ascending aorta	Thoracic Aorta
Ascending palatine artery	Face Artery
Ascending pharyngeal artery	External Carotid Artery, Right
	External Carotid Artery, Left
Atlantoaxial joint	Cervical Vertebral Joint
Atrioventricular node	Conduction Mechanism
Atrium dextrum cordis	Atrium, Right
Atrium pulmonale	Atrium, Left
Auditory tube	Eustachian Tube, Right
	Eustachian Tube, Left
Auerbach's (myenteric) plexus	Abdominal Sympathetic Nerve
Auricle	External Ear, Right
	External Ear, Left
	External Ear, Bilateral
Auricularis muscle	Head Muscle
Axillary fascia	Subcutaneous Tissue and Fascia, Right Upper Arm
	Subcutaneous Tissue and Fascia, Left Upper Arm
Axillary nerve	Brachial Plexus
Bartholin's (greater vestibular) gland	Vestibular Gland
Basal (internal) cerebral vein	Intracranial Vein
Basal nuclei	Basal Ganglia
Basilar artery	Intracranial Artery
Basis pontis	Pons
Biceps brachii muscle	Upper Arm Muscle, Right
	Upper Arm Muscle, Left
Biceps femoris muscle	Upper Leg Muscle, Right
	Upper Leg Muscle, Left
Bicipital aponeurosis	Subcutaneous Tissue and Fascia, Right Lower Arm
	Subcutaneous Tissue and Fascia, Left Lower Arm
Bicuspid valve	Mitral Valve
Body of femur	Femoral Shaft, Right
	Femoral Shaft, Left
Body of fibula	Fibula, Left
	Fibula, Right

Anatomical Term	PCS Description
Bony labyrinth	Inner Ear, Left
	Inner Ear, Right
Bony orbit	Orbit, Left
	Orbit, Right
Bony vestibule	Inner Ear, Left
	Inner Ear, Right
Botallo's duct	Pulmonary Artery, Left
Brachial (lateral) lymph node	Lymphatic, Left Axillary
	Lymphatic, Right Axillary
Brachialis muscle	Upper Arm Muscle, Right
	Upper Arm Muscle, Left
Brachiocephalic trunk or artery	Innominate Artery
	Innominate Artery
Brachiocephalic vein	Innominate Vein, Right
	Innominate Vein, Left
Brachioradialis muscle	Lower Arm and Wrist Muscle, Right
	Lower Arm and Wrist Muscle, Left
Broad ligament	Uterine Supporting Structure
Bronchial artery	Thoracic Aorta
Buccal gland	Buccal Mucosa
Buccinator lymph node	Lymphatic, Head
Buccinator muscle	Facial Muscle
Bulbospongiosus muscle	Perineum Muscle
Bulbourethral (Cowper's) gland	Urethra
Bundle of His	Conduction Mechanism
Bundle of Kent	Conduction Mechanism
Calcaneocuboid ligament	Foot Bursa and Ligament, Right
	Foot Bursa and Ligament, Left
Calcaneocuboid joint	Tarsal Joint, Right
	Tarsal Joint, Left
Calcaneofibular ligament	Ankle Bursa and Ligament, Right
	Ankle Bursa and Ligament, Left
Calcaneus	Tarsal, Left
	Tarsal, Right
Capitate bone	Carpal, Left
	Carpal, Right
Cardia	Esophagogastric Junction
Cardiac plexus	Thoracic Sympathetic Nerve
Cardioesophageal junction	Esophagogastric Junction
Caroticotympanic artery	Internal Carotid Artery, Right
	Internal Carotid Artery, Left
Carotid glomus	Carotid Bodies, Bilateral
	Carotid Body, Right
	Carotid Body, Left
Carotid sinus nerve	Glossopharyngeal Nerve
Carotid sinus	Internal Carotid Artery, Right
	Internal Carotid Artery, Left
Carpometacarpal (CMC) joint	Metacarpocarpal Joint, Right
	Metacarpocarpal Joint, Left

Anatomical Term	PCS Description
Carpometacarpal ligament	Hand Bursa and Ligament, Right
	Hand Bursa and Ligament, Left
Cauda equina	Lumbar Spinal Cord
Cavernous plexus	Head and Neck Sympathetic Nerve
Celiac ganglion	Abdominal Sympathetic Nerve
Celiac (solar) plexus	Abdominal Sympathetic Nerve
Celiac lymph node	Lymphatic, Aortic
Celiac trunk	Celiac Artery
Central axillary lymph node	Lymphatic, Left Axillary
	Lymphatic, Right Axillary
Cerebral aqueduct (Sylvius)	Cerebral Ventricle
Cerebrum	Brain
Cervical esophagus	Esophagus, Upper
Cervical facet joint	Cervical Vertebral Joints, 2 or more
	Cervical Vertebral Joint
Cervical ganglion	Head and Neck Sympathetic Nerve
Cervical intertransverse ligament	Head and Neck Bursa and Ligament
Cervical interspinous ligament	Head and Neck Bursa and Ligament
Cervical ligamentum flavum	Head and Neck Bursa and Ligament
Cervical lymph node	Lymphatic, Left Neck
	Lymphatic, Right Neck
Cervicothoracic facet joint	Cervicothoracic Vertebral Joint
Choana	Nasopharynx
Chondroglossus muscle	Tongue, Palate, Pharynx Muscle
Chorda tympani	Facial Nerve
Choroid plexus	Cerebral Ventricle
Ciliary body	Eye, Left
	Eye, Right
Ciliary ganglion	Head and Neck Sympathetic Nerve
Circle of Willis	Intracranial Artery
Circumflex iliac artery	Femoral Artery, Right
	Femoral Artery, Left
Claustrum	Basal Ganglia
Coccygeal body	Coccygeal Glomus
Coccygeus muscle	Trunk Muscle, Left
Cochlea	Inner Ear, Left
	Inner Ear, Right
Cochlear nerve	Acoustic Nerve
Columella	Nose
Common digital vein	Foot Vein, Left
	Foot Vein, Right
Common facial vein	Face Vein, Left
	Face Vein, Right
Common fibular nerve	Peroneal Nerve
Common hepatic artery	Hepatic Artery
Common iliac (subaortic) lymph node	Lymphatic, Pelvis

Anatomical Term	PCS Description
Common interosseous artery	Ulnar Artery, Right
	Ulnar Artery, Left
Common peroneal nerve	Peroneal Nerve
Condyloid process	Mandible, Left
	Mandible, Right
Conus arteriosus	Ventricle, Right
Conus medullaris	Lumbar Spinal Cord
Coracoacromial ligament	Shoulder Bursa and Ligament, Right
	Shoulder Bursa and Ligament, Left
Coracobrachialis muscle	Upper Arm Muscle, Right
	Upper Arm Muscle, Left
Coracoclavicular ligament	Shoulder Bursa and Ligament, Right
	Shoulder Bursa and Ligament, Left
Coracohumeral ligament	Shoulder Bursa and Ligament, Right
	Shoulder Bursa and Ligament, Left
Coracoid process	Scapula, Left
	Scapula, Right
Corniculate cartilage	Larynx
Corpus callosum	Brain
Corpus cavernosum	Penis
Corpus spongiosum	Penis
Corpus striatum	Basal Ganglia
Corrugator supercilii muscle	Facial Muscle
Costocervical trunk	Subclavian Artery, Right
	Subclavian Artery, Left
Costoclavicular ligament	Shoulder Bursa and Ligament, Right
	Shoulder Bursa and Ligament, Left
Costotransverse joint	Thoracic Vertebral Joints, 8 or more
	Thoracic Vertebral Joints, 2 to 7
	Thoracic Vertebral Joint
Costotransverse ligament	Thorax Bursa and Ligament, Right
	Thorax Bursa and Ligament, Left
Costovertebral joint	Thoracic Vertebral Joints, 8 or more
	Thoracic Vertebral Joints, 2 to 7
	Thoracic Vertebral Joint
Costoxiphoid ligament	Thorax Bursa and Ligament, Right
	Thorax Bursa and Ligament, Left
Cowper's (bulbourethral) gland	Urethra
Cranial dura mater	Dura Mater
Cranial epidural space	Epidural Space
Cranial subarachnoid space	Subarachnoid Space
Cranial subdural space	Subdural Space
Cremaster muscle	Perineum Muscle
Cribriform plate	Ethmoid Bone, Right
	Ethmoid Bone, Left
Cricoid cartilage	Larynx
Cricothyroid artery	Thyroid Artery, Right
	Thyroid Artery, Left

Anatomical Term	PCS Description
Cricothyroid muscle	Neck Muscle, Right
	Neck Muscle, Left
Crural fascia	Subcutaneous Tissue and Fascia, Right Upper Leg
	Subcutaneous Tissue and Fascia, Left Upper Leg
Cubital lymph node	Lymphatic, Left Upper Extremity
	Lymphatic, Right Upper Extremity
Cubital nerve	Ulnar Nerve
Cuboid bone	Tarsal, Left
	Tarsal, Right
Cuboideonavicular joint	Tarsal Joint, Right
	Tarsal Joint, Left
Culmen	Cerebellum
Cuneiform cartilage	Larynx
Cuneonavicular ligament	Foot Bursa and Ligament, Right
	Foot Bursa and Ligament, Left
Cuneonavicular joint	Tarsal Joint, Right
	Tarsal Joint, Left
Cutaneous (transverse) cervical nerve	Cervical Plexus
Deep cervical fascia	Subcutaneous Tissue and Fascia, Anterior Neck
Deep cervical vein	Vertebral Vein, Right
	Vertebral Vein, Left
Deep circumflex iliac artery	External Iliac Artery, Right
	External Iliac Artery, Left
Deep facial vein	Face Vein, Left
	Face Vein, Right
Deep femoral artery	Femoral Artery, Right
	Femoral Artery, Left
Deep femoral (profunda femoris) vein	Femoral Vein, Right
	Femoral Vein, Left
Deep palmar arch	Hand Artery, Right
	Hand Artery, Left
Deep transverse perineal muscle	Perineum Muscle
Deferential artery	Internal Iliac Artery, Right
	Internal Iliac Artery, Left
Deltoid fascia	Subcutaneous Tissue and Fascia, Right Upper Arm
	Subcutaneous Tissue and Fascia, Left Upper Arm
Deltoid ligament	Ankle Bursa and Ligament, Right
	Ankle Bursa and Ligament, Left
Deltoid muscle	Shoulder Muscle, Right
	Shoulder Muscle, Left
Deltopectoral (infraclavicular) lymph node	Lymphatic, Left Upper Extremity
	Lymphatic, Right Upper Extremity
Dentate ligament	Dura Mater
Denticulate ligament	Spinal Cord
Depressor anguli oris muscle	Facial Muscle

Anatomical Term	PCS Description
Depressor labii inferioris muscle	Facial Muscle
Depressor septi nasi muscle	Facial Muscle
Depressor supercilii muscle	Facial Muscle
Dermis	Skin
Descending genicular artery	Femoral Artery, Right
	Femoral Artery, Left
Diaphragma sellae	Dura Mater
Distal radioulnar joint	Wrist Joint, Right
	Wrist Joint, Left
Dorsal digital nerve	Radial Nerve
Dorsal metacarpal vein	Hand Vein, Left
	Hand Vein, Right
Dorsal metatarsal artery	Foot Artery, Right
	Foot Artery, Left
Dorsal metatarsal vein	Foot Vein, Left
	Foot Vein, Right
Dorsal scapular artery	Subclavian Artery, Right
	Subclavian Artery, Left
Dorsal scapular nerve	Brachial Plexus
Dorsal venous arch	Foot Vein, Left
	Foot Vein, Right
Dorsalis pedis artery	Anterior Tibial Artery, Right
	Anterior Tibial Artery, Left
Duct of Santorini	Pancreatic Duct, Accessory
Duct of Wirsung	Pancreatic Duct
Ductus deferens	Vas Deferens, Right
	Vas Deferens, Left
	Vas Deferens, Bilateral
	Vas Deferens
Duodenal ampulla	Ampulla of Vater
Duodenojejunal flexure	Jejunum
Dural venous sinus	Intracranial Vein
Earlobe	External Ear, Right
	External Ear, Left
	External Ear, Bilateral
Eighth cranial nerve	Acoustic Nerve
Ejaculatory duct	Vas Deferens, Right
	Vas Deferens, Left
	Vas Deferens, Bilateral
	Vas Deferens
Eleventh cranial nerve	Accessory Nerve
Encephalon	Brain
Ependyma	Cerebral Ventricle
Epidermis	Skin
Epiploic foramen	Peritoneum
Epithalamus	Thalamus
Epitroclear lymph node	Lymphatic, Left Upper Extremity
	Lymphatic, Right Upper Extremity

Anatomical Term	PCS Description
Erector spinae muscle	Trunk Muscle, Right
	Trunk Muscle, Left
Esophageal artery	Thoracic Aorta
Esophageal plexus	Thoracic Sympathetic Nerve
Ethmoidal air cell	Ethmoid Sinus, Right
	Ethmoid Sinus, Left
Extensor carpi radialis muscle	Lower Arm and Wrist Muscle, Right
Extensor carpi ulnaris muscle	Lower Arm and Wrist Muscle, Right
Extensor digitorum brevis muscle	Foot Muscle, Right
	Foot Muscle, Left
Extensor digitorum longus muscle	Lower Leg Muscle, Right
	Lower Leg Muscle, Left
Extensor hallucis brevis muscle	Foot Muscle, Right
	Foot Muscle, Left
Extensor hallucis longus muscle	Lower Leg Muscle, Right
	Lower Leg Muscle, Left
External anal sphincter	Anal Sphincter
External auditory meatus	External Auditory Canal, Right
	External Auditory Canal, Left
External maxillary artery	Face Artery
External naris	Nose
External oblique aponeurosis	Subcutaneous Tissue and Fascia, Trunk
External oblique muscle	Abdomen Muscle, Right
	Abdomen Muscle, Left
External popliteal nerve	Peroneal Nerve
External pudendal artery	Femoral Artery, Right
	Femoral Artery, Left
External pudendal vein	Greater Saphenous Vein, Right
	Greater Saphenous Vein, Left
External urethral sphincter	Urethra
Extradural space	Epidural Space
Facial artery	Face Artery
False vocal cord	Larynx
Falx cerebri	Dura Mater
Fascia lata	Subcutaneous Tissue and Fascia, Right Upper Leg
	Subcutaneous Tissue and Fascia, Left Upper Leg
Femoral head	Upper Femur, Right
	Upper Femur, Left
Femoral lymph node	Lymphatic, Left Lower Extremity
	Lymphatic, Right Lower Extremity
Femoropatellar joint	Knee Joint, Right
	Knee Joint, Left
Femorotibial joint	Knee Joint, Right
	Knee Joint, Left
Fibular artery	Peroneal Artery, Right
	Peroneal Artery, Left
Fibularis brevis muscle	Lower Leg Muscle, Right
	Lower Leg Muscle, Left
Fibularis longus muscle	Lower Leg Muscle, Right
	Lower Leg Muscle, Left
Fifth cranial nerve	Trigeminal Nerve
First cranial nerve	Olfactory Nerve
First intercostal nerve	Brachial Plexus
Flexor carpi ulnaris muscle	Lower Arm and Wrist Muscle, Left
	Lower Arm and Wrist Muscle, Right
Flexor digitorum brevis muscle	Foot Muscle, Right
	Foot Muscle, Left
Flexor digitorum longus muscle	Lower Leg Muscle, Right
	Lower Leg Muscle, Left
Flexor hallucis brevis muscle	Foot Muscle, Right
	Foot Muscle, Left
Flexor hallucis longus muscle	Lower Leg Muscle, Right
	Lower Leg Muscle, Left
Flexor pollicis longus muscle	Lower Arm and Wrist Muscle, Right
	Lower Arm and Wrist Muscle, Left
Foramen magnum	Occipital Bone, Right
	Occipital Bone, Left
Foramen of Monro (intraventricular)	Cerebral Ventricle
Foreskin	Prepuce
Fossa of Rosenmuller	Nasopharynx
Fourth cranial nerve	Trochlear Nerve
Fourth ventricle	Cerebral Ventricle
Fovea	Retina, Left
	Retina, Right
Frenulum labii inferioris	Lower Lip
Frenulum labii superioris	Upper Lip
Frenulum linguae	Tongue
Frontal lobe	Cerebral Hemisphere
Frontal vein	Face Vein, Left
	Face Vein, Right
Fundus uteri	Uterus
Galea aponeurotica	Subcutaneous Tissue and Fascia, Scalp
Ganglion impar (ganglion of Walther)	Sacral Sympathetic Nerve
Gasserian ganglion	Trigeminal Nerve
Gastric lymph node	Lymphatic, Aortic
Gastric plexus	Abdominal Sympathetic Nerve
Gastrocnemius muscle	Lower Leg Muscle, Right
	Lower Leg Muscle, Left
Gastrocolic ligament	Greater Omentum
Gastrocolic omentum	Greater Omentum
Gastroduodenal artery	Hepatic Artery
Gastroesophageal (GE) junction	Esophagogastric Junction
Gastrohepatic omentum	Lesser Omentum
Gastrophrenic ligament	Greater Omentum

Anatomical Term	PCS Description
Gastrosplenic ligament	Greater Omentum
Gemellus muscle	Hip Muscle, Right
	Hip Muscle, Left
Geniculate ganglion	Facial Nerve
Geniculate nucleus	Thalamus
Genioglossus muscle	Tongue, Palate, Pharynx Muscle
Genitofemoral nerve	Lumbar Plexus
Glans penis	Prepuce
Glenohumeral joint	Shoulder Joint, Right
	Shoulder Joint, Left
Glenohumeral ligament	Shoulder Bursa and Ligament, Right
	Shoulder Bursa and Ligament, Left
Glenoid fossa (of scapula)	Glenoid Cavity, Right
	Glenoid Cavity, Left
Glenoid ligament (labrum)	Shoulder Bursa and Ligament, Right
	Shoulder Bursa and Ligament, Left
Globus pallidus	Basal Ganglia
Glossoepiglottic fold	Epiglottis
Glottis	Larynx
Gluteal lymph node	Lymphatic, Pelvis
Gluteal vein	Hypogastric Vein, Right
	Hypogastric Vein, Left
Gluteus maximus muscle	Hip Muscle, Right
	Hip Muscle, Left
Gluteus medius muscle	Hip Muscle, Right
	Hip Muscle, Left
Gluteus minimus muscle	Hip Muscle, Right
	Hip Muscle, Left
Gracilis muscle	Upper Leg Muscle, Right
	Upper Leg Muscle, Left
Great auricular nerve	Cervical Plexus
Great cerebral vein	Intracranial Vein
Great saphenous vein	Greater Saphenous Vein, Right
	Greater Saphenous Vein, Left
Greater alar cartilage	Nose
Greater occipital nerve	Cervical Nerve
Greater splanchnic nerve	Thoracic Sympathetic Nerve
Greater superficial petrosal nerve	Facial Nerve
Greater trochanter	Upper Femur, Right
	Upper Femur, Left
Greater tuberosity	Humeral Head, Right
	Humeral Head, Left
Greater vestibular (Bartholin's) gland	Vestibular Gland
Greater wing	Sphenoid Bone, Right
	Sphenoid Bone, Left
Hallux	1st Toe, Left
	1st Toe, Right
Hamate bone	Carpal, Left
	Carpal, Right

Anatomical Term	PCS Description
Head of fibula	Fibula, Left
	Fibula, Right
Helix	External Ear, Right
	External Ear, Left
	External Ear, Bilateral
Hepatic artery proper	Hepatic Artery
Hepatic flexure	Ascending Colon
Hepatic lymph node	Lymphatic, Aortic
Hepatic plexus	Abdominal Sympathetic Nerve
Hepatic portal vein	Portal Vein
Hepatogastric ligament	Lesser Omentum
Hepatopancreatic ampulla	Ampulla of Vater
Humeroradial joint	Elbow Joint, Right
	Elbow Joint, Left
Humeroulnar joint	Elbow Joint, Right
	Elbow Joint, Left
Hyoglossus muscle	Tongue, Palate, Pharynx Muscle
Hyoid artery	Thyroid Artery, Right
	Thyroid Artery, Left
Hypogastric artery	Internal Iliac Artery, Right
	Internal Iliac Artery, Left
Hypopharynx	Pharynx
Hypophysis	Pituitary Gland
Hypothenar muscle	Hand Muscle, Right
	Hand Muscle, Left
Ileal artery	Superior Mesenteric Artery
Ileocolic artery	Superior Mesenteric Artery
Ileocolic vein	Colic Vein
Iliac crest	Pelvic Bone, Right
	Pelvic Bone, Left
Iliac fascia	Subcutaneous Tissue and Fascia, Right Upper Leg
	Subcutaneous Tissue and Fascia, Left Upper Leg
Iliac lymph node	Lymphatic, Pelvis
Iliacus muscle	Hip Muscle, Right
	Hip Muscle, Left
Iliofemoral ligament	Hip Bursa and Ligament, Right
	Hip Bursa and Ligament, Left
Iliohypogastric nerve	Lumbar Plexus
Ilioinguinal nerve	Lumbar Plexus
Iliolumbar artery	Internal Iliac Artery, Right
	Internal Iliac Artery, Left
Iliolumbar ligament	Trunk Bursa and Ligament, Right
	Trunk Bursa and Ligament, Left
Iliotibial tract (band)	Subcutaneous Tissue and Fascia, Right Upper Leg
	Subcutaneous Tissue and Fascia, Left Upper Leg
Ilium	Pelvic Bone, Right
	Pelvic Bone, Left

Anatomical Term	PCS Description
Incus	Auditory Ossicle, Right
	Auditory Ossicle, Left
Inferior cardiac nerve	Thoracic Sympathetic Nerve
Inferior cerebellar vein	Intracranial Vein
Inferior cerebral vein	Intracranial Vein
Inferior epigastric artery	External Iliac Artery, Right
	External Iliac Artery, Left
Inferior epigastric lymph node	Lymphatic, Pelvis
Inferior genicular artery	Popliteal Artery, Right
	Popliteal Artery, Left
Inferior gluteal artery	Internal Iliac Artery, Right
	Internal Iliac Artery, Left
Inferior gluteal nerve	Sacral Plexus
Inferior hypogastric plexus	Abdominal Sympathetic Nerve
Inferior labial artery	Face Artery
Inferior longitudinal muscle	Tongue, Palate, Pharynx Muscle
Inferior mesenteric ganglion	Abdominal Sympathetic Nerve
Inferior mesenteric lymph node	Lymphatic, Mesenteric
Inferior mesenteric plexus	Abdominal Sympathetic Nerve
Inferior oblique muscle	Extraocular Muscle, Right
	Extraocular Muscle, Left
Inferior pancreaticoduodenal artery	Superior Mesenteric Artery
Inferior phrenic artery	Abdominal Aorta
Inferior rectus muscle	Extraocular Muscle, Right
	Extraocular Muscle, Left
Inferior suprarenal artery	Renal Artery, Right
	Renal Artery, Left
Inferior tarsal plate	Lower Eyelid, Right
	Lower Eyelid, Left
Inferior thyroid vein	Innominate Vein, Right
	Innominate Vein, Left
Inferior tibiofibular joint	Ankle Joint, Right
	Ankle Joint, Left
Inferior turbinate	Nasal Turbinate
Inferior ulnar collateral artery	Brachial Artery, Right
	Brachial Artery, Left
Inferior vesical artery	Internal Iliac Artery, Right
	Internal Iliac Artery, Left
Infraauricular lymph node	Lymphatic, Head
Infraclavicular (deltopectoral) lymph node	Lymphatic, Left Upper Extremity
	Lymphatic, Right Upper Extremity
Infrahyoid muscle	Neck Muscle, Right
	Neck Muscle, Left
Infraparotid lymph node	Lymphatic, Head

Anatomical Term	PCS Description
Infraspinatus fascia	Subcutaneous Tissue and Fascia, Right Upper Arm
	Subcutaneous Tissue and Fascia, Left Upper Arm
Infraspinatus muscle	Shoulder Muscle, Right
	Shoulder Muscle, Left
Infundibulopelvic ligament	Uterine Supporting Structure
Inguinal canal	Inguinal Region, Right
	Inguinal Region, Left
	Inguinal Region, Bilateral
Inguinal triangle	Inguinal Region, Right
	Inguinal Region, Left
	Inguinal Region, Bilateral
Interatrial septum	Atrial Septum
Intercarpal joint	Carpal Joint, Right
	Carpal Joint, Left
Intercarpal ligament	Hand Bursa and Ligament, Right
	Hand Bursa and Ligament, Left
Interclavicular ligament	Shoulder Bursa and Ligament, Right
	Shoulder Bursa and Ligament, Left
Intercostal lymph node	Lymphatic, Thorax
Intercostal nerve	Thoracic Nerve
Intercostal muscle	Thorax Muscle, Right
	Thorax Muscle, Left
Intercostobrachial nerve	Thoracic Nerve
Intercuneiform ligament	Foot Bursa and Ligament, Right
	Foot Bursa and Ligament, Left
Intercuneiform joint	Tarsal Joint, Right
	Tarsal Joint, Left
Intermediate cuneiform bone	Tarsal, Left
	Tarsal, Right
Internal (basal) cerebral vein	Intracranial Vein
Internal anal sphincter	Anal Sphincter
Internal carotid plexus	Head and Neck Sympathetic Nerve
Internal iliac vein	Hypogastric Vein, Right
	Hypogastric Vein, Left
Internal maxillary artery	External Carotid Artery, Right
	External Carotid Artery, Left
Internal naris	Nose
Internal oblique muscle	Abdomen Muscle, Right
	Abdomen Muscle, Left
Internal pudendal artery	Internal Iliac Artery, Left
	Internal Iliac Artery, Right
Internal pudendal vein	Hypogastric Vein, Right
	Hypogastric Vein, Left
Internal thoracic artery	Internal Mammary Artery, Right
	Internal Mammary Artery, Left
	Subclavian Artery, Right
	Subclavian Artery, Left
Internal urethral sphincter	Urethra

Anatomical Term	PCS Description
Interphalangeal (IP) joint	Finger Phalangeal Joint, Right
	Finger Phalangeal Joint, Left
	Toe Phalangeal Joint, Right
	Toe Phalangeal Joint, Left
Interphalangeal ligament	Foot Bursa and Ligament, Right
	Foot Bursa and Ligament, Left
	Hand Bursa and Ligament, Right
	Hand Bursa and Ligament, Left
Interspinalis muscle	Trunk Muscle, Right
	Trunk Muscle, Left
Interspinous ligament	Trunk Bursa and Ligament, Right
	Trunk Bursa and Ligament, Left
Intertransverse ligament	Trunk Bursa and Ligament, Right
	Trunk Bursa and Ligament, Left
Intertransversarius muscle	Trunk Muscle, Right
	Trunk Muscle, Left
Interventricular foramen (Monro)	Cerebral Ventricle
Interventricular septum	Ventricular Septum
Intestinal lymphatic trunk	Cisterna Chyli
Ischiatic nerve	Sciatic Nerve
Ischiocavernosus muscle	Perineum Muscle
Ischiofemoral ligament	Hip Bursa and Ligament, Right
	Hip Bursa and Ligament, Left
Ischium	Pelvic Bone, Right
	Pelvic Bone, Left
Jejunal artery	Superior Mesenteric Artery
Jugular body	Glomus Jugulare
Jugular lymph node	Lymphatic, Left Neck
	Lymphatic, Right Neck
Labia majora	Vulva
Labia minora	Vulva
Labial gland	Buccal Mucosa
Lacrimal canaliculus	Lacrimal Duct, Right
	Lacrimal Duct, Left
Lacrimal punctum	Lacrimal Duct, Right
	Lacrimal Duct, Left
Lacrimal sac	Lacrimal Duct, Right
	Lacrimal Duct, Left
Laryngopharynx	Pharynx
Lateral (brachial) lymph node	Lymphatic, Left Axillary
	Lymphatic, Right Axillary
Lateral canthus	Upper Eyelid, Right
	Upper Eyelid, Left
Lateral collateral ligament (LCL)	Knee Bursa and Ligament, Right
	Knee Bursa and Ligament, Left
Lateral condyle of femur	Lower Femur, Right
	Lower Femur, Left
Lateral condyle of tibia	Tibia, Left
	Tibia, Right

Anatomical Term	PCS Description
Lateral cuneiform bone	Tarsal, Left
	Tarsal, Right
Lateral epicondyle of femur	Lower Femur, Right
	Lower Femur, Left
Lateral epicondyle of humerus	Humeral Shaft, Right
	Humeral Shaft, Left
Lateral femoral cutaneous nerve	Lumbar Plexus
Lateral malleolus	Fibula, Left
	Fibula, Right
Lateral meniscus	Knee Joint, Right
	Knee Joint, Left
Lateral nasal cartilage	Nose
Lateral plantar artery	Foot Artery, Right
	Foot Artery, Left
Lateral plantar nerve	Tibial Nerve
Lateral rectus muscle	Extraocular Muscle, Right
	Extraocular Muscle, Left
Lateral sacral artery	Internal Iliac Artery, Right
	Internal Iliac Artery, Left
Lateral sacral vein	Hypogastric Vein, Right
	Hypogastric Vein, Left
Lateral sural cutaneous nerve	Peroneal Nerve
Lateral tarsal artery	Foot Artery, Right
	Foot Artery, Left
Lateral temporomandibular ligament	Head and Neck Bursa and Ligament
Lateral thoracic artery	Axillary Artery, Right
	Axillary Artery, Left
Latissimus dorsi muscle	Trunk Muscle, Right
	Trunk Muscle, Left
Least splanchnic nerve	Thoracic Sympathetic Nerve
Left ascending lumbar vein	Hemiazygos Vein
Left atrioventricular valve	Mitral Valve
Left auricular appendix	Atrium, Left
Left colic vein	Colic Vein
Left coronary sulcus	Heart, Left
Left gastric artery	Gastric Artery
Left gastroepiploic artery	Splenic Artery
Left gastroepiploic vein	Splenic Vein
Left inferior phrenic vein	Renal Vein, Left
Left inferior pulmonary vein	Pulmonary Vein, Left
Left jugular trunk	Thoracic Duct
Left lateral ventricle	Cerebral Ventricle
Left ovarian vein	Renal Vein, Left
Left second lumbar vein	Renal Vein, Left
Left subclavian trunk	Thoracic Duct
Left subcostal vein	Hemiazygos Vein

Anatomical Term	PCS Description
Left superior pulmonary vein	Pulmonary Vein, Left
Left suprarenal vein	Renal Vein, Left
Left testicular vein	Renal Vein, Left
Leptomeninges	Cerebral Meninges
	Spinal Meninges
Lesser alar cartilage	Nose
Lesser occipital nerve	Cervical Plexus
Lesser splanchnic nerve	Thoracic Sympathetic Nerve
Lesser trochanter	Upper Femur, Right
	Upper Femur, Left
Lesser tuberosity	Humeral Head, Right
	Humeral Head, Left
Lesser wing	Sphenoid Bone, Right
	Sphenoid Bone, Left
Levator anguli oris muscle	Facial Muscle
Levator ani muscle	Trunk Muscle, Left
Levator labii superioris alaeque nasi muscle	Facial Muscle
Levator labii superioris muscle	Facial Muscle
Levator palpebrae superioris muscle	Upper Eyelid, Right
	Upper Eyelid, Left
Levator scapulae muscle	Neck Muscle, Right
	Neck Muscle, Left
Levator veli palatini muscle	Tongue, Palate, Pharynx Muscle
Levatores costarum muscle	Thorax Muscle, Right
	Thorax Muscle, Left
Ligament of head of fibula	Knee Bursa and Ligament, Right
	Knee Bursa and Ligament, Left
Ligament of the lateral malleolus	Ankle Bursa and Ligament, Right
	Ankle Bursa and Ligament, Left
Ligamentum flavum	Trunk Bursa and Ligament, Right
	Trunk Bursa and Ligament, Left
Lingual artery	External Carotid Artery, Right
	External Carotid Artery, Left
Lingual tonsil	Tongue
Locus ceruleus	Pons
Long thoracic nerve	Brachial Plexus
Lumbar artery	Abdominal Aorta
Lumbar facet joint	Lumbar Vertebral Joints, 2 or more
	Lumbar Vertebral Joint
Lumbar ganglion	Lumbar Sympathetic Nerve
Lumbar lymph node	Lymphatic, Aortic
Lumbar lymphatic trunk	Cisterna Chyli
Lumbar splanchnic nerve	Lumbar Sympathetic Nerve
Lumbosacral facet joint	Lumbosacral Joint
Lumbosacral trunk	Lumbar Nerve
Lunate bone	Carpal, Left
	Carpal, Right

Anatomical Term	PCS Description
Lunotriquetral ligament	Hand Bursa and Ligament, Right
	Hand Bursa and Ligament, Left
Macula	Retina, Left
	Retina, Right
Malleus	Auditory Ossicle, Right
	Auditory Ossicle, Left
Mammary duct	Breast, Bilateral
	Breast, Left
	Breast, Right
Mammary gland	Breast, Bilateral
	Breast, Left
	Breast, Right
Mammillary body	Hypothalamus
Mandibular nerve	Trigeminal Nerve
Mandibular notch	Mandible, Left
	Mandible, Right
Manubrium	Sternum
Masseter muscle	Head Muscle
Masseteric fascia	Subcutaneous Tissue and Fascia, Face
Mastoid (postauricular) lymph node	Lymphatic, Left Neck
	Lymphatic, Right Neck
Mastoid air cells	Mastoid Sinus, Right
	Mastoid Sinus, Left
Mastoid process	Temporal Bone, Right
	Temporal Bone, Left
Maxillary artery	External Carotid Artery, Right
	External Carotid Artery, Left
Maxillary nerve	Trigeminal Nerve
Medial canthus	Lower Eyelid, Right
	Lower Eyelid, Left
Medial collateral ligament (MCL)	Knee Bursa and Ligament, Right
	Knee Bursa and Ligament, Left
Medial condyle of femur	Lower Femur, Right
	Lower Femur, Left
Medial condyle of tibia	Tibia, Left
	Tibia, Right
Medial cuneiform bone	Tarsal, Left
	Tarsal, Right
Medial epicondyle of femur	Lower Femur, Right
	Lower Femur, Left
Medial epicondyle of humerus	Humeral Shaft, Right
	Humeral Shaft, Left
Medial malleolus	Tibia, Left
	Tibia, Right
Medial meniscus	Knee Joint, Right
	Knee Joint, Left
Medial plantar artery	Foot Artery, Right
	Foot Artery, Left
Medial plantar nerve	Tibial Nerve
Medial popliteal nerve	Tibial Nerve

Anatomical Term	PCS Description
Medial rectus muscle	Extraocular Muscle, Right
	Extraocular Muscle, Left
Medial sural cutaneous nerve	Tibial Nerve
Median antebrachial vein	Basilic Vein, Right
	Basilic Vein, Left
Median cubital vein	Basilic Vein, Right
	Basilic Vein, Left
Median sacral artery	Abdominal Aorta
Mediastinal lymph node	Lymphatic, Thorax
Meissner's (submucous) plexus	Abdominal Sympathetic Nerve
Membranous urethra	Urethra
Mental foramen	Mandible, Left
	Mandible, Right
Mentalis muscle	Facial Muscle
Mesoappendix	Mesentery
Mesocolon	Mesentery
Metacarpal ligament	Hand Bursa and Ligament, Right
	Hand Bursa and Ligament, Left
Metacarpophalangeal ligament	Hand Bursa and Ligament, Right
	Hand Bursa and Ligament, Left
Metatarsal ligament	Foot Bursa and Ligament, Right
	Foot Bursa and Ligament, Left
Metatarsophalangeal ligament	Foot Bursa and Ligament, Right
	Foot Bursa and Ligament, Left
Metatarsophalangeal (MTP) joint	Metatarsal-Phalangeal Joint, Right
	Metatarsal-Phalangeal Joint, Left
Metathalamus	Thalamus
Midcarpal joint	Carpal Joint, Right
	Carpal Joint, Left
Middle cardiac nerve	Thoracic Sympathetic Nerve
Middle cerebral artery	Intracranial Artery
Middle cerebral vein	Intracranial Vein
Middle colic vein	Colic Vein
Middle genicular artery	Popliteal Artery, Right
	Popliteal Artery, Left
Middle hemorrhoidal vein	Hypogastric Vein, Right
	Hypogastric Vein, Left
Middle rectal artery	Internal Iliac Artery, Right
	Internal Iliac Artery, Left
Middle suprarenal artery	Abdominal Aorta
Middle temporal artery	Temporal Artery, Right
	Temporal Artery, Left
Middle turbinate	Nasal Turbinate
Mitral annulus	Mitral Valve
Molar gland	Buccal Mucosa
Musculocutaneous nerve	Brachial Plexus
Musculophrenic artery	Internal Mammary Artery, Right
	Internal Mammary Artery, Left
Musculospiral nerve	Radial Nerve
Myelencephalon	Medulla Oblongata

Anatomical Term	PCS Description
Myenteric (Auerbach's) plexus	Abdominal Sympathetic Nerve
Myometrium	Uterus
Nail bed	Finger Nail
	Toe Nail
Nail plate	Finger Nail
	Toe Nail
Nasal cavity	Nose
Nasal concha	Nasal Turbinate
Nasalis muscle	Facial Muscle
Nasolacrimal duct	Lacrimal Duct, Right
	Lacrimal Duct, Left
Navicular bone	Tarsal, Left
	Tarsal, Right
Neck of femur	Upper Femur, Right
	Upper Femur, Left
Neck of humerus (anatomical) (surgical)	Humeral Head, Right
	Humeral Head, Left
Nerve to the stapedius	Facial Nerve
Neurohypophysis	Pituitary Gland
Ninth cranial nerve	Glossopharyngeal Nerve
Nostril	Nose
Obturator artery	Internal Iliac Artery, Right
	Internal Iliac Artery, Left
Obturator lymph node	Lymphatic, Pelvis
Obturator muscle	Hip Muscle, Right
	Hip Muscle, Left
Obturator nerve	Lumbar Plexus
Obturator vein	Hypogastric Vein, Right
	Hypogastric Vein, Left
Obtuse margin	Heart, Left
Occipital artery	External Carotid Artery, Right
	External Carotid Artery, Left
Occipital lobe	Cerebral Hemisphere
Occipital lymph node	Lymphatic, Left Neck
	Lymphatic, Right Neck
Occipitofrontalis muscle	Facial Muscle
Olecranon bursa	Elbow Bursa and Ligament, Right
	Elbow Bursa and Ligament, Left
Olecranon process	Ulna, Left
	Ulna, Right
Olfactory bulb	Olfactory Nerve
Ophthalmic artery	Internal Carotid Artery, Right
	Internal Carotid Artery, Left
Ophthalmic nerve	Trigeminal Nerve
Ophthalmic vein	Intracranial Vein
Optic chiasma	Optic Nerve
Optic disc	Retina, Left
	Retina, Right
Optic foramen	Sphenoid Bone, Right
	Sphenoid Bone, Left

Anatomical Term	PCS Description
Orbicularis oculi muscle	Upper Eyelid, Right
	Upper Eyelid, Left
Orbicularis oris muscle	Facial Muscle
Orbital fascia	Subcutaneous Tissue and Fascia, Face
Orbital portion of ethmoid bone	Orbit, Left
	Orbit, Right
Orbital portion of frontal bone	Orbit, Left
	Orbit, Right
Orbital portion of lacrimal bone	Orbit, Left
	Orbit, Right
Orbital portion of maxilla	Orbit, Left
	Orbit, Right
Orbital portion of palatine bone	Orbit, Left
	Orbit, Right
Orbital portion of sphenoid bone	Orbit, Left
	Orbit, Right
Orbital portion of zygomatic bone	Orbit, Left
	Orbit, Right
Oropharynx	Pharynx
Ossicular chain	Auditory Ossicle, Right
	Auditory Ossicle, Left
Otic ganglion	Head and Neck Sympathetic Nerve
Oval window	Inner Ear, Left
	Inner Ear, Right
Ovarian artery	Abdominal Aorta
Ovarian ligament	Uterine Supporting Structure
Oviduct	Fallopian Tube, Right
	Fallopian Tube, Left
Palatine gland	Buccal Mucosa
Palatine tonsil	Tonsils
Palatine uvula	Uvula
Palatoglossal muscle	Tongue, Palate, Pharynx Muscle
Palatopharyngeal muscle	Tongue, Palate, Pharynx Muscle
Palmar (volar) metacarpal vein	Hand Vein, Right
	Hand Vein, Left
Palmar (volar) digital vein	Hand Vein, Left
	Hand Vein, Right
Palmar cutaneous nerve	Median Nerve
	Radial Nerve
Palmar fascia (aponeurosis)	Subcutaneous Tissue and Fascia, Right Hand
	Subcutaneous Tissue and Fascia, Left Hand
Palmar interosseous muscle	Hand Muscle, Right
	Hand Muscle, Left
Palmar ulnocarpal ligament	Wrist Bursa and Ligament, Right
	Wrist Bursa and Ligament, Left
Palmaris longus muscle	Lower Arm and Wrist Muscle, Right
	Lower Arm and Wrist Muscle, Left
Pancreatic artery	Splenic Artery
Pancreatic plexus	Abdominal Sympathetic Nerve
Pancreatic vein	Splenic Vein

Anatomical Term	PCS Description
Pancreaticosplenic lymph node	Lymphatic, Aortic
Paraaortic lymph node	Lymphatic, Aortic
Pararectal lymph node	Lymphatic, Mesenteric
Parasternal lymph node	Lymphatic, Thorax
Paratracheal lymph node	Lymphatic, Thorax
Paraurethral (Skene's) gland	Vestibular Gland
Parietal lobe	Cerebral Hemisphere
Parotid lymph node	Lymphatic, Head
Parotid plexus	Facial Nerve
Pars flaccida	Tympanic Membrane, Right
	Tympanic Membrane, Left
Patellar ligament	Knee Bursa and Ligament, Right
	Knee Bursa and Ligament, Left
Patellar tendon	Knee Tendon, Right
	Knee Tendon, Left
Pectineus muscle	Upper Leg Muscle, Right
	Upper Leg Muscle, Left
Pectoral (anterior) lymph node	Lymphatic, Left Axillary
	Lymphatic, Right Axillary
Pectoral fascia	Subcutaneous Tissue and Fascia, Chest
Pectoralis major muscle	Thorax Muscle, Left
	Thorax Muscle, Right
Pectoralis minor muscle	Thorax Muscle, Left
	Thorax Muscle, Right
Pelvic fascia	Subcutaneous Tissue and Fascia, Trunk
Pelvic splanchnic nerve	Abdominal Sympathetic Nerve
	Sacral Sympathetic Nerve
Penile urethra	Urethra
Pericardiophrenic artery	Internal Mammary Artery, Right
	Internal Mammary Artery, Left
Perimetrium	Uterus
Peroneus brevis muscle	Lower Leg Muscle, Right
	Lower Leg Muscle, Left
Peroneus longus muscle	Lower Leg Muscle, Right
	Lower Leg Muscle, Left
Petrous part of temporal bone	Temporal Bone, Right
	Temporal Bone, Left
Pharyngeal constrictor muscle	Tongue, Palate, Pharynx Muscle
Pharyngeal plexus	Vagus Nerve
Pharyngeal recess	Nasopharynx
Pharyngeal tonsil	Adenoids
Pharyngotympanic tube	Eustachian Tube, Right
	Eustachian Tube, Left
Pia mater	Cerebral Meninges
	Spinal Meninges
Pinna	External Ear, Right
	External Ear, Left
	External Ear, Bilateral
Piriform recess (sinus)	Pharynx

Anatomical Term	PCS Description
Piriformis muscle	Hip Muscle, Right
	Hip Muscle, Left
Pisiform bone	Carpal, Left
	Carpal, Right
Pisohamate ligament	Hand Bursa and Ligament, Right
	Hand Bursa and Ligament, Left
Pisometacarpal ligament	Hand Bursa and Ligament, Right
	Hand Bursa and Ligament, Left
Plantar digital vein	Foot Vein, Left
	Foot Vein, Right
Plantar fascia (aponeurosis)	Subcutaneous Tissue and Fascia, Right Foot
	Subcutaneous Tissue and Fascia, Left Foot
Plantar metatarsal vein	Foot Vein, Left
	Foot Vein, Right
Plantar venous arch	Foot Vein, Left
	Foot Vein, Right
Platysma muscle	Neck Muscle, Right
	Neck Muscle, Left
Plica semilunaris	Conjunctiva, Right
	Conjunctiva, Left
Pneumogastric nerve	Vagus Nerve
Pneumotaxic center	Pons
Pontine tegmentum	Pons
Popliteal lymph node	Lymphatic, Left Lower Extremity
	Lymphatic, Right Lower Extremity
Popliteal ligament	Knee Bursa and Ligament, Right
	Knee Bursa and Ligament, Left
Popliteal vein	Femoral Vein, Right
	Femoral Vein, Left
Popliteus muscle	Lower Leg Muscle, Right
	Lower Leg Muscle, Left
Postauricular (mastoid) lymph node	Lymphatic, Left Neck
	Lymphatic, Right Neck
Postcava	Inferior Vena Cava
Posterior (subscapular) lymph node	Lymphatic, Left Axillary
	Lymphatic, Right Axillary
Posterior auricular artery	External Carotid Artery, Right
	External Carotid Artery, Left
Posterior auricular nerve	Facial Nerve
Posterior auricular vein	External Jugular Vein, Right
	External Jugular Vein, Left
Posterior cerebral artery	Intracranial Artery
Posterior chamber	Eye, Left
	Eye, Right
Posterior circumflex humeral artery	Axillary Artery, Right
	Axillary Artery, Left
Posterior communicating artery	Intracranial Artery
Posterior cruciate ligament (PCL)	Knee Bursa and Ligament, Right
	Knee Bursa and Ligament, Left

Anatomical Term	PCS Description
Posterior facial (retromandibular) vein	Face Vein, Left
	Face Vein, Right
Posterior femoral cutaneous nerve	Sacral Plexus
Posterior inferior cerebellar artery (PICA)	Intracranial Artery
Posterior interosseous nerve	Radial Nerve
Posterior labial nerve	Pudendal Nerve
Posterior scrotal nerve	Pudendal Nerve
Posterior spinal artery	Vertebral Artery, Right
	Vertebral Artery, Left
Posterior tibial recurrent artery	Anterior Tibial Artery, Right
	Anterior Tibial Artery, Left
Posterior ulnar recurrent artery	Ulnar Artery, Right
	Ulnar Artery, Left
Posterior vagal trunk	Vagus Nerve
Preauricular lymph node	Lymphatic, Head
Precava	Superior Vena Cava
Prepatellar bursa	Knee Bursa and Ligament, Right
	Knee Bursa and Ligament, Left
Pretracheal fascia	Subcutaneous Tissue and Fascia, Anterior Neck
Prevertebral fascia	Subcutaneous Tissue and Fascia, Posterior Neck
Princeps pollicis artery	Hand Artery, Right
	Hand Artery, Left
Procerus muscle	Facial Muscle
Profunda brachii	Brachial Artery, Right
	Brachial Artery, Left
Profunda femoris (deep femoral) vein	Femoral Vein, Right
	Femoral Vein, Left
Pronator quadratus muscle	Lower Arm and Wrist Muscle, Right
	Lower Arm and Wrist Muscle, Left
Pronator teres muscle	Lower Arm and Wrist Muscle, Right
	Lower Arm and Wrist Muscle, Left
Prostatic urethra	Urethra
Proximal radioulnar joint	Elbow Joint, Right
	Elbow Joint, Left
Psoas muscle	Hip Muscle, Right
	Hip Muscle, Left
Pterygoid muscle	Head Muscle
Pterygoid process	Sphenoid Bone, Right
	Sphenoid Bone, Left
Pterygopalatine (sphenopalatine) ganglion	Head and Neck Sympathetic Nerve
Pubic ligament	Trunk Bursa and Ligament, Right
	Trunk Bursa and Ligament, Left
Pubis	Pelvic Bone, Right
	Pelvic Bone, Left

Anatomical Term	PCS Description
Pubofemoral ligament	Hip Bursa and Ligament, Right
	Hip Bursa and Ligament, Left
Pudendal nerve	Sacral Plexus
Pulmoaortic canal	Pulmonary Artery, Left
Pulmonary annulus	Pulmonary Valve
Pulmonary plexus	Thoracic Sympathetic Nerve
	Vagus Nerve
Pulmonic valve	Pulmonary Valve
Pulvinar	Thalamus
Pyloric antrum	Stomach, Pylorus
Pyloric canal	Stomach, Pylorus
Pyloric sphincter	Stomach, Pylorus
Pyramidalis muscle	Abdomen Muscle, Right
	Abdomen Muscle, Left
Quadrangular cartilage	Nasal Septum
Quadrate lobe	Liver
Quadratus femoris muscle	Hip Muscle, Right
	Hip Muscle, Left
Quadratus lumborum muscle	Trunk Muscle, Right
	Trunk Muscle, Left
Quadratus plantae muscle	Foot Muscle, Right
	Foot Muscle, Left
Quadriceps (femoris)	Upper Leg Muscle, Right
	Upper Leg Muscle, Left
	Upper Leg Tendon, Right
	Upper Leg Tendon, Left
Radial collateral ligament	Elbow Bursa and Ligament, Right
	Elbow Bursa and Ligament, Left
Radial collateral carpal ligament	Wrist Bursa and Ligament, Right
	Wrist Bursa and Ligament, Left
Radial notch	Ulna, Left
	Ulna, Right
Radial recurrent artery	Radial Artery, Right
	Radial Artery, Left
Radial vein	Brachial Vein, Right
	Brachial Vein, Left
Radialis indicis	Hand Artery, Right
	Hand Artery, Left
Radiocarpal joint	Wrist Joint, Right
	Wrist Joint, Left
Radiocarpal ligament	Wrist Bursa and Ligament, Right
	Wrist Bursa and Ligament, Left
Rectosigmoid junction	Sigmoid Colon
Radioulnar ligament	Wrist Bursa and Ligament, Right
	Wrist Bursa and Ligament, Left
Rectus abdominis muscle	Abdomen Muscle, Right
	Abdomen Muscle, Left
Rectus femoris muscle	Upper Leg Muscle, Right
	Upper Leg Muscle, Left
Recurrent laryngeal nerve	Vagus Nerve
Renal calyx	Kidney
	Kidney, Left
	Kidney, Right
	Kidneys, Bilateral
Renal capsule	Kidney
	Kidney, Left
	Kidney, Right
	Kidneys, Bilateral
Renal cortex	Kidney
	Kidney, Left
	Kidney, Right
	Kidneys, Bilateral
Renal plexus	Abdominal Sympathetic Nerve
Renal segment	Kidney
	Kidney, Left
	Kidney, Right
	Kidneys, Bilateral
Renal segmental artery	Renal Artery, Right
	Renal Artery, Left
Retroperitoneal lymph node	Lymphatic, Aortic
Retroperitoneal space	Retroperitoneum
Retropharyngeal lymph node	Lymphatic, Left Neck
	Lymphatic, Right Neck
Retropubic space	Pelvic Cavity
Rhinopharynx	Nasopharynx
Rhomboid major muscle	Trunk Muscle, Right
	Trunk Muscle, Left
Rhomboid minor muscle	Trunk Muscle, Right
	Trunk Muscle, Left
Right ascending lumbar vein	Azygos Vein
Right atrioventricular valve	Tricuspid Valve
Right auricular appendix	Atrium, Right
Right colic vein	Colic Vein
Right coronary sulcus	Heart, Right
Right gastric artery	Gastric Artery
Right gastroepiploic vein	Superior Mesenteric Vein
Right inferior phrenic vein	Inferior Vena Cava
Right inferior pulmonary vein	Pulmonary Vein, Right
Right jugular trunk	Lymphatic, Right Neck
Right lateral ventricle	Cerebral Ventricle
Right lymphatic duct	Lymphatic, Right Neck
Right ovarian vein	Inferior Vena Cava
Right second lumbar vein	Inferior Vena Cava
Right subclavian trunk	Lymphatic, Right Neck
Right subcostal vein	Azygos Vein
Right superior pulmonary vein	Pulmonary Vein, Right
Right suprarenal vein	Inferior Vena Cava

Anatomical Term	PCS Description
Right testicular vein	Inferior Vena Cava
Rima glottidis	Larynx
Risorius muscle	Facial Muscle
Round ligament of uterus	Uterine Supporting Structure
Round window	Inner Ear, Left
	Inner Ear, Right
Sacral ganglion	Sacral Sympathetic Nerve
Sacral lymph node	Lymphatic, Pelvis
Sacral splanchnic nerve	Sacral Sympathetic Nerve
Sacrococcygeal ligament	Trunk Bursa and Ligament, Right
	Trunk Bursa and Ligament, Left
Sacrococcygeal symphysis	Sacrococcygeal Joint
Sacroiliac ligament	Trunk Bursa and Ligament, Right
	Trunk Bursa and Ligament, Left
Sacrospinous ligament	Trunk Bursa and Ligament, Right
	Trunk Bursa and Ligament, Left
Sacrotuberous ligament	Trunk Bursa and Ligament, Right
	Trunk Bursa and Ligament, Left
Salpingopharyngeus muscle	Tongue, Palate, Pharynx Muscle
Salpinx	Fallopian Tube, Left
	Fallopian Tube, Right
Saphenous nerve	Femoral Nerve
Sartorius muscle	Upper Leg Muscle, Right
	Upper Leg Muscle, Left
Scalene muscle	Neck Muscle, Right
	Neck Muscle, Left
Scaphoid bone	Carpal, Left
	Carpal, Right
Scapholunate ligament	Hand Bursa and Ligament, Right
	Hand Bursa and Ligament, Left
Scaphotrapezium ligament	Hand Bursa and Ligament, Right
	Hand Bursa and Ligament, Left
Scarpa's (vestibular) ganglion	Acoustic Nerve
Sebaceous gland	Skin
Second cranial nerve	Optic Nerve
Sella turcica	Sphenoid Bone, Right
	Sphenoid Bone, Left
Semicircular canal	Inner Ear, Left
	Inner Ear, Right
Semimembranosus muscle	Upper Leg Muscle, Right
	Upper Leg Muscle, Left
Semitendinosus muscle	Upper Leg Muscle, Right
	Upper Leg Muscle, Left
Septal cartilage	Nasal Septum
Serratus anterior muscle	Thorax Muscle, Right
	Thorax Muscle, Left
Serratus posterior muscle	Trunk Muscle, Right
	Trunk Muscle, Left
Seventh cranial nerve	Facial Nerve
Short gastric artery	Splenic Artery
Sigmoid artery	Inferior Mesenteric Artery
Sigmoid flexure	Sigmoid Colon
Sigmoid vein	Inferior Mesenteric Vein
Sinoatrial node	Conduction Mechanism
Sinus venosus	Atrium, Right
Sixth cranial nerve	Abducens Nerve
Skene's (paraurethral) gland	Vestibular Gland
Small saphenous vein	Lesser Saphenous Vein, Right
	Lesser Saphenous Vein, Left
Solar (celiac) plexus	Abdominal Sympathetic Nerve
Soleus muscle	Lower Leg Muscle, Right
	Lower Leg Muscle, Left
Sphenomandibular ligament	Head and Neck Bursa and Ligament
Sphenopalatine (pterygopalatine) ganglion	Head and Neck Sympathetic Nerve
Spinal dura mater	Dura Mater
Spinal epidural space	Epidural Space
Spinal subarachnoid space	Subarachnoid Space
Spinal subdural space	Subdural Space
Spinous process	Cervical Vertebra
	Lumbar Vertebra
	Thoracic Vertebra
Spiral ganglion	Acoustic Nerve
Splenic flexure	Transverse Colon
Splenic plexus	Abdominal Sympathetic Nerve
Splenius capitis muscle	Head Muscle
Splenius cervicis muscle	Neck Muscle, Right
	Neck Muscle, Left
Stapes	Auditory Ossicle, Right
	Auditory Ossicle, Left
Stellate ganglion	Head and Neck Sympathetic Nerve
Stensen's duct	Parotid Duct, Right
	Parotid Duct, Left
Sternoclavicular ligament	Shoulder Bursa and Ligament, Right
	Shoulder Bursa and Ligament, Left
Sternocleidomastoid artery	Thyroid Artery, Right
	Thyroid Artery, Left
Sternocleidomastoid muscle	Neck Muscle, Right
	Neck Muscle, Left
Sternocostal ligament	Thorax Bursa and Ligament, Right
	Thorax Bursa and Ligament, Left
Styloglossus muscle	Tongue, Palate, Pharynx Muscle
Stylomandibular ligament	Head and Neck Bursa and Ligament
Stylopharyngeus muscle	Tongue, Palate, Pharynx Muscle
Subacromial bursa	Shoulder Bursa and Ligament, Right
	Shoulder Bursa and Ligament, Left

Anatomical Term	PCS Description
Subaortic (common iliac) lymph node	Lymphatic, Pelvis
Subclavicular (apical) lymph node	Lymphatic, Left Axillary
	Lymphatic, Right Axillary
Subclavius muscle	Thorax Muscle, Right
	Thorax Muscle, Left
Subclavius nerve	Brachial Plexus
Subcostal artery	Thoracic Aorta
Subcostal muscle	Thorax Muscle, Right
	Thorax Muscle, Left
Subcostal nerve	Thoracic Nerve
Submandibular ganglion	Facial Nerve
	Head and Neck Sympathetic Nerve
Submandibular gland	Submaxillary Gland, Right
	Submaxillary Gland, Left
Submandibular lymph node	Lymphatic, Head
Submaxillary ganglion	Head and Neck Sympathetic Nerve
Submaxillary lymph node	Lymphatic, Head
Submental artery	Face Artery
Submental lymph node	Lymphatic, Head
Submucous (Meissner's) plexus	Abdominal Sympathetic Nerve
Suboccipital nerve	Cervical Nerve
Suboccipital venous plexus	Vertebral Vein, Right
	Vertebral Vein, Left
Subparotid lymph node	Lymphatic, Head
Subscapular aponeurosis	Subcutaneous Tissue and Fascia, Right Upper Arm
	Subcutaneous Tissue and Fascia, Left Upper Arm
Subscapular artery	Axillary Artery, Right
	Axillary Artery, Left
Subscapular (posterior) lymph node	Lymphatic, Left Axillary
	Lymphatic, Right Axillary
Subscapularis muscle	Shoulder Muscle, Right
	Shoulder Muscle, Left
Substantia nigra	Basal Ganglia
Subtalar (talocalcaneal) joint	Tarsal Joint, Right
	Tarsal Joint, Left
Subtalar ligament	Foot Bursa and Ligament, Right
	Foot Bursa and Ligament, Left
Subthalamic nucleus	Basal Ganglia
Superficial epigastric artery	Femoral Artery, Left
	Femoral Artery, Right
Superficial epigastric vein	Greater Saphenous Vein, Left
	Greater Saphenous Vein, Right
Superficial circumflex iliac vein	Greater Saphenous Vein, Left
	Greater Saphenous Vein, Right
Superficial palmar arch	Hand Artery, Right
	Hand Artery, Left
Superficial palmar venous arch	Hand Vein, Left
	Hand Vein, Right

Anatomical Term	PCS Description
Superficial transverse perineal muscle	Perineum Muscle
Superficial temporal artery	Temporal Artery, Right
	Temporal Artery, Left
Superior cardiac nerve	Thoracic Sympathetic Nerve
Superior cerebellar vein	Intracranial Vein
Superior cerebral vein	Intracranial Vein
Superior clunic (cluneal) nerve	Lumbar Nerve
Superior epigastric artery	Internal Mammary Artery, Right
	Internal Mammary Artery, Left
Superior genicular artery	Popliteal Artery, Right
	Popliteal Artery, Left
Superior gluteal artery	Internal Iliac Artery, Right
	Internal Iliac Artery, Left
Superior gluteal nerve	Lumbar Plexus
Superior hypogastric plexus	Abdominal Sympathetic Nerve
Superior labial artery	Face Artery
Superior laryngeal artery	Thyroid Artery, Right
	Thyroid Artery, Left
Superior laryngeal nerve	Vagus Nerve
Superior longitudinal muscle	Tongue, Palate, Pharynx Muscle
Superior mesenteric ganglion	Abdominal Sympathetic Nerve
Superior mesenteric lymph node	Lymphatic, Mesenteric
Superior mesenteric plexus	Abdominal Sympathetic Nerve
Superior oblique muscle	Extraocular Muscle, Right
	Extraocular Muscle, Left
Superior olivary nucleus	Pons
Superior rectal artery	Inferior Mesenteric Artery
Superior rectal muscle	Extraocular Muscle, Right
	Extraocular Muscle, Left
Superior rectal vein	Inferior Mesenteric Vein
Superior tarsal plate	Upper Eyelid, Right
	Upper Eyelid, Left
Superior thoracic artery	Axillary Artery, Right
	Axillary Artery, Left
Superior thyroid artery	External Carotid Artery, Right
	External Carotid Artery, Left
	Thyroid Artery, Right
	Thyroid Artery, Left
Superior turbinate	Nasal Turbinate
Superior ulnar collateral artery	Brachial Artery, Right
	Brachial Artery, Left
Supraclavicular nerve	Cervical Plexus
Supraclavicular (Virchow's) lymph node	Lymphatic, Left Neck
	Lymphatic, Right Neck
Suprahyoid lymph node	Lymphatic, Head

Anatomical Term	PCS Description
Suprahyoid muscle	Neck Muscle, Right
	Neck Muscle, Left
Suprainguinal lymph node	Lymphatic, Pelvis
Supraorbital vein	Face Vein, Left
	Face Vein, Right
Suprarenal gland	Adrenal Glands, Bilateral
	Adrenal Gland, Right
	Adrenal Gland, Left
	Adrenal Gland
Suprarenal plexus	Abdominal Sympathetic Nerve
Suprascapular nerve	Brachial Plexus
Supraspinatus fascia	Subcutaneous Tissue and Fascia, Right Upper Arm
	Subcutaneous Tissue and Fascia, Left Upper Arm
Supraspinatus muscle	Shoulder Muscle, Right
	Shoulder Muscle, Left
Supraspinous ligament	Trunk Bursa and Ligament, Right
	Trunk Bursa and Ligament, Left
Suprasternal notch	Sternum
Supratrochlear lymph node	Lymphatic, Left Upper Extremity
	Lymphatic, Right Upper Extremity
Sural artery	Popliteal Artery, Right
	Popliteal Artery, Left
Sweat gland	Skin
Talocalcaneal ligament	Foot Bursa and Ligament, Right
	Foot Bursa and Ligament, Left
Talocalcaneal (subtalar) joint	Tarsal Joint, Right
	Tarsal Joint, Left
Talocalcaneonavicular joint	Tarsal Joint, Right
	Tarsal Joint, Left
Talocalcaneonavicular ligament	Foot Bursa and Ligament, Right
	Foot Bursa and Ligament, Left
Talocrural joint	Ankle Joint, Right
	Ankle Joint, Left
Talofibular ligament	Ankle Bursa and Ligament, Right
	Ankle Bursa and Ligament, Left
Talus bone	Tarsal, Left
	Tarsal, Right
Tarsometatarsal joint	Metatarsal-Tarsal Joint, Right
	Metatarsal-Tarsal Joint, Left
Tarsometatarsal ligament	Foot Bursa and Ligament, Right
	Foot Bursa and Ligament, Left
Temporal lobe	Cerebral Hemisphere
Temporalis muscle	Head Muscle
Temporoparietalis muscle	Head Muscle
Tensor fasciae latae muscle	Hip Muscle, Right
	Hip Muscle, Left
Tensor veli palatini muscle	Tongue, Palate, Pharynx Muscle
Tenth cranial nerve	Vagus Nerve

Anatomical Term	PCS Description
Tentorium cerebelli	Dura Mater
Teres major muscle	Shoulder Muscle, Right
	Shoulder Muscle, Left
Teres minor muscle	Shoulder Muscle, Right
	Shoulder Muscle, Left
Testicular artery	Abdominal Aorta
Thenar muscle	Hand Muscle, Right
	Hand Muscle, Left
Third cranial nerve	Oculomotor Nerve
Third occipital nerve	Cervical Nerve
Third ventricle	Cerebral Ventricle
Thoracic aortic plexus	Thoracic Sympathetic Nerve
Thoracic esophagus	Esophagus, Middle
Thoracic facet joint	Thoracic Vertebral Joints, 8 or more
	Thoracic Vertebral Joints, 2 to 7
	Thoracic Vertebral Joint
Thoracic ganglion	Thoracic Sympathetic Nerve
Thoracoacromial artery	Axillary Artery, Right
	Axillary Artery, Left
Thoracolumbar facet joint	Thoracolumbar Vertebral Joint
Thymus gland	Thymus
Thyroarytenoid muscle	Neck Muscle, Right
	Neck Muscle, Left
Thyrocervical trunk	Thyroid Artery, Right
	Thyroid Artery, Left
Thyroid cartilage	Larynx
Tibialis anterior muscle	Lower Leg Muscle, Right
	Lower Leg Muscle, Left
Tibialis posterior muscle	Lower Leg Muscle, Right
	Lower Leg Muscle, Left
Tracheobronchial lymph node	Lymphatic, Thorax
Tragus	External Ear, Right
	External Ear, Left
	External Ear, Bilateral
Transversalis fascia	Subcutaneous Tissue and Fascia, Trunk
Transverse acetabular ligament	Hip Bursa and Ligament, Left
	Hip Bursa and Ligament, Right
Transverse (cutaneous) cervical nerve	Cervical Plexus
Transverse facial artery	Temporal Artery, Right
	Temporal Artery, Left
Transverse humeral ligament	Shoulder Bursa and Ligament, Right
	Shoulder Bursa and Ligament, Left
Transverse ligament of atlas	Head and Neck Bursa and Ligament
Transverse scapular ligament	Shoulder Bursa and Ligament, Right
	Shoulder Bursa and Ligament, Left
Transverse thoracis muscle	Thorax Muscle, Right
	Thorax Muscle, Left

Anatomical Term	PCS Description
Transversospinalis muscle	Trunk Muscle, Right
	Trunk Muscle, Left
Transversus abdominis muscle	Abdomen Muscle, Right
	Abdomen Muscle, Left
Trapezium bone	Carpal, Left
	Carpal, Right
Trapezius muscle	Trunk Muscle, Right
	Trunk Muscle, Left
Trapezoid bone	Carpal, Left
	Carpal, Right
Triceps brachii muscle	Upper Arm Muscle, Right
	Upper Arm Muscle, Left
Tricuspid annulus	Tricuspid Valve
Trifacial nerve	Trigeminal Nerve
Trigone of bladder	Bladder
Triquetral bone	Carpal, Left
	Carpal, Right
Trochanteric bursa	Hip Bursa and Ligament, Right
	Hip Bursa and Ligament, Left
Twelfth cranial nerve	Hypoglossal Nerve
Tympanic cavity	Middle Ear, Right
	Middle Ear, Left
Tympanic nerve	Glossopharyngeal Nerve
Tympanic part of temoporal bone	Temporal Bone, Right
	Temporal Bone, Left
Ulnar collateral ligament	Elbow Bursa and Ligament, Right
	Elbow Bursa and Ligament, Left
Ulnar collateral carpal ligament	Wrist Bursa and Ligament, Right
	Wrist Bursa and Ligament, Left
Ulnar notch	Radius, Left
	Radius, Right
Ulnar vein	Brachial Vein, Right
	Brachial Vein, Left
Umbilical artery	Internal Iliac Artery, Right
	Internal Iliac Artery, Left
Ureteral orifice	Ureter
	Ureter, Left
	Ureter, Right
	Ureters, Bilateral
Ureteropelvic junction (UPJ)	Kidney Pelvis, Right
	Kidney Pelvis, Left
Ureterovesical orifice	Ureter, Left
	Ureter, Right
Uterine artery	Internal Iliac Artery, Right
	Internal Iliac Artery, Left
Uterine cornu	Uterus
Uterine tube	Fallopian Tube, Right
	Fallopian Tube, Left
Uterine vein	Hypogastric Vein, Right
	Hypogastric Vein, Left
Vaginal artery	Internal Iliac Artery, Right
	Internal Iliac Artery, Left
Vaginal vein	Hypogastric Vein, Right
	Hypogastric Vein, Left
Vastus intermedius muscle	Upper Leg Muscle, Right
	Upper Leg Muscle, Left
Vastus lateralis muscle	Upper Leg Muscle, Right
	Upper Leg Muscle, Left
Vastus medialis muscle	Upper Leg Muscle, Right
	Upper Leg Muscle, Left
Ventricular fold	Larynx
Vermiform appendix	Appendix
Vermilion border	Lower Lip
	Upper Lip
Vertebral arch	Cervical Vertebra
	Lumbar Vertebra
	Thoracic Vertebra
Vertebral canal	Spinal Canal
Vertebral foramen	Cervical Vertebra
	Lumbar Vertebra
	Thoracic Vertebra
Vertebral lamina	Cervical Vertebra
	Lumbar Vertebra
	Thoracic Vertebra
Vertebral pedicle	Cervical Vertebra
	Lumbar Vertebra
	Thoracic Vertebra
Vesical vein	Hypogastric Vein, Right
	Hypogastric Vein, Left
Vestibular (Scarpa's) ganglion	Acoustic Nerve
Vestibular nerve	Acoustic Nerve
Vestibulocochlear nerve	Acoustic Nerve
Virchow's (supraclavicular) lymph node	Lymphatic, Left Neck
	Lymphatic, Right Neck
Vitreous body	Vitreous, Left
	Vitreous, Right
Vocal fold	Vocal Cord, Right
	Vocal Cord, Left
Volar (palmar) digital vein	Hand Vein, Left
	Hand Vein, Right
Volar (palmar) metacarpal vein	Hand Vein, Left
	Hand Vein, Right
Vomer bone	Nasal Septum (bone
Xiphoid process	Sternum
Zonule of Zinn	Lens, Left
	Lens, Right
Zygomatic process of frontal bone	Frontal Bone, Right
	Frontal Bone, Left

Anatomical Term	PCS Description
Zygomatic process of temporal bone	Temporal Bone, Right
	Temporal Bone, Left
Zygomaticus muscle	Facial Muscle

Appendix D: Device Key and Aggregation Table

Device Key

Device Term	PCS Description
AbioCor® Total Replacement Heart	Synthetic Substitute
Acellular Hydrated Dermis	Nonautologous Tissue Substitute
ACUITY™ Steerable Lead	Cardiac Lead in Heart and Great Vessels
AMPLATZER® Muscular VSD Occluder	Synthetic Substitute
AMS 800® Urinary Control System	Artificial Sphincter in Urinary System
AneuRx® AAA Advantage®	Intraluminal Device
Annuloplasty ring	Synthetic Substitute
Artificial anal sphincter (AAS)	Artificial Sphincter in Gastrointestinal System
Artificial bowel sphincter (neosphincter)	Artificial Sphincter in Gastrointestinal System
Artificial urinary sphincter (AUS)	Artificial Sphincter in Urinary System
Attain Ability® Lead	Cardiac Lead, Pacemaker for Insertion in Heart and Great Vessels
Attain StarFix® (OTW) Lead	Cardiac Lead in Heart and Great Vessels
Autograft	Autologous Tissue Substitute
Autologous artery graft	Autologous Arterial Tissue in Heart and Great Vessels Autologous Arterial Tissue in Upper Arteries Autologous Arterial Tissue in Lower Arteries Autologous Arterial Tissue in Upper Veins Autologous Arterial Tissue in Lower Veins
Autologous vein graft	Autologous Venous Tissue in Heart and Great Vessels Autologous Venous Tissue in Upper Arteries Autologous Venous Tissue in Lower Arteries Autologous Venous Tissue in Upper Veins Autologous Venous Tissue in Lower Veins
Axial Lumbar Interbody Fusion System	Interbody Fusion Device in Lower Joints
AxiaLIF® System	Interbody Fusion Device in Lower Joints
BAK/C® Interbody Cervical Fusion System	Interbody Fusion Device in Upper Joints
Bard® Composix® (E/X)(LP) mesh	Synthetic Substitute
Bard® Composix® Kugel® patch	Synthetic Substitute
Bard® Dulex™ mesh	Synthetic Substitute
Bard® Ventralex™ Hernia Patch	Synthetic Substitute
Baroreflex Activation Therapy® (BAT®)	Stimulator Lead in Upper Arteries Cardiac Rhythm Related Device in Subcutaneous Tissue and Fascia
Berlin Heart Ventricular Assist Device	Implantable Heart Assist System in Heart and Great Vessels
Bioactive embolization coil(s)	Intraluminal Device, Bioactive in Upper Arteries
Biventricular external heart assist system	External Heart Assist System in Heart and Great Vessels
Blood glucose monitoring system	Monitoring Device
Bone anchored hearing device	Hearing Device, Bone Conduction for Insertion in Ear, Nose, Sinus Hearing Device, Bone Conduction in Head and Facial Bones
Bone bank bone graft	Nonautologous Tissue Substitute
Bone screw (interlocking)(lag)(pedicle)(recessed)	Internal Fixation Device in Head and Facial Bones Internal Fixation Device in Upper Bones Internal Fixation Device in Lower Bones
Bovine pericardial valve	Zooplastic Tissue in Heart and Great Vessels
Bovine pericardium graft	Zooplastic Tissue in Heart and Great Vessels
Brachytherapy seeds	Radioactive Element
BRYAN® Cervical Disc System	Synthetic Substitute
BVS 5000 Ventricular Assist Device	External Heart Assist System in Heart and Great Vessels
Cardiac contractility modulation lead	Cardiac Lead in Heart and Great Vessels
Cardiac resynchronization therapy (CRT) lead	Cardiac Lead in Heart and Great Vessels
CardioMEMS® pressure sensor	Monitoring Device, Pressure Sensor for Insertion in Heart and Great Vessels
Carotid (artery) sinus (baroreceptor) lead	Stimulator Lead in Upper Arteries
Carotid WALLSTENT® Monorail® Endoprosthesis	Intraluminal Device
Centrimag® Blood Pump	Intraluminal Device
Clamp and rod internal fixation system (CRIF)	Internal Fixation Device in Upper Bones Internal Fixation Device in Lower Bones
CoAxia NeuroFlo catheter	Intraluminal Device
Cobalt/chromium head and polyethylene socket	Synthetic Substitute, Metal on Polyethylene for Replacement in Lower Joints

Device Term	PCS Description
Cobalt/chromium head and socket	Synthetic Substitute, Metal for Replacement in Lower Joints
Cochlear implant (CI), multiple channel (electrode)	Hearing Device, Multiple Channel Cochlear Prosthesis for Insertion in Ear, Nose, Sinus
Cochlear implant (CI), single channel (electrode)	Hearing Device, Single Channel Cochlear Prosthesis for Insertion in Ear, Nose, Sinus
COGNIS® CRT-D	Cardiac Resynchronization Defibrillator Pulse Generator for Insertion in Subcutaneous Tissue and Fascia
Colonic Z-Stent®	Intraluminal Device
CONSERVE® PLUS Total Resurfacing Hip System	Resurfacing Device in Lower Joints
CONTAK RENEWAL® 3 RF (HE) CRT-D	Cardiac Resynchronization Defibrillator Pulse Generator for Insertion in Subcutaneous Tissue and Fascia
Continuous Glucose Monitoring (CGM) device	Monitoring Device
Cormet Hip Resurfacing System	Resurfacing Device in Lower Joints
CoRoent® XL	Interbody Fusion Device in Lower Joints
Corox OTW (Bipolar) Lead	Cardiac Lead, Pacemaker for Insertion in Heart and Great Vessels
Cortical strip neurostimulator lead	Neurostimulator Lead in Central Nervous System
Cultured epidermal cell autograft	Autologous Tissue Substitute
CYPHER® Stent	Intraluminal Device, Drug-eluting in Heart and Great Vessels
Cystostomy tube	Drainage Device
DBS lead	Neurostimulator Lead in Central Nervous System
DeBakey Left Ventricular Assist Device	Implantable Heart Assist System in Heart and Great Vessels
Deep brain neurostimulator lead	Neurostimulator Lead in Central Nervous System
Delta frame external fixator	External Fixation Device, Hybrid for Insertion in Upper Bones External Fixation Device, Hybrid for Reposition in Upper Bones External Fixation Device, Hybrid for Insertion in Lower Bones External Fixation Device, Hybrid for Reposition in Lower Bones
Delta III Reverse shoulder prosthesis	Synthetic Substitute, Reverse Ball and Socket for Replacement in Upper Joints
Diaphragmatic pacemaker generator	Stimulator Generator in Subcutaneous Tissue and Fascia
Direct Lateral Interbody Fusion (DLIF) device	Interbody Fusion Device in Lower Joints
DuraHeart Left Ventricular Assist System	Implantable Heart Assist System in Heart and Great Vessels

Device Term	PCS Description
Durata® Defibrillation Lead	Cardiac Lead, Defibrillator for Insertion in Heart and Great Vessels
Dynesys® Dynamic Stabilization System	Spinal Stabilization Device, Pedicle-Based for Insertion in Upper Joints Spinal Stabilization Device, Pedicle-Based for Insertion in Lower Joints
E-Luminexx™ (Biliary)(Vascular) Stent	Intraluminal Device
Electrical bone growth stimulator (EBGS)	Bone Growth Stimulator in Head and Facial Bones Bone Growth Stimulator in Upper Bones Bone Growth Stimulator in Lower Bones
Electrical muscle stimulation (EMS) lead	Stimulator Lead in Muscles
Electronic muscle stimulator lead	Stimulator Lead in Muscles
Embolization coil(s)	Intraluminal Device
Endeavor® (III)(IV) (Sprint) Zotarolimus-eluting Coronary Stent System	Intraluminal Device, Drug-eluting in Heart and Great Vessels
EndoSure® sensor	Monitoring Device, Pressure Sensor for Insertion in Heart and Great Vessels
ENDOTAK RELIANCE® (G) Defibrillation Lead	Cardiac Lead, Defibrillator for Insertion in Heart and Great Vessels
Endotracheal tube (cuffed)(double-lumen)	Intraluminal Device, Endotracheal Airway in Respiratory System
Endurant® Endovascular Stent Graft	Intraluminal Device
Epicel® cultured epidermal autograft	Autologous Tissue Substitute
Epic™ Stented Tissue Valve (aortic)	Zooplastic Tissue in Heart and Great Vessels
Esophageal obturator airway (EOA)	Intraluminal Device, Airway in Gastrointestinal System
Esteem® implantable hearing system	Hearing Device in Ear, Nose, Sinus
Everolimus-eluting coronary stent	Intraluminal Device, Drug-eluting in Heart and Great Vessels
Ex-PRESS™ mini glaucoma shunt	Synthetic Substitute
Express® (LD) Premounted Stent System	Intraluminal Device
Express® Biliary SD Monorail® Premounted Stent System	Intraluminal Device
Express® SD Renal Monorail® Premounted Stent System	Intraluminal Device

Device Term	PCS Description
External fixator	External Fixation Device in Head and Facial Bones External Fixation Device in Upper Bones External Fixation Device in Lower Bones External Fixation Device in Upper Joints External Fixation Device in Lower Joints
EXtreme Lateral Interbody Fusion (XLIF) device	Interbody Fusion Device in Lower Joints
Facet replacement spinal stabilization device	Spinal Stabilization Device, Facet Replacement for Insertion in Upper Joints Spinal Stabilization Device, Facet Replacement for Insertion in Lower Joints
FLAIR® Endovascular Stent Graft	Synthetic Substitute
Flexible Composite Mesh	Synthetic Substitute
Foley catheter	Drainage Device
Formula™ Balloon-Expandable Renal Stent System	Intraluminal Device
Fusion screw (compression)(lag)(locking)	Internal Fixation Device in Upper Joints Internal Fixation Device in Lower Joints
Gastric electrical stimulation (GES) lead	Stimulator Lead in Gastrointestinal System
Gastric pacemaker lead	Stimulator Lead in Gastrointestinal System
GORE® DUALMESH®	Synthetic Substitute
Guedel airway	Intraluminal Device, Airway in Mouth and Throat
HeartMate II® Left Ventricular Assist Device (LVAD)	Implantable Heart Assist System in Heart and Great Vessels
HeartMate XVE® Left Ventricular Assist Device (LVAD)	Implantable Heart Assist System in Heart and Great Vessels
Hip (joint) liner	Liner in Lower Joints
Holter valve ventricular shunt	Synthetic Substitute
Ilizarov external fixator	External Fixation Device, Ring for Insertion in Upper Bones External Fixation Device, Ring for Reposition in Upper Bones External Fixation Device, Ring for Insertion in Lower Bones External Fixation Device, Ring for Reposition in Lower Bones
Ilizarov-Vecklich device	External Fixation Device, Limb Lengthening for Insertion in Upper Bones External Fixation Device, Limb Lengthening for Insertion in Lower Bones
Impella® (2.5)(5.0)(LD) cardiac assist device	Intraluminal Device
Implantable cardioverter-defibrillator (ICD)	Defibrillator Generator for Insertion in Subcutaneous Tissue and Fascia
Implantable gastric pacemaker generator	Stimulator Generator in Subcutaneous Tissue and Fascia
Implantable glucose monitoring device	Monitoring Device
Implantable hemodynamic monitor (IHM)	Monitoring Device, Hemodynamic for Insertion in Subcutaneous Tissue and Fascia
Implantable hemodynamic monitoring system (IHMS)	Monitoring Device, Hemodynamic for Insertion in Subcutaneous Tissue and Fascia
Implantable Miniature Telescope™ (IMT)	Synthetic Substitute, Intraocular Telescope for Replacement in Eye
Implantable pain pump	Infusion Device, Pump in Subcutaneous Tissue and Fascia
Implanted (venous)(access) port	Vascular Access Device, Reservoir in Subcutaneous Tissue and Fascia
Injection reservoir	Vascular Access Device, Reservoir in Subcutaneous Tissue and Fascia
Interbody fusion (spine) cage	Interbody Fusion Device in Upper Joints Interbody Fusion Device in Lower Joints
Interspinous process spinal stabilization device	Spinal Stabilization Device, Interspinous Process for Insertion in Upper Joints Spinal Stabilization Device, Interspinous Process for Insertion in Lower Joints
InterStim® Therapy lead	Neurostimulator Lead in Peripheral Nervous System
InterStim® Therapy neurostimulator	Stimulator Generator in Subcutaneous Tissue and Fascia
Intra-aortic balloon pump	Intraluminal Device
Intramedullary (IM) rod (nail)	Internal Fixation Device, Intramedullary in Upper Bones Internal Fixation Device, Intramedullary in Lower Bones
Intramedullary skeletal kinetic distractor (ISKD)	Internal Fixation Device, Intramedullary in Upper Bones Internal Fixation Device, Intramedullary in Lower Bones
Intrauterine Device (IUD)	Contraceptive Device in Female Reproductive System
Joint fixation plate	Internal Fixation Device in Upper Joints Internal Fixation Device in Lower Joints
Joint liner (insert)	Liner in Lower Joints
Joint spacer (antibiotic)	Spacer in Upper Joints Spacer in Lower Joints
Kinetra® multiple-channel neurostimulator	Stimulator Generator, Multiple Array for Insertion in Subcutaneous Tissue and Fascia

Device Term	PCS Description
Kirschner wire (K-wire)	Internal Fixation Device in Head and Facial Bones Internal Fixation Device in Upper Bones Internal Fixation Device in Lower Bones Internal Fixation Device in Upper Joints Internal Fixation Device in Lower Joints
Knee (implant) insert	Liner in Lower Joints
Kuntscher nail	Internal Fixation Device, Intramedullary in Upper Bones Internal Fixation Device, Intramedullary in Lower Bones
LAP-BAND® Adjustable Gastric Banding System	Extraluminal Device
LifeStent® (Flexstar)(XL) Vascular Stent System	Intraluminal Device
LIVIAN™ CRT-D	Cardiac Resynchronization Defibrillator Pulse Generator for Insertion in Subcutaneous Tissue and Fascia
Mark IV Breathing Pacemaker System	Stimulator Generator in Subcutaneous Tissue and Fascia
Melody® transcatheter pulmonary valve	Zooplastic Tissue in Heart and Great Vessels
Micrus CERECYTE Microcoil	Intraluminal Device, Bioactive in Upper Arteries
MitraClip valve repair system	Synthetic Substitute
Mitroflow® Aortic Pericardial Heart Valve	Zooplastic Tissue in Heart and Great Vessels
Nasopharyngeal airway (NPA)	Intraluminal Device, Airway in Ear, Nose, Sinus
Neuromuscular electrical stimulation (NEMS) lead	Stimulator Lead in Muscles
Neurostimulator generator, multiple channel	Stimulator Generator, Multiple Array for Insertion in Subcutaneous Tissue and Fascia
Neurostimulator generator, multiple channel rechargeable	Stimulator Generator, Multiple Array Rechargeable for Insertion in Subcutaneous Tissue and Fascia
Neurostimulator generator, single channel	Stimulator Generator, Single Array for Insertion in Subcutaneous Tissue and Fascia
Neurostimulator generator, single channel rechargeable	Stimulator Generator, Single Array Rechargeable for Insertion in Subcutaneous Tissue and Fascia
Neutralization plate	Internal Fixation Device in Head and Facial Bones Internal Fixation Device in Upper Bones Internal Fixation Device in Lower Bones
Nitinol framed polymer mesh	Synthetic Substitute
Non-tunneled central venous catheter	Infusion Device
Novacor Left Ventricular Assist Device	Implantable Heart Assist System in Heart and Great Vessels
Novation® Ceramic AHS® (Articulation Hip System)	Synthetic Substitute, Ceramic for Replacement in Lower Joints
Optimizer™ III implantable pulse generator	Contractility Modulation Device for Insertion in Subcutaneous Tissue and Fascia
Oropharyngeal airway (OPA)	Intraluminal Device, Airway in Mouth and Throat
Ovatio™ CRT-D	Cardiac Resynchronization Defibrillator Pulse Generator for Insertion in Subcutaneous Tissue and Fascia
Oxidized zirconium ceramic hip bearing surface	Synthetic Substitute, Ceramic on Polyethylene for Replacement in Lower Joints
Paclitaxel-eluting coronary stent	Intraluminal Device, Drug-eluting in Heart and Great Vessels
Paclitaxel-eluting peripheral stent	Intraluminal Device, Drug-eluting in Upper Arteries Intraluminal Device, Drug-eluting in Lower Arteries
Partially absorbable mesh	Synthetic Substitute
Pedicle-based dynamic stabilization device	Spinal Stabilization Device, Pedicle-Based for Insertion in Upper Joints Spinal Stabilization Device, Pedicle-Based for Insertion in Lower Joints
Percutaneous endoscopic gastrojejunostomy (PEG/J) tube	Feeding Device in Gastrointestinal System
Percutaneous endoscopic gastrostomy (PEG) tube	Feeding Device in Gastrointestinal System
Percutaneous nephrostomy catheter	Drainage Device
Percutaneous tibial nerve stimulation (PTNS) lead	Stimulator Lead in Urinary System
Peripherally inserted central catheter (PICC)	Infusion Device
Pessary ring	Intraluminal Device, Pessary in Female Reproductive System
Phrenic nerve stimulator generator	Stimulator Generator in Subcutaneous Tissue and Fascia
Phrenic nerve stimulator lead	Diaphragmatic Pacemaker Lead in Respiratory System
PHYSIOMESH™ Flexible Composite Mesh	Synthetic Substitute
Pipeline™ Embolization device (PED)	Intraluminal Device
Polyethylene socket	Synthetic Substitute, Polyethylene for Replacement in Lower Joints
Polymethylmethacrylate (PMMA)	Synthetic Substitute
Polypropylene mesh	Synthetic Substitute
Porcine (bioprosthetic) valve	Zooplastic Tissue in Heart and Great Vessels
PRESTIGE® Cervical Disc	Synthetic Substitute

Device Term	PCS Description
PROCEED™ Ventral Patch	Synthetic Substitute
Prodisc-C	Synthetic Substitute
Prodisc-L	Synthetic Substitute
PROLENE Polypropylene Hernia System (PHS)	Synthetic Substitute
Protégé® RX Carotid Stent System	Intraluminal Device
Pump reservoir	Vascular Access Device, Reservoir in Subcutaneous Tissue and Fascia
PVAD™ Ventricular Assist Device	External Heart Assist System in Heart and Great Vessels
REALIZE® Adjustable Gastric Band	Extraluminal Device
Rebound HRD® (Hernia Repair Device)	Synthetic Substitute
Reverse® Shoulder Prosthesis	Synthetic Substitute, Reverse Ball and Socket for Replacement in Upper Joints
Revo MRI™ SureScan® pacemaker	Pacemaker, Dual Chamber for Insertion in Subcutaneous Tissue and Fascia
Rheos® System device	Cardiac Rhythm Related Device in Subcutaneous Tissue and Fascia
Rheos® System lead	Stimulator Lead in Upper Arteries
RNS System lead	Neurostimulator Lead in Central Nervous System
RNS system neurostimulator generator	Neurostimulator Generator in Head and Facial Bones
Sacral nerve modulation (SNM) lead	Stimulator Lead in Urinary System
Sacral neuromodulation lead	Stimulator Lead in Urinary System
SAPIEN transcatheter aortic valve	Zooplastic Tissue in Heart and Great Vessels
Sheffield hybrid external fixator	External Fixation Device, Hybrid for Insertion in Upper Bones External Fixation Device, Hybrid for Reposition in Upper Bones External Fixation Device, Hybrid for Insertion in Lower Bones External Fixation Device, Hybrid for Reposition in Lower Bones
Sheffield ring external fixator	External Fixation Device, Ring for Insertion in Upper Bones External Fixation Device, Ring for Reposition in Upper Bones External Fixation Device, Ring for Insertion in Lower Bones External Fixation Device, Ring for Reposition in Lower Bones
Single lead pacemaker (atrium)(ventricle)	Pacemaker, Single Chamber for Insertion in Subcutaneous Tissue and Fascia
Single lead rate responsive pacemaker (atrium)(ventricle)	Pacemaker, Single Chamber Rate Responsive for Insertion in Subcutaneous Tissue and Fascia
Sirolimus-eluting coronary stent	Intraluminal Device, Drug-eluting in Heart and Great Vessels

Device Term	PCS Description
SJM Biocor® Stented Valve System	Zooplastic Tissue in Heart and Great Vessels
Soletra® single-channel neurostimulator	Stimulator Generator, Single Array for Insertion in Subcutaneous Tissue and Fascia
Spinal cord neurostimulator lead	Neurostimulator Lead in Central Nervous System
Spiration IBV™ Valve System	Intraluminal Device, Endobronchial Valve in Respiratory System
Stent (angioplasty)(embolization)	Intraluminal Device
Stented tissue valve	Zooplastic Tissue in Heart and Great Vessels
Stratos LV	Cardiac Resynchronization Pacemaker Pulse Generator for Insertion in Subcutaneous Tissue and Fascia
Subcutaneous injection reservoir	Vascular Access Device, Reservoir in Subcutaneous Tissue and Fascia
Subdermal progesterone implant	Contraceptive Device in Subcutaneous Tissue and Fascia
SynCardia Total Artificial Heart	Synthetic Substitute
Talent® Abdominal Stent Graft System	Intraluminal Device
Talent® Captiva	Intraluminal Device
Talent® Converter	Intraluminal Device
Talent® Occluder	Intraluminal Device
TandemHeart® System	Intraluminal Device
TAXUS® Liberté® Paclitaxel-eluting Coronary Stent System	Intraluminal Device, Drug-eluting in Heart and Great Vessels
Therapeutic occlusion coil(s)	Intraluminal Device
Thoracostomy tube	Drainage Device
Thoratec IVAD (Implantable Ventricular Assist Device)	Implantable Heart Assist System in Heart and Great Vessels
TigerPaw® system for closure of left atrial appendage	Extraluminal Device
Tissue bank graft	Nonautologous Tissue Substitute
Tissue expander (inflatable)(injectable)	Tissue Expander in Skin and Breast Tissue Expander in Subcutaneous Tissue and Fascia
Titanium Sternal Fixation System (TSFS)	Internal Fixation Device, Rigid Plate for Insertion in Upper Bones Internal Fixation Device, Rigid Plate for Reposition in Upper Bones
Total artificial (replacement) heart	Synthetic Substitute
Tracheostomy tube	Tracheostomy Device in Respiratory System
Trifecta™ Valve (aortic)	Zooplastic Tissue in Heart and Great Vessels
Tunneled central venous catheter	Vascular Access Device in Subcutaneous Tissue and Fascia
Two lead pacemaker	Pacemaker, Dual Chamber for Insertion in Subcutaneous Tissue and Fascia

Device Term	PCS Description
Ultraflex™ Precision Colonic Stent System	Intraluminal Device
ULTRAPRO Hernia System (UHS)	Synthetic Substitute
ULTRAPRO Partially Absorbable Lightweight Mesh	Synthetic Substitute
ULTRAPRO Plug	Synthetic Substitute
Ultrasonic osteogenic stimulator	Bone Growth Stimulator in Head and Facial Bones Bone Growth Stimulator in Upper Bones Bone Growth Stimulator in Lower Bones
Ultrasound bone healing system	Bone Growth Stimulator in Head and Facial Bones Bone Growth Stimulator in Upper Bones Bone Growth Stimulator in Lower Bones
Uniplanar external fixator	External Fixation Device, Monoplanar for Insertion in Upper Bones External Fixation Device, Monoplanar for Reposition in Upper Bones External Fixation Device, Monoplanar for Insertion in Lower Bones External Fixation Device, Monoplanar for Reposition in Lower Bones
Urinary incontinence stimulator lead	Stimulator Lead in Urinary System
Vaginal pessary	Intraluminal Device, Pessary in Female Reproductive System
Valiant Thoracic Stent Graft	Synthetic Substitute
Vectra® Vascular Access Graft	Vascular Access Device in Subcutaneous Tissue and Fascia
Ventrio™ Hernia Patch	Synthetic Substitute
WALLSTENT® Endoprosthesis	Intraluminal Device
X-STOP® Spacer	Spinal Stabilization Device, Interspinous Process for Insertion in Upper Joints Spinal Stabilization Device, Interspinous Process for Insertion in Lower Joints
Xenograft	Zooplastic Tissue in Heart and Great Vessels
XIENCE V Everolimus Eluting Coronary Stent System	Intraluminal Device, Drug-eluting in Heart and Great Vessels
XLIF® System	Interbody Fusion Device in Lower Joints
Zenith Flex® AAA Endovascular Graft	Intraluminal Device
Zenith TX2® TAA Endovascular Graft	Intraluminal Device
Zenith® Renu™ AAA Ancillary Graft	Intraluminal Device
Zilver® PTX® (paclitaxel) Drug-Eluting Peripheral Stent	Intraluminal Device, Drug-eluting in Upper Arteries Intraluminal Device, Drug-eluting in Lower Arteries
Zimmer® NexGen® LPS Mobile Bearing Knee	Synthetic Substitute
Zimmer® NexGen® LPS-Flex Mobile Knee	Synthetic Substitute
Zotarolimus-eluting coronary stent	Intraluminal Device, Drug-eluting in Heart and Great Vessels

Device Aggregation Table

This table crosswalks specific device character value definitions for specific root operations in a specific body system to the more general device character value to be used when the root operation covers a wide range of body parts and the device character represents an entire family of devices.

Specific Device	for Operation	in Body System	General Device
Autologous Arterial Tissue (A)	All applicable	Heart and Great Vessels Lower Arteries Lower Veins Upper Arteries Upper Veins	**7** Autologous Tissue Substitute
Autologous Venous Tissue (9)	All applicable	Heart and Great Vessels Lower Arteries Lower Veins Upper Arteries Upper Veins	**7** Autologous Tissue Substitute
Cardiac Lead, Defibrillator (K)	Insertion	Heart and Great Vessels	**M** Cardiac Lead
Cardiac Lead, Pacemaker (J)	Insertion	Heart and Great Vessels	**M** Cardiac Lead
Cardiac Resynchronization Defibrillator Pulse Generator (9)	Insertion	Subcutaneous Tissue and Fascia	**P** Cardiac Rhythm Related Device
Cardiac Resynchronization Pacemaker Pulse Generator (7)	Insertion	Subcutaneous Tissue and Fascia	**P** Cardiac Rhythm Related Device
Contractility Modulation Device (A)	Insertion	Subcutaneous Tissue and Fascia	**P** Cardiac Rhythm Related Device

Specific Device	for Operation	in Body System	General Device
Defibrillator Generator (8)	Insertion	Subcutaneous Tissue and Fascia	**P** Cardiac Rhythm Related Device
External Fixation Device, Hybrid (D)	Insertion	Lower Bones Upper Bones	**5** External Fixation Device
External Fixation Device, Hybrid (D)	Reposition	Lower Bones Upper Bones	**5** External Fixation Device
External Fixation Device, Limb Lengthening (8)	Insertion	Lower Bones Upper Bones	**5** External Fixation Device
External Fixation Device, Monoplanar (B)	Insertion	Lower Bones Upper Bones	**5** External Fixation Device
External Fixation Device, Monoplanar (B)	Reposition	Lower Bones Upper Bones	**5** External Fixation Device
External Fixation Device, Ring (C)	Insertion	Lower Bones Upper Bones	**5** External Fixation Device
External Fixation Device, Ring (C)	Reposition	Lower Bones Upper Bones	**5** External Fixation Device
Hearing Device, Bone Conduction (S)	All applicable	Head and Facial Bones	**S** Hearing Device, Bone Conduction
Hearing Device, Bone Conduction (4)	Insertion	Ear, Nose, Sinus	**S** Hearing Device
Hearing Device, Multiple Channel Cochlear Prosthesis (6)	Insertion	Ear, Nose, Sinus	**S** Hearing Device
Hearing Device, Single Channel Cochlear Prosthesis (5)	Insertion	Ear, Nose, Sinus	**S** Hearing Device
Internal Fixation Device, Intramedullary (6)	All applicable	Lower Bones Upper Bones	**4** Internal Fixation Device
Internal Fixation Device, Rigid Plate (Ø)	Insertion	Upper Bones	**4** Internal Fixation Device
Internal Fixation Device, Rigid Plate (Ø)	Reposition	Upper Bones	**4** Internal Fixation Device
Intraluminal Device, Pessary (G)	All applicable	Female Reproductive System	**D** Intraluminal Device
Intraluminal Device, Airway (B)	All applicable	Ear, Nose, Sinus Gastrointestinal System Mouth and Throat	**D** Intraluminal Device
Intraluminal Device, Bioactive (B)	All applicable	Upper Arteries	**D** Intraluminal Device
Intraluminal Device, Drug-eluting (4)	All applicable	Heart and Great Vessels Lower Arteries Upper Arteries	**D** Intraluminal Device
Intraluminal Device, Endobronchial Valve (G)	All applicable	Respiratory System	**D** Intraluminal Device
Intraluminal Device, Endotracheal Airway (E)	All applicable	Respiratory System	**D** Intraluminal Device
Intraluminal Device, Radioactive (T)	All applicable	Heart and Great Vessels	**D** Intraluminal Device
Monitoring Device, Hemodynamic (Ø)	Insertion	Subcutaneous Tissue and Fascia	**2** Monitoring Device
Monitoring Device, Pressure Sensor (Ø)	Insertion	Heart and Great Vessels	**2** Monitoring Device
Pacemaker, Dual Chamber (6)	Insertion	Subcutaneous Tissue and Fascia	**P** Cardiac Rhythm Related Device
Pacemaker, Single Chamber (4)	Insertion	Subcutaneous Tissue and Fascia	**P** Cardiac Rhythm Related Device
Pacemaker, Single Chamber Rate Responsive (5)	Insertion	Subcutaneous Tissue and Fascia	**P** Cardiac Rhythm Related Device
Spinal Stabilization Device, Facet Replacement (D)	Insertion	Lower Joints Upper Joints	**4** Internal Fixation Device
Spinal Stabilization Device, Interspinous Process (B)	Insertion	Lower Joints Upper Joints	**4** Internal Fixation Device
Spinal Stabilization Device, Pedicle-Based (C)	Insertion	Lower Joints Upper Joints	**4** Internal Fixation Device
Stimulator Generator, Multiple Array (D)	Insertion	Subcutaneous Tissue and Fascia	**M** Stimulator Generator
Stimulator Generator, Multiple Array Rechargeable (E)	Insertion	Subcutaneous Tissue and Fascia	**M** Stimulator Generator
Stimulator Generator, Single Array (B)	Insertion	Subcutaneous Tissue and Fascia	**M** Stimulator Generator
Stimulator Generator, Single Array Rechargeable (C)	Insertion	Subcutaneous Tissue and Fascia	**M** Stimulator Generator
Synthetic Substitute, Ceramic (3)	Replacement	Lower Joints	**J** Synthetic Substitute
Synthetic Substitute, Ceramic on Polyethylene (4)	Replacement	Lower Joints	**J** Synthetic Substitute
Synthetic Substitute, Intraocular Telescope (Ø)	Replacement	Eye	**J** Synthetic Substitute

Appendix D: Device Key and Aggregation Table

Specific Device	for Operation	in Body System	General Device
Synthetic Substitute, Metal (1)	Replacement	Lower Joints	**J** Synthetic Substitute
Synthetic Substitute, Metal on Polyethylene (2)	Replacement	Lower Joints	**J** Synthetic Substitute
Synthetic Substitute, Polyethylene (Ø)	Replacement	Lower Joints	**J** Synthetic Substitute
Synthetic Substitute, Reverse Ball and Socket (Ø)	Replacement	Upper Joints	**J** Synthetic Substitute

Appendix E: Type and Type Qualifier Definitions Sections B–H

Section B–Imaging

Type (Character 3)	Definition
Computerized Tomography (CT Scan) (2)	Computer reformatted digital display of multiplanar images developed from the capture of multiple exposures of external ionizing radiation
Fluoroscopy (1)	Single plane or bi-plane real time display of an image developed from the capture of external ionizing radiation on a fluorescent screen. The image may also be stored by either digital or analog means
Magnetic Resonance Imaging (MRI) (3)	Computer reformatted digital display of multiplanar images developed from the capture of radiofrequency signals emitted by nuclei in a body site excited within a magnetic field
Plain Radiography (Ø)	Planar display of an image developed from the capture of external ionizing radiation on photographic or photoconductive plate
Ultrasonography (4)	Real time display of images of anatomy or flow information developed from the capture of reflected and attenuated high frequency sound waves

Section C–Nuclear Medicine

Type (Character 3)	Definition
Nonimaging Nuclear Medicine Assay (6)	Introduction of radioactive materials into the body for the study of body fluids and blood elements, by the detection of radioactive emissions
Nonimaging Nuclear Medicine Probe (5)	Introduction of radioactive materials into the body for the study of distribution and fate of certain substances by the detection of radioactive emissions; or, alternatively, measurement of absorption of radioactive emissions from an external source
Nonimaging Nuclear Medicine Uptake (4)	Introduction of radioactive materials into the body for measurements of organ function, from the detection of radioactive emissions
Planar Nuclear Medicine Imaging (1)	Introduction of radioactive materials into the body for single plane display of images developed from the capture of radioactive emissions
Positron Emission Tomographic (PET) Imaging (3)	Introduction of radioactive materials into the body for three dimensional display of images developed from the simultaneous capture, 18Ø degrees apart, of radioactive emissions
Systemic Nuclear Medicine Therapy (7)	Introduction of unsealed radioactive materials into the body for treatment
Tomographic (Tomo) Nuclear Medicine Imaging (2)	Introduction of radioactive materials into the body for three dimensional display of images developed from the capture of radioactive emissions

Section F–Physical Rehabilitation and Diagnostic Audiology

Type (Character 3)	Definition
Activities of Daily Living Assessment (2)	Measurement of functional level for activities of daily living
Activities of Daily Living Treatment (8)	Exercise or activities to facilitate functional competence for activities of daily living
Caregiver Training (F)	Training in activities to support patient's optimal level of function
Cochlear Implant Treatment (B)	Application of techniques to improve the communication abilities of individuals with cochlear implant
Device Fitting (D)	Fitting of a device designed to facilitate or support achievement of a higher level of function
Hearing Aid Assessment (4)	Measurement of the appropriateness and/or effectiveness of a hearing device
Hearing Assessment (3)	Measurement of hearing and related functions

Continued on next page

Section F–Physical Rehabilitation and Diagnostic Audiology

Continued from previous page

Type (Character 3)	Definition
Hearing Treatment (9)	Application of techniques to improve, augment, or compensate for hearing and related functional impairment
Motor Function Assessment/Nerve Function Assessment (1)	Measurement of motor, nerve, and related functions
Motor Treatment (7)	Exercise or activities to increase or facilitate motor function
Speech Assessment (Ø)	Measurement of speech and related functions
Speech Treatment (6)	Application of techniques to improve, augment, or compensate for speech and related functional impairment
Vestibular Assessment (5)	Measurement of the vestibular system and related functions
Vestibular Treatment (C)	Application of techniques to improve, augment, or compensate for vestibular and related functional impairment

Section F–Physical Rehabilitation and Diagnostic Audiology

Type Qualifier (Character 5)	Definition
Acoustic Reflex Decay (J)	Measures reduction in size/strength of acoustic reflex over time Includes/Examples: Includes site of lesion test
Acoustic Reflex Patterns (G)	Defines site of lesion based upon presence/absence of acoustic reflexes with ipsilateral vs. contralateral stimulation
Acoustic Reflex Threshold (H)	Determines minimal intensity that acoustic reflex occurs with ipsilateral and/or contralateral stimulation
Aerobic Capacity and Endurance (7)	Measures autonomic responses to positional changes; perceived exertion, dyspnea or angina during activity; performance during exercise protocols; standard vital signs; and blood gas analysis or oxygen consumption
Alternate Binaural or Monaural Loudness Balance (7)	Determines auditory stimulus parameter that yields the same objective sensation Includes/Examples: Sound intensities that yield same loudness perception
Anthropometric Characteristics (B)	Measures edema, body fat composition, height, weight, length and girth
Aphasia (Assessment) (C)	Measures expressive and receptive speech and language function including reading and writing
Aphasia (Treatment) (3)	Applying techniques to improve, augment, or compensate for receptive/ expressive language impairments
Articulation/Phonology (Assessment) (9)	Measures speech production
Articulation/Phonology (Treatment) (4)	Applying techniques to correct, improve, or compensate for speech productive impairment
Assistive Listening Device (5)	Assists in use of effective and appropriate assistive listening device/system
Assistive Listening System Device Selection (4)	Measures the effectiveness and appropriateness of assistive listening systems/devices
Assistive, Adaptive,Supportive or Protective Devices (9)	Explanation: Devices to facilitate or support achievement of a higher level of function in wheelchair mobility; bed mobility; transfer or ambulation ability; bath and showering ability; dressing; grooming; personal hygiene; play or leisure
Auditory Evoked Potentials (L)	Measures electric responses produced by the VIIIth cranial nerve and brainstem following auditory stimulation
Auditory Processing (Assessment) (Q)	Evaluates ability to receive and process auditory information and comprehension of spoken language
Auditory Processing (Treatment) (2)	Applying techniques to improve the receiving and processing of auditory information and comprehension of spoken language

Continued on next page

Section F–Physical Rehabilitation and Diagnostic Audiology

Continued from previous page

Type Qualifier (Character 5)	Definition
Augmentative/Alternative Communication System (Assessment) (L)	Determines the appropriateness of aids, techniques, symbols, and/or strategies to augment or replace speech and enhance communication Includes/Examples: Includes the use of telephones, writing equipment, emergency equipment, and TDD
Augmentative/Alternative Communication System (Treatment) (3)	Includes/Examples: Includes augmentative communication devices and aids
Aural Rehabilitation (5)	Applying techniques to improve the communication abilities associated with hearing loss
Aural Rehabilitation Status (P)	Measures impact of a hearing loss including evaluation of receptive and expressive communication skills
Bathing/Showering (Ø)	Includes/Examples: Includes obtaining and using supplies; soaping, rinsing, and drying body parts; maintaining bathing position; and transferring to and from bathing positions
Bathing/Showering Techniques (Ø)	Activities to facilitate obtaining and using supplies, soaping, rinsing and drying body parts, maintaining bathing position, and transferring to and from bathing positions
Bed Mobility (Assessment) (B)	Transitional movement within bed
Bed Mobility (Treatment) (5)	Exercise or activities to facilitate transitional movements within bed
Bedside Swallowing and Oral Function (H)	Includes/Examples: Bedside swallowing includes assessment of sucking, masticating, coughing, and swallowing. Oral function includes assessment of musculature for controlled movements, structures, and functions to determine coordination and phonation
Bekesy Audiometry (3)	Uses an instrument that provides a choice of discrete or continuously varying pure tones; choice of pulsed or continuous signal
Binaural Electroacoustic Hearing Aid Check (6)	Determines mechanical and electroacoustic function of bilateral hearing aids using hearing aid test box
Binaural Hearing Aid (Assessment) (3)	Measures the candidacy, effectiveness, and appropriateness of a hearing aid Explanation: Measures bilateral fit
Binaural Hearing Aid (Treatment) (2)	Explanation: Assists in achieving maximum understanding and performance
Bithermal, Binaural Caloric Irrigation (Ø)	Measures the rhythmic eye movements stimulated by changing the temperature of the vestibular system
Bithermal, Monaural Caloric Irrigation (1)	Measures the rhythmic eye movements stimulated by changing the temperature of the vestibular system in one ear
Brief Tone Stimuli (R)	Measures specific central auditory process
Cerumen Management (3)	Includes examination of external auditory canal and tympanic membrane and removal of cerumen from external ear canal
Cochlear Implant (Ø)	Measures candidacy for cochlear implant
Cochlear Implant Rehabilitation (Ø)	Applying techniques to improve the communication abilities of individuals with cochlear implant; includes programming the device, providing patients/families with information
Communicative/Cognitive Integration Skills (Assessment) (G)	Measures ability to use higher cortical functions Includes/Examples: Includes orientation, recognition, attention span, initiation and termination of activity, memory, sequencing, categorizing, concept formation, spatial operations, judgment, problem solving, generalization and pragmatic communication
Communicative/Cognitive Integration Skills (Treatment) (6)	Activities to facilitate the use of higher cortical functions Includes/Examples: Includes level of arousal, orientation, recognition, attention span, initiation and termination of activity, memory sequencing, judgment and problem solving, learning and generalization, and pragmatic communication
Computerized Dynamic Posturography (6)	Measures the status of the peripheral and central vestibular system and the sensory/motor component of balance; evaluates the efficacy of vestibular rehabilitation
Conditioned Play Audiometry (4)	Behavioral measures using nonspeech and speech stimuli to obtain frequency-specific and ear-specific information on auditory status from the patient Explanation: Obtains speech reception threshold by having patient point to pictures of spondaic words

Continued on next page

Section F–Physical Rehabilitation and Diagnostic Audiology

Continued from previous page

Type Qualifier (Character 5)	Definition
Coordination/Dexterity (Assessment) (3)	Measures large and small muscle groups for controlled goal- directed movements Explanation: Dexterity includes object manipulation
Coordination/Dexterity (Treatment) (2)	Exercise or activities to facilitate gross coordination and fine coordination
Cranial Nerve Integrity (9)	Measures cranial nerve sensory and motor functions, including tastes, smell and facial expression
Dichotic Stimuli (T)	Measures specific central auditory process
Distorted Speech (S)	Measures specific central auditory process
Dix-Hallpike Dynamic (5)	Measures nystagmus following Dix-Hallpike maneuver
Dressing (1)	Includes/Examples: Includes selecting clothing and accessories, obtaining clothing from storage, dressing, fastening and adjusting clothing and shoes, and applying and removing personal devices, prosthesis or orthosis
Dressing Techniques (1)	Activities to facilitate selecting clothing and accessories, dressing and undressing, adjusting clothing and shoes, applying and removing devices, prostheses or orthoses
Dynamic Orthosis (6)	Includes/Examples: Includes customized and prefabricated splints, inhibitory casts, spinal and other braces, and protective devices; allows motion through transfer of movement from other body parts or by use of outside forces
Ear Canal Probe Microphone (1)	Real ear measures
Ear Protector Attentuation (7)	Measures ear protector fit and effectiveness
Electrocochleography (K)	Measures the VIIIth cranial nerve action potential
Environmental, Home, Work Barriers (B)	Measures current and potential barriers to optimal function, including safety hazards, access problems and home or office design
Ergonomics and Body Mechanics (C)	Ergonomic measurement of job tasks, work hardening or work conditioning needs; functional capacity; and body mechanics
Eustachian Tube Function (F)	Measures eustachian tube function and patency of eustachian tube
Evoked Otoacoustic Emissions, Diagnostic (N)	Measures auditory evoked potentials in a diagnostic format
Evoked Otoacoustic Emissions, Screening (M)	Measures auditory evoked potentials in a screening format
Facial Nerve Function (7)	Measures electrical activity of the VIIth cranial nerve (facial nerve)
Feeding/Eating (Assessment) (2)	Includes/Examples: Includes setting up food, selecting and using utensils and tableware, bringing food or drink to mouth, cleaning face, hands, and clothing, and management of alternative methods of nourishment
Feeding/Eating (Treatment) (3)	Exercise or activities to facilitate setting up food, selecting and using utensils and tableware, bringing food or drink to mouth, cleaning face, hands, and clothing, and management of alternative methods of nourishment
Filtered Speech (Ø)	Uses high or low pass filtered speech stimuli to assess central auditory processing disorders, site of lesion testing
Fluency (Assessment) (D)	Measures speech fluency or stuttering
Fluency (Treatment) (7)	Applying techniques to improve and augment fluent speech
Gait Training/Functional Ambulation (9)	Exercise or activities to facilitate ambulation on a variety of surfaces and in a variety of environments
Gait/Balance (D)	Measures biomechanical, arthrokinematic and other spatial and temporal characteristics of gait and balance

Continued on next page

Section F–Physical Rehabilitation and Diagnostic Audiology

Continued from previous page

Type Qualifier (Character 5)	Definition
Grooming/Personal Hygiene (Assessment) (3)	Includes/Examples: Includes ability to obtain and use supplies in a sequential fashion, general grooming, oral hygiene, toilet hygiene, personal care devices, including care for artificial airways
Grooming/Personal Hygiene (Treatment) (2)	Activities to facilitate obtaining and using supplies in a sequential fashion: general grooming, oral hygiene, toilet hygiene, cleaning body, and personal care devices, including artificial airways
Hearing and Related Disorders Counseling (Ø)	Provides patients/families/caregivers with information, support, referrals to facilitate recovery from a communication disorder Includes/Examples: Includes strategies for psychosocial adjustment to hearing loss for clients and families/caregivers
Hearing and Related Disorders Prevention (1)	Provides patients/families/caregivers with information and support to prevent communication disorders
Hearing Screening (Ø)	Pass/refer measures designed to identify need for further audiologic assessment
Home Management (Assessment) (4)	Obtaining and maintaining personal and household possessions and environment Includes/Examples: Includes clothing care, cleaning, meal preparation and cleanup, shopping, money management, household maintenance, safety procedures, and childcare/parenting
Home Management (Treatment) (4)	Activities to facilitate obtaining and maintaining personal household possessions and environment Includes/Examples: Includes clothing care, cleaning, meal preparation and clean-up, shopping, money management, household maintenance, safety procedures, childcare/parenting
Instrumental Swallowing and Oral Function (J)	Definition: Measures swallowing function using instrumental diagnostic procedures Explanation: Methods include videofluoroscopy, ultrasound, manometry, endoscopy
Integumentary Integrity (1)	Includes/Examples: Includes burns, skin conditions, ecchymosis, bleeding, blisters, scar tissue, wounds and other traumas, tissue mobility, turgor and texture
Manual Therapy Techniques (7)	Techniques in which the therapist uses his/her hands to administer skilled movements Includes/Examples: Includes connective tissue massage, joint mobilization and manipulation, manual lymph drainage, manual traction, soft tissue mobilization and manipulation
Masking Patterns (W)	Measures central auditory processing status
Monaural Electroacoustic Hearing Aid Check (8)	Determines mechanical and electroacoustic function of one hearing aid using hearing aid test box
Monaural Hearing Aid (Assessment) (2)	Measures the candidacy, effectiveness, and appropriateness of a hearing aid Explanation: Measures unilateral fit
Monaural Hearing Aid (Treatment) (1)	Explanation: Assists in achieving maximum understanding and performance
Motor Function (Assessment) (4)	Measures the body's functional and versatile movement patterns Includes/Examples: Includes motor assessment scales, analysis of head, trunk and limb movement, and assessment of motor learning
Motor Function (Treatment) (3)	Exercise or activities to facilitate crossing midline, laterality, bilateral integration, praxis, neuromuscular relaxation, inhibition, facilitation, motor function and motor learning
Motor Speech (Assessment) (B)	Measures neurological motor aspects of speech production
Motor Speech (Treatment) (B)	Applying techniques to improve and augment the impaired neurological motor aspects of speech production
Muscle Performance (Assessment) (Ø)	Measures muscle strength, power and endurance using manual testing, dynamometry or computer-assisted electromechanical muscle test; functional muscle strength, power and endurance; muscle pain, tone, or soreness; or pelvic-floor musculature Explanation: Muscle endurance refers to the ability to contract a muscle repeatedly over time
Muscle Performance (Treatment) (1)	Exercise or activities to increase the capacity of a muscle to do work in terms of strength, power, and/or endurance Explanation: Muscle strength is the force exerted to overcome resistance in one maximal effort. Muscle power is work produced per unit of time, or the product of strength and speed. Muscle endurance is the ability to contract a muscle repeatedly over time
Neuromotor Development (D)	Measures motor development, righting and equilibrium reactions, and reflex and equilibrium reactions

Continued on next page

Section F–Physical Rehabilitation and Diagnostic Audiology

Continued from previous page

Type Qualifier (Character 5)	Definition
Neurophysiologic Intraoperative (8)	Monitors neural status during surgery
Non-invasive Instrumental Status (N)	Instrumental measures of oral, nasal, vocal, and velopharyngeal functions as they pertain to speech production
Nonspoken Language (Assessment) (7)	Measures nonspoken language (print, sign, symbols) for communication
Nonspoken Language (Treatment) (Ø)	Applying techniques that improve, augment, or compensate spoken communication
Oral Peripheral Mechanism (P)	Structural measures of face, jaw, lips, tongue, teeth, hard and soft palate, pharynx as related to speech production
Orofacial Myofunctional (Assessment) (K)	Measures orofacial myofunctional patterns for speech and related functions
Orofacial Myofunctional (Treatment) (9)	Applying techniques to improve, alter, or augment impaired orofacial myofunctional patterns and related speech production errors
Oscillating Tracking (3)	Measures ability to visually track
Pain (F)	Measures muscle soreness, pain and soreness with joint movement, and pain perception Includes/Examples: Includes questionnaires, graphs, symptom magnification scales or visual analog scales
Perceptual Processing (Assessment) (5)	Measures stereognosis, kinesthesia, body schema, right-left discrimination, form constancy, position in space, visual closure, figure-ground, depth perception, spatial relations and topographical orientation
Perceptual Processing (Treatment) (1)	Exercise and activities to facilitate perceptual processing Explanation: Includes stereognosis, kinesthesia, body schema, right-left discrimination, form constancy, position in space, visual closure, figure-ground, depth perception, spatial relations, and topographical orientation Includes/Examples: Includes stereognosis, kinesthesia, body schema, right-left discrimination, form constancy, position in space, visual closure, figure-ground, depth perception, spatial relations, and topographical orientation
Performance Intensity Phonetically Balanced Speech Discrimination (Q)	Measures word recognition over varying intensity levels
Postural Control (3)	Exercise or activities to increase postural alignment and control
Prosthesis (8)	Explanation: Artificial substitutes for missing body parts that augment performance or function
Psychosocial Skills (Assessment) (6)	The ability to interact in society and to process emotions Includes/Examples: Includes psychological (values, interests, self-concept); social (role performance, social conduct, interpersonal skills, self expression); self-management (coping skills, time management, self-control)
Psychosocial Skills (Treatment) (6)	The ability to interact in society and to process emotions Includes/Examples: Includes psychological (values, interests, self-concept); social (role performance, social conduct, interpersonal skills, self expression); self-management (coping skills, time management, self-control)
Pure Tone Audiometry, Air (1)	Air-conduction pure tone threshold measures with appropriate masking
Pure Tone Audiometry, Air and Bone (2)	Air-conduction and bone-conduction pure tone threshold measures with appropriate masking
Pure Tone Stenger (C)	Measures unilateral nonorganic hearing loss based on simultaneous presentation of pure tones of differing volume
Range of Motion and Joint Integrity (5)	Measures quantity, quality, grade, and classification of joint movement and/or mobility Explanation: Range of Motion is the space, distance or angle through which movement occurs at a joint or series of joints. Joint integrity is the conformance of joints to expected anatomic, biomechanical and kinematic norms
Range of Motion and Joint Mobility (Ø)	Exercise or activities to increase muscle length and joint mobility

Continued on next page

Section F–Physical Rehabilitation and Diagnostic Audiology

Continued from previous page

Type Qualifier (Character 5)	Definition
Receptive/Expressive Language (Assessment) (8)	Measures receptive and expressive language
Receptive/Expressive Language (Treatment) (B)	Applying techniques to improve and augment receptive/expressive language
Reflex Integrity (G)	Measures the presence, absence, or exaggeration of developmentally appropriate, pathologic or normal reflexes
Select Picture Audiometry (5)	Establishes hearing threshold levels for speech using pictures
Sensorineural Acuity Level (4)	Measures sensorineural acuity masking presented via bone conduction
Sensory Aids (5)	Determines the appropriateness of a sensory prosthetic device, other than a hearing aid or assistive listening system/device
Sensory Awareness/ Processing/ Integrity (6)	Includes/Examples: Includes light touch, pressure, temperature, pain, sharp/dull, proprioception, vestibular, visual, auditory, gustatory, and olfactory
Short Increment Sensitivity Index (9)	Measures the ear's ability to detect small intensity changes; site of lesion test requiring a behavioral response
Sinusoidal Vertical Axis Rotational (4)	Measures nystagmus following rotation
Somatosensory Evoked Potentials (9)	Measures neural activity from sites throughout the body
Speech/Language Screening (6)	Identifies need for further speech and/or language evaluation
Speech Threshold (1)	Measures minimal intensity needed to repeat spondaic words
Speech/Word Recognition (2)	Measures ability to repeat/identify single syllable words; scores given as a percentage; includes word recognition/speech discrimination
Speech-Language Pathology and Related Disorders Counseling (1)	Provides patients/families with information, support, referrals to facilitate recovery from a communication disorder
Speech-Language Pathology and Related Disorders Prevention (2)	Applying techniques to avoid or minimize onset and/or development of a communication disorder
Staggered Spondaic Word (3)	Measures central auditory processing site of lesion based upon dichotic presentation of spondaic words
Static Orthosis (7)	Includes/Examples: Includes customized and prefabricated splints, inhibitory casts, spinal and other braces, and protective devices; has no moving parts, maintains joint(s) in desired position
Stenger (B)	Measures unilateral nonorganic hearing loss based on simultaneous presentation of signals of differing volume
Swallowing Dysfunction (D)	Activities to improve swallowing function in coordination with respiratory function Includes/Examples: Includes function and coordination of sucking, mastication, coughing, swallowing
Synthetic Sentence Identification (5)	Measures central auditory dysfunction using identification of third order approximations of sentences and competing messages
Temporal Ordering of Stimuli (V)	Measures specific central auditory process
Therapeutic Exercise (7)	Exercise or activities to facilitate sensory awareness, sensory processing, sensory integration, balance training, conditioning, reconditioning Includes/Examples: Includes developmental activities, breathing exercises, aerobic endurance activities, aquatic exercises, stretching and ventilatory muscle training
Tinnitus Masker (Assessment) (7)	Determines candidacy for tinnitus masker
Tinnitus Masker (Treatment) (Ø)	Explanation: Used to verify physical fit, acoustic appropriateness, and benefit; assists in achieving maximum benefit
Tone Decay (B)	Measures decrease in hearing sensitivity to a tone; site of lesion test requiring a behavioral response
Transfer (5)	Transitional movement from one surface to another

Continued on next page

Section F–Physical Rehabilitation and Diagnostic Audiology

Continued from previous page

Type Qualifier (Character 5)	Definition
Transfer Training (8)	Exercise or activities to facilitate movement from one surface to another
Tympanometry (D)	Measures the integrity of the middle ear; measures ease at which sound flows through the tympanic membrane while air pressure against the membrane is varied
Unithermal Binaural Screen (2)	Measures the rhythmic eye movements stimulated by changing the temperature of the vestibular system in both ears using warm water, screening format
Ventilation/Respiration/Circulation (G)	Measures ventilatory muscle strength, power and endurance, pulmonary function and ventilatory mechanics Includes/Examples: Includes ability to clear airway, activities that aggravate or relieve edema, pain, dyspnea or other symptoms, chest wall mobility, cardiopulmonary response to performance of ADL and IAD, cough and sputum, standard vital signs
Vestibular (Ø)	Applying techniques to compensate for balance disorders; includes habituation, exercise therapy, and balance retraining
Visual Motor Integration (Assessment) (2)	Coordinating the interaction of information from the eyes with body movement during activity
Visual Motor Integration (Treatment) (2)	Exercise or activities to facilitate coordinating the interaction of information from eyes with body movement during activity
Visual Reinforcement Audiometry (6)	Behavioral measures using nonspeech and speech stimuli to obtain frequency/ear-specific information on auditory status Includes/Examples: Includes a conditioned response of looking toward a visual reinforcer (e.g., lights, animated toy) every time auditory stimuli are heard
Vocational Activities and Functional Community or Work Reintegration Skills (Assessment) (H)	Measures environmental, home, work (job/school/play) barriers that keep patients from functioning optimally in their environment Includes/Examples: Includes assessment of vocational skills and interests, environment of work (job/school/play), injury potential and injury prevention or reduction, ergonomic stressors, transportation skills, and ability to access and use community resources
Vocational Activities/Functional Community Skills/Work Reintegration Skills (Treatment) (7)	Activities to facilitate vocational exploration, body mechanics training, job acquisition, and environmental or work (job/school/play) task adaptation Includes/Examples: Includes injury prevention and reduction, ergonomic stressor reduction, job coaching and simulation, work hardening and conditioning, driving training, transportation skills, and use of community resources
Voice (Assessment) (F)	Measures vocal structure, function and production
Voice (Treatment) (C)	Applying techniques to improve voice and vocal function
Voice Prosthetic (Assessment) (M)	Determines the appropriateness of voice prosthetic/adaptive device to enhance or facilitate communication
Voice Prosthetic (Treatment) (4)	Includes/Examples: Includes electrolarynx, and other assistive, adaptive, supportive devices
Wheelchair Mobility (Assessment) (F)	Measures fit and functional abilities within wheelchair in a variety of environments
Wheelchair Mobility (Treatment) (4)	Management, maintenance and controlled operation of a wheelchair, scooter or other device, in and on a variety of surfaces and environments
Wound Management (5)	Includes/Examples: Includes non-selective and selective debridement (enzymes, autolysis, sharp debridement), dressings (wound coverings, hydrogel, vacuum-assisted closure), topical agents, etc.

Section G–Mental Health

Type (Character 3)	Definition
Biofeedback (C)	Provision of information from the monitoring and regulating of physiological processes in conjunction with cognitive-behavioral techniques to improve patient functioning or well-being Includes/Examples: Includes EEG, blood pressure, skin temperature or peripheral blood flow, ECG, electrooculogram, EMG, respirometry or capnometry, GSR/EDR, perineometry to monitor/regulate bowel/bladder activity, electrogastrogram to monitor/regulate gastric motility
Counseling (6)	The application of psychological methods to treat an individual with normal developmental issues and psychological problems in order to increase function, improve well-being, alleviate distress, maladjustment or resolve crises
Crisis Intervention (2)	Treatment of a traumatized, acutely disturbed or distressed individual for the purpose of short-term stabilization Includes/Examples: Includes defusing, debriefing, counseling, psychotherapy and/or coordination of care with other providers or agencies
Electroconvulsive Therapy (B)	The application of controlled electrical voltages to treat a mental health disorder Includes/Examples: Includes appropriate sedation and other preparation of the individual
Family Psychotherapy (7)	Treatment that includes one or more family members of an individual with a mental health disorder by behavioral, cognitive, psychoanalytic, psychodynamic or psychophysiological means to improve functioning or well-being Explanation: Remediation of emotional or behavioral problems presented by one or more family members in cases where psychotherapy with more than one family member is indicated
Group Psychotherapy (H)	Treatment of two or more individuals with a mental health disorder by behavioral, cognitive, psychoanalytic, psychodynamic or psychophysiological means to improve functioning or well-being
Hypnosis (F)	Induction of a state of heightened suggestibility by auditory, visual and tactile techniques to elicit an emotional or behavioral response
Individual Psychotherapy (5)	Treatment of an individual with a mental health disorder by behavioral, cognitive, psychoanalytic, psychodynamic or psychophysiological means to improve functioning or well-being
Light Therapy (J)	Application of specialized light treatments to improve functioning or well-being
Medication Management (3)	Monitoring and adjusting the use of medications for the treatment of a mental health disorder
Narcosynthesis (G)	Administration of intravenous barbiturates in order to release suppressed or repressed thoughts
Psychological Tests (1)	The administration and interpretation of standardized psychological tests and measurement instruments for the assessment of psychological function

Section G–Mental Health

Type Qualifier (Character 4)	Definition
Behavioral (1)	Primarily to modify behavior Includes/Examples: Includes modeling and role playing, positive reinforcement of target behaviors, response cost, and training of self-management skills
Cognitive (2)	Primarily to correct cognitive distortions and errors
Cognitive-Behavioral (8)	Combining cognitive and behavioral treatment strategies to improve functioning Explanation: Maladaptive responses are examined to determine how cognitions relate to behavior patterns in response to an event. Uses learning principles and information-processing models
Developmental (Ø)	Age-normed developmental status of cognitive, social and adaptive behavior skills
Intellectual and Psychoeducational (2)	Intellectual abilities, academic achievement and learning capabilities (including behaviors and emotional factors affecting learning)

Continued on next page

Section G–Mental Health

Continued from previous page

Type Qualifier (Character 4)	Definition
Interactive (Ø)	Uses primarily physical aids and other forms of non-oral interaction with a patient who is physically, psychologically or developmentally unable to use ordinary language for communication Includes/Examples: Includes the use of toys in symbolic play
Interpersonal (3)	Helps an individual make changes in interpersonal behaviors to reduce psychological dysfunction Includes/Examples: Includes exploratory techniques, encouragement of affective expression, clarification of patient statements, analysis of communication patterns, use of therapy relationship and behavior change techniques
Neurobehavioral Status/Cognitive Status (4)	Includes neurobehavioral status exam, interview(s), and observation for the clinical assessment of thinking, reasoning and judgment, acquired knowledge, attention, memory, visual spatial abilities, language functions, and planning
Neuropsychological (3)	Thinking, reasoning and judgment, acquired knowledge, attention, memory, visual spatial abilities, language functions, planning
Personality and Behavioral (1)	Mood, emotion, behavior, social functioning, psychopathological conditions, personality traits and characteristics
Psychoanalysis (4)	Methods of obtaining a detailed account of past and present mental and emotional experiences to determine the source and eliminate or diminish the undesirable effects of unconscious conflicts Explanation: Accomplished by making the individual aware of their existence, origin, and inappropriate expression in emotions and behavior
Psychodynamic (5)	Exploration of past and present emotional experiences to understand motives and drives using insight-oriented techniques to reduce the undesirable effects of internal conflicts on emotions and behavior Explanation: Techniques include empathetic listening, clarifying self-defeating behavior patterns, and exploring adaptive alternatives
Psychophysiological (9)	Monitoring and alteration of physiological processes to help the individual associate physiological reactions combined with cognitive and behavioral strategies to gain improved control of these processes to help the individual cope more effectively
Supportive (6)	Formation of therapeutic relationship primarily for providing emotional support to prevent further deterioration in functioning during periods of particular stress Explanation: Often used in conjunction with other therapeutic approaches
Vocational (1)	Exploration of vocational interests, aptitudes and required adaptive behavior skills to develop and carry out a plan for achieving a successful vocational placement Includes/Examples: Includes enhancing work related adjustment and/or pursuing viable options in training education or preparation

Section H - Substance Abuse Treatment

Type (Character 3)	Definition
Detoxification Services (2)	Detoxification from alcohol and/or drugs Explanation: Not a treatment modality, but helps the patient stabilize physically and psychologically until the body becomes free of drugs and the effects of alcohol
Family Counseling (6)	The application of psychological methods that includes one or more family members to treat an individual with addictive behavior Explanation: Provides support and education for family members of addicted individuals. Family member participation is seen as a critical area of substance abuse treatment
Group Counseling (4)	The application of psychological methods to treat two or more individuals with addictive behavior Explanation: Provides structured group counseling sessions and healing power through the connection with others
Individual Counseling (3)	The application of psychological methods to treat an individual with addictive behavior Explanation: Comprised of several different techniques, which apply various strategies to address drug addiction
Individual Psychotherapy (5)	Treatment of an individual with addictive behavior by behavioral, cognitive, psychoanalytic, psychodynamic or psychophysiological means
Medication Management (8)	Monitoring and adjusting the use of replacement medications for the treatment of addiction
Pharmacotherapy (9)	The use of replacement medications for the treatment of addiction

Appendix F: Components of the Medical and Surgical Approach Definitions

Approach	Definition	Access Location	Method	Type of Instrumentation	Example
Open (Ø)	Cutting through the skin or mucous membrane and any other body layers necessary to expose the site of the procedure.	Skin or mucous membraneany other body layers	Cutting	None	Abdominal hysterectomy
Percutaneous (3)	Entry, by puncture or minor incision, of instrumentation through the skin or mucous membrane and/or any other body layers necessary to reach the site of the procedure	Skin or mucous membrane, any other body layers	Puncture or minor incision	Without visualization	Needle biopsy of liver, Liposuction
Percutaneous endoscopic (4)	Entry, by puncture or minor incision, of instrumentation through the skin or mucous membrane and/or any other body layers necessary to reach and visualize the site of the procedure	Skin or mucous membrane, any other body layers	Puncture or minor incision	With visualization	Arthroscopy, Laparoscopic cholecystectomy
Via natural or artificial opening (7)	Entry of instrumentation through a natural or artificial external opening to reach the site of the procedure	Natural or artificial external opening	Direct entry	Without visualization	Endotracheal tube insertion, Foley catheter placement
Via natural or artificial opening endoscopic (8)	Entry of instrumentation through a natural or artificial external opening to reach and visualize the site of the procedure	Natural or artificial external opening	Direct entry with puncture or minor incision for instrumentation only	With visualization	Sigmoidoscopy, EGD, ERCP
Via natural or artificial opening with percutaneous endoscopic assistance (F)	Entry of instrumentation through a natural or artificial external opening and entry, by puncture or minor incision, of instrumentation through the skin or mucous membrane and any other body layers necessary to aid in the performance of the procedure	Skin or mucous membrane, any other body layers	Cutting	With visualization	Laparoscopic-assisted vaginal hysterectomy
External (X)	Procedures performed directly on the skin or mucous membrane and procedures performed indirectly by the application of external force through the skin or mucous membrane	Skin or mucous membrane	Direct or indirect application	None	Closed fracture reduction, Resection of tonsils

Appendix G: Character Meanings

Ø: Medical and Surgical

Ø: Central Nervous System

Operation–Character 3	Body Part–Character 4	Approach–Character 5	Device–Character 6	Qualifier–Character 7
1 Bypass	Ø Brain	Ø Open	Ø Drainage Device	Ø Nasopharynx
2 Change	1 Cerebral Meninges	3 Percutaneous	2 Monitoring Device	1 Mastoid Sinus
5 Destruction	2 Dura Mater	4 Percutaneous Endoscopic	3 Infusion Device	2 Atrium
8 Division	3 Epidural Space	X External	7 Autologous Tissue Substitute	3 Blood Vessel
9 Drainage	4 Subdural Space		J Synthetic Substitute	4 Pleural Cavity
B Excision	5 Subarachnoid Space		K Nonautologous Tissue Substitute	5 Intestine
C Extirpation	6 Cerebral Ventricle		M Electrode	6 Peritoneal Cavity
D Extraction	7 Cerebral Hemisphere		Y Other Device	7 Urinary Tract
F Fragmentation	8 Basal Ganglia		Z No Device	8 Bone Marrow
H Insertion	9 Thalamus			9 Fallopian Tube
J Inspection	A Hypothalamus			B Cerebral Cisterns
K Map	B Pons			F Olfactory Nerve
N Release	C Cerebellum			G Optic Nerve
P Removal	D Medulla Oblongata			H Oculomotor Nerve
Q Repair	E Cranial Nerve			J Trochlear Nerve
S Reposition	F Olfactory Nerve			K Trigeminal Nerve
T Resection	G Optic Nerve			L Abducens Nerve
U Supplement	H Oculomotor Nerve			M Facial Nerve
W Revision	J Trochlear Nerve			N Acoustic Nerve
X Transfer	K Trigeminal Nerve			P Glossopharyngeal Nerve
	L Abducens Nerve			Q Vagus Nerve
	M Facial Nerve			R Accessory Nerve
	N Acoustic Nerve			S Hypoglossal Nerve
	P Glossopharyngeal Nerve			X Diagnostic
	Q Vagus Nerve			Z No Qualifier
	R Accessory Nerve			
	S Hypoglossal Nerve			
	T Spinal Meninges			
	U Spinal Canal			
	V Spinal Cord			
	W Cervical Spinal Cord			
	X Thoracic Spinal Cord			
	Y Lumbar Spinal Cord			

Ø: Medical and Surgical

1: Peripheral Nervous System

Operation–Character 3	Body Part–Character 4	Approach–Character 5	Device–Character 6	Qualifier–Character 7
2 Change	Ø Cervical Plexus	Ø Open	Ø Drainage Device	1 Cervical Nerve
5 Destruction	1 Cervical Nerve	3 Percutaneous	2 Monitoring Device	2 Phrenic Nerve
8 Division	2 Phrenic Nerve	4 Percutaneous Endoscopic	7 Autologous Tissue Substitute	4 Ulnar Nerve
9 Drainage	3 Brachial Plexus	X External	M Neurostimulator Lead	5 Median Nerve
B Excision	4 Ulnar Nerve		Y Other Device	6 Radial Nerve
C Extirpation	5 Median Nerve		Z No Device	8 Thoracic Nerve
D Extraction	6 Radial Nerve			B Lumbar Nerve
H Insertion	8 Thoracic Nerve			C Perineal Nerve
J Inspection	9 Lumbar Plexus			D Femoral Nerve
N Release	A Lumbosacral Plexus			F Sciatic Nerve
P Removal	B Lumbar Nerve			G Tibial Nerve
Q Repair	C Pudendal Nerve			H Peroneal Nerve
S Reposition	D Femoral Nerve			X Diagnostic
U Supplement	F Sciatic Nerve			Z No Qualifier
W Revision	G Tibial Nerve			
X Transfer	H Peroneal Nerve			
	K Head and Neck Sympathetic Nerve			
	L Thoracic Sympathetic Nerve			
	M Abdominal Sympathetic Nerve			
	N Lumbar Sympathetic Nerve			
	P Sacral Sympathetic Nerve			
	Q Sacral Plexus			
	R Sacral Nerve			
	Y Peripheral Nerve			

Ø: Medical and Surgical

2: Heart and Great Vessels

Operation–Character 3	Body Part–Character 4	Approach–Character 5	Device–Character 6	Qualifier–Character 7
1 Bypass	Ø Coronary Artery, One Site	Ø Open	Ø Monitoring Device, Pressure Sensor	Ø Allogeneic
5 Destruction	1 Coronary Artery, Two Sites	3 Percutaneous	2 Monitoring Device	1 Syngeneic
7 Dilation	2 Coronary Artery, Three Sites	4 Percutaneous Endoscopic	3 Infusion Device	2 Zooplastic
8 Division	3 Coronary Artery, Four or More Sites	X External	4 Intraluminal Device, Drug-eluting	3 Coronary Artery
B Excision	4 Coronary Vein		7 Autologous Tissue Substitute	4 Coronary Vein
C Extirpation	5 Atrial Septum		8 Zooplastic Tissue	5 Coronary Circulation
F Fragmentation	6 Atrium, Right		9 Autologous Venous Tissue	6 Bifurcation
H Insertion	7 Atrium, Left		A Autologous Arterial Tissue	7 Atrium, Left
J Inspection	8 Conduction Mechanism		C Extraluminal Device	8 Internal Mammary, Right
K Map	9 Chordae Tendineae		D Intraluminal Device	9 Internal Mammary, Left
L Occlusion	A Heart		J Synthetic Substitute OR Cardiac Lead, Pacemaker (for root operation INSERTION only)	A Pacemaker Lead
N Release	B Heart, Right		K Nonautologous Tissue Substitute OR Cardiac Lead, Defibrillator (for root operation INSERTION only)	B Subclavian
P Removal	C Heart, Left		M Cardiac Lead	C Thoracic Artery
Q Repair	D Papillary Muscle		Q Implantable Heart Assist System	D Carotid
R Replacement	F Aortic Valve		R External Heart Assist System	E Defibrillator Lead
S Reposition	G Mitral Valve		T Intraluminal Device, Radioactive	F Abdominal Artery
T Resection	H Pulmonary Valve		Z No Device	G Pressure Sensor
				H Transapical
				J Temporary
				K Left Atrial Appendage
U Supplement	J Tricuspid Valve			P Pulmonary Trunk
V Restriction	K Ventricle, Right			Q Pulmonary Artery, Right
W Revision	L Ventricle, Left			R Pulmonary Artery, Left
Y Transplantation	M Ventricular Septum			S Biventricular
	N Pericardium			T Ductus Arteriosus
	P Pulmonary Trunk			W Aorta
	Q Pulmonary Artery, Right			X Diagnostic
	R Pulmonary Artery, Left			Z No Qualifier
	S Pulmonary Vein, Right			
	T Pulmonary Vein, Left			
	V Superior Vena Cava			
	W Thoracic Aorta			
	Y Great Vessel			

Ø: Medical and Surgical

3: Upper Arteries

Operation–Character 3	Body Part–Character 4	Approach–Character 5	Device–Character 6	Qualifier–Character 7
1 Bypass	Ø Internal Mammary Artery, Right	Ø Open	Ø Drainage Device	Ø Upper Arm Artery, Right
5 Destruction	1 Internal Mammary Artery, Left	3 Percutaneous	2 Monitoring Device	1 Upper Arm Artery, Left
7 Dilation	2 Innominate Artery	4 Percutaneous Endoscopic	3 Infusion Device	2 Upper Arm Artery, Bilateral
9 Drainage	3 Subclavian Artery, Right	X External	4 Intraluminal Device, Drug-eluting	3 Lower Arm Artery, Right
B Excision	4 Subclavian Artery, Left		7 Autologous Tissue Substitute	4 Lower Arm Artery, Left
C Extirpation	5 Axillary Artery, Right		9 Autologous Venous Tissue	5 Lower Arm Artery, Bilateral
H Insertion	6 Axillary Artery, Left		A Autologous Arterial Tissue	6 Upper Leg Artery, Right
J Inspection	7 Brachial Artery, Right		B Intraluminal Device, Bioactive	7 Upper Leg Artery, Left
L Occlusion	8 Brachial Artery, Left		C Extraluminal Device	8 Upper Leg Artery, Bilateral
N Release	9 Ulnar Artery, Right		D Intraluminal Device	9 Lower Leg Artery, Right
P Removal	A Ulnar Artery, Left		J Synthetic Substitute	B Lower Leg Artery, Left
Q Repair	B Radial Artery, Right		K Nonautologous Tissue Substitute	C Lower Leg Artery, Bilateral
R Replacement	C Radial Artery, Left		M Stimulator Lead	D Upper Arm Vein
S Reposition	D Hand Artery, Right		Z No Device	F Lower Arm Vein
U Supplement	F Hand Artery, Left			G Intracranial Artery
V Restriction	G Intracranial Artery			J Extracranial Artery, Right
W Revision	H Common Carotid Artery, Right			K Extracranial Artery, Left
	J Common Carotid Artery, Left			M Pulmonary Artery, Right
	K Internal Carotid Artery, Right			N Pulmonary Artery, Left
	L Internal Carotid Artery, Left			X Diagnostic
	M External Carotid Artery, Right			Z No Qualifier
	N External Carotid Artery, Left			
	P Vertebral Artery, Right			
	Q Vertebral Artery, Left			
	R Face Artery			
	S Temporal Artery, Right			
	T Temporal Artery, Left			
	U Thyroid Artery, Right			
	V Thyroid Artery, Left			
	Y Upper Artery			

Ø: Medical and Surgical

4: Lower Arteries

Operation–Character 3	Body Part–Character 4	Approach–Character 5	Device–Character 6	Qualifier–Character 7
1 Bypass	Ø Abdominal Aorta	Ø Open	Ø Drainage Device	Ø Abdominal Aorta
5 Destruction	1 Celiac Artery	3 Percutaneous	1 Radioactive Element	1 Celiac Artery
7 Dilation	2 Gastric Artery	4 Percutaneous Endoscopic	2 Monitoring Device	2 Mesenteric Artery
9 Drainage	3 Hepatic Artery	X External	3 Infusion Device	3 Renal Artery, Right
B Excision	4 Splenic Artery		4 Intraluminal Device, Drug-eluting	4 Renal Artery, Left
C Extirpation	5 Superior Mesenteric Artery		7 Autologous Tissue Substitute	5 Renal Artery, Bilateral
H Insertion	6 Colic Artery, Right		9 Autologous Venous Tissue	6 Common Iliac Artery, Right
J Inspection	7 Colic Artery, Left		A Autologous Arterial Tissue	7 Common Iliac Artery, Left
L Occlusion	8 Colic Artery, Middle		C Extraluminal Device	8 Common Iliac Arteries, Bilateral
N Release	9 Renal Artery, Right		D Intraluminal Device	9 Internal Iliac Artery, Right
P Removal	A Renal Artery, Left		J Synthetic Substitute	B Internal Iliac Artery, Left
Q Repair	B Inferior Mesenteric Artery		K Nonautologous Tissue Substitute	C Internal Iliac Arteries, Bilateral
R Replacement	C Common Iliac Artery, Right		Z No Device	D External Iliac Artery, Right
S Reposition	D Common Iliac Artery, Left			F External Iliac Artery, Left
U Supplement	E Internal Iliac Artery, Right			G External Iliac Arteries, Bilateral
V Restriction	F Internal Iliac Artery, Left			H Femoral Artery, Right
W Revision	H External Iliac Artery, Right			J Femoral Artery, Left
	J External Iliac Artery, Left			K Femoral Arteries, Bilateral
	K Femoral Artery, Right			L Popliteal Artery
	L Femoral Artery, Left			M Peroneal Artery
	M Popliteal Artery, Right			N Posterior Tibial Artery
	N Popliteal Artery, Left			P Foot Artery
	P Anterior Tibial Artery, Right			Q Lower Extremity Artery
	Q Anterior Tibial Artery, Left			R Lower Artery
	R Posterior Tibial Artery, Right			S Lower Extremity Vein
	S Posterior Tibial Artery, Left			T Uterine Artery, Right
	T Peroneal Artery, Right			U Uterine Artery, Left
	U Peroneal Artery, Left			X Diagnostic
	V Foot Artery, Right			Z No Qualifier
	W Foot Artery, Left			
	Y Lower Artery			

Ø: Medical and Surgical

5: Upper Veins

Operation–Character 3	Body Part–Character 4	Approach–Character 5	Device–Character 6	Qualifier–Character 7
1 Bypass	Ø Azygos Vein	Ø Open	Ø Drainage Device	X Diagnostic
5 Destruction	1 Hemiazygos Vein	3 Percutaneous	2 Monitoring Device	Y Upper Vein
7 Dilation	3 Innominate Vein, Right	4 Percutaneous Endoscopic	3 Infusion Device	Z No Qualifier
9 Drainage	4 Innominate Vein, Left	X External	7 Autologous Tissue Substitute	
B Excision	5 Subclavian Vein, Right		9 Autologous Venous Tissue	
C Extirpation	6 Subclavian Vein, Left		A Autologous Arterial Tissue	
D Extraction	7 Axillary Vein, Right		C Extraluminal Device	
H Insertion	8 Axillary Vein, Left		D Intraluminal Device	
J Inspection	9 Brachial Vein, Right		J Synthetic Substitute	
L Occlusion	A Brachial Vein, Left		K Nonautologous Tissue Substitute	
N Release	B Basilic Vein, Right		Z No Device	
P Removal	C Basilic Vein, Left			
Q Repair	D Cephalic Vein, Right			
R Replacement	F Cephalic Vein, Left			
S Reposition	G Hand Vein, Right			
U Supplement	H Hand Vein, Left			
V Restriction	L Intracranial Vein			
W Revision	M Internal Jugular Vein, Right			
	N Internal Jugular Vein, Left			
	P External Jugular Vein, Right			
	Q External Jugular Vein, Left			
	R Vertebral Vein, Right			
	S Vertebral Vein, Left			
	T Face Vein, Right			
	V Face Vein, Left			
	Y Upper Vein			

Ø: Medical and Surgical

6: Lower Veins

Operation–Character 3	Body Part–Character 4	Approach–Character 5	Device–Character 6	Qualifier–Character 7
1 Bypass	Ø Inferior Vena Cava	Ø Open	Ø Drainage Device	5 Superior Mesenteric Vein
5 Destruction	1 Splenic Vein	3 Percutaneous	2 Monitoring Device	6 Inferior Mesenteric Vein
7 Dilation	2 Gastric Vein	4 Percutaneous Endoscopic	3 Infusion Device	9 Renal Vein, Right
9 Drainage	3 Esophageal Vein	X External	7 Autologous Tissue Substitute	B Renal Vein, Left
B Excision	4 Hepatic Vein		9 Autologous Venous Tissue	C Hemorrhoidal Plexus
C Extirpation	5 Superior Mesenteric Vein		A Autologous Arterial Tissue	T Via Umbilical Vein
D Extraction	6 Inferior Mesenteric Vein		C Extraluminal Device	X Diagnostic
H Insertion	7 Colic Vein		D Intraluminal Device	Y Lower Vein
J Inspection	8 Portal Vein		J Synthetic Substitute	Z No Qualifier
L Occlusion	9 Renal Vein, Right		K Nonautologous Tissue Substitute	
N Release	B Renal Vein, Left		Z No Device	
P Removal	C Common Iliac Vein, Right			
Q Repair	D Common Iliac Vein, Left			
R Replacement	F External Iliac Vein, Right			
S Reposition	G External Iliac Vein, Left			
U Supplement	H Hypogastric Vein, Right			
V Restriction	J Hypogastric Vein, Left			
W Revision	M Femoral Vein, Right			
	N Femoral Vein, Left			
	P Greater Saphenous Vein, Right			
	Q Greater Saphenous Vein, Left			
	R Lesser Saphenous Vein, Right			
	S Lesser Saphenous Vein, Left			
	T Foot Vein, Right			
	V Foot Vein, Left			
	Y Lower Vein			

Ø: Medical and Surgical

7: Lymphatic and Hemic Systems*

Operation–Character 3	Body Part–Character 4	Approach–Character 5	Device–Character 6	Qualifier–Character 7
2 Change	Ø Lymphatic, Head	Ø Open	Ø Drainage Device	Ø Allogeneic
5 Destruction	1 Lymphatic, Right Neck	3 Percutaneous	3 Infusion Device	1 Syngeneic
9 Drainage	2 Lymphatic, Left Neck	4 Percutaneous Endoscopic	7 Autologous Tissue Substitute	2 Zooplastic
B Excision	3 Lymphatic, Right Upper Extremity	X External	C Extraluminal Device	X Diagnostic
C Extirpation	4 Lymphatic, Left Upper Extremity		D Intraluminal Device	Z No Qualifier
D Extraction	5 Lymphatic, Right Axillary		J Synthetic Substitute	
H Insertion	6 Lymphatic, Left Axillary		K Nonautologous Tissue Substitute	
J Inspection	7 Lymphatic, Thorax		Y Other Device	
L Occlusion	8 Lymphatic, Internal Mammary, Right		Z No Device	
N Release	9 Lymphatic, Internal Mammary, Left			
P Removal	B Lymphatic, Mesenteric			
Q Repair	C Lymphatic, Pelvis			
S Reposition	D Lymphatic, Aortic			
T Resection	F Lymphatic, Right Lower Extremity			
U Supplement	G Lymphatic, Left Lower Extremity			
V Restriction	H Lymphatic, Right Inguinal			
W Revision	J Lymphatic, Left Inguinal			
Y Transplantation	K Thoracic Duct			
	L Cisterna Chyli			
	M Thymus			
	N Lymphatic			
	P Spleen			
	Q Bone Marrow, Sternum			
	R Bone Marrow, Iliac			
	S Bone Marrow, Vertebral			
	T Bone Marrow			

* Includes lymph vessels and lymph nodes.

Ø: Medical and Surgical

8: Eye

Operation–Character 3	Body Part–Character 4	Approach–Character 5	Device–Character 6	Qualifier–Character 7
Ø Alteration	Ø Eye, Right	Ø Open	Ø Drainage Device OR Synthetic Substitute, Intraocular Telescope (for root operation REPLACEMENT only)	3 Nasal Cavity
1 Bypass	1 Eye, Left	3 Percutaneous	1 Radioactive Element	4 Sclera
2 Change	2 Anterior Chamber, Right	7 Via Natural or Artificial Opening	3 Infusion Device	X Diagnostic
5 Destruction	3 Anterior Chamber, Left	8 Via Natural or Artificial Opening Endoscopic	7 Autologous Tissue Substitute	Z No Qualifier
7 Dilation	4 Vitreous, Right	X External	C Extraluminal Device	
9 Drainage	5 Vitreous, Left		D Intraluminal Device	
B Excision	6 Sclera, Right		J Synthetic Substitute	
C Extirpation	7 Sclera, Left		K Nonautologous Tissue Substitute	
D Extraction	8 Cornea, Right		Y Other Device	
F Fragmentation	9 Cornea, Left		Z No Device	
H Insertion	A Choroid, Right			
J Inspection	B Choroid, Left			
L Occlusion	C Iris, Right			
M Reattachment	D Iris, Left			
N Release	E Retina, Right			
P Removal	F Retina, Left			
Q Repair	G Retinal Vessel, Right			
R Replacement	H Retinal Vessel, Left			
S Reposition	J Lens, Right			
T Resection	K Lens, Left			
U Supplement	L Extraocular Muscle, Right			
V Restriction	M Extraocular Muscle, Left			
W Revision	N Upper Eyelid, Right			
X Transfer	P Upper Eyelid, Left			
	Q Lower Eyelid, Right			
	R Lower Eyelid, Left			
	S Conjunctiva, Right			
	T Conjunctiva, Left			
	V Lacrimal Gland, Right			
	W Lacrimal Gland, Left			
	X Lacrimal Duct, Right			
	Y Lacrimal Duct, Left			

Ø: Medical and Surgical

9: Ear, Nose, Sinus*

Operation–Character 3	Body Part–Character 4	Approach–Character 5	Device–Character 6	Qualifier–Character 7
Ø Alteration	Ø External Ear, Right	Ø Open	Ø Drainage Device	Ø Endolymphatic
1 Bypass	1 External Ear, Left	3 Percutaneous	4 Hearing Device, Bone Conduction	X Diagnostic
2 Change	2 External Ear, Bilateral	4 Percutaneous Endoscopic	5 Hearing Device, Single Channel Cochlear Prosthesis	Z No Qualifier
5 Destruction	3 External Auditory Canal, Right	7 Via Natural or Artificial Opening	6 Hearing Device, Multiple Channel Cochlear Prosthesis	
7 Dilation	4 External Auditory Canal, Left	8 Via Natural or Artificial Opening Endoscopic	7 Autologous Tissue Substitute	
8 Division	5 Middle Ear, Right	X External	B Intraluminal Device, Airway	
9 Drainage	6 Middle Ear, Left		D Intraluminal Device	
B Excision	7 Tympanic Membrane, Right		J Synthetic Substitute	
C Extirpation	8 Tympanic Membrane, Left		K Nonautologous Tissue Substitute	
D Extraction	9 Auditory Ossicle, Right		S Hearing Device	
H Insertion	A Auditory Ossicle, Left		Y Other Device	
J Inspection	B Mastoid Sinus, Right		Z No Device	
M Reattachment	C Mastoid Sinus, Left			
N Release	D Inner Ear, Right			
P Removal	E Inner Ear, Left			
Q Repair	F Eustachian Tube, Right			
R Replacement	G Eustachian Tube, Left			
S Reposition	H Ear, Right			
T Resection	J Ear, Left			
U Supplement	K Nose			
W Revision	L Nasal Turbinate			
	M Nasal Septum			
	N Nasopharynx			
	P Accessory Sinus			
	Q Maxillary Sinus, Right			
	R Maxillary Sinus, Left			
	S Frontal Sinus, Right			
	T Frontal Sinus, Left			
	U Ethmoid Sinus, Right			
	V Ethmoid Sinus, Left			
	W Sphenoid Sinus, Right			
	X Sphenoid Sinus, Left			
	Y Sinus			

* Includes sinus ducts.

Ø: Medical and Surgical

B: Respiratory System

Operation–Character 3	Body Part–Character 4	Approach–Character 5	Device–Character 6	Qualifier–Character 7
1 Bypass	Ø Tracheobronchial Tree	Ø Open	Ø Drainage Device	Ø Allogeneic
2 Change	1 Trachea	3 Percutaneous	1 Radioactive Element	1 Syngeneic
5 Destruction	2 Carina	4 Percutaneous Endoscopic	2 Monitoring Device	2 Zooplastic
7 Dilation	3 Main Bronchus, Right	7 Via Natural or Artificial Opening	3 Infusion Device	4 Cutaneous
9 Drainage	4 Upper Lobe Bronchus, Right	8 Via Natural or Artificial Opening Endoscopic	7 Autologous Tissue Substitute	6 Esophagus
B Excision	5 Middle Lobe Bronchus, Right	X External	C Extraluminal Device	X Diagnostic
C Extirpation	6 Lower Lobe Bronchus, Right		D Intraluminal Device	Z No Qualifier
D Extraction	7 Main Bronchus, Left		E Intraluminal Device, Endotracheal Airway	
F Fragmentation	8 Upper Lobe Bronchus, Left		F Tracheostomy Device	
H Insertion	9 Lingula Bronchus		G Intraluminal Endobronchial Valve	
J Inspection	B Lower Lobe Bronchus, Left		J Synthetic Substitute	
L Occlusion	C Upper Lung Lobe, Right		K Nonautologous Tissue Substitute	
M Reattachment	D Middle Lung Lobe, Right		M Diaphragmatic Pacemaker Lead	
N Release	F Lower Lung Lobe, Right		Y Other Device	
P Removal	G Upper Lung Lobe, Left		Z No Device	
Q Repair	H Lung Lingula			
S Reposition	J Lower Lung Lobe, Left			
T Resection	K Lung, Right			
U Supplement	L Lung, Left			
V Restriction	M Lungs, Bilateral			
W Revision	N Pleura, Right			
Y Transplantation	P Pleura, Left			
	Q Pleura			
	R Diaphragm, Right			
	S Diaphragm, Left			
	T Diaphragm			

Ø: Medical and Surgical

C: Mouth and Throat

Operation–Character 3	Body Part–Character 4	Approach–Character 5	Device–Character 6	Qualifier–Character 7
Ø Alteration	Ø Upper Lip	Ø Open	Ø Drainage Device	Ø Single
2 Change	1 Lower Lip	3 Percutaneous	1 Radioactive Element	1 Multiple
5 Destruction	2 Hard Palate	4 Percutaneous Endoscopic	5 External Fixation Device	2 All
7 Dilation	3 Soft Palate	7 Via Natural or Artificial Opening	7 Autologous Tissue Substitute	X Diagnostic
9 Drainage	4 Buccal Mucosa	8 Via Natural or Artificial Opening Endoscopic	B Intraluminal Device, Airway	Z No Qualifier
B Excision	5 Upper Gingiva	X External	C Extraluminal Device	
C Extirpation	6 Lower Gingiva		D Intraluminal Device	
D Extraction	7 Tongue		J Synthetic Substitute	
F Fragmentation	8 Parotid Gland, Right		K Nonautologous Tissue Substitute	
H Insertion	9 Parotid Gland, Left		Y Other Device	
J Inspection	A Salivary Gland		Z No Device	
L Occlusion	B Parotid Duct, Right			
M Reattachment	C Parotid Duct, Left			
N Release	D Sublingual Gland, Right			
P Removal	F Sublingual Gland, Left			
Q Repair	G Submaxillary Gland, Right			
R Replacement	H Submaxillary Gland, Left			
S Reposition	J Minor Salivary Gland			
T Resection	M Pharynx			
U Supplement	N Uvula			
V Restriction	P Tonsils			
W Revision	Q Adenoids			
X Transfer	R Epiglottis			
	S Larynx			
	T Vocal Cord, Right			
	V Vocal Cord, Left			
	W Upper Tooth			
	X Lower Tooth			
	Y Mouth and Throat			

Appendix G: Character Meanings

Ø: Medical and Surgical

D: Gastrointestinal System

Operation–Character 3	Body Part–Character 4	Approach–Character 5	Device–Character 6	Qualifier–Character 7
1 Bypass	Ø Upper Intestinal Tract	Ø Open	Ø Drainage Device	Ø Allogeneic
2 Change	1 Esophagus, Upper	3 Percutaneous	1 Radioactive Element	1 Syngeneic
5 Destruction	2 Esophagus, Middle	4 Percutaneous Endoscopic	2 Monitoring Device	2 Zooplastic
7 Dilation	3 Esophagus, Lower	7 Via Natural or Artificial Opening	3 Infusion Device	3 Vertical
8 Division	4 Esophagogastric Junction	8 Via Natural or Artificial Opening Endoscopic	7 Autologous Tissue Substitute	4 Cutaneous
9 Drainage	5 Esophagus	X External	B Intraluminal Device, Airway	5 Esophagus
B Excision	6 Stomach		C Extraluminal Device	6 Stomach
C Extirpation	7 Stomach, Pylorus		D Intraluminal Device	9 Duodenum
F Fragmentation	8 Small Intestine		J Synthetic Substitute	A Jejunum
H Insertion	9 Duodenum		K Nonautologous Tissue Substitute	B Ileum
J Inspection	A Jejunum		L Artificial Sphincter	H Cecum
L Occlusion	B Ileum		M Stimulator Lead	K Ascending Colon
M Reattachment	C Ileocecal Valve		U Feeding Device	L Transverse Colon
N Release	D Lower Intestinal Tract		Y Other Device	M Descending Colon
P Removal	E Large Intestine		Z No Device	N Sigmoid Colon
Q Repair	F Large Intestine, Right			P Rectum
R Replacement	G Large Intestine, Left			Q Anus
S Reposition	H Cecum			X Diagnostic
T Resection	J Appendix			Z No Qualifier
U Supplement	K Ascending Colon			
V Restriction	L Transverse Colon			
W Revision	M Descending Colon			
X Transfer	N Sigmoid Colon			
Y Transplantation	P Rectum			
	Q Anus			
	R Anal Sphincter			
	S Greater Omentum			
	T Lesser Omentum			
	U Omentum			
	V Mesentery			
	W Peritoneum			

Ø: Medical and Surgical

F: Hepatobiliary System and Pancreas

Operation–Character 3	Body Part–Character 4	Approach–Character 5	Device–Character 6	Qualifier–Character 7
1 Bypass	Ø Liver	Ø Open	Ø Drainage Device	Ø Allogeneic
2 Change	1 Liver, Right Lobe	3 Percutaneous	1 Radioactive Element	1 Syngeneic
5 Destruction	2 Liver, Left Lobe	4 Percutaneous Endoscopic	2 Monitoring Device	2 Zooplastic
7 Dilation	4 Gallbladder	7 Via Natural or Artificial Opening	3 Infusion Device	3 Duodenum
8 Division	5 Hepatic Duct, Right	8 Via Natural or Artificial Opening Endoscopic	7 Autologous Tissue Substitute	4 Stomach
9 Drainage	6 Hepatic Duct, Left	X External	C Extraluminal Device	5 Hepatic Duct, Right
B Excision	8 Cystic Duct		D Intraluminal Device	6 Hepatic Duct, Left
C Extirpation	9 Common Bile Duct		J Synthetic Substitute	7 Hepatic Duct, Caudate
F Fragmentation	B Hepatobiliary Duct		K Nonautologous Tissue Substitute	8 Cystic Duct
H Insertion	C Ampulla of Vater		Y Other Device	9 Common Bile Duct
J Inspection	D Pancreatic Duct		Z No Device	B Small Intestine
L Occlusion	F Pancreatic Duct, Accessory			C Large Intestine
M Reattachment	G Pancreas			X Diagnostic
N Release				Z No Qualifier
P Removal				
Q Repair				
R Replacement				
S Reposition				
T Resection				
U Supplement				
V Restriction				
W Revision				
Y Transplantation				

Ø: Medical and Surgical

G: Endocrine System

Operation–Character 3	Body Part–Character 4	Approach–Character 5	Device–Character 6	Qualifier–Character 7
2 Change	Ø Pituitary Gland	Ø Open	Ø Drainage Device	X Diagnostic
5 Destruction	1 Pineal Body	3 Percutaneous	2 Monitoring Device	Z No Qualifier
8 Division	2 Adrenal Gland, Left	4 Percutaneous Endoscopic	3 Infusion Device	
9 Drainage	3 Adrenal Gland, Right	X External	Y Other Device	
B Excision	4 Adrenal Glands, Bilateral		Z No Device	
C Extirpation	5 Adrenal Gland			
H Insertion	6 Carotid Body, Left			
J Inspection	7 Carotid Body, Right			
M Reattachment	8 Carotid Bodies, Bilateral			
N Release	9 Para-aortic Body			
P Removal	B Coccygeal Glomus			
Q Repair	C Glomus Jugulare			
S Reposition	D Aortic Body			
T Resection	F Paraganglion Extremity			
W Revision	G Thyroid Gland Lobe, Left			
	H Thyroid Gland Lobe, Right			
	J Thyroid Gland Isthmus			
	K Thyroid Gland			
	L Superior Parathyroid Gland, Right			
	M Superior Parathyroid Gland, Left			
	N Inferior Parathyroid Gland, Right			
	P Inferior Parathyroid Gland, Left			
	Q Parathyroid Glands, Multiple			
	R Parathyroid Gland			
	S Endocrine Gland			

Ø: Medical and Surgical

H: Skin and Breast*

Operation–Character 3	Body Part–Character 4	Approach–Character 5	Device–Character 6	Qualifier–Character 7
Ø Alteration	Ø Skin, Scalp	Ø Open	Ø Drainage Device	3 Full Thickness
2 Change	1 Skin, Face	3 Percutaneous	1 Radioactive Element	4 Partial Thickness
5 Destruction	2 Skin, Right Ear	7 Via Natural or Artificial Opening	7 Autologous Tissue Substitute	5 Latissimus Dorsi Myocutaneous Flap
8 Division	3 Skin, Left Ear	8 Via Natural or Artificial Opening Endoscopic	J Synthetic Substitute	6 Transverse Rectus Abdominis Myocutaneous Flap
9 Drainage	4 Skin, Neck	X External	K Nonautologous Tissue Substitute	7 Deep Inferior Epigastric Artery Perforator Flap
B Excision	5 Skin, Chest		N Tissue Expander	8 Superficial Inferior Epigastric Artery Flap
C Extirpation	6 Skin, Back		Y Other Device	9 Gluteal Artery Perforator Flap
D Extraction	7 Skin, Abdomen		Z No Device	D Multiple
H Insertion	8 Skin, Buttock			X Diagnostic
J Inspection	9 Skin, Perineum			Z No Qualifier
M Reattachment	A Skin, Genitalia			
N Release	B Skin, Right Upper Arm			
P Removal	C Skin, Left Upper Arm			
Q Repair	D Skin, Right Lower Arm			
R Replacement	E Skin, Left Lower Arm			
S Reposition	F Skin, Right Hand			
T Resection	G Skin, Left Hand			
U Supplement	H Skin, Right Upper Leg			
W Revision	J Skin, Left Upper Leg			
X Transfer	K Skin, Right Lower Leg			
	L Skin, Left Lower Leg			
	M Skin, Right Foot			
	N Skin, Left Foot			
	P Skin			
	Q Finger Nail			
	R Toe Nail			
	S Hair			
	T Breast, Right			
	U Breast, Left			
	V Breast, Bilateral			
	W Nipple, Right			
	X Nipple, Left			
	Y Supernumerary Breast			

* Includes skin and breast glands and ducts.

Ø: Medical and Surgical

J: Subcutaneous Tissue and Fascia

Operation–Character 3	Body Part–Character 4	Approach–Character 5	Device–Character 6	Qualifier–Character 7
Ø Alteration	Ø Subcutaneous Tissue and Fascia, Scalp	Ø Open	Ø Monitoring Device, Hemodynamic	B Skin and Subcutaneous Tissue
2 Change	1 Subcutaneous Tissue and Fascia, Face	3 Percutaneous	1 Radioactive Element	C Skin, Subcutaneous Tissue and Fascia
5 Destruction	4 Subcutaneous Tissue and Fascia, Anterior Neck	X External	2 Monitoring Device	X Diagnostic
8 Division	5 Subcutaneous Tissue and Fascia, Posterior Neck		3 Infusion Device	Z No Qualifier
9 Drainage	6 Subcutaneous Tissue and Fascia, Chest		4 Pacemaker, Single Chamber	
B Excision	7 Subcutaneous Tissue and Fascia, Back		5 Pacemaker, Single Chamber Rate Responsive	
C Extirpation	8 Subcutaneous Tissue and Fascia, Abdomen		6 Pacemaker, Dual Chamber	
D Extraction	9 Subcutaneous Tissue and Fascia, Buttock		7 Autologous Tissue Substitute OR Cardiac Resynchronization Pacemaker Pulse Generator (for root operation INSERTION only)	
H Insertion	B Subcutaneous Tissue and Fascia, Perineum		8 Defibrillator Generator	
J Inspection	C Subcutaneous Tissue and Fascia, Pelvic Region		9 Cardiac Resynchronization Defibrillator Pulse Generator	
N Release	D Subcutaneous Tissue and Fascia, Right Upper Arm		A Contractility Modulation Device	
P Removal	F Subcutaneous Tissue and Fascia, Left Upper Arm		B Stimulator Generator, Single Array	
Q Repair	G Subcutaneous Tissue and Fascia, Right Lower Arm		C Stimulator Generator, Single Array Rechargeable	
R Replacement	H Subcutaneous Tissue and Fascia, Left Lower Arm		D Stimulator Generator, Multiple Array	
W Revision	J Subcutaneous Tissue and Fascia, Right Hand		E Stimulator Generator, Multiple Array Rechargea	
X Transfer	K Subcutaneous Tissue and Fascia, Left Hand		H Contraceptive Device	
	L Subcutaneous Tissue and Fascia, Right Upper Leg		J Synthetic Substitute	
	M Subcutaneous Tissue and Fascia, Left Upper Leg		K Nonautologous Tissue Substitute	
	N Subcutaneous Tissue and Fascia, Right Lower Leg		M Stimulator Generator	
	P Subcutaneous Tissue and Fascia, Left Lower Leg		N Tissue Expander	
	Q Subcutaneous Tissue and Fascia, Right Foot		P Cardiac Rhythm Related Device	
	R Subcutaneous Tissue and Fascia, Left Foot		V Infusion Pump	
	S Subcutaneous Tissue and Fascia, Head and Neck		W Reservoir	
	T Subcutaneous Tissue and Fascia, Trunk		X Vascular Access Device	
	V Subcutaneous Tissue and Fascia, Upper Extremity		Y Other Device	
	W Subcutaneous Tissue and Fascia, Lower Extremity		Z No Device	

Ø: Medical and Surgical

K: Muscles

Operation–Character 3	Body Part–Character 4	Approach–Character 5	Device–Character 6	Qualifier–Character 7
2 Change	Ø Head Muscle	Ø Open	Ø Drainage Device	Ø Skin
5 Destruction	1 Facial Muscle	3 Percutaneous	7 Autologous Tissue Substitute	1 Subcutaneous Tissue
8 Division	2 Neck Muscle, Right	4 Percutaneous Endoscopic	J Synthetic Substitute	2 Skin and Subcutaneous Tissue
9 Drainage	3 Neck Muscle, Left	X External	K Nonautologous Tissue Substitute	6 Transverse Rectus Abdominis Myocutaneous Flap
B Excision	4 Tongue, Palate, Pharynx Muscle		M Stimulator Lead	X Diagnostic
C Extirpation	5 Shoulder Muscle, Right		Y Other Device	Z No Qualifier
H Insertion	6 Shoulder Muscle, Left		Z No Device	
J Inspection	7 Upper Arm Muscle, Right			
M Reattachment	8 Upper Arm Muscle, Left			
N Release	9 Lower Arm and Wrist Muscle, Right			
P Removal	B Lower Arm and Wrist Muscle, Left			
Q Repair	C Hand Muscle, Right			
S Reposition	D Hand Muscle, Left			
T Resection	F Trunk Muscle, Right			
U Supplement	G Trunk Muscle, Left			
W Revision	H Thorax Muscle, Right			
X Transfer	J Thorax Muscle, Left			
	K Abdomen Muscle, Right			
	L Abdomen Muscle, Left			
	M Perineum Muscle			
	N Hip Muscle, Right			
	P Hip Muscle, Left			
	Q Upper Leg Muscle, Right			
	R Upper Leg Muscle, Left			
	S Lower Leg Muscle, Right			
	T Lower Leg Muscle, Left			
	V Foot Muscle, Right			
	W Foot Muscle, Left			
	X Upper Muscle			
	Y Lower Muscle			

Ø: Medical and Surgical

L: Tendons*

Operation–Character 3	Body Part–Character 4	Approach–Character 5	Device–Character 6	Qualifier–Character 7
2 Change	Ø Head and Neck Tendon	Ø Open	Ø Drainage Device	X Diagnostic
5 Destruction	1 Shoulder Tendon, Right	3 Percutaneous	7 Autologous Tissue Substitute	Z No Qualifier
8 Division	2 Shoulder Tendon, Left	4 Percutaneous Endoscopic	J Synthetic Substitute	
9 Drainage	3 Upper Arm Tendon, Right	X External	K Nonautologous Tissue Substitute	
B Excision	4 Upper Arm Tendon, Left		Y Other Device	
C Extirpation	5 Lower Arm and Wrist Tendon, Right		Z No Device	
J Inspection	6 Lower Arm and Wrist Tendon, Left			
M Reattachment	7 Hand Tendon, Right			
N Release	8 Hand Tendon, Left			
P Removal	9 Trunk Tendon, Right			
Q Repair	B Trunk Tendon, Left			
R Replacement	C Thorax Tendon, Right			
S Reposition	D Thorax Tendon, Left			
T Resection	F Abdomen Tendon, Right			
U Supplement	G Abdomen Tendon, Left			
W Revision	H Perineum Tendon			
X Transfer	J Hip Tendon, Right			
	K Hip Tendon, Left			
	L Upper Leg Tendon, Right			
	M Upper Leg Tendon, Left			
	N Lower Leg Tendon, Right			
	P Lower Leg Tendon, Left			
	Q Knee Tendon, Right			
	R Knee Tendon, Left			
	S Ankle Tendon, Right			
	T Ankle Tendon, Left			
	V Foot Tendon, Right			
	W Foot Tendon, Left			
	X Upper Tendon			
	Y Lower Tendon			

* Includes synovial membrane.

Ø: Medical and Surgical

M: Bursae and Ligaments*

Operation–Character 3	Body Part–Character 4	Approach–Character 5	Device–Character 6	Qualifier–Character 7
2 Change	Ø Head and Neck Bursa and Ligament	Ø Open	Ø Drainage Device	X Diagnostic
5 Destruction	1 Shoulder Bursa and Ligament, Right	3 Percutaneous	7 Autologous Tissue Substitute	Z No Qualifier
8 Division	2 Shoulder Bursa and Ligament, Left	4 Percutaneous Endoscopic	J Synthetic Substitute	
9 Drainage	3 Elbow Bursa and Ligament, Right	X External	K Nonautologous Tissue Substitute	
B Excision	4 Elbow Bursa and Ligament, Left		Y Other Device	
C Extirpation	5 Wrist Bursa and Ligament, Right		Z No Device	
D Extraction	6 Wrist Bursa and Ligament, Left			
J Inspection	7 Hand Bursa and Ligament, Right			
M Reattachment	8 Hand Bursa and Ligament, Left			
N Release	9 Upper Extremity Bursa and Ligament, Right			
P Removal	B Upper Extremity Bursa and Ligament, Left			
Q Repair	C Trunk Bursa and Ligament, Right			
S Reposition	D Trunk Bursa and Ligament, Left			
T Resection	F Thorax Bursa and Ligament, Right			
U Supplement	G Thorax Bursa and Ligament, Left			
W Revision	H Abdomen Bursa and Ligament, Right			
X Transfer	J Abdomen Bursa and Ligament, Left			
	K Perineum Bursa and Ligament			
	L Hip Bursa and Ligament, Right			
	M Hip Bursa and Ligament, Left			
	N Knee Bursa and Ligament, Right			
	P Knee Bursa and Ligament, Left			
	Q Ankle Bursa and Ligament, Right			
	R Ankle Bursa and Ligament, Left			
	S Foot Bursa and Ligament, Right			
	T Foot Bursa and Ligament, Left			
	V Lower Extremity Bursa and Ligament, Right			
	W Lower Extremity Bursa and Ligament, Left			
	X Upper Bursa and Ligament			
	Y Lower Bursa and Ligament			

* Includes synovial membrane.

Ø: Medical and Surgical

N: Head and Facial Bones

Operation–Character 3	Body Part–Character 4	Approach–Character 5	Device–Character 6	Qualifier–Character 7
2 Change	Ø Skull	Ø Open	Ø Drainage Device	X Diagnostic
5 Destruction	1 Frontal Bone, Right	3 Percutaneous	4 Internal Fixation Device	Z No Qualifier
8 Division	2 Frontal Bone, Left	4 Percutaneous Endoscopic	5 External Fixation Device	
9 Drainage	3 Parietal Bone, Right	X External	7 Autologous Tissue Substitute	
B Excision	4 Parietal Bone, Left		J Synthetic Substitute	
C Extirpation	5 Temporal Bone, Right		K Nonautologous Tissue Substitute	
H Insertion	6 Temporal Bone, Left		M Bone Growth Stimulator	
J Inspection	7 Occipital Bone, Right		N Neurostimulator Generator	
N Release	8 Occipital Bone, Left		S Hearing Device, Bone Conduction	
P Removal	B Nasal Bone		Y Other Device	
Q Repair	C Sphenoid Bone, Right		Z No Device	
R Replacement	D Sphenoid Bone, Left			
S Reposition	F Ethmoid Bone, Right			
T Resection	G Ethmoid Bone, Left			
U Supplement	H Lacrimal Bone, Right			
W Revision	J Lacrimal Bone, Left			
	K Palatine Bone, Right			
	L Palatine Bone, Left			
	M Zygomatic Bone, Right			
	N Zygomatic Bone, Left			
	P Orbit, Right			
	Q Orbit, Left			
	R Maxilla, Right			
	S Maxilla, Left			
	T Mandible, Right			
	V Mandible, Left			
	W Facial Bone			
	X Hyoid Bone			

Ø: Medical and Surgical

P: Upper Bones

Operation–Character 3	Body Part–Character 4	Approach–Character 5	Device–Character 6	Qualifier–Character 7
2 Change	Ø Sternum	Ø Open	Ø Drainage Device OR Internal Fixation Device, Rigid Plate (for root operation INSERTION only)	X Diagnostic
5 Destruction	1 Rib, Right	3 Percutaneous	4 Internal Fixation Device	Z No Qualifier
8 Division	2 Rib, Left	4 Percutaneous Endoscopic	5 External Fixation Device	
9 Drainage	3 Cervical Vertebra	X External	6 Internal Fixation Device, Intramedullary	
B Excision	4 Thoracic Vertebra		7 Autologous Tissue Substitute	
C Extirpation	5 Scapula, Right		8 External Fixation Device, Limb Lengthening	
H Insertion	6 Scapula, Left		B External Fixation Device, Monoplanar	
J Inspection	7 Glenoid Cavity, Right		C External Fixation Device, Ring	
N Release	8 Glenoid Cavity, Left		D External Fixation Device, Hybrid	
P Removal	9 Clavicle, Right		J Synthetic Substitute	
Q Repair	B Clavicle, Left		K Nonautologous Tissue Substitute	
R Replacement	C Humeral Head, Right		M Bone Growth Stimulator	
S Reposition	D Humeral Head, Left		Y Other Device	
T Resection	F Humeral Shaft, Right		Z No Device	
U Supplement	G Humeral Shaft, Left			
W Revision	H Radius, Right			
	J Radius, Left			
	K Ulna, Right			
	L Ulna, Left			
	M Carpal, Right			
	N Carpal, Left			
	P Metacarpal, Right			
	Q Metacarpal, Left			
	R Thumb Phalanx, Right			
	S Thumb Phalanx, Left			
	T Finger Phalanx, Right			
	V Finger Phalanx, Left			
	Y Upper Bone			

Ø: Medical and Surgical

Q: Lower Bones

Operation–Character 3	Body Part–Character 4	Approach–Character 5	Device–Character 6	Qualifier–Character 7
2 Change	Ø Lumbar Vertebra	Ø Open	Ø Drainage Device	X Diagnostic
5 Destruction	1 Sacrum	3 Percutaneous	4 Internal Fixation Device	Z No Qualifier
8 Division	2 Pelvic Bone, Right	4 Percutaneous Endoscopic	5 External Fixation Device	
9 Drainage	3 Pelvic Bone, Left	X External	6 Internal Fixation Device, Intramedullary	
B Excision	4 Acetabulum, Right		7 Autologous Tissue Substitute	
C Extirpation	5 Acetabulum, Left		8 External Fixation Device, Limb Lengthening	
H Insertion	6 Upper Femur, Right		B External Fixation Device, Monoplanar	
J Inspection	7 Upper Femur, Left		C External Fixation Device, Ring	
N Release	8 Femoral Shaft, Right		D External Fixation Device, Hybrid	
P Removal	9 Femoral Shaft, Left		J Synthetic Substitute	
Q Repair	B Lower Femur, Right		K Nonautologous Tissue Substitute	
R Replacement	C Lower Femur, Left		M Bone Growth Stimulator	
S Reposition	D Patella, Right		Y Other Device	
T Resection	F Patella, Left		Z No Device	
U Supplement	G Tibia, Right			
W Revision	H Tibia, Left			
	J Fibula, Right			
	K Fibula, Left			
	L Tarsal, Right			
	M Tarsal, Left			
	N Metatarsal, Right			
	P Metatarsal, Left			
	Q Toe Phalanx, Right			
	R Toe Phalanx, Left			
	S Coccyx			
	Y Lower Bone			

Ø: Medical and Surgical

R: Upper Joints*

Operation–Character 3	Body Part–Character 4	Approach–Character 5	Device–Character 6	Qualifier–Character 7
2 Change	Ø Occipital-cervical Joint	Ø Open	Ø Drainage Device OR Synthetic Substitute, Reverse Ball and Socket (for root operation REPLACEMENT only)	Ø Anterior Approach, Anterior Column
5 Destruction	1 Cervical Vertebral Joint	3 Percutaneous	3 Infusion Device	1 Posterior Approach, Posterior Column
9 Drainage	2 Cervical Vertebral Joint, 2 or more	4 Percutaneous Endoscopic	4 Internal Fixation Device	6 Humeral Surface
B Excision	3 Cervical Vertebral Disc	X External	5 External Fixation Device	7 Glenoid Surface
C Extirpation	4 Cervicothoracic Vertebral Joint		7 Autologous Tissue Substitute	J Posterior Approach, Anterior Column
G Fusion	5 Cervicothoracic Vertebral Disc		8 Spacer	X Diagnostic
H Insertion	6 Thoracic Vertebral Joint		A Interbody Fusion	Z No Qualifier
J Inspection	7 Thoracic Vertebral Joint, 2 to 7		B Spinal Stabilization Device, Interspinous Process	
N Release	8 Thoracic Vertebral Joint, 8 or more		C Spinal Stabilization Device, Pedicle-Based	
P Removal	9 Thoracic Vertebral Disc		D Spinal Stabilization Device, Facet Replacement	
Q Repair	A Thoracolumbar Vertebral Joint		J Synthetic Substitute	
R Replacement	B Thoracolumbar Vertebral Disc		K Nonautologous Tissue Substitute	
S Reposition	C Temporomandibular Joint, Right		Y Other Device	
T Resection	D Temporomandibular Joint, Left		Z No Device	
U Supplement	E Sternoclavicular Joint, Right			
W Revision	F Sternoclavicular Joint, Left			
	G Acromioclavicular Joint, Right			
	H Acromioclavicular Joint, Left			
	J Shoulder Joint, Right			
	K Shoulder Joint, Left			
	L Elbow Joint, Right			
	M Elbow Joint, Left			
	N Wrist Joint, Right			
	P Wrist Joint, Left			
	Q Carpal Joint, Right			
	R Carpal Joint, Left			
	S Metacarpocarpal Joint, Right			
	T Metacarpocarpal Joint, Left			
	U Metacarpophalangeal Joint, Right			
	V Metacarpophalangeal Joint, Left			
	W Finger Phalangeal Joint, Right			
	X Finger Phalangeal Joint, Left			
	Y Upper Joint			

* Includes synovial membrane.

Ø: Medical and Surgical

S: Lower Joints*

Operation–Character 3	Body Part–Character 4	Approach–Character 5	Device–Character 6	Qualifier–Character 7
2 Change	Ø Lumbar Vertebral Joint	Ø Open	Ø Drainage Device OR Synthetic Substitute, Polyethylene (for root operation REPLACEMENT only)	Ø Anterior Approach, Anterior Column
5 Destruction	1 Lumbar Vertebral Joint, 2 or more	3 Percutaneous	1 Synthetic Substitute, Metal	1 Approach, Posterior Posterior Column
9 Drainage	2 Lumbar Vertebral Disc	4 Percutaneous Endoscopic	2 Synthetic Substitute, Metal on Polyethylene	9 Cemented
B Excision	3 Lumbosacral Joint	X External	3 Synthetic Substitute, Ceramic	A Uncemented
C Extirpation	4 Lumbosacral Disc		4 Internal Fixation Device OR Synthetic Substitute, Ceramic on Polyethylene (for root operation REPLACEMENT only)	C Patellar Surface
G Fusion	5 Sacrococcygeal Joint		5 External Fixation Device	J Posterior Approach, Anterior Column
H Insertion	6 Coccygeal Joint		7 Autologous Tissue Substitute	X Diagnostic
J Inspection	7 Sacroiliac Joint, Right		8 Spacer	Z No Qualifier
N Release	8 Sacroiliac Joint, Left		9 Liner	
P Removal	9 Hip Joint, Right		A Interbody Fusion Device	
Q Repair	B Hip Joint, Left		B Resurfacing Device OR Spinal Stabilization Device, Interspinous Process (for root operation INSERTION only)	
R Replacement	C Knee Joint, Right		C Spinal Stabilization Device, Pedicle-Based	
S Reposition	D Knee Joint, Left		D Spinal Stabilization Device, Facet Replacement	
T Resection	F Ankle Joint, Right		J Synthetic Substitute	
U Supplement	G Ankle Joint, Left		K Nonautologous Tissue Substitute	
W Revision	H Tarsal Joint, Right		Y Other Device	
	J Tarsal Joint, Left		Z No Device	
	K Metatarsal-Tarsal Joint, Right			
	L Metatarsal-Tarsal Joint, Left			
	M Metatarsal-Phalangeal Joint, Right			
	N Metatarsal-Phalangeal Joint, Left			
	P Toe Phalangeal Joint, Right			
	Q Toe Phalangeal Joint, Left			
	Y Lower Joint			

* Includes synovial membrane.

Ø: Medical and Surgical

T: Urinary System

Operation–Character 3	Body Part–Character 4	Approach–Character 5	Device–Character 6	Qualifier–Character 7
1 Bypass	Ø Kidney, Right	Ø Open	Ø Drainage Device	Ø Allogeneic
2 Change	1 Kidney, Left	3 Percutaneous	2 Monitoring Device	1 Syngeneic
5 Destruction	2 Kidneys, Bilateral	4 Percutaneous Endoscopic	3 Infusion Device	2 Zooplastic
7 Dilation	3 Kidney Pelvis, Right	7 Via Natural or Artificial Opening	7 Autologous Tissue Substitute	3 Kidney Pelvis, Right
8 Division	4 Kidney Pelvis, Left	8 Via Natural or Artificial Opening Endoscopic	C Extraluminal Device	4 Kidney Pelvis, Left
9 Drainage	5 Kidney	X External	D Intraluminal Device	6 Ureter, Right
B Excision	6 Ureter, Right		J Synthetic Substitute	7 Ureter, Left
C Extirpation	7 Ureter, Left		K Nonautologous Tissue Substitute	8 Colon
D Extraction	8 Ureters, Bilateral		L Artificial Sphincter	9 Colocutaneous
F Fragmentation	9 Ureter		M Stimulator Lead	A Ileum
H Insertion	B Bladder		Y Other Device	B Bladder
J Inspection	C Bladder Neck		Z No Device	C Ileocutaneous
L Occlusion	D Urethra			D Cutaneous
M Reattachment				X Diagnostic
N Release				Z No Qualifier
P Removal				
Q Repair				
R Replacement				
S Reposition				
T Resection				
U Supplement				
V Restriction				
W Revision				
X Transfer				
Y Transplantation				

Ø: Medical and Surgical

U: Female Reproductive System

Operation–Character 3	Body Part–Character 4	Approach–Character 5	Device–Character 6	Qualifier–Character 7
1 Bypass	Ø Ovary, Right	Ø Open	Ø Drainage Device	Ø Allogeneic
2 Change	1 Ovary, Left	3 Percutaneous	1 Radioactive Element	1 Syngeneic
5 Destruction	2 Ovaries, Bilateral	4 Percutaneous Endoscopic	3 Infusion Device	2 Zooplastic
7 Dilation	3 Ovary	7 Via Natural or Artificial Opening	7 Autologous Tissue Substitute	5 Fallopian Tube, Right
8 Division	4 Uterine Supporting Structure	8 Via Natural or Artificial Opening Endoscopic	C Extraluminal Device	6 Fallopian Tube, Left
9 Drainage	5 Fallopian Tube, Right	F Via Natural or Artificial Opening With Percutaneous Endoscopic Assistance	D Intraluminal Device	9 Uterus
B Excision	6 Fallopian Tube, Left	X External	G Intraluminal Device, Pessary	X Diagnostic
C Extirpation	7 Fallopian Tubes, Bilateral		H Contraceptive Device	Z No Qualifier
D Extraction	8 Fallopian Tube		J Synthetic Substitute	
F Fragmentation	9 Uterus		K Nonautologous Tissue Substitute	
H Insertion	B Endometrium		Y Other Device	
J Inspection	C Cervix		Z No Device	
L Occlusion	D Uterus and Cervix			
M Reattachment	F Cul-de-sac			
N Release	G Vagina			
P Removal	H Vagina and Cul-de-sac			
Q Repair	J Clitoris			
S Reposition	K Hymen			
T Resection	L Vestibular Gland			
U Supplement	M Vulva			
V Restriction	N Ova			
W Revision				
X Transfer				
Y Transplantation				

Ø: Medical and Surgical

V: Male Reproductive System

Operation–Character 3	Body Part–Character 4	Approach–Character 5	Device–Character 6	Qualifier–Character 7
1 Bypass	Ø Prostate	Ø Open	Ø Drainage Device	J Epididymis, Right
2 Change	1 Seminal Vesicle, Right	3 Percutaneous	1 Radioactive Element	K Epididymis, Left
5 Destruction	2 Seminal Vesicle, Left	4 Percutaneous Endoscopic	3 Infusion Device	N Vas Deferens, Right
7 Dilation	3 Seminal Vesicles, Bilateral	7 Via Natural or Artificial Opening	7 Autologous Tissue Substitute	P Vas Deferens, Left
9 Drainage	4 Prostate and Seminal Vesicles	8 Via Natural or Artificial Opening Endoscopic	C Extraluminal Device	X Diagnostic
B Excision	5 Scrotum	X External	D Intraluminal Device	Z No Qualifier
C Extirpation	6 Tunica Vaginalis, Right		J Synthetic Substitute	
H Insertion	7 Tunica Vaginalis, Left		K Nonautologous Tissue Substitute	
J Inspection	8 Scrotum and Tunica Vaginalis		Y Other Device	
L Occlusion	9 Testis, Right		Z No Device	
M Reattachment	B Testis, Left			
N Release	C Testes, Bilateral			
P Removal	D Testis			
Q Repair	F Spermatic Cord, Right			
R Replacement	G Spermatic Cord, Left			
S Reposition	H Spermatic Cords, Bilateral			
T Resection	J Epididymis, Right			
U Supplement	K Epididymis, Left			
W Revision	L Epididymis, Bilateral			
	M Epididymis and Spermatic Cord			
	N Vas Deferens, Right			
	P Vas Deferens, Left			
	Q Vas Deferens, Bilateral			
	R Vas Deferens			
	S Penis			
	T Prepuce			
	V Male External Genitalia			

Ø: Medical and Surgical

W: Anatomical Regions, General

Operation–Character 3	Body Region–Character 4	Approach–Character 5	Device–Character 6	Qualifier–Character 7
Ø Alteration	Ø Head	Ø Open	Ø Drainage Device	Ø Vagina
1 Bypass	1 Cranial Cavity	3 Percutaneous	1 Radioactive Element	1 Penis
2 Change	2 Face	4 Percutaneous Endoscopic	3 Infusion Device	2 Stoma
3 Control	3 Oral Cavity and Throat	7 Via Natural or Artificial Opening	7 Autologous Tissue Substitute	4 Cutaneous
4 Creation	4 Upper Jaw	8 Via Natural or Artificial Opening Endoscopic	J Synthetic Substitute	9 Pleural Cavity, Right
8 Division	5 Lower Jaw	X External	K Nonautologous Tissue Substitute	B Pleural Cavity, Left
9 Drainage	6 Neck		Y Other Device	G Peritoneal Cavity
B Excision	8 Chest Wall		Z No Device	J Pelvic Cavity
C Extirpation	9 Pleural Cavity, Right			X Diagnostic
F Fragmentation	B Pleural Cavity, Left			Y Lower Vein
H Insertion	C Mediastinum			Z No Qualifier
J Inspection	D Pericardial Cavity			
M Reattachment	F Abdominal Wall			
P Removal	G Peritoneal Cavity			
Q Repair	H Retroperitoneum			
U Supplement	J Pelvic Cavity			
W Revision	K Upper Back			
	L Lower Back			
	M Perineum, Male			
	N Perineum, Female			
	P Gastrointestinal Tract			
	Q Respiratory Tract			
	R Genitourinary Tract			

Ø: Medical and Surgical

X: Anatomical Regions, Upper Extremities

Operation–Character 3	Body Part–Character 4	Approach–Character 5	Device–Character 6	Qualifier–Character 7
Ø Alteration	Ø Forequarter, Right	Ø Open	Ø Drainage Device	Ø Complete
2 Change	1 Forequarter, Left	3 Percutaneous	1 Radioactive Element	1 High
3 Control	2 Shoulder Region, Right	4 Percutaneous Endoscopic	3 Infusion Device	2 Mid
6 Detachment	3 Shoulder Region, Left	X External	7 Autologous Tissue Substitute	3 Low
9 Drainage	4 Axilla, Right		J Synthetic Substitute	4 Complete 1st Ray
B Excision	5 Axilla, Left		K Nonautologous Tissue Substitute	5 Complete 2nd Ray
H Insertion	6 Upper Extremity, Right		Y Other Device	6 Complete 3rd Ray
J Inspection	7 Upper Extremity, Left		Z No Device	7 Complete 4th Ray
M Reattachment	8 Upper Arm, Right			8 Complete 5th Ray
P Removal	9 Upper Arm, Left			9 Partial 1st Ray
Q Repair	B Elbow Region, Right			B Partial 2nd Ray
R Replacement	C Elbow Region, Left			C Partial 3rd Ray
U Supplement	D Lower Arm, Right			D Partial 4th Ray
W Revision	F Lower Arm, Left			F Partial 5th Ray
X Transfer	G Wrist Region, Right			L Thumb, Right
	H Wrist Region, Left			M Thumb, Left
	J Hand, Right			N Toe, Right
	K Hand, Left			P Toe, Left
	L Thumb, Right			X Diagnostic
	M Thumb, Left			Z No Qualifier
	N Index Finger, Right			
	P Index Finger, Left			
	Q Middle Finger, Right			
	R Middle Finger, Left			
	S Ring Finger, Right			
	T Ring Finger, Left			
	V Little Finger, Right			
	W Little Finger, Left			

Ø: Medical and Surgical

Y: Anatomical Regions, Lower Extremities

Operation–Character 3	Body Part–Character 4	Approach–Character 5	Device–Character 6	Qualifier–Character 7
Ø Alteration	Ø Buttock, Right	Ø Open	Ø Drainage Device	Ø Complete
2 Change	1 Buttock, Left	3 Percutaneous	1 Radioactive Element	1 High
3 Control	2 Hindquarter, Right	4 Percutaneous Endoscopic	3 Infusion Device	2 Mid
6 Detachment	3 Hindquarter, Left	X External	7 Autologous Tissue Substitute	3 Low
9 Drainage	4 Hindquarter, Bilateral		J Synthetic Substitute	4 Complete 1st Ray
B Excision	5 Inguinal Region, Right		K Nonautologous Tissue Substitute	5 Complete 2nd Ray
H Insertion	6 Inguinal Region, Left		Y Other Device	6 Complete 3rd Ray
J Inspection	7 Femoral Region, Right		Z No Device	7 Complete 4th Ray
M Reattachment	8 Femoral Region, Left			8 Complete 5th Ray
P Removal	9 Lower Extremity, Right			9 Partial 1st Ray
Q Repair	A Inguinal Region, Bilateral			B Partial 2nd Ray
U Supplement	B Lower Extremity, Left			C Partial 3rd Ray
W Revision	C Upper Leg, Right			D Partial 4th Ray
	D Upper Leg, Left			F Partial 5th Ray
	E Femoral Region, Bilateral			X Diagnostic
	F Knee Region, Right			Z No Qualifier
	G Knee Region, Left			
	H Lower Leg, Right			
	J Lower Leg, Left			
	K Ankle Region, Right			
	L Ankle Region, Left			
	M Foot, Right			
	N Foot, Left			
	P 1st Toe, Right			
	Q 1st Toe, Left			
	R 2nd Toe, Right			
	S 2nd Toe, Left			
	T 3rd Toe, Right			
	U 3rd Toe, Left			
	V 4th Toe, Right			
	W 4th Toe, Left			
	X 5th Toe, Right			
	Y 5th Toe, Left			

1: Obstetrics

Ø: Pregnancy

Operation–Character 3	Body Part–Character 4	Approach–Character 5	Device–Character 6	Qualifier–Character 7
2 Change	Ø Products of Conception	Ø Open	3 Monitoring Electrode	Ø Classical
9 Drainage	1 Products of Conception, Retained	3 Percutaneous	Y Other Device	1 Low Cervical
A Abortion	2 Products of Conception, Ectopic	4 Percutaneous Endoscopic	Z No Device	2 Extraperitoneal
D Extraction		7 Via Natural or Artificial Opening		3 Low Forceps
E Delivery		8 Via Natural or Artificial Opening Endoscopic		4 Mid Forceps
H Insertion		X External		5 High Forceps
J Inspection				6 Vacuum
P Removal				7 Internal Version
Q Repair				8 Other
S Reposition				9 Fetal Blood
T Resection				A Fetal Cerebrospinal Fluid
Y Transplantation				B Fetal Fluid, Other
				C Amniotic Fluid, Therapeutic
				D Fluid, Other
				E Nervous System
				F Cardiovascular System
				G Lymphatics & Hemic
				H Eye
				J Ear, Nose & Sinus
				K Respiratory System
				L Mouth & Throat
				M Gastrointestinal System
				N Hepatobiliary & Pancreas
				P Endocrine System
				Q Skin
				R Musculoskeletal System
				S Urinary System
				T Female Reproductive System
				U Amniotic Fluid, Diagnostic
				V Male Reproductive System
				W Laminaria
				X Abortifacient
				Y Other Body Systems
				Z No Qualifier

2: Placement

W: Anatomical Regions

Operation–Character 3	Body Region Character 4	Approach–Character 5	Device–Character 6	Qualifier–Character 7
0 Change	0 Head	X External	0 Traction Apparatus	Z No Qualifier
1 Compression	1 Face		1 Splint	
2 Dressing	2 Neck		2 Cast	
3 Immobilization	3 Abdominal Wall		3 Brace	
4 Packing	4 Chest Wall		4 Bandage	
5 Removal	5 Back		5 Packing Material	
6 Traction	6 Inguinal Region, Right		6 Pressure Dressing	
	7 Inguinal Region, Left		7 Intermittent Pressure Device	
	8 Upper Extremity, Right		8 Stereotatic Apparatus	
	9 Upper Extremity, Left		9 Wire	
	A Upper Arm, Right		Y Other Device	
	B Upper Arm, Left		Z No Device	
	C Lower Arm, Right			
	D Lower Arm, Left			
	E Hand, Right			
	F Hand, Left			
	G Thumb, Right			
	H Thumb, Left			
	J Finger, Right			
	K Finger, Left			
	L Lower Extremity, Right			
	M Lower Extremity, Left			
	N Upper Leg, Right			
	P Upper Leg, Left			
	Q Lower Leg, Right			
	R Lower Leg, Left			
	S Foot, Right			
	T Foot, Left			
	U Toe, Right			
	V Toe, Left			

2: Placement

Y: Anatomical Orifices

Operation–Character 3	Body Orifice–Character 4	Approach Character–5	Device Character–6	Qualifier Character–7
0 Change	0 Mouth and Pharynx	X External	5 Packing Material	Z No Qualifier
4 Packing	1 Nasal			
5 Removal	2 Ear			
	3 Anorectal			
	4 Female Genital Tract			
	5 Urethra			

3: Administration

Ø: Circulatory

Operation–Character 3	Body System/Region Character 4	Approach–Character 5	Substance–Character 6	Qualifier–Character 7
2 Transfusion	3 Peripheral Vein	Ø Open	A Stem Cells, Embryonic	Ø Autologous
	4 Central Vein	3 Percutaneous	G Bone Marrow	1 Nonautologous
	5 Peripheral Artery	7 Via Natural or Artificial Opening	H Whole Blood	Z No Qualifier
	6 Central Artery		J Serum Albumin	
	7 Products of Conception, Circulatory		K Frozen Plasma	
			L Fresh Plasma	
			M Plasma Cryoprecipitate	
			N Red Blood Cells	
			P Frozen Red Cells	
			Q White Cells	
			R Platelets	
			S Globulin	
			T Fibrinogen	
			V Antihemophilic Factors	
			W Factor IX	
			X Stem Cells, Cord Blood	
			Y Stem Cells, Hematopoietic	

3: Administration

C: Indwelling Device

Operation–Character 3	Body System/Region Character 4	Approach–Character 5	Substance–Character 6	Qualifier–Character 7
1 Irrigation	Z None	X External	8 Irrigating Substance	Z No Qualifier

3: Administration

E: Physiological Systems and Anatomical Regions

Operation–Character 3	Body System/Region–Character 4	Approach–Character 5	Substance–Character 6	Qualifier–Character 7
Ø Introduction	Ø Skin and Mucous Membranes	Ø Open	Ø Antineoplastic	Ø Autologous
1 Irrigation	1 Subcutaneous Tissue	3 Percutaneous	1 Thrombolytic	1 Nonautologous
	2 Muscle	7 Via Natural or Artificial Opening	2 Anti-infective	2 High-dose Interleukin-2
	3 Peripheral Vein	8 Via Natural or Artificial Opening Endoscopic	3 Anti-inflammatory	3 Low-dose Interleukin-2
	4 Central Vein	X External	4 Serum, Toxoid and Vaccine	4 Liquid Brachytherapy Radioisotope
	5 Peripheral Artery		5 Adhesion Barrier	5 Other Antineoplastic
	6 Central Artery		6 Nutritional Substance	6 Recombinant Human-activated Protein C
	7 Coronary Artery		7 Electrolytic and Water Balance Substance	7 Other Thrombolytic
	8 Heart		8 Irrigating Substance	8 Oxazolidinones
	9 Nose		9 Dialysate	9 Other Anti-infective
	A Bone Marrow		A Stem Cells, Embryonic	A Anit-infective Envelope
	B Ear		B Local Anesthetic	B Recombinant Bone Morphogenetic Protein
	C Eye		C Regional Anesthetic	C Other Substance
	D Mouth and Pharynx		D Inhalation Anesthetic	D Nitric Oxide
	E Products of Conception		E Stem Cells, Somatic	F Other Gas
	F Respiratory Tract		F Intracirculatory Anesthetic	G Insulin
	G Upper GI		G Other Therapeutic Substance	H Human B-type Natriuretic Peptide
	H Lower GI		H Radioactive Substance	J Other Hormone
	J Biliary and Pancreatic Tract		K Other Diagnostic Substance	K Immunostimulator
	K Genitourinary Tract		L Sperm	L Immunosuppressive
	L Pleural Cavity		M Pigment	M Monoclonal Antibody
	M Peritoneal Cavity		N Analgesics, Hypnotics, Sedatives	N Blood Brain Barrier Disruption
	N Male Reproductive		P Platelet Inhibitor	P Clofarabine
	P Female Reproductive		Q Fertilized Ovum	X Diagnostic
	Q Cranial Cavity and Brain		R Antiarrhythmic	Z No Qualifier
	R Spinal Canal		S Gas	
	S Epidural Space		T Destructive Agent	
	T Peripheral Nerves and Plexi		U Pancreatic Islet Cells	
	U Joints		V Hormone	
	V Bones		W Immunotherapeutic	
	W Lymphatics		X Vasopressor	
	X Cranial Nerves			
	Y Pericardial Cavity			

4: Measurement and Monitoring

A: Physiological Systems

Operation–Character 3	Body System–Character 4	Approach–Character 5	Function/Device–Character 6	Qualifier–Character 7
Ø Measurement	Ø Central Nervous	Ø Open	Ø Acuity	Ø Central
1 Monitoring	1 Peripheral Nervous	3 Percutaneous	1 Capacity	1 Peripheral
	2 Cardiac	4 Percutaneous Endoscopic	2 Conductivity	2 Portal
	3 Arterial	7 Via Natural or Artificial Opening	3 Contractility	3 Pulmonary
	4 Venous	8 Via Natural or Artificial Opening Endoscopic	4 Electrical Activity	4 Stress
	5 Circulatory	X External	5 Flow	5 Ambulatory
	6 Lymphatic		6 Metabolism	6 Right Heart
	7 Visual		7 Mobility	7 Left Heart
	8 Olfactory		8 Motility	8 Bilateral
	9 Respiratory		9 Output	9 Sensory
	B Gastrointestinal		B Pressure	A Guidance
	C Biliary		C Rate	B Motor
	D Urinary		D Resistance	C Coronary
	F Musculoskeletal		F Rhythm	D Intracranial
	H Products of Conception, Cardiac		G Secretion	F Other Thoracic
	J Products of Conception, Nervous		H Sound	G Intraoperative
	Z None		J Pulse	Z No Qualifier
			K Temperature	
			L Volume	
			M Total Activity	
			N Sampling and Pressure	
			P Action Currents	
			Q Sleep	
			R Saturation	

4: Measurement and Monitoring

B: Physiological Devices

Operation–Character 3	Body System–Character 4	Approach–Character 5	Function/Device–Character 6	Qualifier–Character 7
Ø Measurement	Ø Central Nervous	X External	S Pacemaker	Z No Qualifier
	1 Peripheral Nervous		T Defibrillator	
	2 Cardiac		V Stimulator	
	9 Respiratory			
	F Musculoskeletal			

5: Extracorporeal Assistance and Performance

A: Physiological Systems

Operation–Character 3	Body System–Character 4	Duration–Character 5	Function–Character 6	Qualifier–Character 7
Ø Assistance	2 Cardiac	Ø Single	Ø Filtration	Ø Balloon Pump
1 Performance	5 Circulatory	1 Intermittent	1 Output	1 Hyperbaric
2 Restoration	9 Respiratory	2 Continuous	2 Oxygenation	2 Manual
	C Biliary	3 Less than 24 Consecutive Hours	3 Pacing	3 Membrane
	D Urinary	4 24-96 Consecutive Hours	4 Rhythm	4 Nonmechanical
		5 Greater than 96 Consecutive Hours	5 Ventilation	5 Pulsatile Compression
		6 Multiple		6 Other Pump
				7 Continuous Positive Airway Pressure
				8 Intermittent Positive Airway Pressure
				9 Continuous Negative Airway Pressure
				B Intermittent Negative Airway Pressure
				C Supersaturated
				D Impeller Pump
				Z No Qualifier

6: Extracorporeal Therapies

A: Physiological Systems

Operation–Character 3	Body System–Character 4	Duration–Character 5	Qualifier–Character 6	Qualifier–Character 7
Ø Atmospheric Control	Ø Skin	Ø Single	Z No Qualifier	Ø Erythrocytes
1 Decompression	1 Urinary	1 Multiple		1 Leukocytes
2 Electromagnetic Therapy	2 Central Nervous			2 Platelets
3 Hyperthermia	3 Musculoskeletal			3 Plasma
4 Hypothermia	5 Circulatory			4 Head and Neck Vessels
5 Pheresis	Z None			5 Heart
6 Phototherapy				6 Peripheral Vessels
7 Ultrasound Therapy				7 Other Vessels
8 Ultraviolet Light Therapy				T Stem Cells, Cord Blood
9 Shock Wave Therapy				V Stem Cells, Hematopoietic
				Z No Qualifier

7: Osteopathic

W: Anatomical Regions

Operation–Character 3	Body Region–Character 4	Approach–Character 5	Method–Character 6	Qualifier–Character 7
Ø Treatment	Ø Head	X External	Ø Articulatory-Raising	Z None
	1 Cervical		1 Fascial Release	
	2 Thoracic		2 General Mobilization	
	3 Lumbar		3 High Velocity-Low Amplitude	
	4 Sacrum		4 Indirect	
	5 Pelvis		5 Low Velocity-High Amplitude	
	6 Lower Extremities		6 Lymphatic Pump	
	7 Upper Extremities		7 Muscle Energy-Isometric	
	8 Rib Cage		8 Muscle Energy-Isotonic	
	9 Abdomen		9 Other Method	

8: Other Procedures

C: Indwelling Devices

Operation–Character 3	Body Region–Character 4	Approach–Character 5	Method–Character 6	Qualifier–Character 7
Ø Other procedures	1 Nervous System	X External	6 Collection	J Cerebrospinal Fluid
	2 Circulatory System			K Blood
				L Other Fluid

8: Other Procedures

E: Physiological Systems and Anatomical Regions

Operation–Character 3	Body Region–Character 4	Approach–Character 5	Method–Character 6	Qualifier–Character 7
Ø Other Procedures	1 Nervous System	Ø Open	Ø Acupuncture	Ø Anesthesia
	2 Circulatory System	3 Percutaneous	1 Therapeutic Massage	1 In Vitro Fertilization
	9 Head and Neck Region	4 Percutaneous Endoscopic	6 Collection	2 Breast Milk
	H Integumentary System and Breast	7 Via Natural or Artificial Opening	B Computer Assisted Procedure	3 Sperm
	K Musculoskeletal System	8 Via Natural or Artificial Opening Endoscopic	C Robotic Assisted Procedure	4 Yoga Therapy
	U Female Reproductive System	X External	D Near Infrared Spectroscopy	5 Meditation
	V Male Reproductive System		Y Other Method	6 Isolation
	W Trunk Region			7 Examination
	X Upper Extremity			8 Suture Removal
	Y Lower Extremity			9 Piercing
	Z None			C Prostate
				D Rectum
				F With Fluoroscopy
				G With Computerized Tomography
				H With Magnetic Resonance Imaging
				Z No Qualifier

9: Chiropractic

W: Anatomical Regions

Operation–Character 3	Body Region–Character 4	Approach–Character 5	Method–Character 6	Qualifier–Character 7
B Manipulation	Ø Head	X External	B Non-Manual	Z None
	1 Cervical		C Indirect Visceral	
	2 Thoracic		D Extra-Articular	
	3 Lumbar		F Direct Visceral	
	4 Sacrum		G Long Lever Specific Contact	
	5 Pelvis		H Short Lever Specific Contact	
	6 Lower Extremities		J Long and Short Lever Specific Contact	
	7 Upper Extremities		K Mechanically Assisted	
	8 Rib Cage		L Other Method	
	9 Abdomen			

B: Imaging

Body System–Character 2	Type–Character 3	Meanings–Character 4	Contrast–Character 5	Qualifier–Character 6	Qualifier–Character 7
Ø Central Nervous System	Ø Plain Radiography	See next page	Ø High Osmolar	Ø Unenhanced and Enhanced	Ø Intraoperative
2 Heart	1 Fluoroscopy		1 Low Osmolar	1 Laser	1 Densitometry
3 Upper Arteries	2 Computerized Tomography (CT Scan)		Y Other Contrast	2 Intravascular Optical Coherence	3 Intravascular
4 Lower Arteries	3 Magnetic Resonance Imaging (MRI)		Z None	Z None	4 Transesophageal
5 Veins	4 Ultrasonography				A Guidance
7 Lymphatic System					Z None
8 Eye					
9 Ear, Nose, Mouth and Throat					
B Respiratory System					
D Gastrointestinal System					
F Hepatobiliary System and Pancreas					
G Endocrine System					
H Skin, Subcutaneous Tissue and Breast					
L Connective Tissue					
N Skull and Facial Bones					
P Non-Axial Upper Bones					
Q Non-Axial Lower Bones					
R Axial Skeleton, Except Skull and Facial Bones					
T Urinary System					
U Female Reproductive System					
V Male Reproductive System					
W Anatomical Regions					
Y Fetus and Obstetrical					

B: Imaging

Body Part—Character 4 Meanings

Body System–Character 2	Body Part–Character 4
Ø Central Nervous System	Ø Brain 7 Cisterna 8 Cerebral Ventricle(s) 9 Sella Turcica/Pituitary Gland B Spinal Cord C Acoustic Nerves
2 Heart	Ø Coronary Artery, Single 1 Coronary Arteries, Multiple 2 Coronary Artery Bypass Graft, Single 3 Coronary Artery Bypass Grafts, Multiple 4 Heart, Right 5 Heart, Left 6 Heart, Right and Left 7 Internal Mammary Bypass Graft, Right 8 Internal Mammary Bypass Graft, Left B Heart with Aorta C Pericardium D Pediatric Heart F Bypass Graft, Other
3 Upper Arteries	Ø Thoracic Aorta 1 Brachiocephalic-Subclavian Artery, Right 2 Subclavian Artery, Left 3 Common Carotid Artery, Right 4 Common Carotid Artery, Left 5 Common Carotid Arteries, Bilateral 6 Internal Carotid Artery, Right 7 Internal Carotid Artery, Left 8 Internal Carotid Arteries, Bilateral 9 External Carotid Artery, Right B External Carotid Artery, Left C External Carotid Arteries, Bilateral D Vertebral Artery, Right F Vertebral Artery, Left G Vertebral Arteries, Bilateral H Upper Extremity Arteries, Right J Upper Extremity Arteries, Left K Upper Extremity Arteries, Bilateral L Intercostal and Bronchial Arteries M Spinal Arteries N Upper Arteries, Other P Thoraco-Abdominal Aorta Q Cervico-Cerebral Arch R Intracranial Arteries S Pulmonary Artery, Right T Pulmonary Artery, Left V Ophthalmic Arteries

Continued on next page

B: Imaging

Body Part—Character 4 Meanings

Continued from previous page

Body System–Character 2	Body Part–Character 4
4 Lower Arteries	Ø Abdominal Aorta
	1 Celiac Artery
	2 Hepatic Artery
	3 Splenic Arteries
	4 Superior Mesenteric Artery
	5 Inferior Mesenteric Artery
	6 Renal Artery, Right
	7 Renal Artery, Left
	8 Renal Arteries, Bilateral
	9 Lumbar Arteries
	B Intra-Abdominal Arteries, Other
	C Pelvic Arteries
	D Aorta and Bilateral Lower Extremity Arteries
	F Lower Extremity Arteries, Right
	G Lower Extremity Arteries, Left
	H Lower Extremity Arteries, Bilateral
	J Lower Arteries, Other
	K Celiac and Mesenteric Arteries
	L Femoral Artery
	M Renal Artery Transplant
	N Penile Arteries
5 Veins	Ø Epidural Veins
	1 Cerebral and Cerebellar Veins
	2 Intracranial Sinuses
	3 Jugular Veins, Right
	4 Jugular Veins, Left
	5 Jugular Veins, Bilateral
	6 Subclavian Vein, Right
	7 Subclavian Vein, Left
	8 Superior Vena Cava
	9 Inferior Vena Cava
	B Lower Extremity Veins, Right
	C Lower Extremity Veins, Left
	D Lower Extremity Veins, Bilateral
	F Pelvic (Iliac) Veins, Right
	G Pelvic (Iliac) Veins, Left
	H Pelvic (Iliac) Veins, Bilateral
	J Renal Vein, Right
	K Renal Vein, Left
	L Renal Veins, Bilateral
	M Upper Extremity Veins, Right
	N Upper Extremity Veins, Left
	P Upper Extremity Veins, Bilateral
	Q Pulmonary Vein, Right
	R Pulmonary Vein, Left
	S Pulmonary Veins, Bilateral
	T Portal and Splanchnic Veins
	V Veins, Other
	W Dialysis Shunt/Fistula
7 Lymphatic System	Ø Abdominal/Retroperitoneal Lymphatics, Unilateral
	1 Abdominal/Retroperitoneal Lymphatics, Bilateral
	4 Lymphatics, Head and Neck
	5 Upper Extremity Lymphatics, Right
	6 Upper Extremity Lymphatics, Left
	7 Upper Extremity Lymphatics, Bilateral
	8 Lower Extremity Lymphatics, Right
	9 Lower Extremity Lymphatics, Left
	B Lower Extremity Lymphatics, Bilateral
	C Lymphatics, Pelvic

Continued on next page

B: Imaging

Body Part—Character 4 Meanings

Continued from previous page

Body System–Character 2		Body Part–Character 4	
8	Eye	Ø	Lacrimal Duct, Right
		1	Lacrimal Duct, Left
		2	Lacrimal Ducts, Bilateral
		3	Optic Foramina, Right
		4	Optic Foramina, Left
		5	Eye, Right
		6	Eye, Left
		7	Eyes, Bilateral
9	Ear, Nose, Mouth and Throat	Ø	Ear
		2	Paranasal Sinuses
		4	Parotid Gland, Right
		5	Parotid Gland, Left
		6	Parotid Glands, Bilateral
		7	Submandibular Gland, Right
		8	Submandibular Gland, Left
		9	Submandibular Glands, Bilateral
		B	Salivary Gland, Right
		C	Salivary Gland, Left
		D	Salivary Glands, Bilateral
		F	Nasopharynx/Oropharynx
		G	Pharynx and Epiglottis
		H	Mastoids
		J	Larynx
B	Respiratory System	2	Lung, Right
		3	Lung, Left
		4	Lungs, Bilateral
		6	Diaphragm
		7	Tracheobronchial Tree, Right
		8	Tracheobronchial Tree, Left
		9	Tracheobronchial Trees, Bilateral
		B	Pleura
		C	Mediastinum
		D	Upper Airways
		F	Trachea/Airways
		G	Lung Apices
D	Gastrointestinal System	1	Esophagus
		2	Stomach
		3	Small Bowel
		4	Colon
		5	Upper GI
		6	Upper GI and Small Bowel
		7	Gastrointestinal Tract
		8	Appendix
		9	Duodenum
		B	Mouth/Oropharynx
		C	Rectum
F	Hepatobiliary System and Pancreas	Ø	Bile Ducts
		1	Biliary and Pancreatic Ducts
		2	Gallbladder
		3	Gallbladder and Bile Ducts
		4	Gallbladder, Bile Ducts and Pancreatic Ducts
		5	Liver
		6	Liver and Spleen
		7	Pancreas
		8	Pancreatic Ducts
		C	Hepatobiliary System, All
G	Endocrine System	Ø	Adrenal Gland, Right
		1	Adrenal Gland, Left
		2	Adrenal Glands, Bilateral
		3	Parathyroid Glands
		4	Thyroid Gland

Continued on next page

B: Imaging

Body Part—Character 4 Meanings

Continued from previous page

Body System–Character 2		Body Part–Character 4	
H	Skin, Subcutaneous Tissue and Breast	Ø	Breast, Right
		1	Breast, Left
		2	Breasts, Bilateral
		3	Single Mammary Duct, Right
		4	Single Mammary Duct, Left
		5	Multiple Mammary Ducts, Right
		6	Multiple Mammary Ducts, Left
		7	Extremity, Upper
		8	Extremity, Lower
		9	Abdominal Wall
		B	Chest Wall
		C	Head and Neck
		D	Subcutaneous Tissue, Head/Neck
		F	Subcutaneous Tissue, Upper Extremity
		G	Subcutaneous Tissue, Thorax
		H	Subcutaneous Tissue, Abdomen and Pelvis
		J	Subcutaneous Tissue, Lower Extremity
L	Connective Tissue	Ø	Connective Tissue, Upper Extremity
		1	Connective Tissue, Lower Extremity
		2	Tendons, Upper Extremity
		3	Tendons, Lower Extremity
N	Skull and Facial Bones	Ø	Skull
		1	Orbit, Right
		2	Orbit, Left
		3	Orbits, Bilateral
		4	Nasal Bones
		5	Facial Bones
		6	Mandible
		7	Temporomandibular Joint, Right
		8	Temporomandibular Joint, Left
		9	Temporomandibular Joints, Bilateral
		B	Zygomatic Arch, Right
		C	Zygomatic Arch, Left
		D	Zygomatic Arches, Bilateral
		F	Temporal Bones
		G	Tooth, Single
		H	Teeth, Multiple
		J	Teeth, All
P	Non-Axial Upper Bones	Ø	Sternoclavicular Joint, Right
		1	Sternoclavicular Joint, Left
		2	Sternoclavicular Joints, Bilateral
		3	Acromioclavicular Joints, Bilateral
		4	Clavicle, Right
		5	Clavicle, Left
		6	Scapula, Right
		7	Scapula, Left
		8	Shoulder, Right
		9	Shoulder, Left
		A	Humerus, Right
		B	Humerus, Left
		C	Hand/Finger Joint, Right
		D	Hand/Finger Joint, Left
		E	Upper Arm, Right
		F	Upper Arm, Left
		G	Elbow, Right
		H	Elbow, Left
		J	Forearm, Right
		K	Forearm, Left

Continued on next page

B: Imaging

Body Part—Character 4 Meanings

Continued from previous page

Body System–Character 2		Body Part–Character 4	
P	Non-Axial Upper Bones	L	Wrist, Right
		M	Wrist, Left
		N	Hand, Right
		P	Hand, Left
		Q	Hands and Wrists, Bilateral
		R	Finger(s), Right
		S	Finger(s), Left
		T	Upper Extremity, Right
		U	Upper Extremity, Left
		V	Upper Extremities, Bilateral
		W	Thorax
		X	Ribs, Right
		Y	Ribs, Left
Q	Non-Axial Lower Bones	Ø	Hip, Right
		1	Hip, Left
		2	Hips, Bilateral
		3	Femur, Right
		4	Femur, Left
		7	Knee, Right
		8	Knee, Left
		9	Knees, Bilateral
		B	Tibia/Fibula, Right
		C	Tibia/Fibula, Left
		D	Lower Leg, Right
		F	Lower Leg, Left
		G	Ankle, Right
		H	Ankle, Left
		J	Calcaneus, Right
		K	Calcaneus, Left
		L	Foot, Right
		M	Foot, Left
		P	Toe(s), Right
		Q	Toe(s), Left
		R	Lower Extremity, Right
		S	Lower Extremity, Left
		V	Patella, Right
		W	Patella, Left
		X	Foot/Toe Joint, Right
		Y	Foot/Toe Joint, Left

Continued on next page

B: Imaging

Body Part—Character 4 Meanings

Continued from previous page

Body System–Character 2		Body Part–Character 4	
R	Axial Skeleton, Except Skull and Facial Bones	Ø	Cervical Spine
		1	Cervical Disc(s)
		2	Thoracic Disc(s)
		3	Lumbar Disc(s)
		4	Cervical Facet Joint(s)
		5	Thoracic Facet Joint(s)
		6	Lumbar Facet Joint(s)
		7	Thoracic Spine
		8	Thoracolumbar Joint
		9	Lumbar Spine
		B	Lumbosacral Joint
		C	Pelvis
		D	Sacroiliac Joints
		F	Sacrum and Coccyx
		G	Whole Spine
		H	Sternum
T	Urinary System	Ø	Bladder
		1	Kidney, Right
		2	Kidney, Left
		3	Kidneys, Bilateral
		4	Kidneys, Ureters and Bladder
		5	Urethra
		6	Ureter, Right
		7	Ureter, Left
		8	Ureters, Bilateral
		9	Kidney Transplant
		B	Bladder and Urethra
		C	Ileal Diversion Loop
		D	Kidney, Ureter and Bladder, Right
		F	Kidney, Ureter and Bladder, Left
		G	Ileal Loop, Ureters and Kidneys
		J	Kidneys and Bladder
U	Female Reproductive System	Ø	Fallopian Tube, Right
		1	Fallopian Tube, Left
		2	Fallopian Tubes, Bilateral
		3	Ovary, Right
		4	Ovary, Left
		5	Ovaries, Bilateral
		6	Uterus
		8	Uterus and Fallopian Tubes
		9	Vagina
		B	Pregnant Uterus
		C	Uterus and Ovaries
V	Male Reproductive System	Ø	Corpora Cavernosa
		1	Epididymis, Right
		2	Epididymis, Left
		3	Prostate
		4	Scrotum
		5	Testicle, Right
		6	Testicle, Left
		7	Testicles, Bilateral
		8	Vasa Vasorum
		9	Prostate and Seminal Vesicles
		B	Penis

Continued on next page

B: Imaging

Body Part—Character 4 Meanings

Continued from previous page

Body System–Character 2		Body Part–Character 4	
W	Anatomical Regions	Ø	Abdomen
		1	Abdomen and Pelvis
		3	Chest
		4	Chest and Abdomen
		5	Chest, Abdomen and Pelvis
		8	Head
		9	Head and Neck
		B	Long Bones, All
		C	Lower Extremity
		F	Neck
		G	Pelvic Region
		H	Retroperitoneum
		J	Upper Extremity
		K	Whole Body
		L	Whole Skeleton
		M	Whole Body, Infant
		P	Brachial Plexus
Y	Fetus and Obstetrical	Ø	Fetal Head
		1	Fetal Heart
		2	Fetal Thorax
		3	Fetal Abdomen
		4	Fetal Spine
		5	Fetal Extremities
		6	Whole Fetus
		7	Fetal Umbilical Cord
		8	Placenta
		9	First Trimester, Single Fetus
		B	First Trimester, Multiple Gestation
		C	Second Trimester, Single Fetus
		D	Second Trimester, Multiple Gestation
		F	Third Trimester, Single Fetus
		G	Third Trimester, Multiple Gestation

C: Nuclear Medicine

Body System–Character 2	Type–Character 3	Meanings–Character 4	Radionuclide–Character 5	Qualifier–Character 6	Qualifier–Character 7
0 Central Nervous System	1 Planar Nuclear Medicine Imaging	See next Page	1 Technetium 99m (Tc-99m)	Z None	Z None
2 Heart	2 Tomographic (Tomo) Nuclear Medicine Imaging		7 Cobalt 58 (Co-58)		
5 Veins	3 Positron Emission Tomographic (PET) Imaging		8 Samarium 153 (Sm-153)		
7 Lymphatic and Hematologic System	4 Nonimaging Nuclear Medicine Uptake		9 Krypton (Kr-81m)		
8 Eye	5 Nonimaging Nuclear Medicine Probe		B Carbon 11 (C-11)		
9 Ear, Nose, Mouth and Throat	6 Nonimaging Nuclear Medicine Assay		C Cobalt 57 (Co-57)		
B Respiratory System	7 Systemic Nuclear Medicine Therapy		D Indium 111 (In-111)		
D Gastrointestinal System			F Iodine 123 (I-123)		
F Hepatobiliary System and Pancreas			G Iodine 131 (I-131)		
G Endocrine System			H Iodine 125 (I-125)		
H Skin, Subcutaneous Tissue and Breast			K Fluorine 18 (F-18)		
P Musculoskeletal System			L Gallium 67 (Ga-67)		
T Urinary System			M Oxygen 15 (O-15)		
V Male Reproductive System			N Phosphorus 32 (P-32)		
W Anatomical Regions			P Strontium 89 (Sr-89)		
			Q Rubidium 82 (Rb-82)		
			R Nitrogen 13 (N-13)		
			S Thallium 201 (Tl-201)		
			T Xenon 127 (Xe-127)		
			V Xenon 133 (Xe-133)		
			W Chromium (Cr-51)		
			Y Other Radionuclide		
			Z None		

C: Nuclear Medicine

Body Part—Character 4 Meanings

Body System–Character 2	Body Part–Character 4
Ø Central Nervous System	Ø Brain 5 Cerebrospinal Fluid Y Central Nervous System
2 Heart	6 Heart, Right and Left G Myocardium Y Heart
5 Veins	B Lower Extremity Veins, Right C Lower Extremity Veins, Left D Lower Extremity Veins, Bilateral N Upper Extremity Veins, Right P Upper Extremity Veins, Left Q Upper Extremity Veins, Bilateral R Central Veins Y Veins
7 Lymphatic and Hematologic System	Ø Bone Marrow 2 Spleen 3 Blood 5 Lymphatics, Head and Neck D Lymphatics, Pelvic J Lymphatics, Head K Lymphatics, Neck L Lymphatics, Upper Chest M Lymphatics, Trunk N Lymphatics, Upper Extremity P Lymphatics, Lower Extremity Y Lymphatic and Hematologic System
8 Eye	9 Lacrimal Ducts, Bilateral Y Eye
9 Ear, Nose, Mouth and Throat	B Salivary Glands, Bilateral Y Ear, Nose, Mouth and Throat
B Respiratory System	2 Lungs and Bronchi Y Respiratory System
D Gastrointestinal System	5 Upper Gastrointestinal Tract 7 Gastrointestinal Tract Y Digestive System
F Hepatobiliary System and Pancreas	4 Gallbladder 5 Liver 6 Liver and Spleen C Hepatobiliary System, All Y Hepatobiliary System and Pancreas
G Endocrine System	1 Parathyroid Glands 2 Thyroid Gland 4 Adrenal Glands, Bilateral Y Endocrine System
H Skin, Subcutaneous Tissue and Breast	Ø Breast, Right 1 Breast, Left 2 Breasts, Bilateral Y Skin, Subcutaneous Tissue and Breast

Continued on next page

C: Nuclear Medicine

Body Part—Character 4 Meanings

Continued from previous page

Body System–Character 2		Body Part–Character 4	
P	Musculoskeletal System	1	Skull
		2	Cervical Spine
		3	Skull and Cervical Spine
		4	Thorax
		5	Spine
		6	Pelvis
		7	Spine and Pelvis
		8	Upper Extremity, Right
		9	Upper Extremity, Left
		B	Upper Extremities, Bilateral
		C	Lower Extremity, Right
		D	Lower Extremity, Left
		F	Lower Extremities, Bilateral
		G	Thoracic Spine
		H	Lumbar Spine
		J	Thoracolumbar Spine
		N	Upper Extremities
		P	Lower Extremities
		Y	Musculoskeletal System, Other
		Z	Musculoskeletal System, All
T	Urinary System	3	Kidneys, Ureters and Bladder
		H	Bladder and Ureters
		Y	Urinary System
V	Male Reproductive System	9	Testicles, Bilateral
		Y	Male Reproductive System
W	Anatomical Regions	Ø	Abdomen
		1	Abdomen and Pelvis
		3	Chest
		4	Chest and Abdomen
		6	Chest and Neck
		B	Head and Neck
		D	Lower Extremity
		G	Thyroid
		J	Pelvic Region
		M	Upper Extremity
		N	Whole Body
		Y	Anatomical Regions, Multiple
		Z	Anatomical Region, Other

D: Radiation Oncology

Body System–Character 2	Modality–Character 3	Meanings–Character 4	Modality–Qualifier Character 5	Isotope–Character 6	Qualifier–Character 7
Ø Central and Peripheral Nervous System	Ø Beam Radiation	See next Page	Ø Photons <1 MeV	7 Cesium 137 (Cs-137)	Ø Intraoperative
7 Lymphatic and Hematologic System	1 Brachytherapy		1 Photons 1 - 1Ø MeV	8 Iridium 192 (Ir-192)	Z None
8 Eye	2 Stereotactic Radiosurgery		2 Photons >1Ø MeV	9 Iodine 125 (I-125)	
9 Ear, Nose, Mouth and Throat	Y Other Radiation		3 Electrons	B Palladium 1Ø3 (Pd-1Ø3)	
B Respiratory System			4 Heavy Particles (Protons, Ions)	C Californium 252 (Cf-252)	
D Gastrointestinal System			5 Neutrons	D Iodine 131 (I-131)	
F Hepatobiliary System and Pancreas			6 Neutron Capture	F Phosphorus 32 (P-32)	
G Endocrine System			7 Contact Radiation	G Strontium 89 (Sr-89)	
H Skin			8 Hyperthermia	H Strontium 9Ø (Sr-9Ø)	
M Breast			9 High Dose Rate (HDR)	Y Other Isotope	
P Musculoskeletal System			B Low Dose Rate (LDR)	Z None	
T Urinary System			C Intraoperative Radiation Therapy (IORT)		
U Female Reproductive System			D Stereotactic Other Photon Radiosurgery		
V Male Reproductive System			F Plaque Radiation		
W Anatomical Regions			G Isotope Administration		
			H Stereotactic Particulate Radiosurgery		
			J Stereotactic Gamma Beam Radiosurgery		
			K Laser Interstitial Thermal Therapy		

D. Radiation Oncology

Treatment Site—Character 4 Meanings

Body System–Character 2		Treatment Site–Character 4	
Ø	Central and Peripheral Nervous System	Ø	Brain
		1	Brain Stem
		6	Spinal Cord
		7	Peripheral Nerve
7	Lymphatic and Hematologic System	Ø	Bone Marrow
		1	Thymus
		2	Spleen
		3	Lymphatics, Neck
		4	Lymphatics, Axillary
		5	Lymphatics, Thorax
		6	Lymphatics, Abdomen
		7	Lymphatics, Pelvis
		8	Lymphatics, Inguinal
8	Eye	Ø	Eye
9	Ear, Nose, Mouth and Throat	Ø	Ear
		1	Nose
		3	Hypopharynx
		4	Mouth
		5	Tongue
		6	Salivary Glands
		7	Sinuses
		8	Hard Palate
		9	Soft Palate
		B	Larynx
		C	Pharynx
		D	Nasopharynx
		F	Oropharynx
B	Respiratory System	Ø	Trachea
		1	Bronchus
		2	Lung
		5	Pleura
		6	Mediastinum
		7	Chest Wall
		8	Diaphragm
D	Gastrointestinal System	Ø	Esophagus
		1	Stomach
		2	Duodenum
		3	Jejunum
		4	Ileum
		5	Colon
		7	Rectum
		8	Anus
F	Hepatobiliary System and Pancreas	Ø	Liver
		1	Gallbladder
		2	Bile Ducts
		3	Pancreas
G	Endocrine System	Ø	Pituitary Gland
		1	Pineal Body
		2	Adrenal Glands
		4	Parathyroid Glands
		5	Thyroid

Continued on next page

D. Radiation Oncology

Treatment Site—Character 4 Meanings

Continued from previous page

Body System–Character 2		Treatment Site–Character 4	
H	Skin	2	Skin, Face
		3	Skin, Neck
		4	Skin, Arm
		5	Skin, Hand
		6	Skin, Chest
		7	Skin, Back
		8	Skin, Abdomen
		9	Skin, Buttock
		B	Skin, Leg
		C	Skin, Foot
M	Breast	Ø	Breast, Left
		1	Breast, Right
P	Musculoskeletal System	Ø	Skull
		2	Maxilla
		3	Mandible
		4	Sternum
		5	Rib(s)
		6	Humerus
		7	Radius/Ulna
		8	Pelvic Bones
		9	Femur
		B	Tibia/Fibula
		C	Other Bone
T	Urinary System	Ø	Kidney
		1	Ureter
		2	Bladder
		3	Urethra
U	Female Reproductive System	Ø	Ovary
		1	Cervix
		2	Uterus
V	Male Reproductive System	Ø	Prostate
		1	Testis
W	Anatomical Regions	1	Head and Neck
		2	Chest
		3	Abdomen
		4	Hemibody
		5	Whole Body
		6	Pelvic Region

F: Physical Rehabilitation and Diagnostic Audiology

0: Rehabilitation

See next page for Character 5 Meanings

Type–Character 3	Body System–Body Region–Character 4	Equipment – Character 6	Qualifier–Character 7
0 Speech Assessment	0 Neurological System - Head and Neck	1 Audiometer	Z None
1 Motor and/or Nerve Function Assessment	1 Neurological System - Upper Back / Upper Extremity	2 Sound Field / Booth	
2 Activities of Daily Living Assessment	2 Neurological System - Lower Back / Lower Extremity	4 Electroacoustic Immitance / Acoustic Reflex	
6 Speech Treatment	3 Neurological System - Whole Body	5 Hearing Aid Selection / Fitting / Test	
7 Motor Treatment	4 Circulatory System - Head and Neck	7 Electrophysiologic	
8 Activities of Daily Living Treatment	5 Circulatory System - Upper Back / Upper Extremity	8 Vestibular / Balance	
9 Hearing Treatment	6 Circulatory System - Lower Back / Lower Extremity	9 Cochlear Implant	
B Cochlear Implant Treatment	7 Circulatory System - Whole Body	B Physical Agents	
C Vestibular Treatment	8 Respiratory System - Head and Neck	C Mechanical	
D Device Fitting	9 Respiratory System - Upper Back / Upper Extremity	D Electrotherapeutic	
F Caregiver Training	B Respiratory System - Lower Back / Lower Extremity	E Orthosis	
	C Respiratory System - Whole Body	F Assistive, Adaptive, Supportive or Protective	
	D Integumentary System - Head and Neck	G Aerobic Endurance and Conditioning	
	F Integumentary System - Upper Back / Upper Extremity	H Mechanical or Electromechanical	
	G Integumentary System - Lower Back / Lower Extremity	J Somatosensory	
	H Integumentary System - Whole Body	K Audiovisual	
	J Musculoskeletal System - Head and Neck	L Assistive Listening	
	K Musculoskeletal System - Upper Back / Upper Extremity	M Augmentative / Alternative Communication	
	L Musculoskeletal System - Lower Back / Lower Extremity	N Biosensory Feedback	
	M Musculoskeletal System - Whole Body	P Computer	
	N Genitourinary System	Q Speech Analysis	
	Z None	S Voice Analysis	
		T Aerodynamic Function	
		U Prosthesis	
		V Speech Prosthesis	
		W Swallowing	
		X Cerumen Management	
		Y Other Equipment	
		Z None	

F: Physical Rehabilitation and Diagnostic Audiology

0: Rehabilitation

Type Qualifier—Character 5 Meanings

Type–Character 3	Type Qualifier–Character 5
Ø Speech Assessment	Ø Filtered Speech
	1 Speech Threshold
	2 Speech/Word Recognition
	3 Staggered Spondaic Word
	4 Sensorineural Acuity Level
	5 Synthetic Sentence Identification
	6 Speech and/or Language Screening
	7 Nonspoken Language
	8 Receptive/Expressive Language
	9 Articulation/Phonology
	B Motor Speech
	C Aphasia
	D Fluency
	F Voice
	G Communicative/Cognitive Integration Skills
	H Bedside Swallowing and Oral Function
	J Instrumental Swallowing and Oral Function
	K Orofacial Myofunctional
	L Augmentative/Alternative Communication System
	M Voice Prosthetic
	N Non-invasive Instrumental Status
	P Oral Peripheral Mechanism
	Q Performance Intensity Phonetically Balanced Speech Discrimination
	R Brief Tone Stimuli
	S Distorted Speech
	T Dichotic Stimuli
	V Temporal Ordering of Stimuli
	W Masking Patterns
	X Other Specified Central Auditory Processing
1 Motor and/or Nerve Function Assessment	Ø Muscle Performance
	1 Integumentary Integrity
	2 Visual Motor Integration
	3 Coordination/Dexterity
	4 Motor Function
	5 Range of Motion and Joint Integrity
	6 Sensory Awareness/Processing/Integrity
	7 Facial Nerve Function
	9 Somatosensory Evoked Potentials
	B Bed Mobility
	C Transfer
	D Gait and/or Balance
	F Wheelchair Mobility
	G Reflex Integrity
2 Activities of Daily Living Assessment	Ø Bathing/Showering
	1 Dressing
	2 Feeding/Eating
	3 Grooming/Personal Hygiene
	4 Home Management
	5 Perceptual Processing
	6 Psychosocial Skills
	7 Aerobic Capacity and Endurance
	8 Anthropometric Characteristics
	9 Cranial Nerve Integrity
	B Environmental, Home and Work Barriers
	C Ergonomics and Body Mechanics
	D Neuromotor Development
	F Pain
	G Ventilation, Respiration and Circulation
	H Vocational Activities and Functional Community or Work Reintegration Skills

Continued on next page

F: Physical Rehabilitation and Diagnostic Audiology

0: Rehabilitation

Type Qualifier—Character 5 Meanings

Continued from previous page

Type–Character 3		Type Qualifier–Character 5	
6	Speech Treatment	0	Nonspoken Language
		1	Speech-Language Pathology and Related Disorders Counseling
		2	Speech-Language Pathology and Related Disorders Prevention
		3	Aphasia
		4	Articulation/Phonology
		5	Aural Rehabilitation
		6	Communicative/Cognitive Integration Skills
		7	Fluency
		8	Motor Speech
		9	Orofacial Myofunctional
		B	Receptive/Expressive Language
		C	Voice
		D	Swallowing Dysfunction
7	Motor Treatment	0	Range of Motion and Joint Mobility
		1	Muscle Performance
		2	Coordination/Dexterity
		3	Motor Function
		4	Wheelchair Mobility
		5	Bed Mobility
		6	Therapeutic Exercise
		7	Manual Therapy Techniques
		8	Transfer Training
		9	Gait Training/Functional Ambulation
8	Activities of Daily Living Treatment	0	Bathing/Showering Techniques
		1	Dressing Techniques
		2	Grooming/Personal Hygiene
		3	Feeding/Eating
		4	Home Management
		5	Wound Management
		6	Psychosocial Skills
		7	Vocational Activities and Functional Community or Work Reintegration Skills
9	Hearing Treatment	0	Hearing and Related Disorders Counseling
		1	Hearing and Related Disorders Prevention
		2	Auditory Processing
		3	Cerumen Management
B	Cochlear Implant Treatment	0	Cochlear Implant Rehabilitation
C	Vestibular Treatment	0	Vestibular
		1	Perceptual Processing
		2	Visual Motor Integration
		3	Postural Control
D	Device Fitting	0	Tinnitus Masker
		1	Monaural Hearing Aid
		2	Binaural Hearing Aid
		3	Augmentative/Alternative Communication System
		4	Voice Prosthetic
		5	Assistive Listening Device
		6	Dynamic Orthosis
		7	Static Orthosis
		8	Prosthesis
		9	Assistive, Adaptive, Supportive or Protective Devices

Continued on next page

F: Physical Rehabilitation and Diagnostic Audiology

0: Rehabilitation

Type Qualifier—Character 5 Meanings

Continued from previous page

Type–Character 3	Type Qualifier–Character 5
F Caregiver Training	Ø Bathing/Showering Technique 1 Dressing 2 Feeding and Eating 3 Grooming/Personal Hygiene 4 Bed Mobility 5 Transfer 6 Wheelchair Mobility 7 Therapeutic Exercise 8 Airway Clearance Techniques 9 Wound Management B Vocational Activities and Functional Community or Work Reintegration Skills C Gait Training/Functional Ambulation D Application, Proper Use and Care of Assistive, Adaptive, Supportive or Protective Devices F Application, Proper Use and Care of Orthoses G Application, Proper Use and Care of Prosthesis H Home Management J Communication Skills

F: Physical Rehabilitation and Diagnostic Audiology

1: Diagnostic Audiology

Type–Character 3	Body System–Body Region–Character 4	Meanings–Character 5	Equipment–Character 6	Qualifer–Character 7
3 Hearing Assessment 4 Hearing Aid Assessment 5 Vestibular Assessment	Z None	See next page	Ø Occupational Hearing 1 Audiometer 2 Sound Field / Booth 3 Tympanometer 4 Electroacoustic Immitance / Acoustic Reflex 5 Hearing Aid Selection / Fitting / Test 6 Otoacoustic Emission (OAE) 7 Electrophysiologic 8 Vestibular / Balance 9 Cochlear Implant K Audiovisual L Assistive Listening P Computer Y Other Equipment Z None	Z None

F: Physical Rehabilitation and Diagnostic Audiology

1: Diagnostic Audiology

Type Qualifier—Character 5 Meanings

Type–Character 3	Type Qualifier–Character 5
3 Hearing Assessment	Ø Hearing Screening
	1 Pure Tone Audiometry, Air
	2 Pure Tone Audiometry, Air and Bone
	3 Bekesy Audiometry
	4 Conditioned Play Audiometry
	5 Select Picture Audiometry
	6 Visual Reinforcement Audiometry
	7 Alternate Binaural or Monaural Loudness Balance
	8 Tone Decay
	9 Short Increment Sensitivity Index
	B Stenger
	C Pure Tone Stenger
	D Tympanometry
	F Eustachian Tube Function
	G Acoustic Reflex Patterns
	H Acoustic Reflex Threshold
	J Acoustic Reflex Decay
	K Electrocochleography
	L Auditory Evoked Potentials
	M Evoked Otoacoustic Emissions, Screening
	N Evoked Otoacoustic Emissions, Diagnostic
	P Aural Rehabilitation Status
	Q Auditory Processing
4 Hearing Aid Assessment	Ø Cochlear Implant
	1 Ear Canal Probe Microphone
	2 Monaural Hearing Aid
	3 Binaural Hearing Aid
	4 Assistive Listening System/Device Selection
	5 Sensory Aids
	6 Binaural Electroacoustic Hearing Aid Check
	7 Ear Protector Attentuation
	8 Monaural Electroacoustic Hearing Aid Check
5 Vestibular Assessment	Ø Bithermal, Bionaural Caloric Irrigation
	1 Bithermal, Monaural Caloric Irrigation
	2 Unithermal Binaural Screen
	3 Oscillating Tracking
	4 Sinusoidal Vertical Axis Rotational
	5 Dix-Hallpike Dynamic
	6 Computerized Dynamic Posturography
	7 Tinnitus Masker

G: Mental Health

Z: Body System—None

Type–Character 3	Type Qualifier –Character 4	Qualifier–Character 5	Qualifier–Character 6	Qualifier–Character 7
1 Psychological Tests	Ø Developmental 1 Personality and Behavioral 2 Intellectual and Psychoeducational 3 Neuropsychological 4 Neurobehavioral and Cognitive Status	Z None	Z None	Z None
2 Crisis Intervention	Z None			
3 Medication Management	Z None			
5 Individual Psychotherapy	Ø Interactive 1 Behavioral 2 Cognitive 3 Interpersonal 4 Psychoanalysis 5 Psychodynamic 6 Supportive 8 Cognitive-Behavioral 9 Psychophysiological			
6 Counseling	Ø Educational 1 Vocational 3 Other Counseling			
7 Family Psychotherapy	2 Other Family Psychotherapy			
B Electroconvulsive Therapy	Ø Unilateral-Single Seizure 1 Unilateral-Multiple Seizure 2 Bilateral-Single Seizure 3 Bilateral-Multiple Seizure 4 Other Electroconvulsive Therapy			
C Biofeedback	9 Other Biofeedback			
F Hypnosis	Z None			
G Narcosynthesis	Z None			
H Group Psychotherapy	Z None			
J Light Therapy	Z None			

H: Substance Abuse Treatment

Z: Body System—None

Type–Character 3	Type Qualifier–Character 4	Qualifier–Character 5	Qualifier–Character 6	Qualifier–Character 7
2 Detoxification Services	Z None	Z None	Z None	Z None
3 Individual Counseling	0 Cognitive 1 Behavioral 2 Cognitive-Behavioral 3 12-Step 4 Interpersonal 5 Vocational 6 Psychoeducation 7 Motivational Enhancement 8 Confrontational 9 Continuing Care B Spiritual C Pre/Post-Test Infectious Disease			
4 Group Counseling	0 Cognitive 1 Behavioral 2 Cognitive-Behavioral 3 12-Step 4 Interpersonal 5 Vocational 6 Psychoeducation 7 Motivational Enhancement 8 Confrontational 9 Continuing Care B Spiritual C Pre/Post-Test Infectious Disease			
5 Individual Psychotherapy	0 Cognitive 1 Behavioral 2 Cognitive-Behavioral 3 12-Step 4 Interpersonal 5 Interactive 6 Psychoeducation 7 Motivational Enhancement 8 Confrontational 9 Supportive B Psychoanalysis C Psychodynamic D Psychophysiological			
6 Family Counseling	3 Other Family Counseling			
8 Medication Management	0 Nicotine Replacement 1 Methadone Maintenance 2 Levo-alpha-acetyl-methadol (LAAM) 3 Antabuse 4 Naltrexone 5 Naloxone 6 Clonidine 7 Bupropion 8 Psychiatric Medication 9 Other Replacement Medication			
9 Pharmacotherapy	0 Nicotine Replacement 1 Methadone Maintenance 2 Levo-alpha-acetyl-methadol (LAAM) 3 Antabuse 4 Naltrexone 5 Naloxone 6 Clonidine 7 Bupropion 8 Psychiatric Medication 9 Other Replacement Medication			

Appendix H: Answers to Coding Exercises

Medical Surgical Section

Procedure	Code
Excision of malignant melanoma from skin of right ear	ØHB2XZZ
Laparoscopy with excision of endometrial implant from left ovary	ØUB14ZZ
Percutaneous needle core biopsy of right kidney	ØTBØ3ZX
EGD with gastric biopsy	ØDB68ZX
Open endarterectomy of left common carotid artery	Ø3CJØZZ
Excision of basal cell carcinoma of lower lip	ØCB1XZZ
Open excision of tail of pancreas	ØFBGØZZ
Percutaneous biopsy of right gastrocnemius muscle	ØKBS3ZX
Sigmoidoscopy with sigmoid polypectomy	ØDBN8ZZ
Open excision of lesion from right Achilles tendon	ØLBNØZZ
Open resection of cecum	ØDTHØZZ
Total excision of pituitary gland, open	ØGTØØZZ
Explantation of left failed kidney, open	ØTT1ØZZ
Open left axillary total lymphadenectomy	Ø7T6ØZZ (RESECTION is coded for cutting out a chain of lymph nodes.)
Laparoscopic-assisted total vaginal hysterectomy	ØUT9FZZ
Right total mastectomy, open	ØHTTØZZ
Open resection of papillary muscle	Ø2TDØZZ (The papillary muscle refers to the heart and is found in the *Heart and Great Vessels* body system.)
Radical retropubic prostatectomy, open	ØVTØØZZ
Laparoscopic cholecystectomy	ØFT44ZZ
Endoscopic bilateral total maxillary sinusectomy	Ø9TQ4ZZ, Ø9TR4ZZ
Amputation at right elbow level	ØX6BØZZ
Right below-knee amputation, proximal tibia/fibula	ØY6HØZ1 (The qualifier *High* here means the portion of the tib/fib closest to the knee.)
Fifth ray carpometacarpal joint amputation, left hand	ØX6KØZ8 (A *complete* ray amputation is through the carpometacarpal joint.)
Right leg and hip amputation through ischium	ØY62ØZZ (The *Hindquarter* body part includes amputation along any part of the hip bone.)
DIP joint amputation of right thumb	ØX6LØZ3 (The qualifier *low* here means through the distal interphalangeal joint.)
Right wrist joint amputation	ØX6JØZØ (Amputation at the wrist joint is actually complete amputation of the hand.)
Trans-metatarsal amputation of foot at left big toe	ØY6NØZ9 (A *partial* amputation is through the shaft of the metatarsal bone.)
Mid-shaft amputation, right humerus	ØX68ØZ2
Left fourth toe amputation, mid-proximal phalanx	ØY6WØZ1 (The qualifier *High* here means anywhere along the proximal phalanx.)
Right above-knee amputation, distal femur	ØY6CØZ3
Cryotherapy of wart on left hand	ØH5GXZZ
Percutaneous radiofrequency ablation of right vocal cord lesion	ØC5T3ZZ
Left heart catheterization with laser destruction of arrhythmogenic focus, A-V node	Ø2583ZZ
Cautery of nosebleed	Ø95KXZZ
Transurethral endoscopic laser ablation of prostate	ØV5Ø8ZZ
Cautery of oozing varicose vein, left calf	Ø65Y3ZZ (The approach is coded *Percutaneous* because that is the normal route to a vein. No mention is made of approach, because likely the skin has eroded at that spot.)
Laparoscopy with destruction of endometriosis, bilateral ovaries	ØU524ZZ
Laser coagulation of right retinal vessel hemorrhage, percutaneous	Ø85G3ZZ (The *Retinal Vessel* body-part values are in the *Eye* body system.)
Thoracoscopic talc instillation pleurodesis, left side	ØB5P4ZZ (See section 3, *Administration*, for applicable injection code.)
Percutaneous talc injection pleurodesis, left side	ØB5PZZ (See section 3, *Administration*, for applicable injection code.)
Sclerotherapy of brachial plexus lesion, alcohol injection	Ø1533ZZ (See section 3, *Administration*, for applicable injection code.)

Procedure	Code
Forceps total mouth extraction, upper and lower teeth	ØCDWXZ2, ØCDXXZ2
Removal of left thumbnail	ØHDQXZZ (No separate body-part value is given for thumbnail, so this is coded to *Fingernail*.)
Extraction of right intraocular lens without replacement, percutaneous	Ø8DJ3ZZ
Laparoscopy with needle aspiration of ova for in vitro fertilization	ØUDN4ZZ
Nonexcisional debridement of skin ulcer, right foot	ØHDMXZZ
Open stripping of abdominal fascia, right side	ØJD8ØZZ
Hysteroscopy with D&C, diagnostic	ØUDB8ZX
Liposuction for medical purposes, left upper arm	ØJDF3ZZ (The *Percutaneous* approach is inherent in the liposuction technique.)
Removal of tattered right ear drum fragments with tweezers	Ø9D77ZZ
Microincisional phlebectomy of spider veins, right lower leg	Ø6DY3ZZ
Routine Foley catheter placement	ØT9B7ØZ
Incision and drainage of external perianal abscess	ØD9QXZZ
Percutaneous drainage of ascites	ØW9G3ZZ (This is drainage of the cavity and not the peritoneal membrane itself.)
Laparoscopy with left ovarian cystotomy and drainage	ØU914ZZ
Laparotomy with hepatotomy and drain placement for liver abscess, right lobe	ØF91ØØZ
Right knee arthrotomy with drain placement	ØS9CØØZ
Thoracentesis of left pleural effusion	ØW9B3ZZ This is drainage of the pleural cavity
Phlebotomy of left median cubital vein for polycythemia vera	Ø59F3ZZ This median cubital vein is a branch of the cephalic vein
Percutaneous chest tube placement for right pneumothorax	ØW993ØZ
Endoscopic drainage of left ethmoid sinus	Ø99V4ZZ
Removal of foreign body, right cornea	Ø8C8XZZ
Percutaneous mechanical thrombectomy, left brachial artery	Ø3C83ZZ
Esophagogastroscopy with removal of bezoar from stomach	ØDC68ZZ
Foreign body removal, skin of left thumb	ØHCGXZZ (There is no specific value for thumb skin, so the procedure is coded to *Hand*.)
Transurethral cystoscopy with removal of bladder stone	ØTCB8ZZ
Forceps removal of foreign body in right nostril	Ø9CKXZZ (Nostril is coded to the *Nose* body-part value.)

Procedure	Code
Laparoscopy with excision of old suture from mesentery	ØDCV4ZZ
Incision and removal of right lacrimal duct stone	Ø8CXØZZ
Nonincisional removal of intraluminal foreign body from vagina	ØUCG7ZZ (The approach *External* is also a possibility. It is assumed here that since the patient went to the doctor to have the object removed, that it was not in the vaginal orifice.)
Open excision of retained sliver, subcutaneous tissue of left foot	ØJCRØZZ
Extracorporeal shockwave lithotripsy (ESWL), bilateral ureters	ØTF6XZZ, ØTF7XZZ (The *Bilateral Ureter* body-part value is not available for the root operation FRAGMENTATION, so the procedures are coded separately.)
Endoscopic retrograde cholangiopancreatography (ERCP) with lithotripsy of common bile duct stone	ØFF98ZZ (ERCP is performed through the mouth to the biliary system via the duodenum, so the approach value is *Via Natural or Artificial Opening Endoscopic*.)
Thoracotomy with crushing of pericardial calcifications	Ø2FNØZZ
Transurethral cystoscopy with fragmentation of bladder calculus	ØTFB8ZZ
Hysteroscopy with intraluminal lithotripsy of left fallopian tube calcification	ØUF68ZZ
Division of right foot tendon, percutaneous	ØL8V3ZZ
Left heart catheterization with division of bundle of HIS	Ø2883ZZ
Open osteotomy of capitate, left hand	ØP8NØZZ (The capitate is one of the carpal bones of the hand.)
EGD with esophagotomy of esophagogastric junction	ØD848ZZ
Sacral rhizotomy for pain control, percutaneous	Ø18R3ZZ
Laparotomy with exploration and adhesiolysis of right ureter	ØTN6ØZZ
Incision of scar contracture, right elbow	ØHNDXZZ (The skin of the elbow region is coded to *Lower Arm*.)
Frenulotomy for treatment of tongue-tie syndrome	ØCN7XZZ (The frenulum is coded to the body-part value *Tongue*.)
Right shoulder arthroscopy with coracoacromial ligament release	ØMN14ZZ
Mitral valvulotomy for release of fused leaflets, open approach	Ø2NGØZZ
Percutaneous left Achilles tendon release	ØLNP3ZZ

Procedure	Code
Laparoscopy with lysis of peritoneal adhesions	0DNW4ZZ
Manual rupture of right shoulder joint adhesions under general anesthesia	0RNJXZZ
Open posterior tarsal tunnel release	01NG0ZZ (The nerve released in the posterior tarsal tunnel is the tibial nerve.)
Laparoscopy with freeing of left ovary and fallopian tube	0UN14ZZ, 0UN64ZZ
Liver transplant with donor matched liver	0FY00Z0
Orthotopic heart transplant using porcine heart	02YA0Z2 (The donor heart comes from an animal [pig], so the qualifier value is *Zooplastic.*)
Right lung transplant, open, using organ donor match	0BYK0Z0
Left kidney/pancreas organ bank transplant	0FYG0Z0, 0TY10Z0
Replantation of avulsed scalp	0HM0XZZ
Reattachment of severed right ear	09M0XZZ
Reattachment of traumatic left gastrocnemius avulsion, open	0KMT0ZZ
Closed replantation of three avulsed teeth, lower jaw	0CMXXZ1
Reattachment of severed left hand	0XMK0ZZ
Right hand open palmaris longus tendon transfer	0LX70ZZ
Endoscopic radial to median nerve transfer	01X64Z5
Fasciocutaneous flap closure of left thigh, open	0JXM0ZC (The qualifier identifies the body layers in addition to fascia included in the procedure.)
Transfer left index finger to left thumb position, open	0XXP0ZM
Percutaneous fascia transfer to fill defect, anterior neck	0JX43ZZ
Trigeminal to facial nerve transfer, percutaneous endoscopic	00XK4ZM
Endoscopic left leg flexor hallucis longus tendon transfer	0LXP4ZZ
Right scalp advancement flap to right temple	0HX0XZZ
Bilateral TRAM pedicle flap reconstruction status post mastectomy, muscle only, open	0KXK0Z6, 0KXL0Z6 (The transverse rectus abdominus muscle (TRAM) flap is coded for each flap developed.)
Skin transfer flap closure of complex open wound, left lower back	0HX6XZZ
Open fracture reduction, right tibia	0QSG0ZZ
Laparoscopy with gastropexy for malrotation	0DS64ZZ
Left knee arthroscopy with reposition of anterior cruciate ligament	0MSP4ZZ
Open transposition of ulnar nerve	01S40ZZ
Closed reduction with percutaneous internal fixation of right femoral neck fracture	0QS634Z
Trans-vaginal intraluminal cervical cerclage	0UVC7DZ
Cervical cerclage using Shirodkar technique	0UVC7ZZ
Thoracotomy with banding of left pulmonary artery using extraluminal device	02VR0CZ
Restriction of thoracic duct with intraluminal stent, percutaneous	07VK3DZ
Craniotomy with clipping of cerebral aneurysm	03VG0CZ (The clip is placed lengthwise on the outside wall of the widened portion of the vessel.)
Nonincisional, trans-nasal placement of restrictive stent in right lacrimal duct	08VX7DZ
Percutaneous ligation of esophageal vein	06L33ZZ
Percutaneous embolization of left internal carotid-cavernous fistula	03LL3DZ
Laparoscopy with bilateral occlusion of fallopian tubes using Hulka extraluminal clips	0UL74CZ
Open suture ligation of failed AV graft, left brachial artery	03L80ZZ
Percutaneous embolization of vascular supply, intracranial meningioma	03LG3DZ
ERCP with balloon dilation of common bile duct	0F798ZZ
PTCA of two coronary arteries, LAD with stent placement, RCA with no stent	02703DZ, 02703ZZ (A separate procedure is coded for each artery dilated, since the device value differs for each artery.)
Cystoscopy with intraluminal dilation of bladder neck stricture	0T7C8ZZ
Open dilation of old anastomosis, left femoral artery	047L0ZZ
Dilation of upper esophageal stricture, direct visualization, with Bougie sound	0D717ZZ
PTA of right brachial artery stenosis	03773ZZ
Transnasal dilation and stent placement in right lacrimal duct	087X7DZ
Hysteroscopy with balloon dilation of bilateral fallopian tubes	0U778ZZ
Tracheoscopy with intraluminal dilation of tracheal stenosis	0B718ZZ
Cystoscopy with dilation of left ureteral stricture, with stent placement	0T778DZ
Open gastric bypass with Roux-en-Y limb to jejunum	0D160ZA
Right temporal artery to intracranial artery bypass using Gore-Tex graft, open	031S0JG
Tracheostomy formation with tracheostomy tube placement, percutaneous	0B113F4
PICVA (percutaneous in situ coronary venous arterialization) of single coronary artery	02103D4
Open left femoral-popliteal artery bypass using cadaver vein graft	041L0KL
Shunting of intrathecal cerebrospinal fluid to peritoneal cavity using synthetic shunt	00160J6
Colostomy formation, open, transverse colon to abdominal wall	0D1L0Z4

Procedure	Code
Open urinary diversion, left ureter, using ileal conduit to skin	0T170ZC
CABG of LAD using left internal mammary artery, open off-bypass	02100Z9
Open pleuroperitoneal shunt, right pleural cavity, using synthetic device	0W190JG
End-of-life replacement of spinal neurostimulator generator, multiple array, in lower abdomen	0JH80DZ (Taking out of the old generator is coded separately to the root operation REMOVAL)
Percutaneous insertion of spinal neurostimulator lead, lumbar spinal cord	00HV3MZ
Percutaneous placement of broken pacemaker lead in left atrium	02H73MZ
Open placement of dual chamber pacemaker generator in chest wall	0JH606Z
Percutaneous placement of venous central line in right internal jugular	05HM33Z
Open insertion of multiple channel cochlear implant, left ear	09HE06Z
Percutaneous placement of Swan-Ganz catheter in superior vena cava	02HV32Z (The Swan-Ganz catheter is coded to the device value *Monitoring Device* because it monitors pulmonary artery output.)
Bronchoscopy with insertion of brachytherapy seeds, right main bronchus	0BH081Z
Placement of intrathecal infusion pump for pain management, percutaneous	0JH73VZ (The device resides principally in the subcutaneous tissue of the back, so it is coded to body system *Subcutaneous Tissue and Fascia*.)
Open placement of bone growth stimulator, left femoral shaft	0QHY0MZ
Cystoscopy with placement of brachytherapy seeds in prostate gland	0VH081Z
Full-thickness skin graft to right lower arm, autograft (do not code graft harvest for this exercise)	0HRDX73
Excision of necrosed left femoral head with bone bank bone graft to fill the defect, open	0QR70KZ
Penetrating keratoplasty of right cornea with donor matched cornea, percutaneous approach	08R83KZ
Bilateral mastectomy with concomitant saline breast implants, open	0HRV0JZ
Excision of abdominal aorta with Gore-Tex graft replacement, open	04R00JZ
Total right knee arthroplasty with insertion of total knee prosthesis	0SRC0JZ
Bilateral mastectomy with free TRAM flap reconstruction	0HRV076
Tenonectomy with graft to right ankle using cadaver graft, open	0LRS0KZ

Procedure	Code
Mitral valve replacement using porcine valve, open	02RG08Z
Percutaneous phacoemulsification of right eye cataract with prosthetic lens insertion	08RJ3JZ
Aortic valve annuloplasty using ring, open	02UF0JZ
Laparoscopic repair of left inguinal hernia with marlex plug	0YU64JZ
Autograft nerve graft to right median nerve, percutaneous endoscopic (do not code graft harvest for this exercise)	01U547Z
Exchange of liner in femoral component of previous left hip replacement, open approach	0SUS09Z (Taking out of the old liner is coded separately to the root operation REMOVAL)
Anterior colporrhaphy with polypropylene mesh reinforcement, open approach	0UUG0JZ
Implantation of CorCap cardiac support device, open approach	02UA0JZ
Abdominal wall herniorrhaphy, open, using synthetic mesh	0WUF0JZ
Tendon graft to strengthen injured left shoulder using autograft, open (do not code graft harvest for this exercise)	0LU207Z
Onlay lamellar keratoplasty of left cornea using autograft, external approach	08U9X7Z
Resurfacing procedure on right femoral head, open approach	0SUR0BZ
Exchange of drainage tube from right hip joint	0S2YX0Z
Tracheostomy tube exchange	0B21XFZ
Change chest tube for left pneumothorax	0W2BX0Z
Exchange of cerebral ventriculostomy drainage tube	0020X0Z
Foley urinary catheter exchange	0T2BX0Z (This is coded to *Drainage Device* because urine is being drained.)
Open removal of lumbar sympathetic neurostimulator lead	01PY0MZ
Nonincisional removal of Swan-Ganz catheter from right pulmonary artery	02PYX2Z
Laparotomy with removal of pancreatic drain	0FPG00Z
Extubation, endotracheal tube	0BP1XFZ
Nonincisional PEG tube removal	0DP6XUZ
Transvaginal removal of extraluminal cervical cerclage	0UPD7CZ
Incision with removal of K-wire fixation, right first metatarsal	0QPN04Z
Cystoscopy with retrieval of left ureteral stent	0TP98DZ
Removal of nasogastric drainage tube for decompression	0DP6X0Z
Removal of external fixator, left radial fracture	0PPJX5Z
Reposition of Swan-Ganz catheter insertion in superior vena cava	02WYX2Z
Open revision of right hip replacement, with readjustment of prosthesis	0SW90JZ

Procedure	Code
Adjustment of position, pacemaker lead in left ventricle, percutaneous	02WA3MZ
External repositioning of Foley catheter to bladder	0TWBX0Z
Revision of VAD reservoir placement in chest wall, causing patient discomfort, open	0JWT0WZ
Thoracotomy with exploration of right pleural cavity	0WJ90ZZ
Diagnostic laryngoscopy	0CJS8ZZ
Exploratory arthrotomy of left knee	0SJD0ZZ
Colposcopy with diagnostic hysteroscopy	0UJD8ZZ
Digital rectal exam	0DJD7ZZ
Diagnostic arthroscopy of right shoulder	0RJJ4ZZ
Endoscopy of maxillary sinus	09JY4ZZ
Laparotomy with palpation of liver	0FJ00ZZ
Transurethral diagnostic cystoscopy	0TJB8ZZ
Colonoscopy, discontinued at sigmoid colon	0DJD8ZZ
Percutaneous mapping of basal ganglia	00K83ZZ
Heart catheterization with cardiac mapping	02K83ZZ
Intraoperative whole brain mapping via craniotomy	00K00ZZ
Mapping of left cerebral hemisphere, percutaneous endoscopic	00K74ZZ
Intraoperative cardiac mapping during open heart surgery	02K80ZZ
Hysteroscopy with cautery of post-hysterectomy oozing and evacuation of clot	0W3R8ZZ
Open exploration and ligation of post-op arterial bleeder, left forearm	0X3F0ZZ
Control of post-operative retroperitoneal bleeding via laparotomy	0W3H0ZZ
Reopening of thoracotomy site with drainage and control of post-op hemopericardium	0W3C0ZZ
Arthroscopy with drainage of hemarthrosis at previous operative site, right knee	0Y3F4ZZ
Radiocarpal fusion of left hand with internal fixation, open	0RGP04Z
Posterior spinal fusion at L1-L3 level with BAK cage interbody fusion device, open	0SG10A1
Intercarpal fusion of right hand with bone bank bone graft, open	0RGQ0KZ
Sacrococcygeal fusion with bone graft from same operative site, open	0SG507Z
Interphalangeal fusion of left great toe, percutaneous pin fixation	0SGQ34Z
Suture repair of left radial nerve laceration	01Q60ZZ (The approach value is *Open*, though the surgical exposure may have been created by the wound itself.)
Laparotomy with suture repair of blunt force duodenal laceration	0DQ90ZZ
Perineoplasty with repair of old obstetric laceration, open	0WQN0ZZ

Procedure	Code
Suture repair of right biceps tendon laceration, open	0LQ30ZZ
Closure of abdominal wall stab wound	0WQF0ZZ
Cosmetic face lift, open, no other information available	0W020ZZ
Bilateral breast augmentation with silicone implants, open	0H0V0JZ
Cosmetic rhinoplasty with septal reduction and tip elevation using local tissue graft, open	090K07Z
Abdominoplasty (tummy tuck), open	0W0F0ZZ
Liposuction of bilateral thighs	0J0L3ZZ, 0J0M3ZZ
Creation of penis in female patient using tissue bank donor graft	0W4N0K1
Creation of vagina in male patient using synthetic material	0W4M0J0

Obstetrics

Procedure	Code
Abortion by dilation and evacuation following laminaria insertion	10A07ZW
Manually assisted spontaneous abortion	10E0XZZ (Since the pregnancy was not artificially terminated, this is coded to *Delivery* because it captures the procedure objective. The fact that it was an abortion will be identified in the diagnosis code.)
Abortion by abortifacient insertion	10A07ZX
Bimanual pregnancy examination	10J07ZZ
Extraperitoneal C-section, low transverse incision	10D00Z2
Fetal spinal tap, percutaneous	10903ZA
Fetal kidney transplant, laparoscopic	10Y04ZS
Open in utero repair of congenital diaphragmatic hernia	10Q00ZK (Diaphragm is classified to the *Respiratory* body system in the *Medical and Surgical* section.)
Laparoscopy with total excision of tubal pregnancy	10T24ZZ
Transvaginal removal of fetal monitoring electrode	10P073Z

Placement

Procedure	Code
Placement of packing material, right ear	2Y42X5Z
Mechanical traction of entire left leg	2W6MXØZ
Removal of splint, right shoulder	2W5AX1Z
Placement of neck brace	2W32X3Z
Change of vaginal packing	2YØ4X5Z
Packing of wound, chest wall	2W44X5Z
Sterile dressing placement to left groin region	2W27X4Z
Removal of packing material from pharynx	2Y5ØX5Z
Placement of intermittent pneumatic compression device, covering entire right arm	2W18X7Z
Exchange of pressure dressing to left thigh	2WØPX6Z

Administration

Procedure	Code
Peritoneal dialysis via indwelling catheter	3E1M39Z
Transvaginal artificial insemination	3EØP7LZ
Infusion of total parenteral nutrition via central venous catheter	3EØ436Z
Esophagogastroscopy with Botox injection into esophageal sphincter	3EØG8GC (Botulinum toxin is a paralyzing agent with temporary effects; it does not sclerose or destroy the nerve.)
Percutaneous irrigation of knee joint	3E1U38Z
Epidural injection of mixed steroid and local anesthetic for pain control	3EØS33Z (This is coded to the substance value *Anti-inflammatory*. The anesthetic is added only to lessen the pain of the injection.)
Chemical pleurodesis using injection of tetracycline	3EØL3TZ
Transfusion of antihemophilic factor, (nonautologous) via arterial central line	3Ø263V1
Transabdominal in vitro fertilization, implantation of donor ovum	3EØP3Q1
Autologous bone marrow transplant via central venous line	3Ø243GØ

Measurement and Monitoring

Procedure	Code
Cardiac stress test, single measurement	4AØ2XM4
EGD with biliary flow measurement	4AØC85Z
Temperature monitoring, rectal	4A1Z7KZ
Peripheral venous pulse, external, single measurement	4AØ4XJ1
Holter monitoring	4A12X45
Respiratory rate, external, single measurement	4AØ9XCZ
Fetal heart rate monitoring, transvaginal	4A1H7CZ
Visual mobility test, single measurement	4AØ7X7Z
Pulmonary artery wedge pressure monitoring from Swan-Ganz catheter	4A133B3
Olfactory acuity test, single measurement	4AØ8XØZ

Extracorporeal Assistance and Performance

Procedure	Code
Mechanical ventilation, 16 hours	5A1935Z
Liver dialysis, single encounter	5A1CØØZ
Cardiac countershock with successful conversion to sinus rhythm	5A22Ø4Z
IPPB (intermittent positive pressure breathing) for mobilization of secretions, 22 hours	5AØ9358
Renal dialysis, series of encounters	5A1D6ØZ
IABP (intra-aortic balloon pump) continuous	5AØ221Ø (The procedure to insert the balloon pump is coded to the root operation INSERTION in the *Medical and Surgical* section).
Intra-operative cardiac pacing, continuous	5A1223Z
ECMO (extracorporeal membrane oxygenation), continuous	5A15223
Controlled mechanical ventilation (CMV), 45 hours	5A1945Z (The endotracheal tube associated with the mechanical ventilation procedure is considered a component of the equipment used in performing the procedure and is not coded separately.)
Pulsatile compression boot with intermittent inflation	5AØ2115 (This is coded to the function value *Cardiac Output*, because the purpose of such compression devices is to return blood to the heart faster.)

Extracorporeal Therapies

Procedure	Code
Donor thrombocytapheresis, single encounter	6A550Z2
Bili-lite UV phototherapy, series treatment	6A801ZZ
Whole body hypothermia, single treatment	6A4Z0ZZ
Circulatory phototherapy, single encounter	6A650ZZ
Shock wave therapy of plantar fascia, single treatment	6A930ZZ
Antigen-free air conditioning, series treatment	6A0Z1ZZ
TMS (transcranial magnetic stimulation), series treatment	6A221ZZ
Therapeutic ultrasound of peripheral vessels, single treatment	6A750ZZ
Plasmapheresis, series treatment	6A551Z3
Extracorporeal electromagnetic stimulation (EMS) for urinary incontinence, single treatment	6A210ZZ

Osteopathic

Procedures	Code
Isotonic muscle energy treatment of right leg	7W06X8Z
Low velocity-high amplitude osteopathic treatment of head	7W00X5Z
Lymphatic pump osteopathic treatment of left axilla	7W07X6Z
Indirect osteopathic treatment of sacrum	7W04X4Z
Articulatory osteopathic treatment of cervical region	7W01X0Z

Other Procedures

Procedure	Code
Near infrared spectroscopy of leg vessels	8E023DZ
CT computer assisted sinus surgery	8E09XBG (The primary procedure is coded separately.)
Suture removal, abdominal wall	8E0WXY8
Isolation after infectious disease exposure	8E0ZXY6
Robotic assisted open prostatectomy	8E0W0CZ (The primary procedure is coded separately.)

Chiropractic

Procedure	Code
Chiropractic treatment of lumbar region using long lever specific contact	9WB3XGZ
Chiropractic manipulation of abdominal region, indirect visceral	9WB9XCZ
Chiropractic extra-articular treatment of hip region	9WB6XDZ
Chiropractic treatment of sacrum using long and short lever specific contact	9WB4XJZ
Mechanically-assisted chiropractic manipulation of head	9WB0XKZ

Imaging

Procedure	Code
Noncontrast CT of abdomen and pelvis	BW21ZZZ
Intravascular ultrasound, left subclavian artery	B342ZZ3
Chest x-ray, AP/PA and lateral views	BW03ZZZ
Endoluminal ultrasound of gallbladder and bile ducts	BF43ZZZ
MRI of thyroid gland, contrast unspecified	BG34YZZ
Esophageal videofluoroscopy study with oral barium contrast	BD11YZZ
Portable x-ray study of right radius/ulna shaft, standard series	BP0JZZZ
Routine fetal ultrasound, second trimester twin gestation	BY4DZZZ
CT scan of bilateral lungs, high osmolar contrast with densitometry	BB240ZZ
Fluoroscopic guidance for percutaneous transluminal angioplasty (PTA) of left common femoral artery, low osmolar contrast	B41G1ZZ

Nuclear Medicine

Procedure	Code
Tomo scan of right and left heart, unspecified radiopharmaceutical, qualitative gated rest	C226YZZ
Technetium pentetate assay of kidneys, ureters, and bladder	CT631ZZ
Uniplanar scan of spine using technetium oxidronate, with first-pass study	CP151ZZ
Thallous chloride tomographic scan of bilateral breasts	CH22SZZ
PET scan of myocardium using rubidium	C23GQZZ
Gallium citrate scan of head and neck, single plane imaging	CW1BLZZ
Xenon gas nonimaging probe of brain	C050VZZ
Upper GI scan, radiopharmaceutical unspecified, for gastric emptying	CD15YZZ
Carbon 11 PET scan of brain with quantification	C030BZZ
Iodinated albumin nuclear medicine assay, blood plasma volume study	C763HZZ

Radiation Oncology

Procedure	Code
Plaque radiation of left eye, single port	D8YØFZZ
8 MeV photon beam radiation to brain	DØØ11ZZ
IORT of colon, 3 ports	DDY5CZZ
HDR brachytherapy of prostate using palladium-1Ø3	DV1Ø9BZ
Electron radiation treatment of right breast, with custom device	DMØ13ZZ
Hyperthermia oncology treatment of pelvic region	DWY68ZZ
Contact radiation of tongue	D9Y57ZZ
Heavy particle radiation treatment of pancreas, four risk sites	DFØ34ZZ
LDR brachytherapy to spinal cord using iodine	DØ16B9Z
Whole body Phosphorus 32 administration with risk to hematopoetic system	DWY5GFZ

Physical Rehabilitation and Diagnostic Audiology

Procedure	Code
Bekesy assessment using audiometer	F13Z31Z
Individual fitting of left eye prosthesis	FØDZ8UZ
Physical therapy for range of motion and mobility, patient right hip, no special equipment	FØ7LØZZ
Bedside swallow assessment using assessment kit	FØØZHYZ
Caregiver training in airway clearance techniques	FØFZ8ZZ
Application of short arm cast in rehabilitation setting	FØDZ7EZ (Inhibitory cast is listed in the equipment reference table under E, *Orthosis*.)
Verbal assessment of patient's pain level	FØ2ZFZZ
Caregiver training in communication skills using manual communication board	FØFZJMZ (Manual communication board is listed in the equipment reference table under M, *Augmentative/ Alternative Communication.*)
Group musculoskeletal balance training exercises, whole body, no special equipment	FØ7M6ZZ (Balance training is included in the motor treatment reference table under *Therapeutic Exercise*.)
Individual therapy for auditory processing using tape recorder	FØ9Z2KZ (Tape recorder is listed in the equipment reference table under *Audiovisual Equipment*.)

Mental Health

Procedure	Code
Cognitive-behavioral psychotherapy, individual	GZ58ZZZ
Narcosynthesis	GZGZZZZ
Light therapy	GZJZZZZ
ECT (electroconvulsive therapy), unilateral, multiple seizure	GZB1ZZZ
Crisis intervention	GZ2ZZZZ
Neuropsychological testing	GZ13ZZZ
Hypnosis	GZFZZZZ
Developmental testing	GZ1ØZZZ
Vocational counseling	GZ61ZZZ
Family psychotherapy	GZ72ZZZ

Substance Abuse Treatment

Procedure	Code
Naltrexone treatment for drug dependency	HZ94ZZZ
Substance abuse treatment family counseling	HZ63ZZZ
Medication monitoring of patient on methadone maintenance	HZ81ZZZ
Individual interpersonal psychotherapy for drug abuse	HZ54ZZZ
Patient in for alcohol detoxification treatment	HZ2ZZZZ
Group motivational counseling	HZ47ZZZ
Individual 12-step psychotherapy for substance abuse	HZ53ZZZ
Post-test infectious disease counseling for IV drug abuser	HZ3CZZZ
Psychodynamic psychotherapy for drug dependent patient	HZ5CZZZ
Group cognitive-behavioral counseling for substance abuse	HZ42ZZZ

